AF707249

Using VitalSource® eBook

Access to the VitalBook™ eBook accompanying this title is via VitalSource® Bookshelf – an eBook reader that allows you to make and share notes and highlights and search across all of the eBooks on your VitalSource Bookshelf. You can access your eBook on- or offline on your smartphone, tablet or PC/Mac and your notes and highlights will automatically stay in sync no matter where you make them.

1. Create a VitalSource Bookshelf account at https://online.vitalsource.com/user/new or login to your existing account if you already have one.

2. Redeem the code provided in the panel below to access your eBook. Login to Bookshelf and click the **Account** menu at the top right of the screen. Select **Redeem** and enter the redemption code shown on the scratch-off panel below in the **Code To Redeem** box. Press **Redeem**. Once the code has been redeemed your eBook will download and appear in your library.

Download and read offline

To use your eBook offline, download Bookshelf to your PC, Mac, iOS device, Android device or Kindle Fire, and login to your Bookshelf account.

On your PC/Mac

Go to http://bookshelf.vitalsource.com/ and follow the instructions to download the free VitalSource Bookshelf app to your PC or Mac and login to your Bookshelf account.

On your iPhone/iPod Touch/iPad

Download the free **VitalSource Bookshelf** App available via the iTunes App Store and login to your Bookshelf account. You can find more information at https://support.vitalsource.com/hc/en-us/categories/200134217-Bookshelf-for-iOS

On your Android™ smartphone, tablet or Kindle Fire

Download the free VitalSource Bookshelf App available via Google Play or Amazon and login to your Bookshelf account. You can find more information at https://support.vitalsource.com/hc/en-us/categories/200139976-Bookshelf-for-Android-and-Kindle-Fire

Support

If you have any questions about downloading Bookshelf, creating your account or accessing and using your eBook edition, please visit http://support.vitalsource.com/

N.B. The code in the scratch-off panel can only be used once. When you have created a Bookshelf account and redeemed the code you will be able to access the eBook online or offline on your smartphone tablet or PC/Mac.

BOVINE PATHOLOGY

A TEXT AND COLOR ATLAS

FSC
www.fsc.org
MIX
Paper from responsible sources
FSC® C022174

BOVINE PATHOLOGY

A TEXT AND COLOR ATLAS

Claus D. Buergelt, DVM, PhD, DACVP
Professor Emeritus of Veterinary Pathology
Department of Comparative,
Diagnostic and Population Medicine
College of Veterinary Medicine
University of Florida, USA

Edward G. Clark, DVM, MVSc, DACVP
Veterinary Diagnostic Pathology Consultant
Calgary, Canada
Adjunct Professor
University of Calgary Faculty of Veterinary Medicine
Calgary, Canada

Fabio Del Piero, DVM, PhD, DACVP
Professor
Department of Pathobiological Sciences
School of Veterinary Medicine
Louisiana State University, USA

CABI

CABI is a trading name of CAB International

CABI
Nosworthy Way
Wallingford
Oxfordshire OX10 8DE
UK

Tel: +44 (0)1491 832111
Fax: +44 (0)1491 833508
E-mail: info@cabi.org
Website: www.cabi.org

CABI
745 Atlantic Avenue
8th Floor
Boston, MA 02111
USA

Tel: +1 (617)682-9015
E-mail: cabi-nao@cabi.org

A catalogue record for this book is available from the British Library, London, UK.

Library of Congress Cataloging-in-Publication Data

Names: Buergelt, Claus D., author. | Clark, Edward G., author. | Del Piero, Fabio, author. | C.A.B. International, issuing body.
Title: Bovine pathology : a text and color atlas / Claus D. Buergelt, Edward G. Clark, Fabio Del Piero.
Description: Wallingford, Oxfordshire ; Boston, MA : CABI, [2017] | Includes bibliographical references and index.
Identifiers: LCCN 2017015883 (print) | LCCN 2017029213 (ebook) | ISBN 9781780646725 (ebook) | ISBN 9781780646732 (epub) | ISBN 9781780646718 (hardcover : alk. paper)
Subjects: | MESH: Cattle Diseases--pathology | Atlases
Classification: LCC SF961 (ebook) | LCC SF961 .B86 2017 (print) | NLM SF 961 | DDC 636.2/089--dc23
LC record available at https://lccn.loc.gov/2017015883

ISBN-13: 9781780646718

Commissioning editor: Caroline Makepeace
Editorial assistant: Alexandra Lainsbury
Production editor: James Bishop

Typeset by SPi, Pondicherry, India
Printed and bound in India

CONTENTS

Contributors vii
Preface ix
Authors' Acknowledgments xi

1 Diseases of Neonates and Calves 1
2 Diseases of the Nervous System 31
3 Diseases of the Respiratory System 57
4 Diseases of the Cardiovascular System 93
5 Diseases of the Gastrointestinal Tract 111
6 Diseases of the Hepatobiliary System and Pancreas 161
7 Diseases of the Urinary System 177
8 Diseases of the Musculoskeletal System 195
9 Diseases of the Endocrine System 217
10 Diseases of the Reproductive System 223
11 Diseases of the Hematopoietic and Hemolymphatic System 261
12 Diseases of the Integument 289
13 Diseases of the Claw and Foot Skin 343
14 Diseases of the Udder and Teats 357
15 Diseases of Eye and Ear 367
16 The Pathology of Select Poisonous Plant-induced Diseases in Cattle 381
17 Bovine Diseases Without Lesions 417

Index 423

CONTRIBUTORS

Mark L. Anderson, DVM, PhD, DACVP, Professor, California Animal Health & Food Safety Laboratory, School of Veterinary Medicine, University of California, Davis, California, USA

Jennifer L. Davies, DVM, MVSc, DACVP, Adjunct Assistant Professor, Director of Diagnostic Services, Department of Ecosystem and Public Health, Faculty of Veterinary Medicine, University of Calgary, Calgary, Alberta, Canada

Ingeborg Maria Langohr, DVM, PhD, DACVP, Professor, Department of Pathobiological Sciences, School of Veterinary Medicine, Louisiana State University, Baton Rouge, Louisiana, USA

Jan K. Shearer, DVM, MS, Professor and Extension Veterinarian, College of Veterinary Medicine, Iowa State University, Ames, Iowa, USA

Bryan L. Stegelmeier, DVM, PhD, DACVP, USDA/ARS, Poisonous Plant Research Laboratory, Logan, Utah, USA

Keith G. Thompson, BVSc, PhD, DACVP, Emeritus Professor, Institute of Veterinary, Animal and Biomedical Sciences, Massey University, Palmerston North, New Zealand

Amy L. Warren, BSc, BVSc, PhD, DACVP, Assistant Professor, Department of Ecosystem and Public Health, Faculty of Veterinary Medicine, University of Calgary, Calgary, Alberta, Canada

PREFACE

This atlas is the reflection of the authors' professional exposure to bovine pathology for a combined total of over 100 years. It is intended to be shared as a legacy with future generations of veterinary pathologists and practitioners. The atlas contains pathologic examples of major bovine diseases encountered in both dairy and beef cattle breeds, with some emphasis on the pathology of diseases occurring in feedlot operations. The atlas is not intended to represent the pathology of global diseases. Most of the diseases listed are from the western hemisphere, with some recent additions from other continents.

We feel the need to convey the following to our readers: the atlas does not claim to represent every disease entity occurring in cattle. We may have omitted some by chance, or simply did not see them in our practice. Not all of our images are of top digital quality as they were scanned from archival entities.

For very unique bovine diseases, contributions from colleagues in the field were solicited. We gratefully acknowledge their willingness to share their material and expertise. We made every effort to obtain appropriate copyright permissions.

The bovine diseases are structured along organ systems. Some presentation overlaps could not be avoided in the specific organ chapters. Our goal was to focus on the gross aspects of bovine pathology, but we added microscopic images to cover a specific morphologic diagnosis and immunohistochemistry for a specific etiologic diagnosis.

Images are the main focus of the atlas, with a legend of lesion description for each transparency. We incorporated a succinct text with topic introduction, aspects of pathogenesis, key clinical signs, and listing of differential diagnoses without creating a textbook. Readers are directed to textbooks for more details.

We aim to bring the atlas to the attention of not only veterinary pathologists and trainees in veterinary pathology but also practitioners performing necropsies in the field, livestock and dairy operation managers, and inspectors working at slaughterhouse facilities. A short list of references at the end of each chapter is intended to encourage detailed reading.

Bovine pathology is a vanishing specialty in many of the teaching institutions, and no longer is on the top of the list for trainees in veterinary medicine. This development motivated us to venture the project so that valuable illustrative material would not languish in institutional archives or our own files.

Finally, we thank our bovine patients for providing us with the material needed for putting the atlas together.

Claus D. Buergelt, Gainesville, Florida, USA
Edward G. Clark, Calgary, Alberta, Canada
Fabio Del Piero, Baton Rouge, Louisiana, USA

AUTHORS' ACKNOWLEDGMENTS

The core collection presented in this atlas stems from our personal files and files from our institutions: the University of Florida, the University of Calgary, Louisiana State University, University of Pennsylvania School of Veterinary Medicine and Cornell University. Other sources to recognize for their contributions are the Department of Pathology, Western College of Veterinary Medicine, University of Saskatchewan, and the Government of Alberta, Canada.

Deep gratitude is expressed to my co-authors, Edward G. Clark and Fabio Del Piero, for their tireless support, advice, critique, suggestions, and expertise to address scientific and technical problems encountered along the way.

Personal thanks are expressed by EGC to the colleagues in the Department of Veterinary Pathology and Prairie Diagnostic Services who, over 30 years at the Western College of Veterinary Medicine, contributed to the collection of images used in this atlas. Many thanks are owed to Drs Eugene Janzen and Debbie Haines for their enormous contribution, through specimen submissions and immunohistochemistry, to the knowledge of feedlot pathology.

Thanks and appreciation are extended to those experts in the field contributing special chapters to the atlas: Mark Anderson, Jennifer Davies, Ingeborg Langohr, Jan Shearer, Bryan Stegelmeier, Keith Thompson, and Amy Warren.

It is with sadness that we had to part with one of the main individual contributors while working on the project: Dr John M. King, Cornell University, a cherished friend, mentor, teacher, and pillar of veterinary pathology. His images presented in the atlas are a reflection of his legacy to veterinary pathology.

Individual colleagues from around the world have generously, and without hesitation, shared their images for inclusion in the contents of the atlas. We received transparencies and copyright approvals from many individuals, acknowledging with gratitude and appreciation their support and generosity. Any omission of contributors' names in the listing is unintentional.

The following individuals and sources contributed:

Argentina: Dr L. Minatel.
Australia: Dr P. Chenoweth.
Brazil: Drs C. Barros, D. Cagnini, D. Driemeier, E. Facury Filho, F. Furlan, G. Kommers, W. Panziera.
Canada: Drs T. Bollinger, J. Caswell, R. Farley, S. Greenwood, E. Janzen, M. Jelinski, C. Knight, C. Legge, G. McGregor, M. Ngeleka, Ontario Veterinary College, R. Postey, A. Saplethun, G. Searcy, E. Waters, J. Webb, D. Well.
Germany: Dr M. Bruegmann.
Italy: Drs F. Guarda, E. Lepri, E. Scanziani.
New Zealand: Drs S. Atkinson, A. Campbell, R. Fairley, K. Thompson.
St Kitts: Dr O. Illanes.
Switzerland: Dr Ch. Griot.
Uruguay: Dr F. Riet-Correa.
USA: Drs A. Berkewitz, P. Blanchard, B. Brodersen, N. Crossland, S. Diab, M. Drost, R. Dubielzig, J. Edwards, P. Habecker, M. Hines, A. Knight, W. Layton, R. Moeller, P. Mouser, D. O'Toole, R. Panciera, P. Pesavento, K. Potter, M. Rebellato, G. Rimoldi, J. Roberts, M. Roberson, G. Saunders, J. Schleining, B. Summers, F. Uzal, H. Van Kruinigen, R. Whitlock, L. Woods.

Publishers/journals: Elsevier, Wiley-Blackwell and the *Journal of Veterinary Diagnostic Investigation.*

Department of Comparative, Diagnostic and Population Medicine, University of Florida: Dr G. Abbot for digital imaging improvement, Dr W. Craft for providing references, Dr M. Dark for computer programming.
Mrs Nancy Buergelt for computer support, encouragement and sharing interest in the project.
Ms Caroline Makepeace, Ms Alexandra Lainsbury, James Bishop and staff, CAB International, for patience, editorial assistance, and making the atlas possible.

CDB, EGC, FDP

CHAPTER 1

Diseases of Neonates and Calves

1.1 Congenital Anomalies

1.2 Nervous System
- 1.2.1 Edema and inflammation
  - 1.2.1.1 Cerebellar herniation (coning)
  - 1.2.1.2 Meningitis
- 1.2.2 Neoplasia
- 1.2.3 Inherited metabolic disorders
  - 1.2.3.1 Bovine maple syrup urine disease
  - 1.2.3.2 Bovine citrullinemia

1.3 Respiratory Disorders
- 1.3.1 Larynx
  - 1.3.1.1 Necrotic laryngitis
- 1.3.2 Lung
  - 1.3.2.1 Bronchopneumonia

1.4 Gastrointestinal Disorders
- 1.4.1 Displacements
- 1.4.2 Inflammation
  - 1.4.2.1 Viruses
  - 1.4.2.2 Bacteria
  - 1.4.2.3 Protozoa
  - 1.4.2.4 Fungi
  - 1.4.2.5 Parasites

1.5 Additional Gastric Conditions
- 1.5.1 Abomasal foreign body formations
- 1.5.2 Abomasal ulceration
- 1.5.3 Hemorrhagic abomasitis
- 1.5.4 Calf sepsis (formerly septicemia)

1.6 Musculoskeletal Disorders
- 1.6.1 Muscular system
  - 1.6.1.1 White muscle disease (WMD)
- 1.6.2 Skeletal system
  - 1.6.2.1 Congenital chondrodysplasia
  - 1.6.2.2 Arthritis

1.7 Neoplasia

1.8 Miscellaneous
- 1.8.1 Bovine neonatal pancytopenia (BNP)
- 1.8.2 Floppy ear syndrome

INTRODUCTION

Success in calf rearing requires good husbandry for steady health maintenance. Many risk factors interfere with the health status of the neonate and the calf in the first weeks of life. Imposing factors include compromised immune status, poor sanitation and ventilation, inadequate nutrition, overcrowding, lack of vaccination and wet and cold weather conditions. The goal of calf rearing should be the creation and maintenance of a protective environment.

Two organ systems of the growing calf are particularly susceptible to disease: the respiratory and the alimentary systems. Most topics in this chapter will deal with infectious agents responsible for the entities of calf pneumonia and calf scours. Additional topics include examples of more common congenital anomalies, nutritional and metabolic enzymatic deficits, as well as two iatrogenic-induced disorders: bovine neonatal pancytopenia (BNP) and floppy ear syndrome.

In this chapter, diseases and disorders of dairy and beef calves are considered arbitrarily up to the age of 3–4 months.

1.1 CONGENITAL ANOMALIES

Introduction. Many of the congenital anomalies occur spontaneously; some of them are the result of genetic mutants and chromosomal abnormalities, and some are the result of environmental factors such as teratogenic toxic plants or transplacentally transmitted teratogenic viruses. Calves with congenital defects are frequently stillborn. This segment presents examples of the more common abnormalities; a few additional defects are listed with the respective organ system chapters in which they occur (ocular, skeletal, reproductive, and dermal).

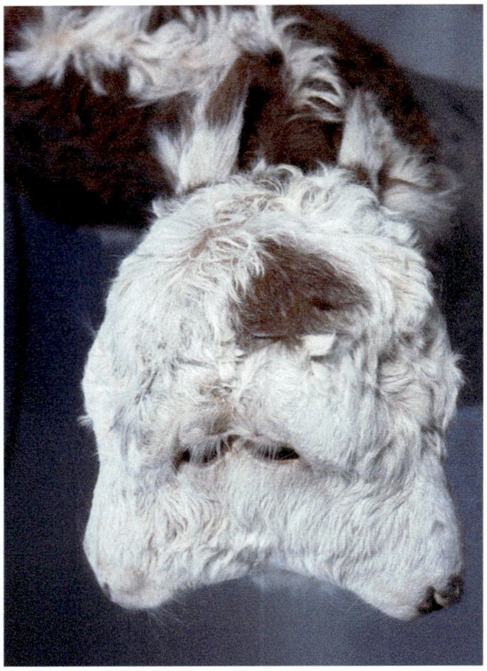

Fig. 1.1. Ox. Conjoined neonate twins. Diprosopus. Craniofacial duplication is a rare form of a conjoined monozygotic twin. Duplication consists of two heads (bicephalic or dicephalic, or polycephalic) and necks, and includes the oral and respiratory anatomic structures associated with these two heads (double tongue, esophagus, trachea). (Courtesy of Department of Pathology, WCVM, University of Saskatchewan, Saskatoon, Canada.)

Diprosopus

Clinical complication: Dystocia

Hydrocephalus

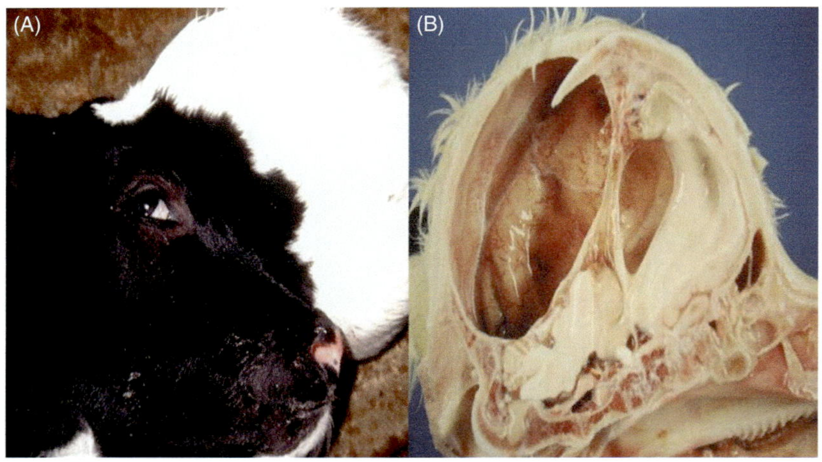

Fig. 1.2. Ox. Head. Hydrocephalus. Inherited forms are found in Hereford, Charolais and Holstein breeds. Grossly, a marked doming (A) of the forehead is visible. (B) A midsagittal section reveals a loss of cerebral tissue and marked distension of the ventricles by excessive CNS fluid (drained in the image) contained by leptomeninges. Transplacental teratogenic viruses such as bluetongue, bovine viral diarrhea virus, Akabane and other bunyaviruses have to be considered as a cause of the condition. Also, vitamin A deficiency may be a cause.

Clinical sign. Dystocia.
Differential diagnoses. Exencephaly, meningocele.

Hydranencephaly

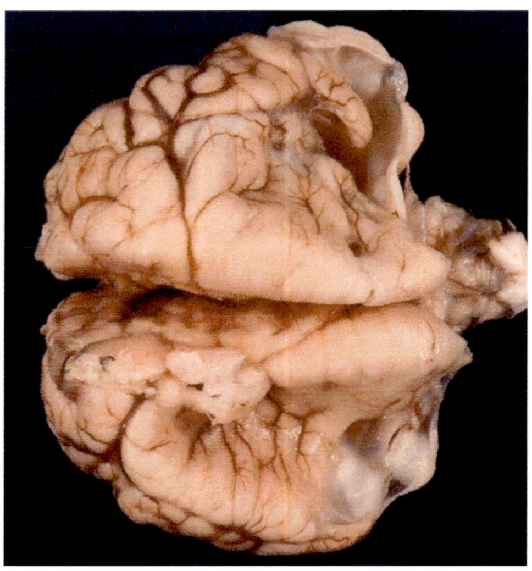

Fig. 1.3. Ox. Head. Hydranencephaly and cerebellar hypoplasia. There is evidence of complete loss of the cerebral parenchyma. The cerebral tissue is replaced by fluid accumulating (drained) within a sac covered by intact leptomeninges. The cerebellum is significantly reduced in size. Transplacental teratogenic viruses may be involved in the pathogenesis.

Aplasia/hypoplasia

Clinical signs. Incoordination, ataxia, blindness.
Differential diagnosis. Genetic induction in Angus and Scottish Highland calves.

Spina bifida

Cranium bifidum is defined as a neural tube defect associated with the cranium.
Clinical signs. Hind-leg paresis, sometimes with anal and tail malfunction and/or arthrogryposis.
Differential diagnoses. Trauma, epitheliogenesis imperfecta.

Cleft palate (Palatoschisis)

Clinical signs. Nasal discharge, regurgitation of milk.

Segmental aplasia

The hypothesis that this defect is iatrogenically introduced during early pregnancy (40–42 days) via rectal palpation has been disproved.
Clinical signs. Abdominal distension, mucinous defecation.
Differential diagnoses. Jejunal volvulus, intussusception, atresia ani.

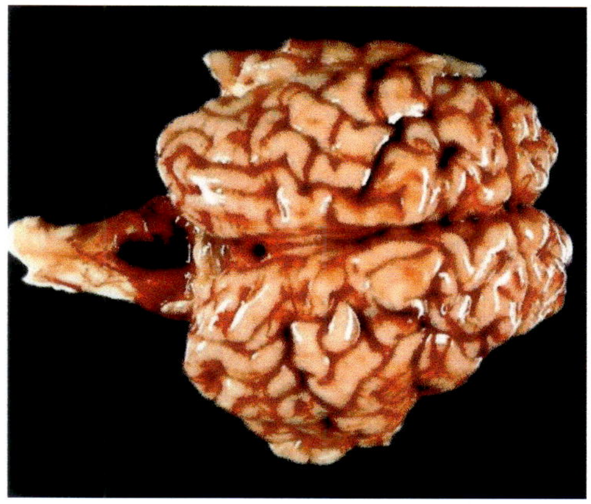

Fig. 1.4. Ox. Cerebellum. Aplasia/hypoplasia. Caused by *in-utero* infection of the dam at days 100–200 of gestation by the bovine viral diarrhea virus, all parts of the cerebellum or portions of the vermis and lateral lobes can be involved. The transmitted virus selectively causes cytolysis of neuroblast precursors interfering with differentiation of the permanent cerebellar cell population.

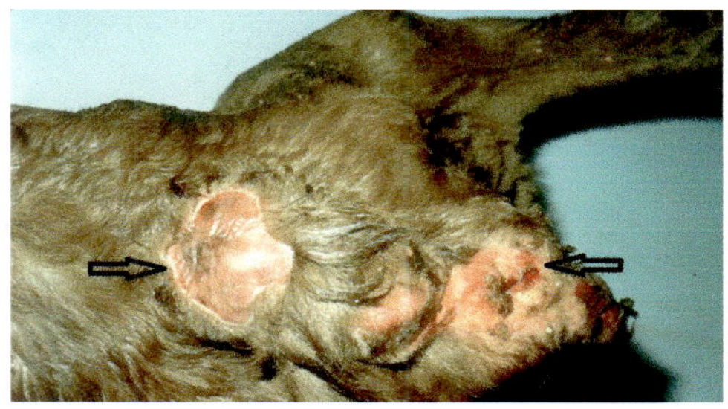

Fig. 1.5. Ox. Spinal cord. Spina bifida. Myelodysplasia (also known as spinal dysraphism) associated with spina bifida is an example of a neurotubal defect and usually occurs in Holstein neonates. Protrusions (arrows) of the spinal cord and meninges are visible at the site of the lumbosacral skin due to a defect of the dorsal spine. The spinal cord directly connects to the skin. (Courtesy of Dr J.M. King and the Section of Anatomic Pathology, Cornell University, USA.)

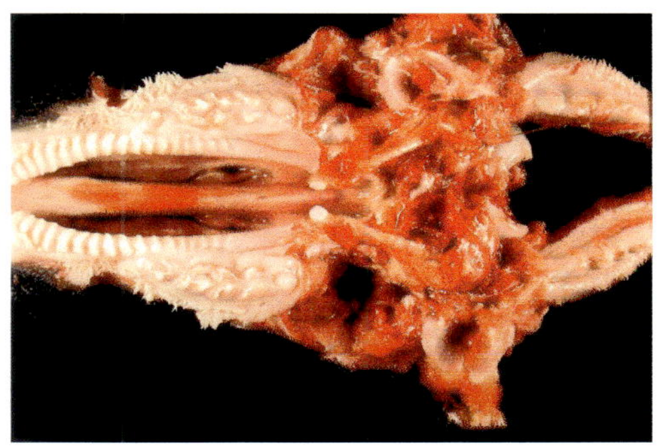

Fig. 1.6. Ox. Palate. Palatoschisis. A cleft affecting soft and hard palates exposes nasal turbinates. Aspiration pneumonia is a fatal complication.

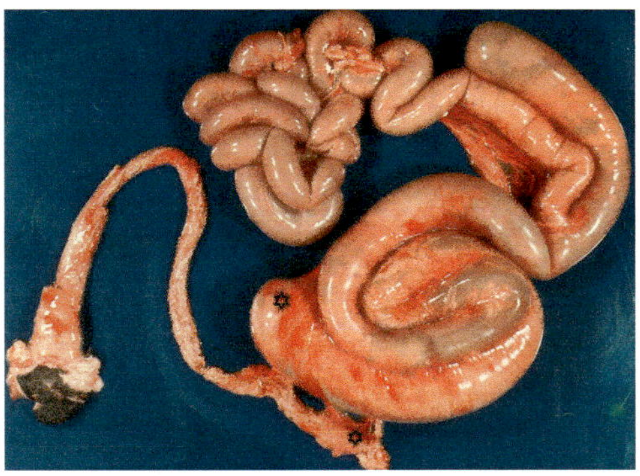

Fig. 1.7. Ox. Colon. Segmental aplasia. Blindly ending segments of the intestinal tract are indicated by asterisks. The proximal segment is markedly distended by digesta, while the distal segment is small and contains only mucus. The jejunum is another site for segmental aplasia in calves.

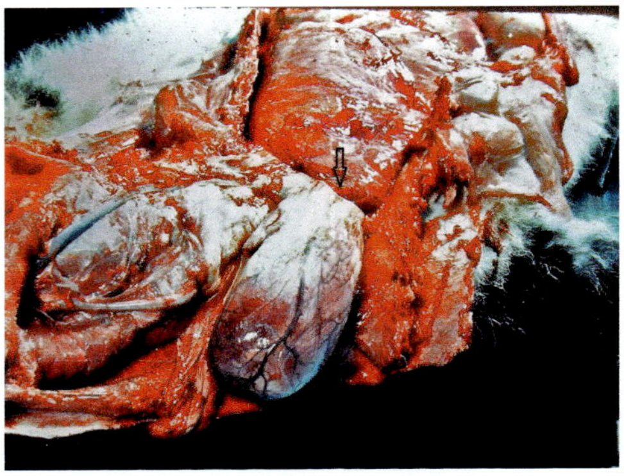

Fig. 1.8. Ox. Ventral neck. Ectopic heart (ectopia cordis). The exposed heart is located within the subcutis of the ventral neck (arrow). It is connected to the major vessels located in the thorax. Other ectopic cardiac locations are the subcutis of the sternum and the inside of the cranial abdomen. The subcutaneous location is often prone to trauma, leading to cardiac tamponade.

Ectopic heart

Clinical sign. Dermal pulsation.
Differential diagnosis. Venous congestion secondary to chronic heart failure.

Ventricular septal defect

Clinical signs. Lack of exercise, depression, respiratory distress.
Differential diagnoses. Tetralogy of Fallot, transposition of greater vessels.

Polycystic kidney

Clinical signs. Anuria, dysuria, or none.
Differential diagnosis. Obstruction of lower urinary system, e.g. hydronephrosis.

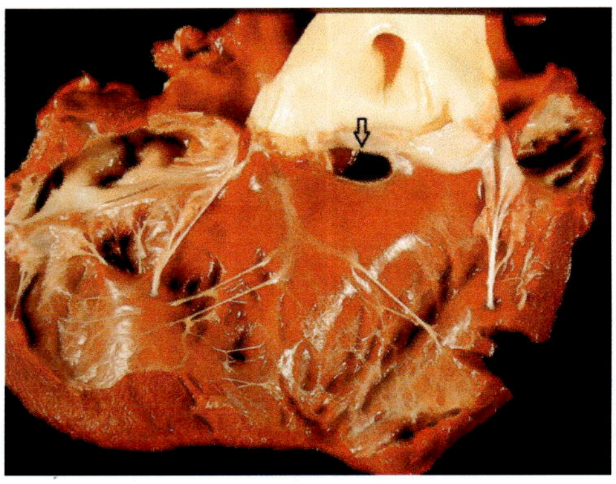

Fig. 1.9. Ox. Heart. Ventricular septal defect (VSD). It is the most common cardiovascular anomaly in ruminants. A cleft (arrow) is present in the membranous part of the ventricle (high VSD). Depending on the size of the defect and on the time of survival, a reversal of the original left-to-right shunt to right-to-left may lead to passive congestion, with cyanosis.

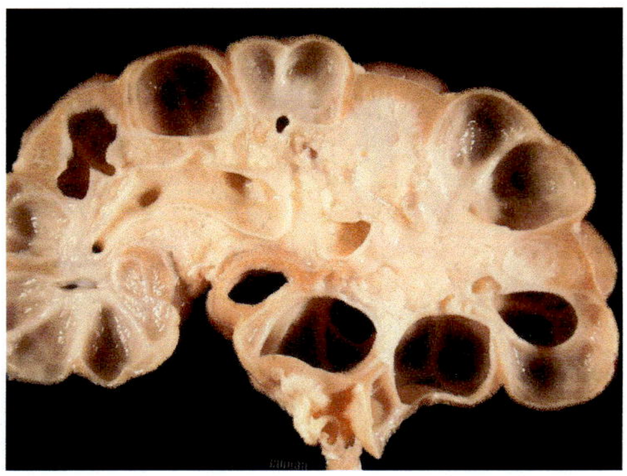

Fig. 1.10. Ox. Kidney. Polycystic kidney. A transverse section shows multiple cysts in the cortex, but also in the medulla, affecting more than 50% of the kidney parenchyma. The condition, when congenital, is the result of a failure of tubulogenesis during renal embryogenesis. Acquired hydronephrosis also has to be considered.

Hypospadia

Clinical signs. Abnormal urination and urine staining.

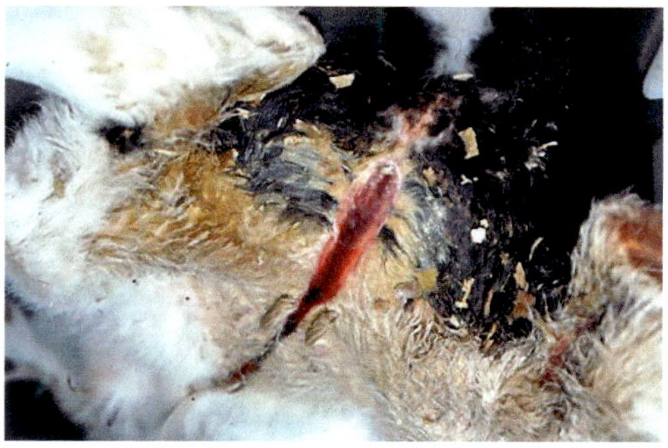

Fig. 1.11. Ox. Perineum. Hypospadia. Seen in neonatal male calves, it is the result of an incomplete ventral closure of the urethral fold and abnormal perianal or scrotal location of the urethra.

Omphalocele

Clinical signs. None.
Differential diagnosis. Amorphous globosus.

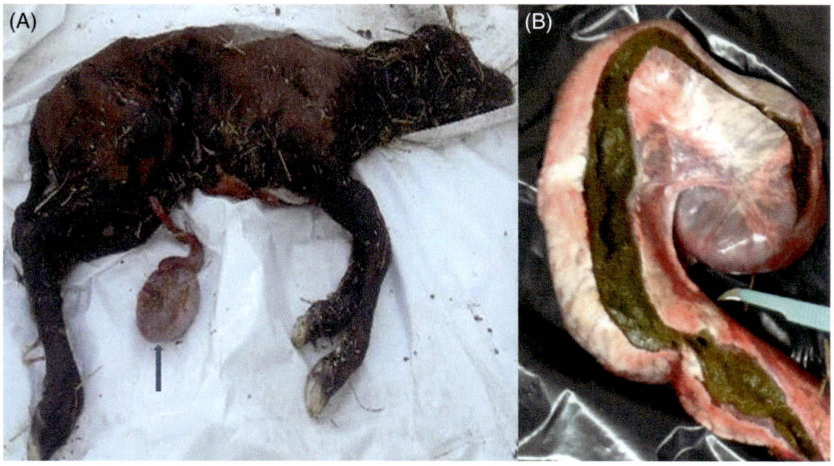

Fig. 1.12. Ox. Stillborn. Omphalocele (umbilical hernia). (A) Connected to the umbilical cord is a blindly ending attachment (arrow). (B).When opened, it shows a tubular organ filled with green, pasty material, indicating meconium. (Courtesy of Dr M. Drost, Drost Project, University of Florida, USA.)

Pulmonary dysplasia

Clinical signs. Respiratory shortness.
Differential diagnosis. Pulmonary emphysema and edema.

There are many additional abnormalities affecting various organ systems and sometimes occurring as multiple defects, including developmental duplications. Genetic, environmental, nutritional, plants, and infectious agents should be taken into consideration in the understanding of the etiology (see list of teratogenic viruses and plants).

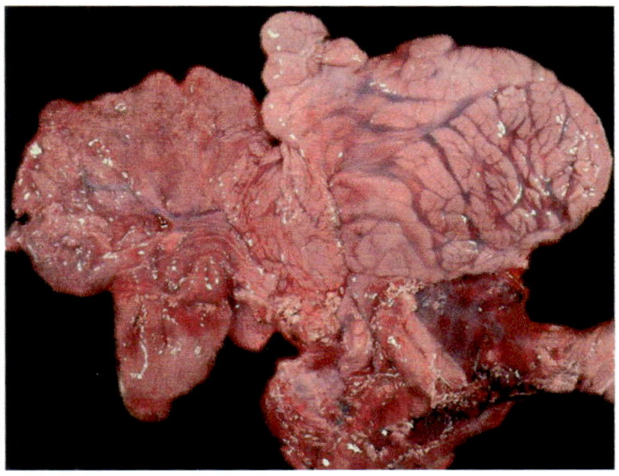

Fig. 1.13. Ox. Lung. Pulmonary dysplasia (hamartoma). A pseudolobulated. bulbous, enlarged gray lung is present on the right. The part on the left represents fetal lung. The dysplasia is histologically characterized by disorganized airway structures missing an alveolar component. This lesion has been hypothesized to be associated with an *in-utero* infection with the bovine viral diarrhea virus.

List of Teratogenic Viruses
- Bluetongue virus (Orbivirus)
- Bovine viral diarrhea virus (BVDV) (Pestivirus)
- Akabane virus (Bunyavirus)
- Schmallenberg virus (Bunyavirus)

List of Teratogenic Plants
- Lupine (*Lupinus caudatus*)
- Locoweed (*Astragalus* spp./*Oxytropis* spp.)
- Poison hemlock (*Conium maculatum*)

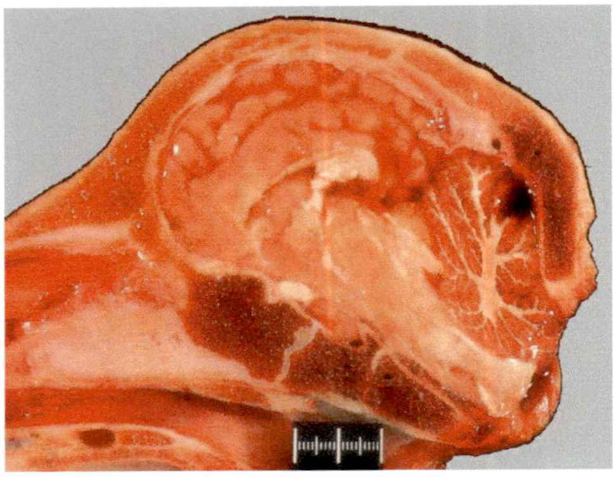

Fig. 1.14. Ox. Cerebrum, cerebellum. Edema. Coning. The cerebrum is markedly edematous. The edematous cerebellum is extremely compressed within the calvaria. It is partially located within the foramen magnum.

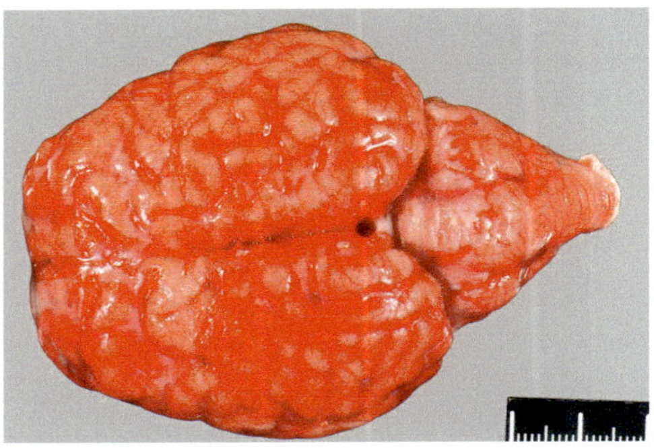

Fig. 1.15. Ox. Cerebrum, cerebellum. Acute meningitis. Meninges are markedly reddened. There is evidence of cerebellar coning.

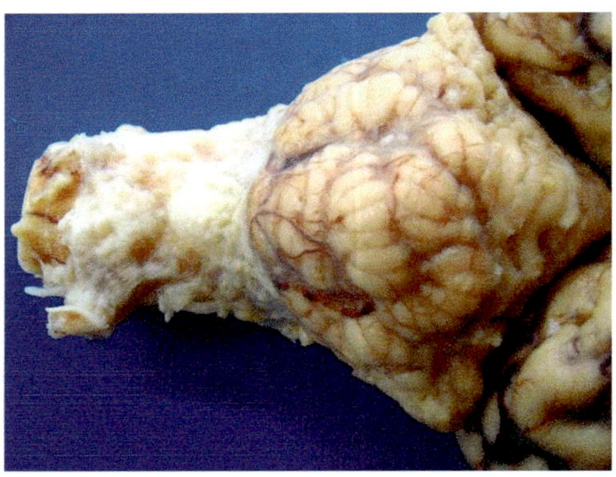

Fig. 1.16. Ox. Cerebellum and brainstem. Purulent meningitis. The brainstem, and to a lesser degree the cerebellar surfaces, are covered by pus. Gram-negative bacteria are frequently involved, including *Escherichia coli* and *Salmonella* spp.

1.2 NERVOUS SYSTEM

1.2.1 Edema and inflammation

1.2.1.1 Cerebellar herniation (coning)

Introduction. If intracranial pressure increases, such as in edema, acute inflammation, hematoma or expending neoplasia, the cerebellar vermis herniates through the foramen magnum, resulting in hemorrhage and sometimes pressure necrosis.

Clinical signs. Ataxia, pain.

Differential diagnosis. Hypovitaminosis A.

1.2.1.2 Meningitis

Introduction. Commonly associated with septicemia, and usually bacterial in origin, it causes behavioral and postural changes in the calf.

Clinical signs. Incoordination, dullness, head pressing, recumbency.

Differential diagnoses. Viral encephalitis, otitis media.

1.2.2 Neoplasia

Introduction. A rare embryonal tumor involving the cerebellum of calves is defined as medulloblastoma.

Clinical signs. Ataxia, opisthotonos.

Differential diagnoses. Cerebellar, abscess.

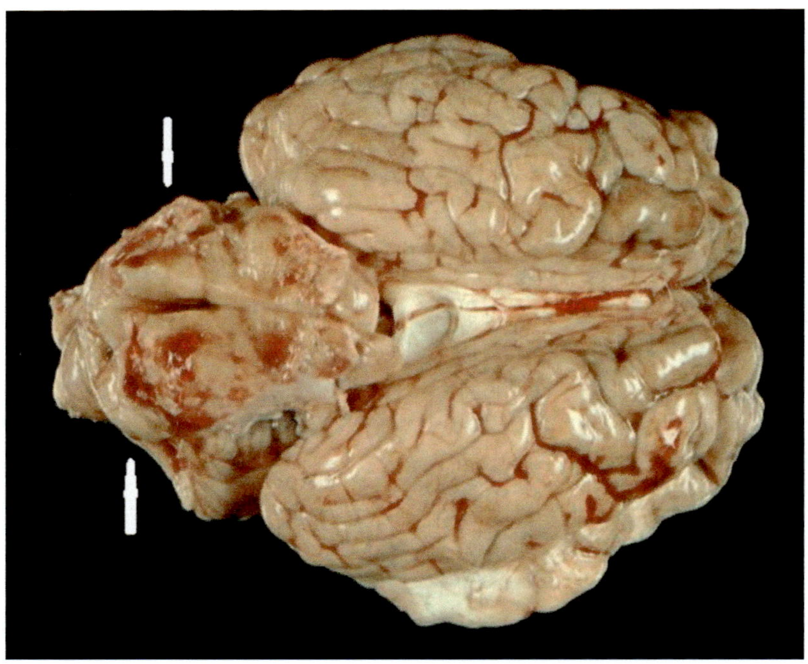

Fig. 1.17. Ox. Cerebellum. Medulloblastoma. A circumscribed gray growth with hemorrhage covers the midline of the vermis (arrows).

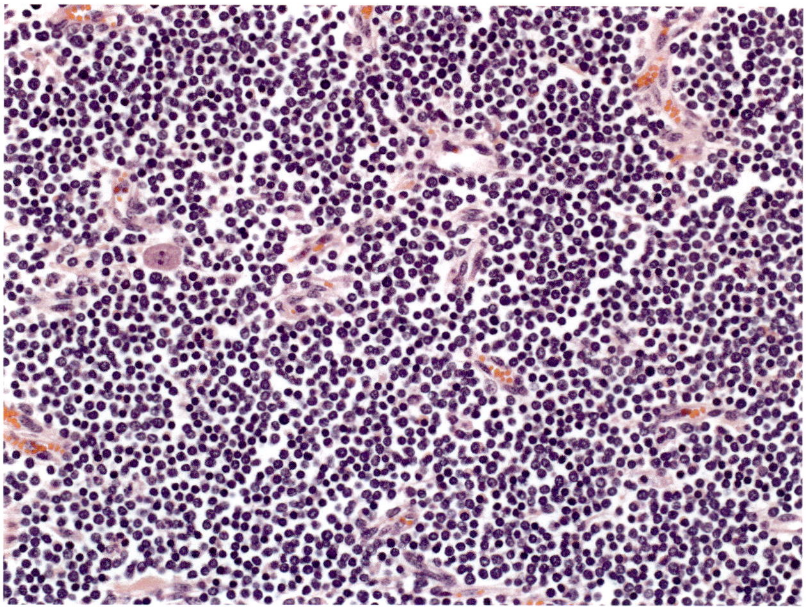

Fig. 1.18. Ox. Cerebellum. Medulloblastoma. The microscopic appearance is that of a densely cellular, basophilic growth with bundles of ovoid and elongated small tumor cells (Hematoxylin and eosin (H&E)).

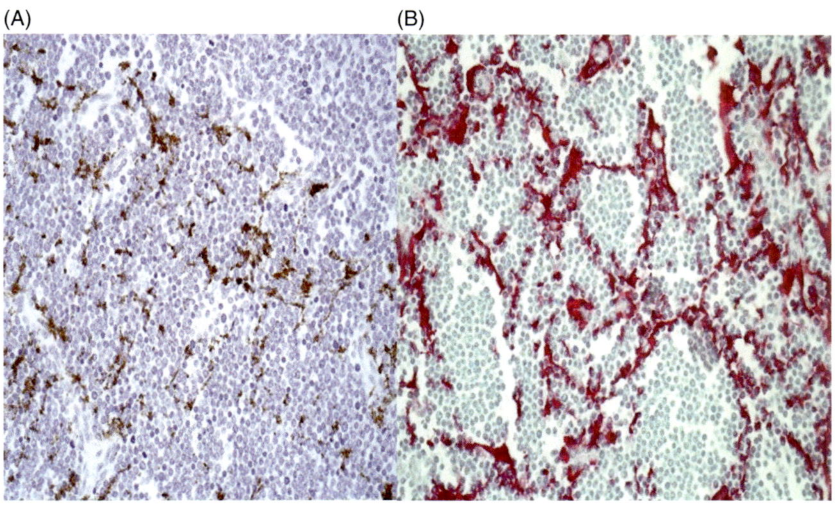

Fig. 1.19. Ox. Cerebellum. Medulloblastoma. Immunoreactivity is positive for fibrillar-oriented synaptophysin (A) and glial fibrillary acid protein (GFAP (B). Other tumor markers are neuron-specific enolase (NSE) and S-100. (Indirect immunohistochemistry (IHC)).

1.2.3 Inherited metabolic disorders

Introduction. Being the result of inherited enzyme deficiencies, the conditions are rare in cattle.

1.2.3.1 Bovine maple syrup urine disease

The disease occurs as an autosomal recessive trait in neonates and calves. It is the result of a branched-chain ketoacid dehydrogenase (BCKAD) complex deficiency. The histologic changes are that of spongiform encephalopathy with spheroids, gitter cells and mild astrogliosis.
Clinical signs. Dullness, recumbency, opisthotonos.
Differential diagnosis. Polioencephalomalacia.

1.2.3.2 Bovine citrullinemia

The progressive central nervous disease is caused by an autosomally inherited dysfunction of the urea cycle enzyme, arginine-succinate synthetase. Edema of the cerebral cortex is a consistent histopathological finding. The defect has been described in Australian and New Zealand Holstein-Friesian cattle. Affected animals appear healthy at birth, but die with acute onset neurologic disease within 1–4 days.
Clinical signs. Disorientation, depression, head pressing, convulsion.
Differential diagnosis. BVDV-induced cerebellar hypoplasia.

1.3 RESPIRATORY DISORDERS

1.3.1 Larynx

1.3.1.1 Necrotic laryngitis

Introduction. The larynx can be the portal of entry and reservoir for some pulmonary pathogens such as *Histophilus somni* and *Mycoplasma bovis*. Another pathogen consistently isolated is *Fusobacterium necrophorum*, causing laryngeal necrosis (calf diphtheria).
Clinical signs. Salivation, dyspnea, stretched neck, odor in breath.
Differential diagnoses. *Histophilus somni* necrohemorrhagic laryngitis, infectious bovine rhinotracheitis (IBR), fungi, trauma (drenching tube) or balling gun.

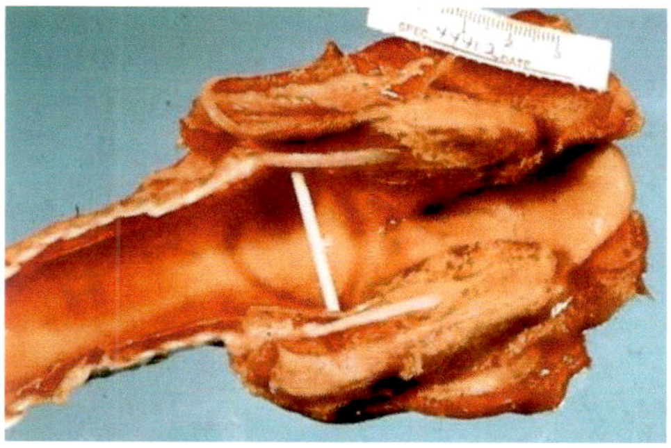

Fig. 1.20. Ox. Larynx. Necrocaseous laryngitis (calf diphtheria). Diphtheritic membranes are present on both sides of the larynx and vocal cords. The inflammation resulting from *Fusobacterium necrophorum* is secondary to the trauma to the region.

1.3.2 Lung

1.3.2.1 Bronchopneumonia

Introduction. Bronchopneumonia in calves is the result of multiple viruses and bacteria leading to the disease entity of enzootic pneumonia affecting dairy calves. Viruses predispose to bacterial infection in many instances. Morbidity is high. Risk factors such as lack of colostrum, poor hygienic management, overcrowded housing, faulty ventilation conditions, and inadequate nutrition are contributors to the entity of enzootic calf pneumonia.
Clinical signs. Nasal discharge, coughing, dyspnea, poor growth.
Differential diagnosis. Aspiration pneumonia.

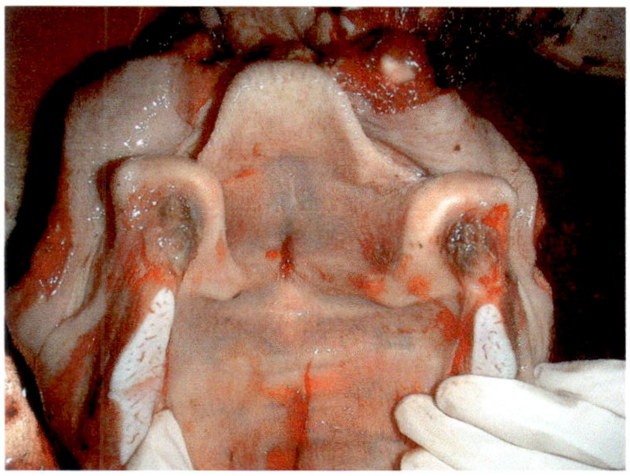

Fig. 1.21. Ox. Larynx. Fibrinonecrotic laryngitis. *Histophilus somni*. Focal mucosal necrosis is present next to the arytenoid cartilage. Early foci of infection may show vesiculopapular changes on the surface of cartilage.

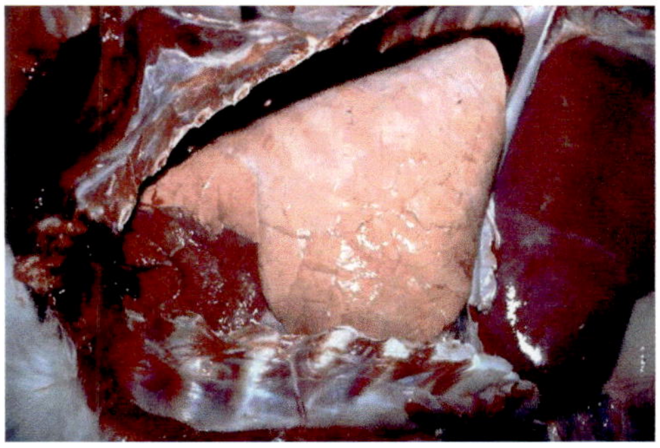

Fig. 1.22. Ox. Lung. Cranioventral necrosuppurative bronchopneumonia. Focal apical areas of consolidated lung lobules are characterized by purple discoloration. A variety of viral agents and some bacterial pathogens are responsible for the lesion.

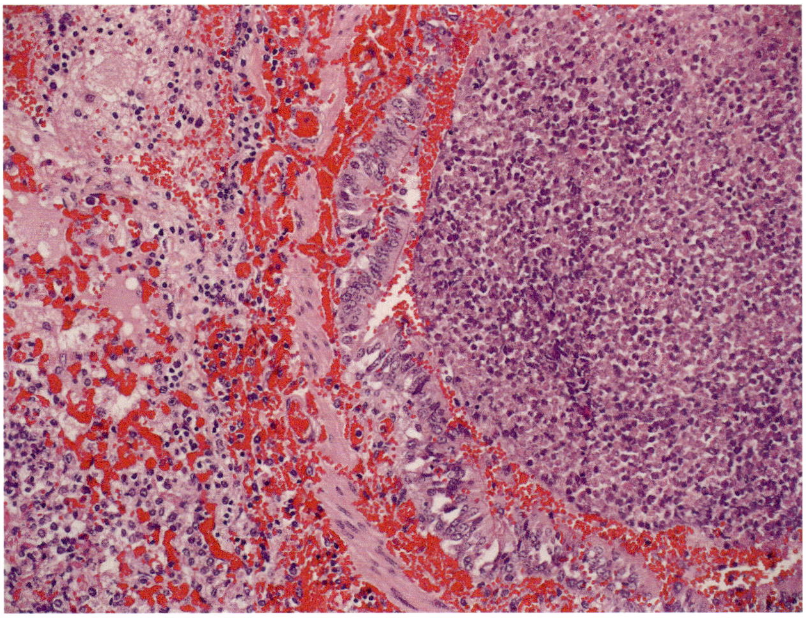

Fig. 1.23. Ox. Lung. Coronavirus pneumonia. Fibrinolymphocytic bronchitis. The bronchus is obstructed by a plug composed of fibrin, neutrophils and lymphocytes, many of which are degenerate. Adjacent alveoli are filled with a proteinaceous exudate and some lymphocytes. Coronavirus can be found in healthy animals in the respiratory tract (H&E). (Courtesy of Dr J. Caswell, University of Guelph, Canada.)

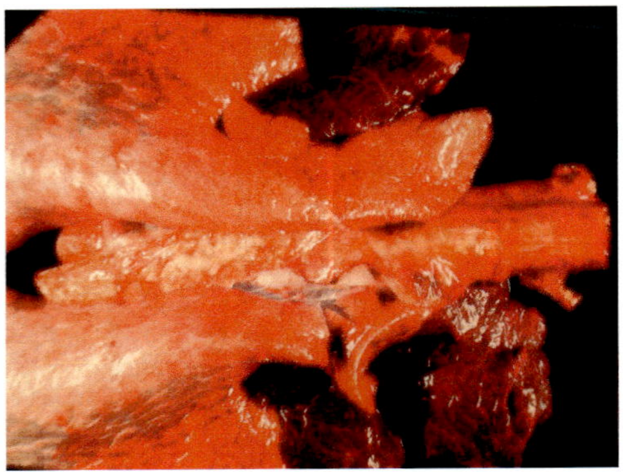

Fig. 1.25. Ox. Lung. Cranioventral suppurative bronchopneumonia. There is consolidation of both apical lobes. Adenovirus was isolated. The virus also causes enteritis in calves, resulting in watery diarrhea. If both organs are involved, the condition is called pneumoenteritis.

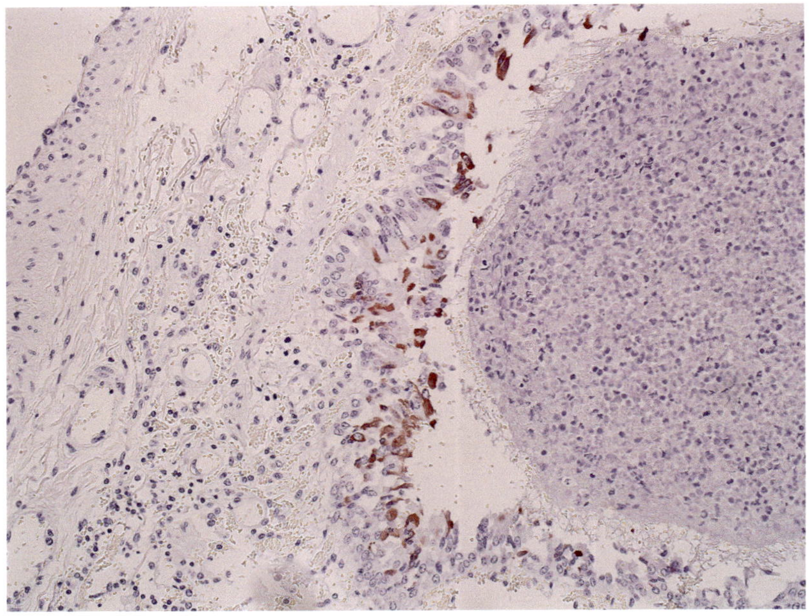

Fig. 1.24. Ox. Lung. Coronavirus pneumonia. Detection of viral antigen in the cytoplasm of respiratory epithelial cells (IHC). (Courtesy of Dr J. Caswell, University of Guelph, Canada.)

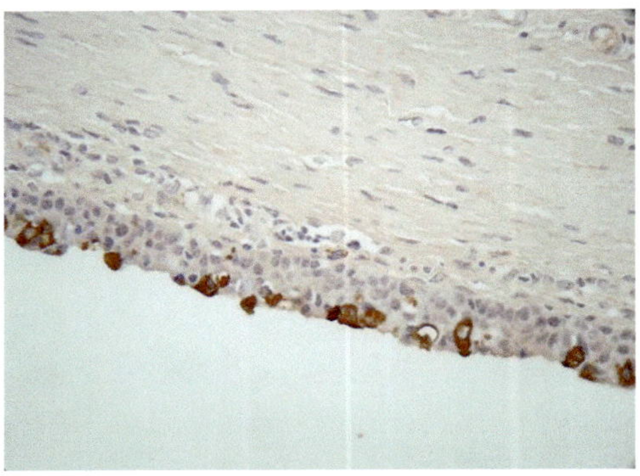

Fig. 1.26. Ox. Trachea. Adenovirus. Identification of viral antigen by indirect immunohistochemistry in the nuclei of epithelial respiratory cells (IHC).

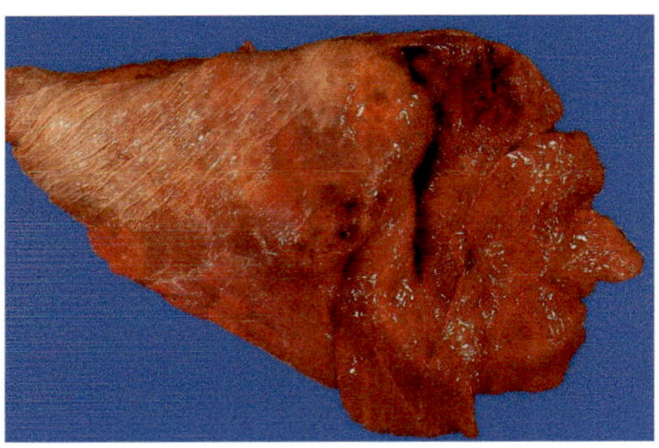

Fig. 1.27. Ox. Lung. Parainfluenza-3. Necrosuppurative bronchopneumonia. Apical, middle and diaphragmatic lobes are affected by brown consolidation.

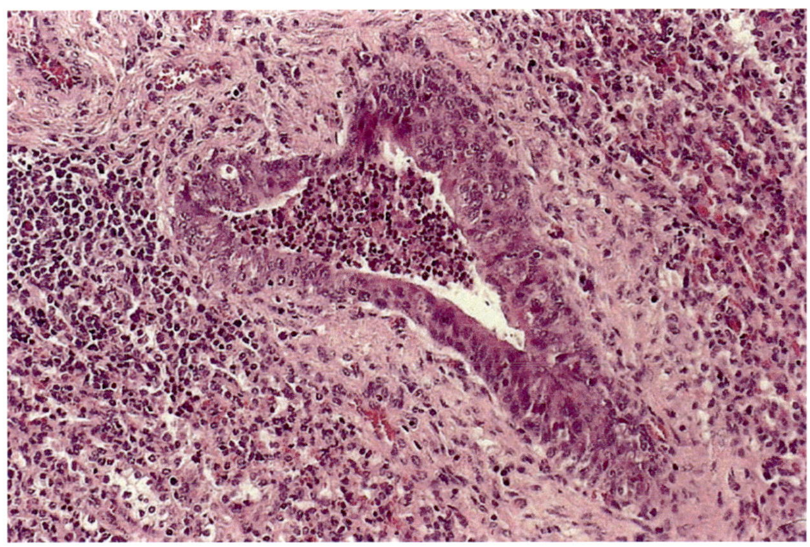

Fig. 1.28. Ox. Lung. Parainfluenza-3. Necrolymphocytic bronchopneumonia. Microscopically, the bronchiole is characterized by degeneration, sequestration and hyperplasia of respiratory epithelial cells. Fibrin and degenerate lymphocytes are present in the lumen. Adjacent alveoli are distended by lymphocytes (H&E).

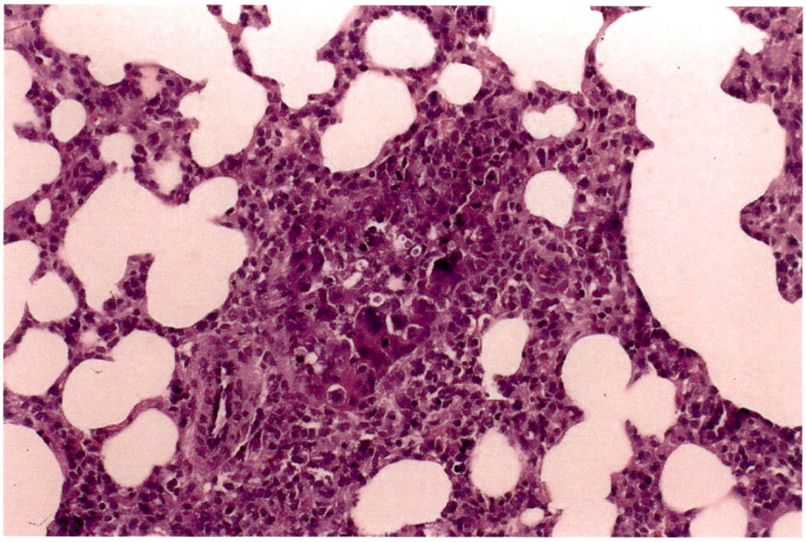

Fig. 1.29. Ox. Lung. Parainfluenza-3. Alveoli contain a focus of lymphocytes mixed with occasional multinucleated giant cells in the center (H&E).

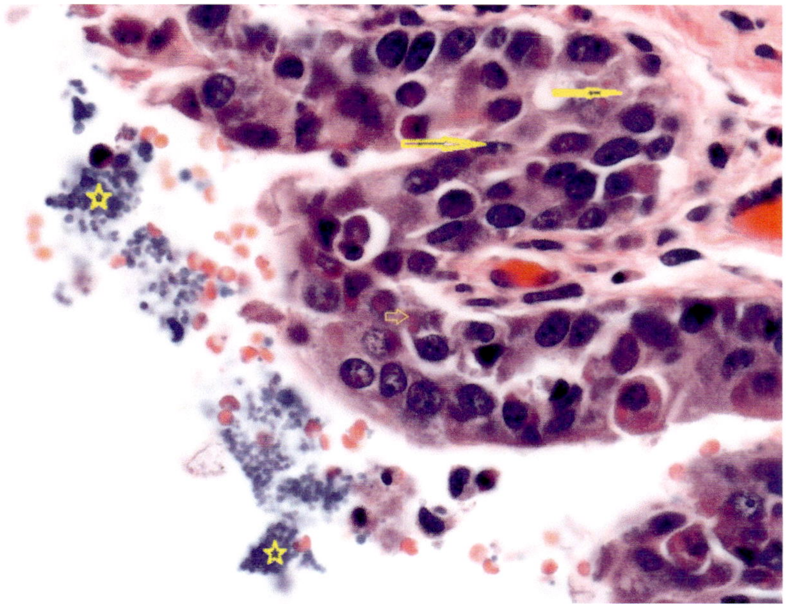

Fig. 1.30. Ox. Lung. Parainfluenza-3. Bronchus. Several eosinophilic viral inclusions (arrows) are visible in the cytoplasm of the respiratory epithelial cells. The lumen contains clusters of *Candida* yeast (asterisk) (H&E).

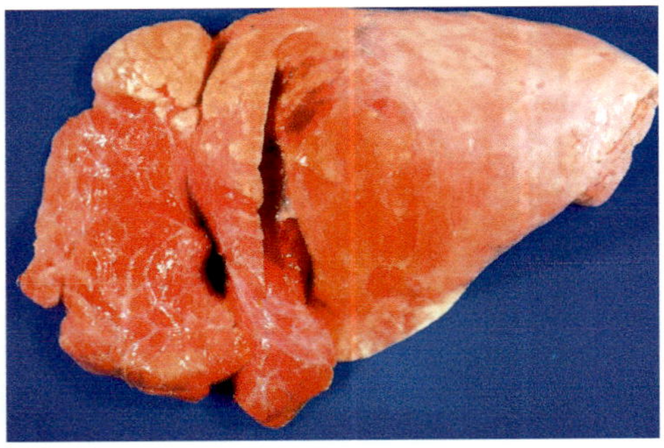

Fig. 1.32. Ox. Lung. Bovine respiratory syncytial virus (BRSV). Suppurative bronchopneumonia. Cranial and middle lung lobes are consolidated. Lobular distribution, diffuse edema and emphysema are characteristic of BRSV. More examples are demonstrated in Chapter 3: Diseases of the Respiratory System.

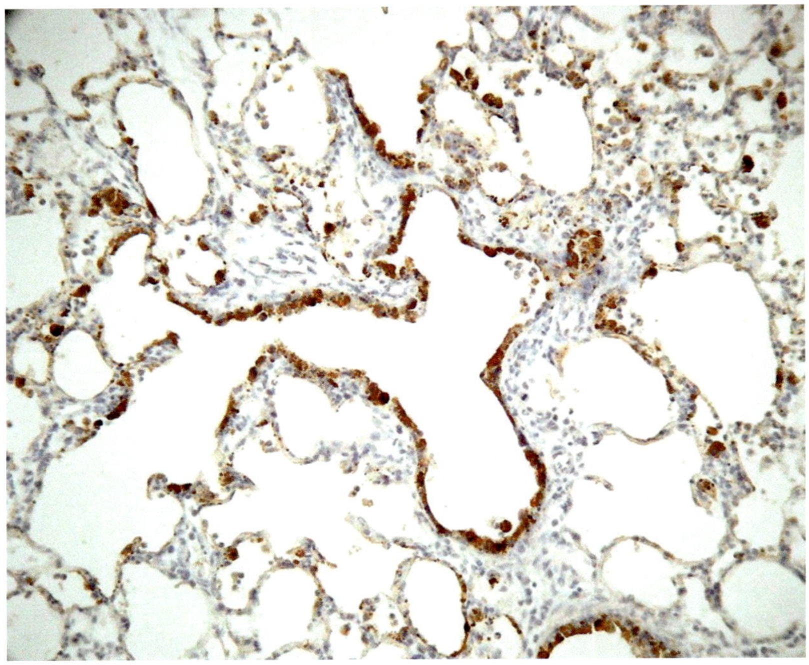

Fig. 1.31. Ox. Lung. Parainfluenza-3. Viral antigen is identified in the cytoplasm of bronchiolar lining cell, bronchi, multinucleate giant cells and macrophages (IHC).

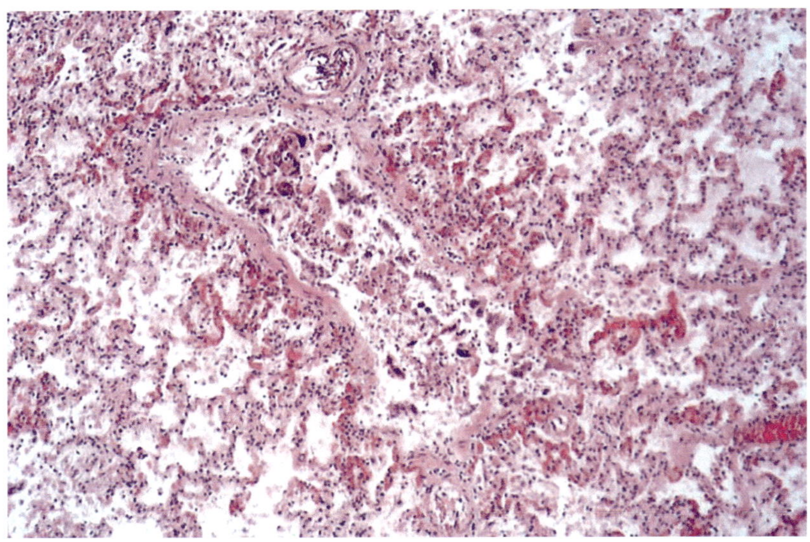

Fig. 1.33. Ox. Lung. Bovine respiratory syncytial virus (BRSV). Necrotizing bronchiolitis. Respiratory epithelium has sloughed into lumen, so are endothelial cells in the upper blood vessel. Alveoli are filled with fluid and loosely arranged, variably sized mononuclear cells (H&E).

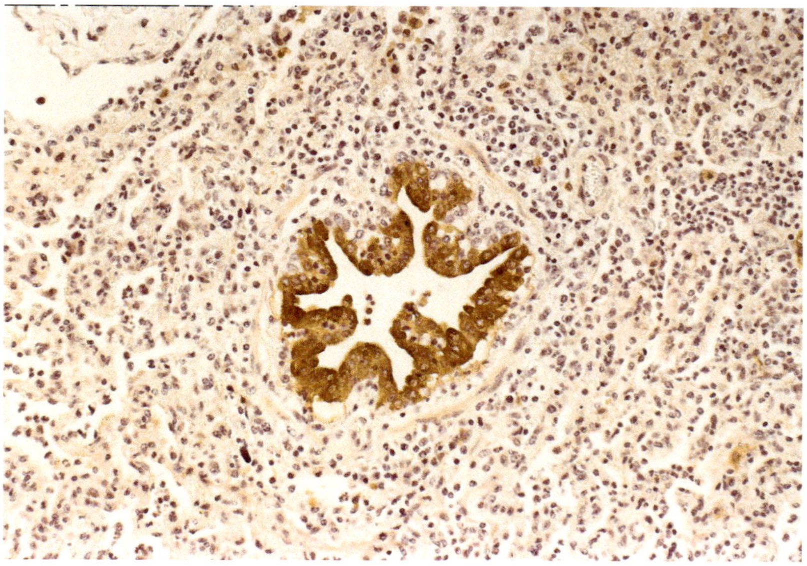

Fig. 1.34. Ox. Lung. Bovine respiratory syncytial virus (BRSV). The virus replicates in epithelial lining cells of the airways and viral antigen is demonstrated in the cytoplasm (IHC).

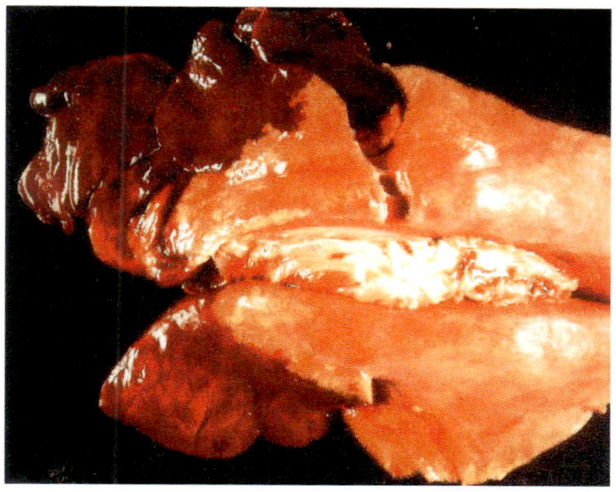

Fig. 1.35. Ox. Lung. Pasteurellosis. Anteroventral suppurative bronchopneumonia. An example of secondary bacterial infection to preceding viral pneumonia, it leads to consolidation without associated overlying pleural fibrin. *Pasteurella multocida* can sometimes be involved as the primary pathogen.

Fact Sheet: Enzootic Calf Pneumonia

Definition

Outbreak of pulmonary infection on dairy premises covering a broad spectrum of pulmonary pathogens and risk factors. The usual age range of affected dairy calves is up to 4 months.

Pathogens

- Primary
  Coronavirus
  Adenovirus
  Parainfluenza-3 virus
  Bovine respiratory syncytial virus
  Bovine viral diarrhea virus (BVDV) (immunosuppressive)
- Secondary
  Pasteurella multocida
  Mannheimia haemolytica
  Trueperella pyogenes
  Bibersteinia trehalosi

Risk Factors

Overcrowding
Poor ventilation
Lack of ventilation
Pre-exposure to BVD virus
Wide fluctuation of weather

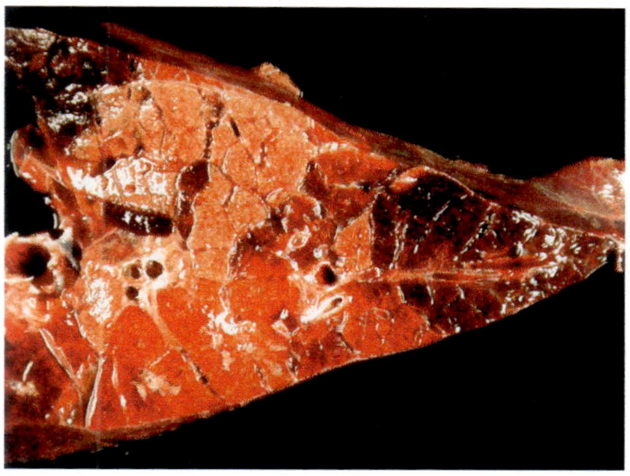

Fig. 1.36. Ox. Lung. Pasteurellosis. Necropurulent bronchopneumonia. The mottled appearance of the lobules on the cut section reflects various phases of inflammation and is a good indicator of *Pasteurella multocida* infection.

Another virus occasionally involved in enzootic calf pneumonia is bovine herpesvirus type 1 (BHV-1), which will be discussed in Chapter 3: Diseases of the Respiratory System.

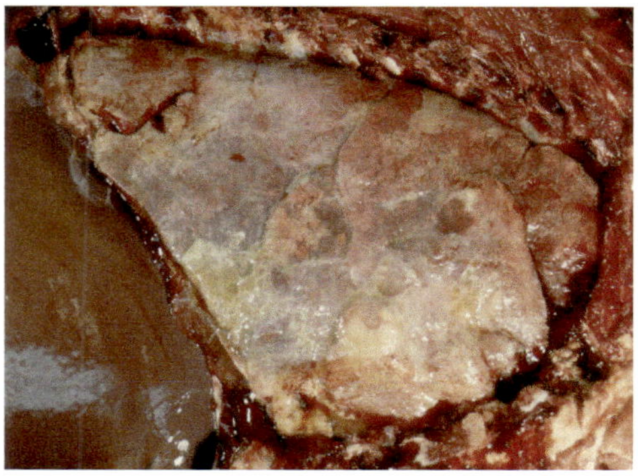

Fig. 1.37. Ox. Lung. *Mannheimia haemolytica*. Fibrinous pleuropneumonia. Severe consolidation of all lung lobes, with fibrin covering the pleura.

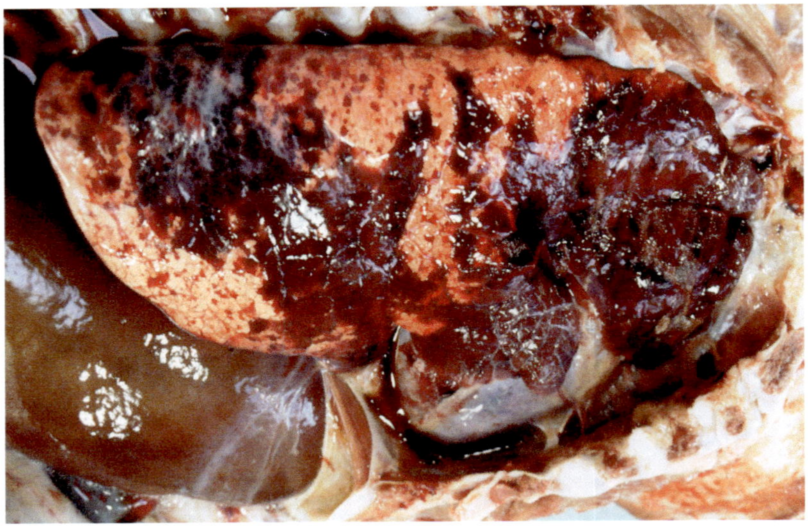

Fig. 1.38. Ox. Lung. *Mannheimia haemolytica*. Hemorrhagic bronchopneumonia with venous thrombosis. Marked necrosis and hemorrhage secondary to vasculitis are indicated by deep red discoloration of multiple lobules, with locally extensive distribution.

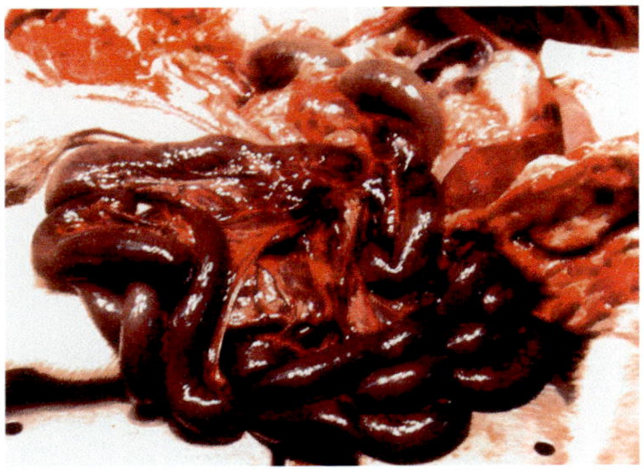

Fig. 1.39. Ox. Small intestine. Volvulus. Hemorrhagic jejunitis. Loops of jejunum are severely reddened due to a twist around the mesenteric attachment.

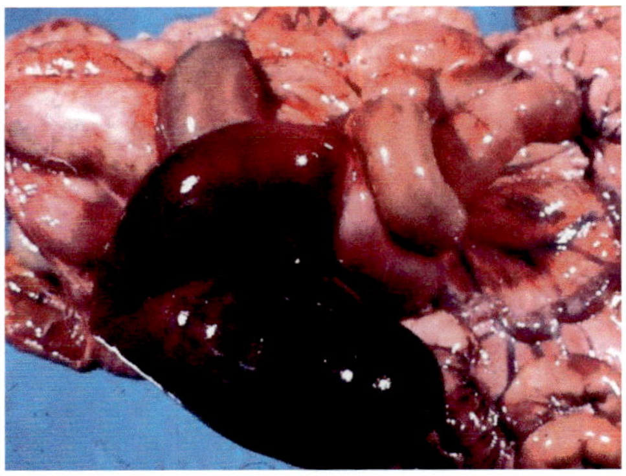

Fig. 1.40. Ox. Cecum. Torsion. Hemorrhagic typhlitis. The entire cecum has rotated around its longitudinal axis and is devitalized.

1.4 GASTROINTESTINAL DISORDERS

1.4.1 Displacements

Introduction. These are sporadic events and involve small and large intestines. Rotations (volvulus, torsion) or intestinal telescoping (intussusception) result in severe toxic necrosis of the tissue segments involved, due to obstruction of blood flow.

Clinical signs. Obstruction, pain, shock.

Differential diagnosis. Acute enteric pathogens (clostridial disease).

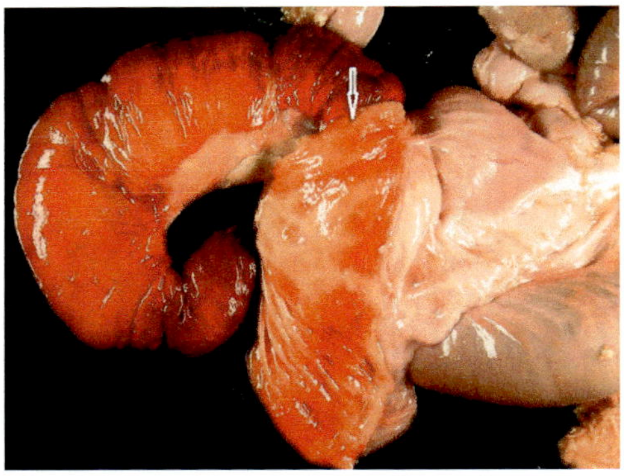

Fig. 1.41. Ox. Cecum. Intussusception. Necrohemorrhagic typhlitis. The entire cecum has telescoped into the colon. Point of invagination is depicted by arrow.

1.4.2 Inflammation

Introduction. Gastrointestinal inflammation in calves is frequently the result of infection. Infectious pathogens are of significant economic consequences and comprise virus, bacteria, protozoa, and occasional fungi and endoparasites. Dual etiology is common as one type of agent predisposes to another.

Clinical signs. Diarrhea, weight loss, dehydration, perineal pasting.

Differential diagnoses. Intestinal displacements, starvation.

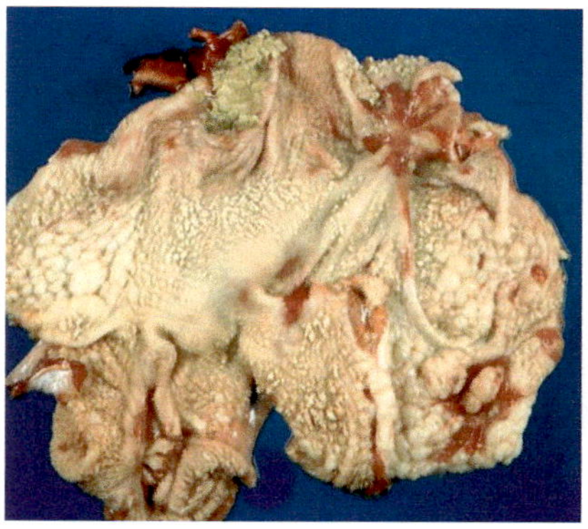

Fig. 1.43. Ox. Rumen. Candidiasis. Parakeratosis. Multifocal dry nodules on the mucosa develop from yeast infection. Similar changes can be encountered on the tongue and in the mucosa of the esophagus. Affected animals are usually immunocompromised. Excessive use of antibiotics can cause ruminal candidiasis as well.

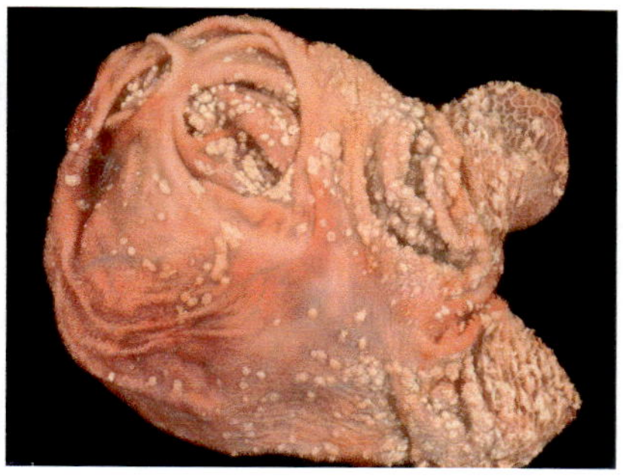

Fig. 1.44. Ox. Rumen. Infectious bovine rhinotracheitis (IBR). Exudative and proliferative rumenitis. Curdled exudate and parakeratosis are features of the alimentary form of IBR in the calf (BHV-1). With this form, lesions would also be expected in the oral cavity and esophagus.

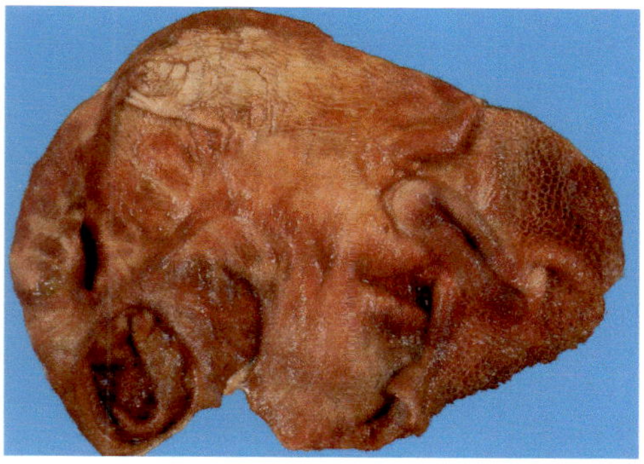

Fig. 1.42. Ox. Rumen/reticulum. Toxic rumenitis/reticulitis. The condition is known as 'ruminal drinking' of suckling calves when a faulty esophageal groove reflux results in the ingestion of milk into the reticulum/rumen. The formation of toxic metabolic fermentation products leads to tympany, mucosal hyperemia, necrosis, and ulceration

Calf scours

Acute enteric diseases of calves are a major cause of mortality in the first weeks of life, and of economic importance for producers replacing livestock with their own progeny. A variety of pathogens are involved, single or in concert with each other. The failure of passive transfer, lack of vaccination, poor hygiene, crowding, inadequate nutrition, and wet, cold conditions are major risk factors. Profuse diarrhea and dehydration are the clinical signs of pathologic intestinal damage. Responsible pathogens can be classified into viral, bacterial, and protozoal.

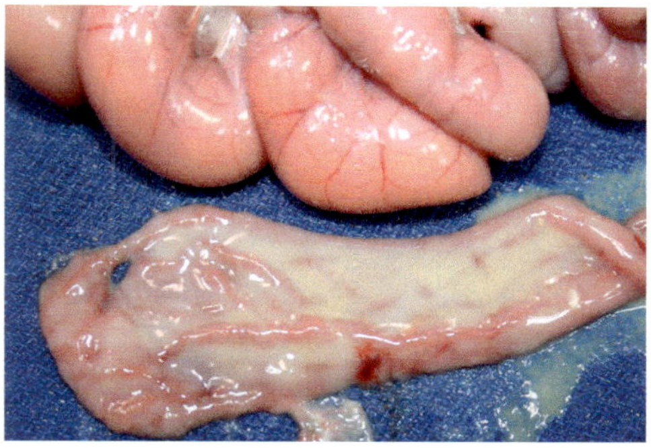

Fig. 1.45. Ox. Jejunum. Coronavirus. Catarrhal enteritis. Loops of jejunum are dilated and extended by milky fluid. When opened, the mucosa is covered by a mucous exudate. Rotavirus infection grossly induces similar changes. Also, intestinal content is identical in a very young calf on a high milk diet.

1.4.2.1 Viruses

Introduction. The viruses responsible for outbreaks of enteritis with severe clinical complications are rotavirus (*Reoviridae*) and coronavirus (*Coronaviridae*). Most infections occur during the first weeks of life. Diagnosis is made via enzyme-linked immunosorbent assay (ELISA), fluorescense microscopy (FM), PCR, immunohistochemistry (IHC), or detection of viral particles in negatively stained feces by transmission electron microscopy (TEM). Other enteric viruses with lesser clinical impact are enteric parvovirus, adenovirus and torovirus (Breda virus) infecting older calves. The role of bovine viral diarrhea virus (BVDV) and IBR in primary calf enteritis is less defined.

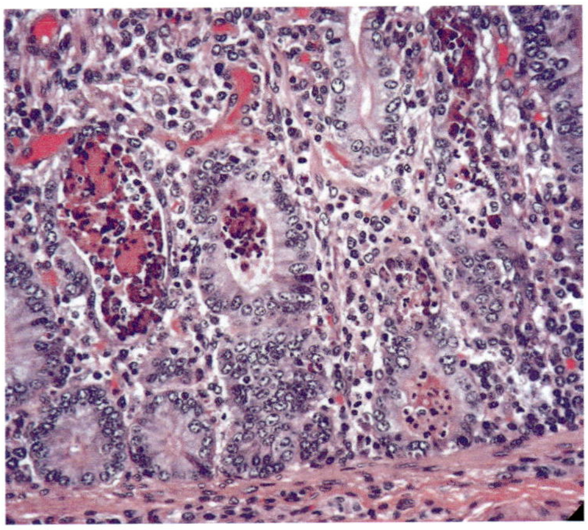

Fig. 1.46. Ox. Jejunum. Coronavirus. Crypt abscesses. Necrotic cellular debris with some fibrin is located within crypts. The lamina propria is infiltrated moderately by lymphocytes and some plasma cells (normal) (H&E).

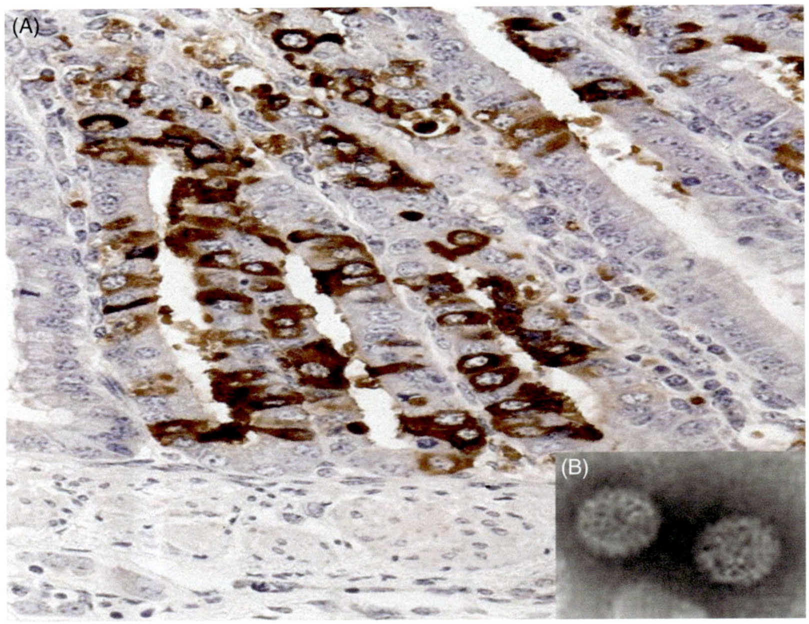

Fig. 1.47. Ox. Colon. Coronavirus. (A) Viral antigen is identified diffusely in the cytoplasm by indirect immunohistochemistry (IHC). (B) (inset) Negatively stained coronavirus particles demonstrated by transmission electron microscopy (TEM). (Courtesy of Dr M. Hines II, University of Georgia, USA.)

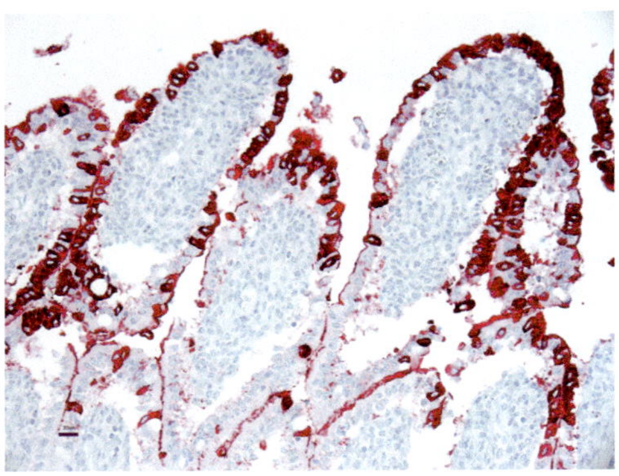

Fig. 1.49. Ox. Small intestine. Rotavirus. Viral antigen is located diffusely in cytoplasm of superficial enterocytes (IHC). (Courtesy of Dr B. Brodersen, University of Nebraska-Lincoln, USA.)

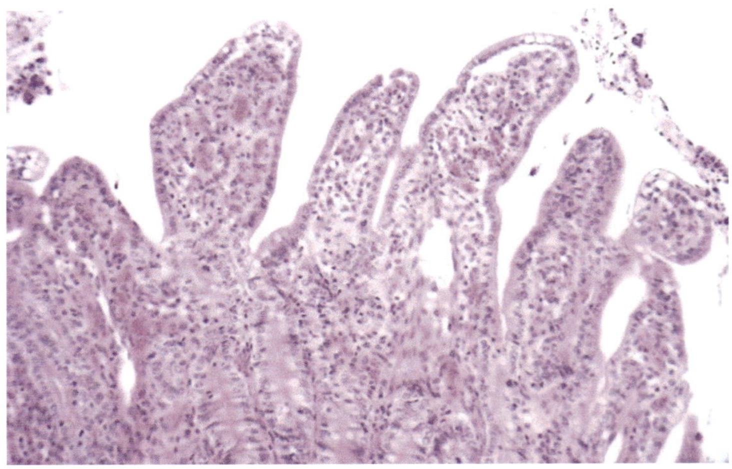

Fig. 1.48. Ox. Small intestine. Rotavirus. Villous atrophy. Villi are slightly shortened and clubbed. The lamina propria contains a normal number of lymphocytes (H&E).

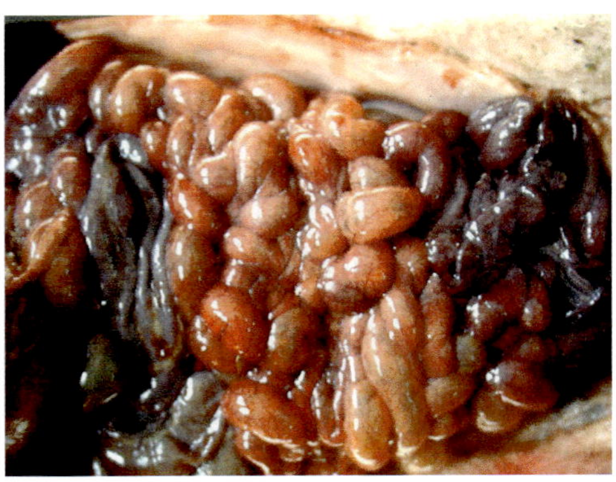

Fig. 1.50. Ox. Small intestine. Colibacillosis. Catarrhal enteritis. Loops of small intestine are markedly distended by watery fluid; some segments have a reddened wall.

1.4.2.2 Bacteria

Introduction. The main types of contagious bacterial enteric pathogens are *Escherichia coli* and *Clostridium perfringens* in the first 2 weeks and *Salmonella enterica* in the first 1–3 months of life. The highly virulent pathogens are associated with high mortality, and in the case of *E. coli*, lead to sepsis (septicemic colibacillosis).

Clinical signs. Watery diarrhea, dehydration, depression, sunken eyes, recumbency.

Differential diagnoses. Protozoa, viruses.

Escherichia coli (E. coli). Various strains of *Escherichia coli* are involved in disease outbreaks, with some of them often fatal (enterotoxigenic *E. coli*). *E. coli* bacteria occur as non-virulent and virulent strains. Non-virulent strains are part of the normal intestinal flora. Virulent strains are classified as to serotypes, composition of antigens and the damage they cause in the intestinal tract. Major strains involved in enteric colibacillosis are the enterotoxigenic (ETEC) strain, the enterohemorrhagic (EHEC) strain, the attachment and effacing (AEEC) strain, a subset of the enteropathogenic, enteroinvasive (EPEC) strain, and the necrotoxigenic strain (NTEC), producing cytotoxic necrotizing factors. The enterohemorrhagic strain produces a Shiga-toxin (verotoxin), damaging intestinal epithelium and vascular endothelium, causing erosive fibrinohemorrhagic enterocolitis. The strain contributes to foodborne illness in humans. Enterotoxigenic *E. coli* produces enterotoxin and colonizes the intestinal epithelium via fimbriae, also known as pili. Immunohistochemical stains for fimbrial adhesin is helpful for the diagnosis, especially of K99 *E. coli*. Culture can be attempted if the animal has not been treated extensively with antibiotics. Microscopic lesions are usually minimal for this strain. Enteroinvasive strains disseminate systemically and are responsible for calf sepsis (septicemic colibacillosis).

Enterotoxemia. Clostridial disease, caused by *Clostridium perfringens*, type A (90% of cases) and type C (5% of cases), secretes enterotoxins, alpha in the case of type A and alpha and beta in the case of type C, causes hemorrhage and ischemic necrosis of small intestinal tissue, leading to gas production, bloat, colic, toxic shock and death.

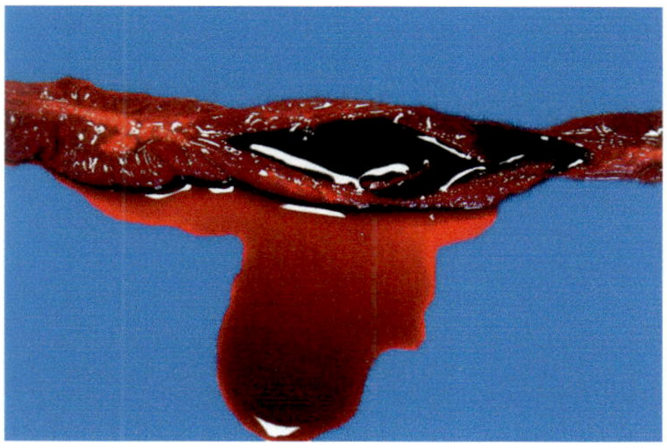

Fig. 1.51. Ox. Small intestine. Clostridial disease. Catarrhal hemorrhagic enteritis. Excessive blood-tinged watery fluid is released from the intestinal lumen. *Clostridium perfringens* sp. (Courtesy of Dr D. O'Toole, University of Wyoming, USA.)

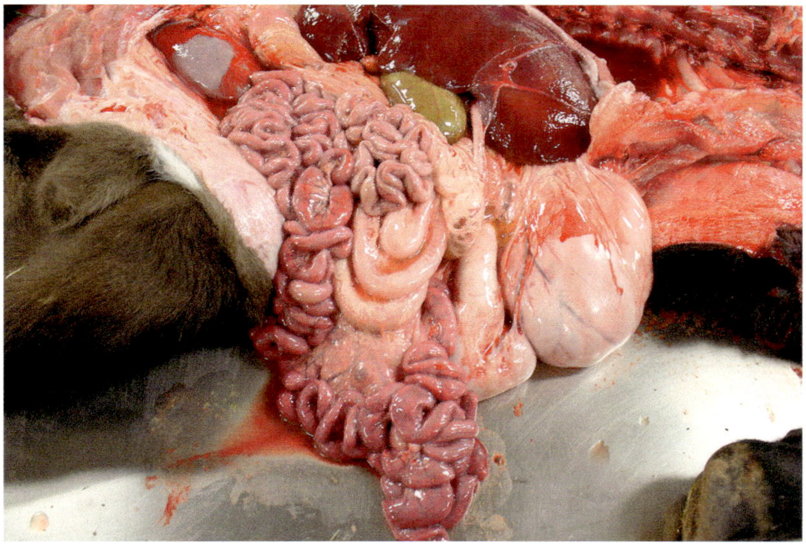

Fig. 1.52. Ox. Small intestine. Clostridial disease. Catarrhal, hemorrhagic enteritis. 'Purple gut'. Distinct purple discoloration of intestine. *Clostridium perfringens* type C is usually isolated. (Courtesy of Dr D. O'Toole, University of Wyoming, USA.)

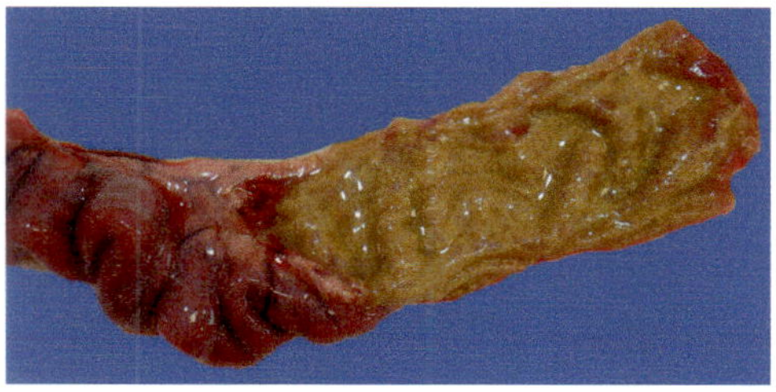

Fig. 1.53. Ox. Small intestine. Clostridial disease. Necrotizing, fibrinous, hemorrhagic enteritis. What looks like digesta is an adherent exudate with a distinctive green tinge which does not wash off. (Courtesy of Dr D. O'Toole, University of Wyoming, USA.)

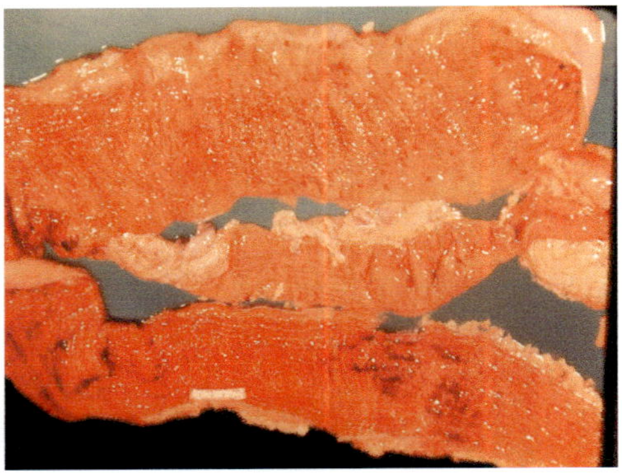

Fig. 1.54. Ox. Small intestine. Acute salmonellosis. Multifocal hemorrhagic enteritis. Petechiae cover the mucosa.

Salmonellosis. Salmonella is an intracellular, gram-negative pathogen with zoonotic potential, and infects both calves and adult cattle. Infection phases range from peracute to chronic, with a pathologic spectrum ranging from minimal punctuate focal hemorrhage in the intestinal mucosa in acute cases to inspissated diphtheritic membranes covering the mucosa of small and large intestines in chronic cases. The species of Salmonella involved in the majority of infections is *Salmonella enterica* with six subspecies. Two capabilities allow *Salmonella* spp. to cause inflammation: penetration of the intestinal epithelium (M-cells); survival in macrophages.

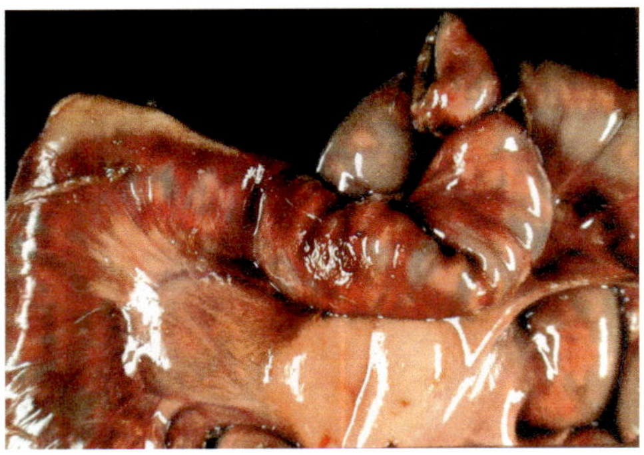

Fig. 1.55. Ox. Colon. Subacute salmonellosis. Transmural necrohemorrhagic enteritis. The entire wall of the intestine is friable, discolored and contains multiple pale foci of necrosis.

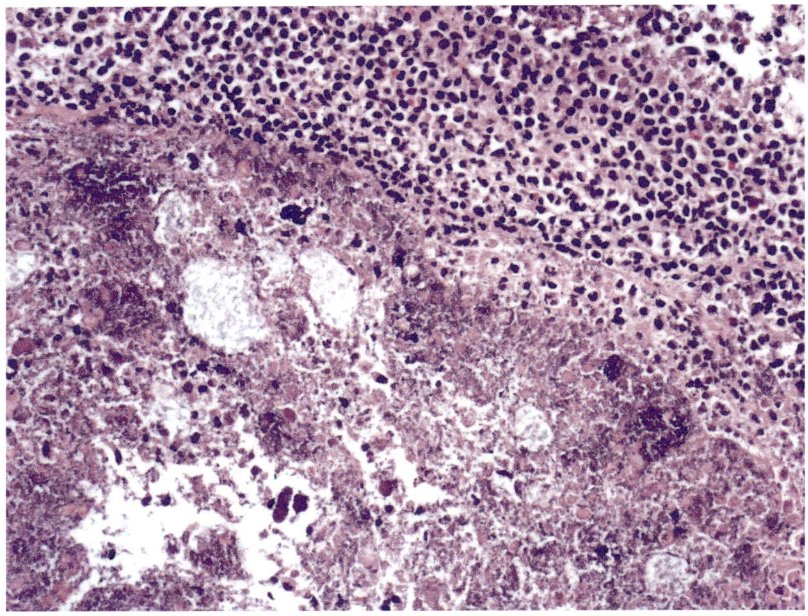

Fig. 1.56. Ox. Intestine. Salmonellosis. Fibrinonecrotic enteritis. The mucosa denuded from its enterocyte lining is covered by fibrin and degenerate, necrotic inflammatory cells. Intermingled are numerous bacterial colonies. Fibrin thrombi in small lamina propria capillaries are suggestive indicators of the disease, although clostridiosis has also been associated with thrombi (H&E).

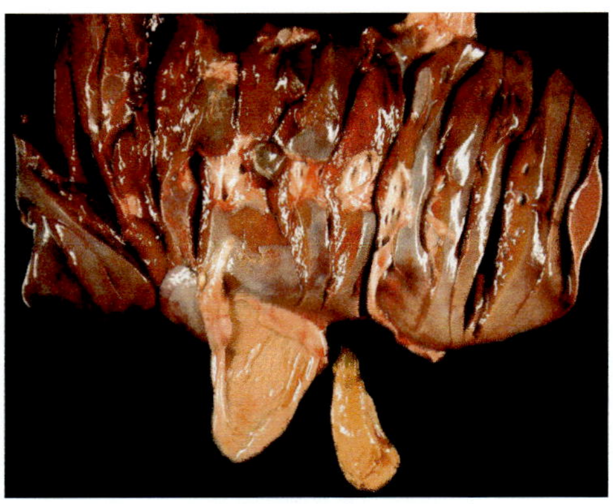

Fig. 1.57. Ox. Gall bladder. Salmonellosis. Fibrin plug. A yellow fibrin cast contained within the gall bladder is highly suggestive of infection with *Salmonella* spp.

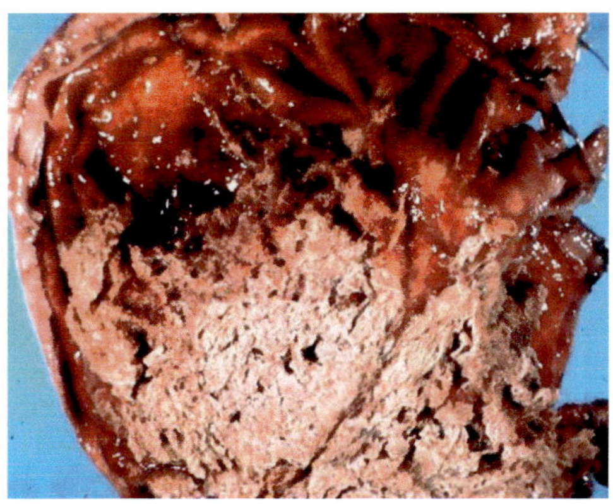

Fig. 1.58. Ox. Abomasum. Salmonellosis. Fibrinous abomasitis. The mucosa is covered with sheaths of fibrin, resembling curdled milk. Differential diagnosis should include infection with the bovine rhinotracheitis virus (IBR), clostridial abomasitis.

1.4.2.3 Protozoa

Introduction. Cryptosporidiosis, giardiasis and coccidiosis are all enteric diseases involved in calf scours and morbidity.
Clinical signs. Profuse watery or bloody diarrhea.
Differential diagnoses. *E. coli*, *Salmonella* spp., bovine rotavirus, bovine coronavirus.

Cryptosporidiosis. Two species are prevalent in calves, *Cryptosporidium parvum* and *Cryptosporidium andersoni*. *C. andersoni* resides in the abomasum, whereas *C. parvum*, a zoonotic pathogen, resides within the intestinal brush border. The agents are intracellular and extracytoplasmic. Transmission is via the oral–fecal route from contaminated environments, water or sewage. Grossly, the intestinal mucosa may be mildly reddened and may be covered by mucous fluid.

Giardiasis. Caused by *Giardia duodenalis*, the flagellated organism attaches to the microvilli of the intestinal epithelium with a ventral sucker interfering with membrane function to induce malabsorption. There are usually no gross changes in infected animals.

Coccidiosis. Infestation in calves with *Eimeria bovis*, but more often with *Eimeria zuernii*, causes severe profuse bloody diarrhea associated with tenesmus, dysentery, rectal prolapse, and weight loss. Small and large intestine are involved. The nervous form of coccidiosis has been reported from northern America due to a potential toxin produced by the parasite.

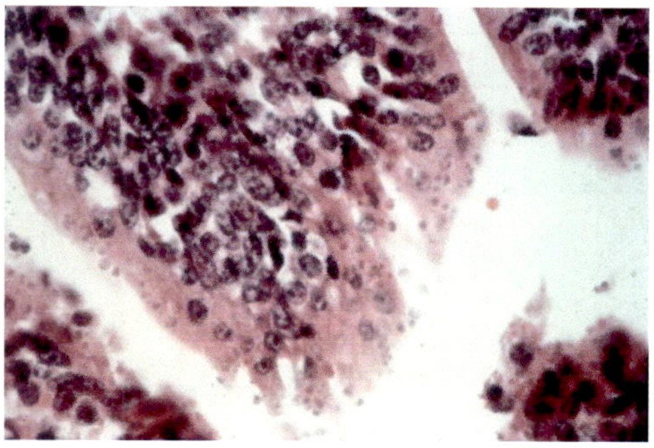

Fig. 1.59. Ox. Jejunum. Cryptosporidiosis. Ruptured brush border. The brush border is discontinuous and contains multiple intracellular, small basophilic structures, 1–2 microns in diameter (H&E)

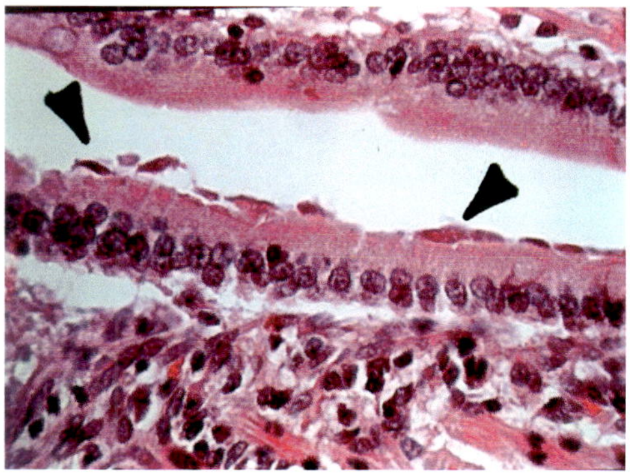

Fig. 1.60. Ox. Jejunum. Giardiasis. Protozoal attachment. Flagellated, banana-shaped structures (arrow heads) phagocytize the intestinal brush border (H&E).

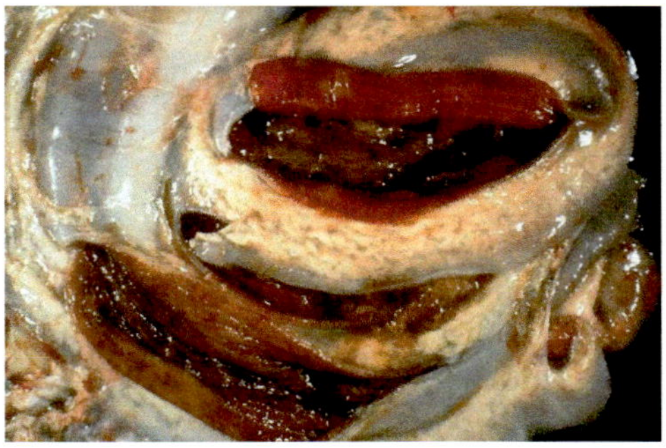

Fig. 1.61. Ox. Colon. Coccidiosis. Hemorrhagic colitis. Segments of the colonic mucosa are deeply red and thickened, and contain a luminal necrotic cast and/or fibrin.

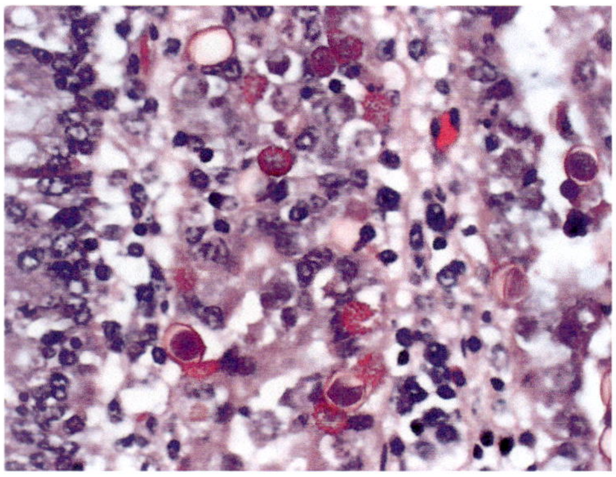

Fig. 1.62. Ox. Colon. Coccidiosis. Lymphocytic colitis with gametogony. Various forms of gametes are lodged within the villous tips of the mucosa (H&E).

1.4.2.4 Fungi

Introduction. Mycotic enteritis is a sporadic individual event and can be predisposed by excessive antibiotic treatment. It needs to be considered in the differential diagnosis of diarrhea when individual animals are affected.

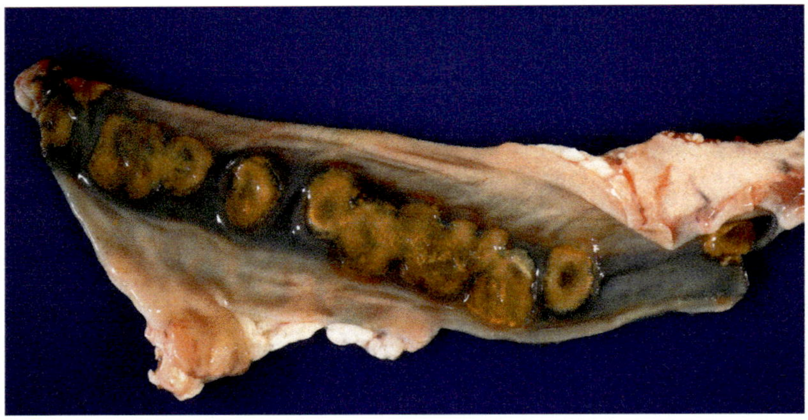

Fig. 1.63. Ox. Jejunum. Mycosis. Multifocal angiocentric fibrinonecrotic enteritis. Elevated plaques with a tan, friable center and dark rim suggest fungal involvement. (Courtesy of the Government of Alberta, Canada.)

1.4.2.5 Parasites

Introduction. Infestation with endoparasites in calves is usually asymptomatic and their presence an incidental finding at necropsy. Endoparasites involved are nematodes and cestodes.

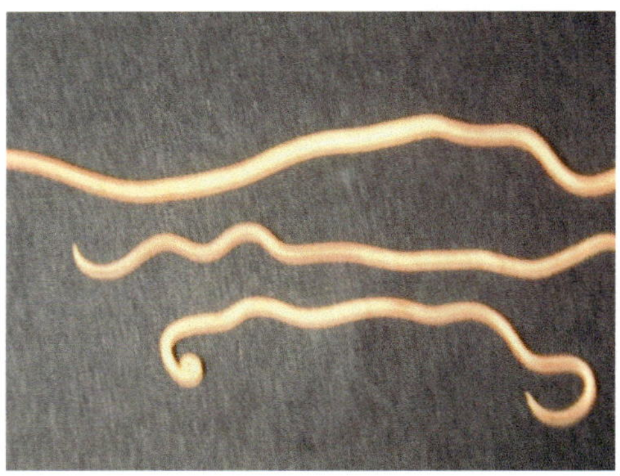

Fig. 1.64. Ox. Ascarids. Adults of *Toxocara vitulorum* collected from the small intestine.

1.5 ADDITIONAL GASTRIC CONDITIONS

1.5.1 Abomasal foreign body formations

These are known as trichobezoars (pilobezoars, hairballs) and incidental findings at necropsy. They develop from self-suckling and swallowing of hair and become entrapped in the abomasum without causing clinical signs. This is particularly common in veal calves. Calves may occasionally be born with hairballs. If the conglomerate is made of plant material, the formations are called phytobezoars. The combination of plant and hair material is called phytotrichobezoars.

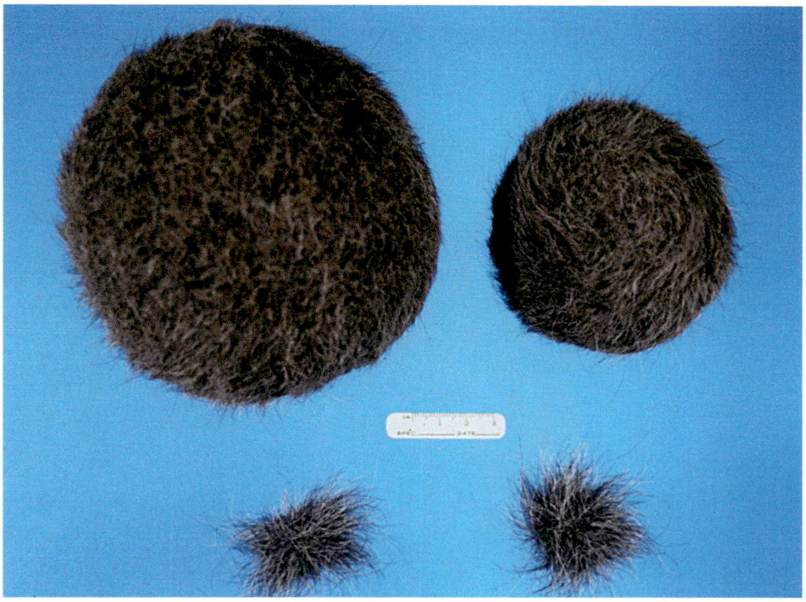

Fig. 1.65. Ox. Abomasal trichobezoars. Multiple, different-sized hairballs were retrieved from the abomasum of an individual or multiple calves.

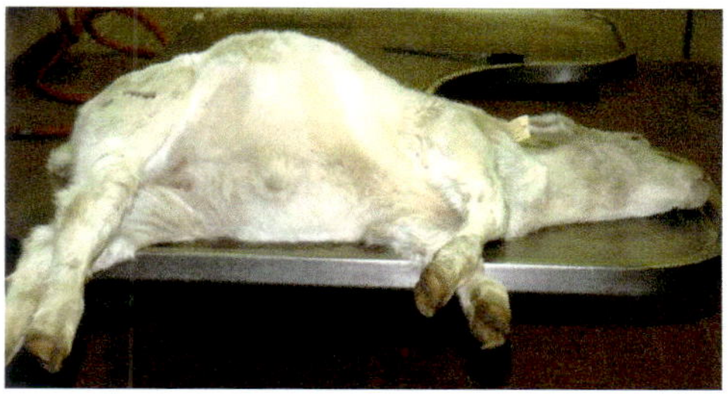

Fig. 1.66. Ox. Whole body. Abomasal tympany (bloat) due to perforated abomasal ulcer. The abdomen is markedly distended by severe antemortem gaseous accumulation (bloat) in the abomasum.

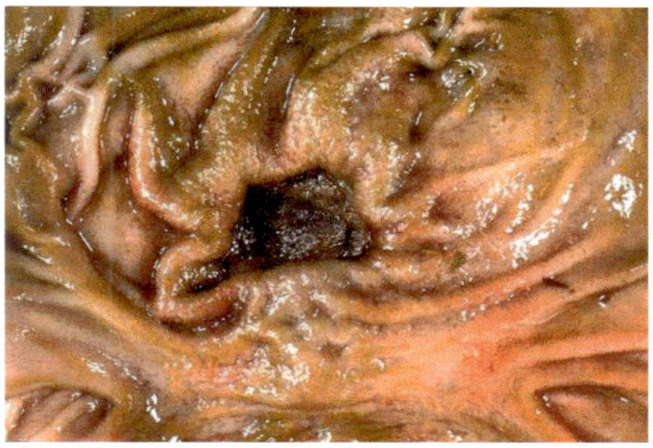

Fig. 1.67. Ox. Abomasum. Chronic, non-perforating ulcer. The ulcer bed is covered by blood and fibrin. The rounded mucosal edges suggest chronicity.

1.5.2 Abomasal ulceration

Introduction. Commonly seen in the abomasum in feedlot cattle. May perforate, especially in young beef calves 2–4 months of age on pasture. In dairy calves, they develop secondarily to stress, poor milk quality, coarse feed, grain overload and subsequent overgrowth of *C. perfringens* type A, rarely type C. A preceding infection with BVDV cannot be confirmed. A small outbreak of abomasal ulcers in dairy calves has been associated with rotavirus infection.

A research project in Canada devoted to finding a cause in pastured beef calves failed to do so.

Clinical signs. Bloat, colic, shock.

Differential diagnoses. Intestinal displacement, peritonitis.

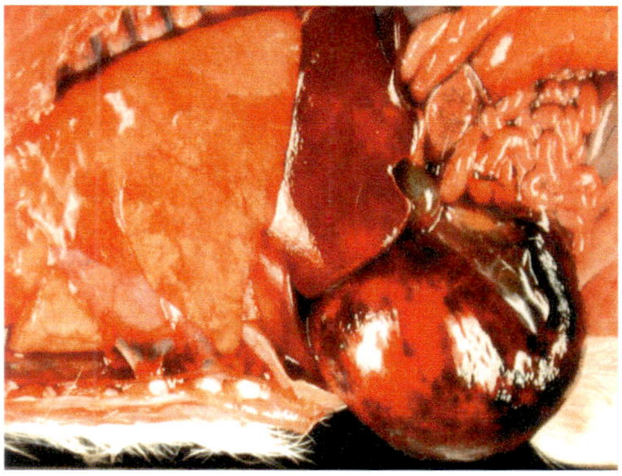

Fig. 1.68. Ox. Abomasum. Braxy-like hemorrhagic abomasitis Transmural hemorrhage in slightly distended abomasum. *Clostridium septicum* was isolated. The condition in sheep is known as braxy.

1.5.3 Hemorrhagic abomasitis

Introduction. Sporadic cases have been incriminated to be caused by infectious agents, such *Clostridium septicum* (braxy), *C. perfringens* type A, *Sarcina ventriculi* or *Salmonella* spp.

Clinical signs. Abdominal pain, tympany, shock.

Differential diagnosis. Abomasal torsion.

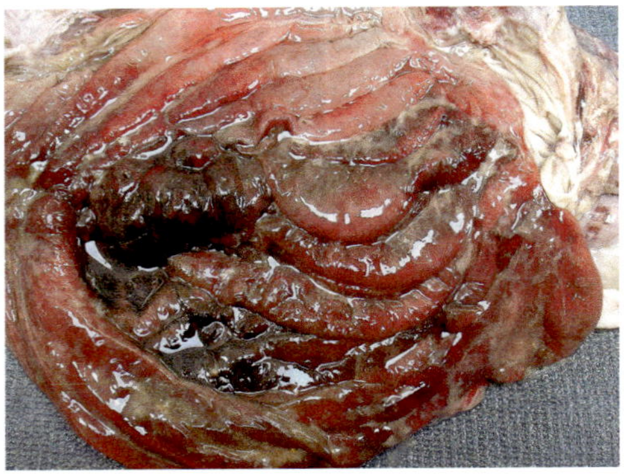

Fig. 1.70. Ox. Abomasum. Braxy-like hemorrhagic necrosis. The abomasal wall is markedly thickened by edema and hemorrhage. The weakened wall is susceptible to perforation. *Clostridium* spp. and *Sarcina* spp. are possible etiologic agents.

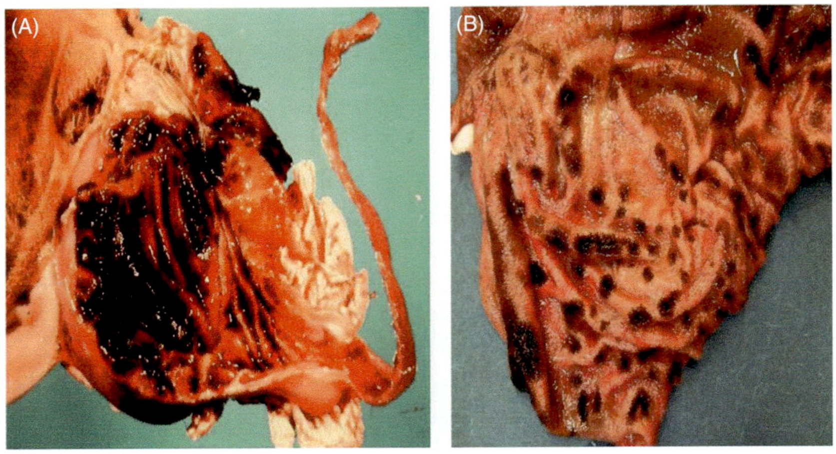

Fig. 1.69. Ox. Abomasum. Multifocal hemorrhagic abomasitis. (A) Large foci of a thickened mucosa are affected by severe hemorrhage. *Clostridium perfringens* type A was isolated. (B) Punctuate foci of hemorrhage are scattered throughout the mucosa. *Salmonella* spp. was isolated.

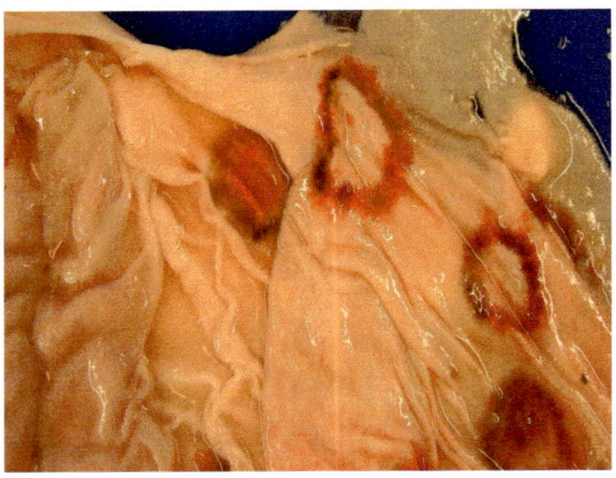

Fig. 1.72. Ox. Abomasum. Mycosis. Angiocentric hemorrhagic abomasitis. Patches of red rings cover the mucosa, suggesting vascular invasion by systemic fungi such as *Aspergillus* spp. Fungal invasion is frequently a sequel to excessive antibiotic treatment or salmonellosis.

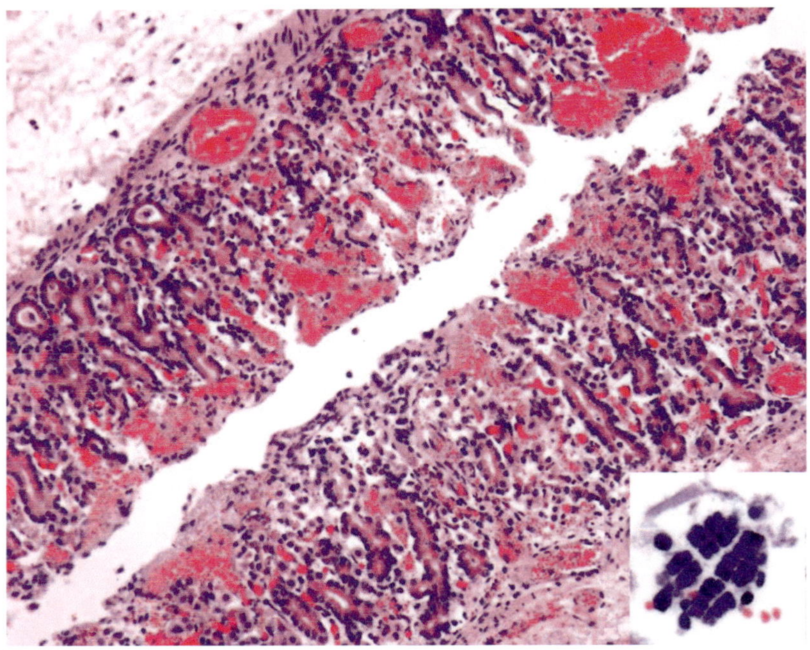

Fig. 1.71. Ox. Abomasum. Fibrinonecrotic hemorrhagic abomasitis. Superficial mucosal cells are necrotic with some fibrin on the surface. There is some lymphocytic infiltration in the lamina propria which is of no significance. Lamina propria blood vessels are markedly congested, partially thrombosed and have perivascular lymphocytic inflammation (H&E). Inset: packet-forming *Sarcina ventriculi* cocci. These may be found on the mucosal surface in calves with abomasal bloat and abomasitis (Giemsa stain).

1.5.4 Calf sepsis (formerly septicemia)

Introduction. Neonatal calves are most susceptible to sepsis following infection with *E. coli*, *Salmonella* spp. and other gram-negative bacteria. Risk factors are weather fluctuations, minimal shelter, lack of colostrum, poor birth hygiene, and umbilical infection as the portal of entry. The term 'septicemia' is now rarely used and has been replaced with sepsis. Sepsis is a life-threatening condition that arises when the body's response to infection injures its own tissues and organs. Sepsis is defined as the systemic inflammatory response syndrome (SIRS) in response to an infectious process. SIRS constitutes the presence of two or more of the following: abnormal body temperature, heart rate, respiratory rate or blood gas, and white blood cell count.

Clinical signs. Fever, depression, anorexia, disorientation, lameness, sudden death.

Differential diagnoses. Congenital abnormalities affecting individual vital organs, cold (freezer) artefact, BVDV infection (see Chapter 15: Diseases of Eye and Ear).

Figures 1.74–1.78 exhibit the frequent gross pathologic changes encountered with septic calves.

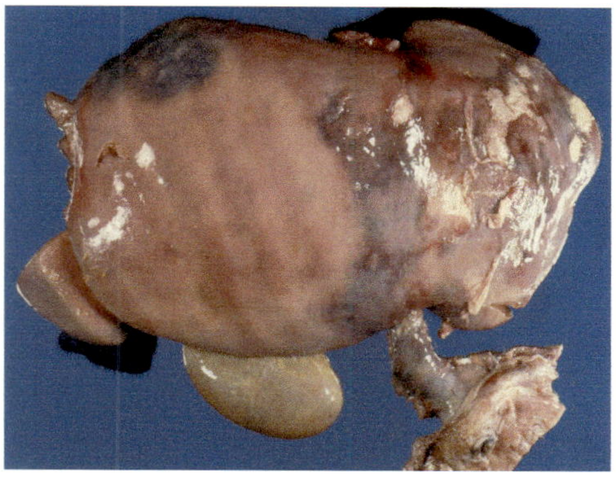

Fig. 1.73. Ox. Umbilicus. Suppurative omphalophlebitis. The umbilicus and ductus venosus are markedly distended by pus, serving as the perfect portal of entry for opportunistic pathogens to translocate hematogenously to various organ systems such as the liver, which contains multiple abscesses.

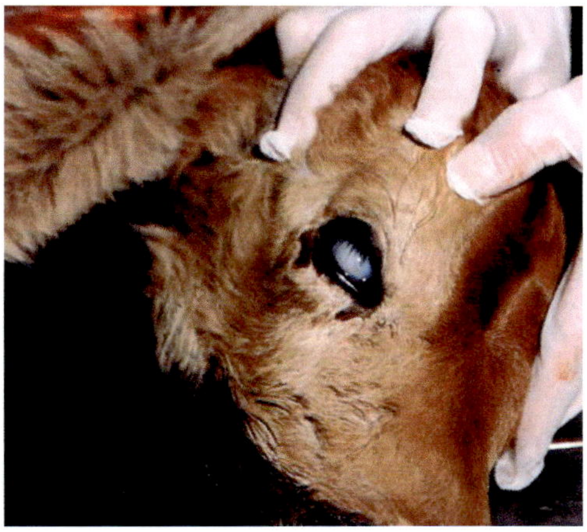

Fig. 1.76. Ox. Eye. Calf sepsis. Hypopyon. A cloudy fibrinosuppurative exudate occupies the anterior eye chamber.

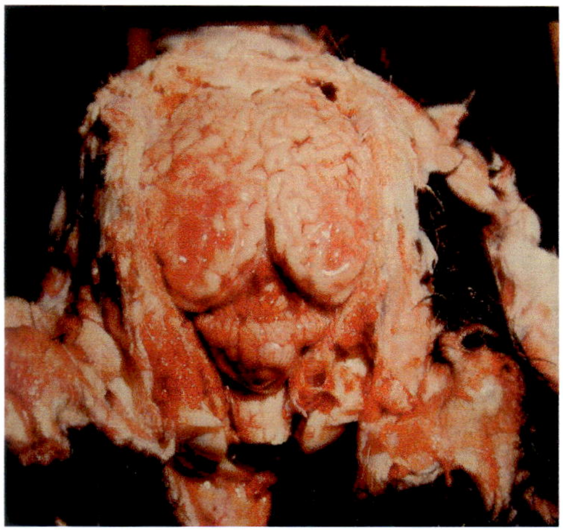

Fig. 1.74. Ox. Brain. Calf sepsis. Hemorrhagic meningitis. The meningeal surface exhibits ecchymotic hemorrhage over occipital lobes and cerebellum.

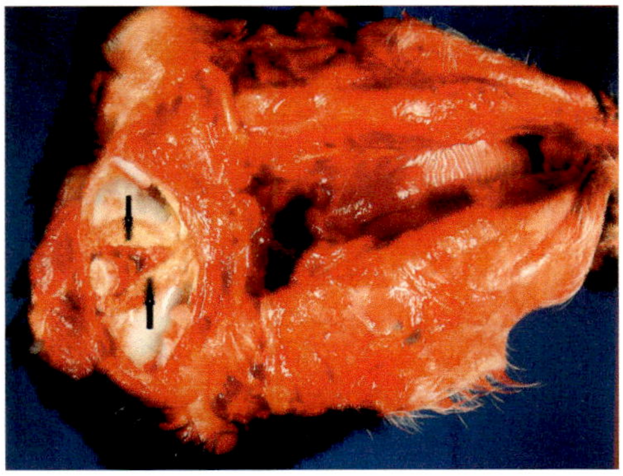

Fig. 1.77. Ox. Atlanto-occipital joint. Calf sepsis. Fibrinous arthritis. Fibrin plugs (arrows) close to the condyles are good indicators for the diagnosis of calf sepsis.

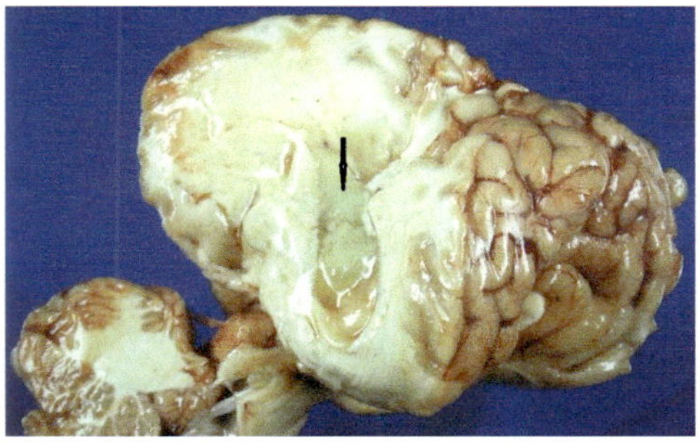

Fig. 1.75. Ox. Brain. Calf sepsis. Purulent ventriculitis. The lateral ventricle (arrow) is filled with viscous pus.

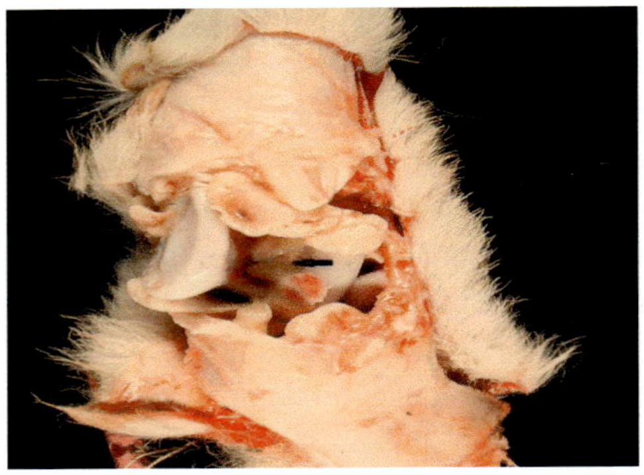

Fig. 1.78. Ox. Hock joint. Calf sepsis. Fibrinous arthritis. Fibrin casts (arrow) cover the articular cartilage. They should not be confused with fat. The hock joints should always be cultured in cases of calf sepsis, with the intent to isolate the pathogen. An antibiotic resistance test should be performed at the same time.

Fact Sheet: Calf Sepsis

Definition

Inflammatory response of various organs to embolic dissemination of gram-negative bacteria from a primary source (nidus) or to toxins (sepsis) produced by the gram-negative bacteria.

Primary source

- Umbilicus
- Digestive tract
- Tonsil

Organ systems involved in gross pathology

- Joints
- Meninges
- Brain
- Eyes
- Gall bladder

Infectious agents isolated

- Coliforms
- *Salmonella* spp.
- *Clostridium perfringens*

Co-infection

- Rotavirus
- Coronavirus
- *Cryptosporidium parvum*
- *Giardia duodenalis*

Risk factors

- Poor umbilical hygiene
- Failure of passive transfer of immunoglobulins
- Nutritional imbalance
- Management practices

1.6 MUSCULOSKELETAL DISORDERS

1.6.1 Muscular system

1.6.1.1 White muscle disease (WMD)

Introduction. The disorder is an example of a nutritional myodegeneration and the result of vitamin E/selenium deficiency observed in many vertebrates. It is responsive to selenium treatment. It typically occurs in fast-growing animals and affects multiple striated muscle groups, principally the most active muscles, and the heart. Sources of nutrient deficiency are selenium-deficient soil or moldy feed (hay). In newborn calves, severe vitamin E deficiency (drought) with no selenium deficiency cause white muscle disease. There is more on WMD in Chapter 8: Diseases of the Musculoskeletal System.

Clinical signs. Lameness, stiff gait, myoglobinuria, aspiration pneumonia, respiratory distress.

Differential diagnoses. Toxic myodegeneration (plants, ionophore antimicrobial), tetanus, hemolytic disorders.

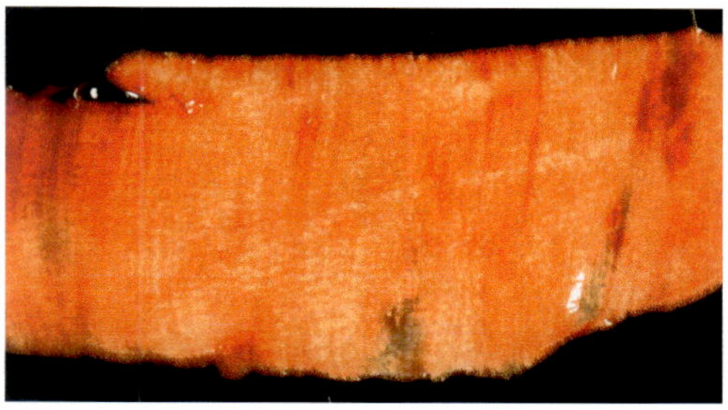

Fig. 1.79. Ox. Diaphragm. White muscle disease (WMD). Myodegeneration. A paintbrush linear arrangement of streaks is distributed along the length of muscle fibers.

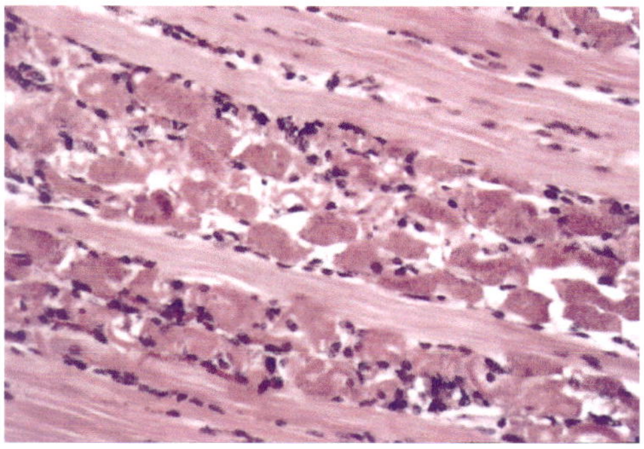

Fig. 1.80. Ox. Skeletal muscle. White muscle disease (WMD). Myonecrosis with mineralization. Swollen muscle fibers have undergone coagulative necrosis with heavy mineralization. Mild lymphocytic inflammation is present adjacent to dense sarcolemmal cells (H&E).

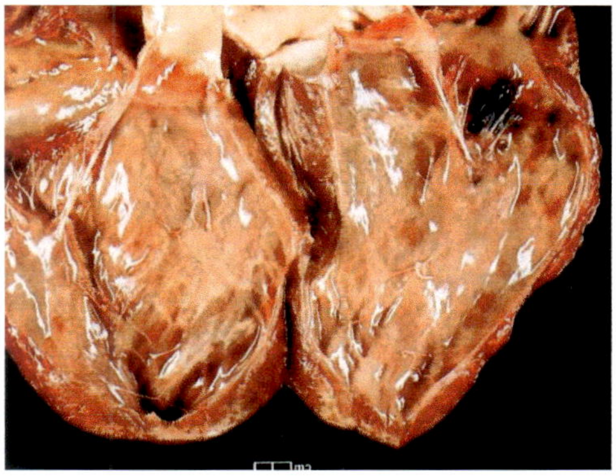

Fig. 1.81. Ox. Heart. White muscle disease (WMD). Cardiac myodegeneration. There is diffuse pallor affecting a thin left ventricle. The presentation of cardiac WMD is unusually extensive in this case.

1.6.2 Skeletal system

Introduction. Skeletal abnormalities may be genetic, teratogenic (viruses), or nutritional in origin.

Clinical signs. Lameness of various degrees; stunted limbs; disproportionate body parts; recumbency.

Differential diagnosis. Acquired locomotor disorders

1.6.2.1 Congenital chondrodysplasia

The condition occurs mainly in beef cattle breeds and produces disproportionate calves (bovine dwarfism). Depending on the breed, a genetic etiology is often involved, with the mode of inheritance either autosomal dominant or autosomal recessive. In some cases, mineral deficiency (zinc, manganese) is hypothesized as being the cause of the deformities. The deformity involves various anatomic parts of the skeletal system (see Chapter 8: Diseases of the Musculoskeletal System).

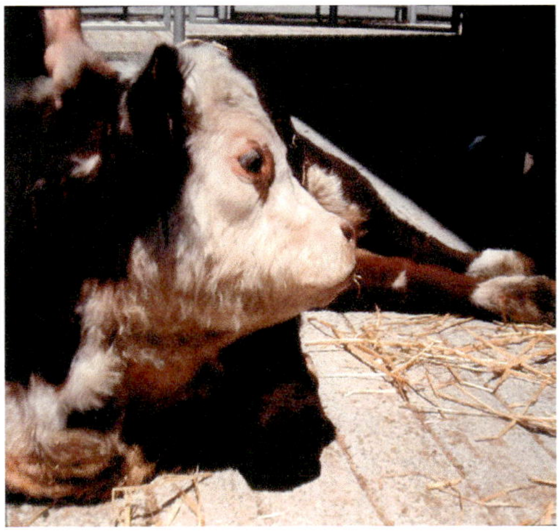

Fig. 1.82. Ox. Head. Chondrodysplasia. A shortening of the cervical vertebral column of the neck with a relatively large head has created the phenotypical appearance of a 'bull nose'.

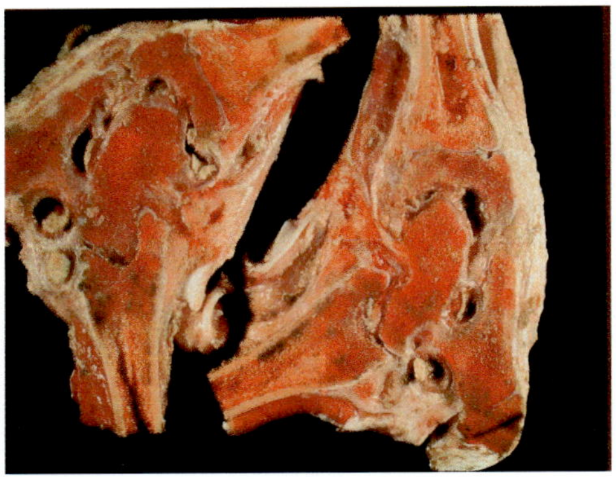

Fig. 1.84. Ox. Joint. Tarsal joint. Septic arthritis. The joint is filled with purulent exudate. Trauma and subsequent infection can be considered a cause if a single joint only is involved.

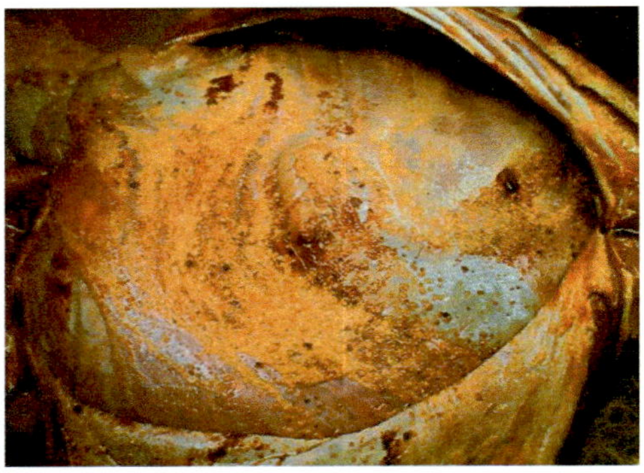

Fig. 1.85. Ox. Peritoneum. Mesothelioma. The serosal surface of the rumen and the abdominal peritoneum are covered by white to yellow, nodular neoplastic growths, many of which are confluent. Calves may be born with the condition.

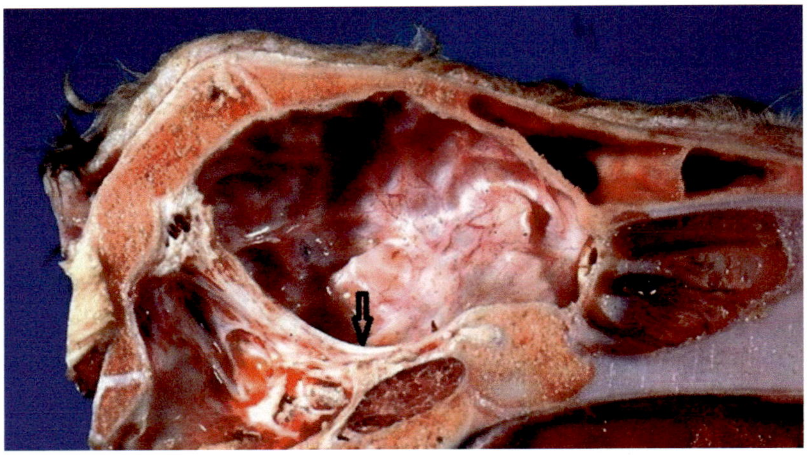

Fig. 1.83. Ox. Skull. Bovine dwarfism. Wing of basisphenoid bone. The accentuation of a sharp, bony proliferation (arrow) is a good anatomic indictor of bovine dwarfism. (Courtesy of Dr J.M. King and Section of Anatomic Pathology, Cornell University, USA.)

1.6.2.2 Arthritis

More examples will be presented in Chapter 8: Diseases of the Musculoskeletal System.

1.7 NEOPLASIA

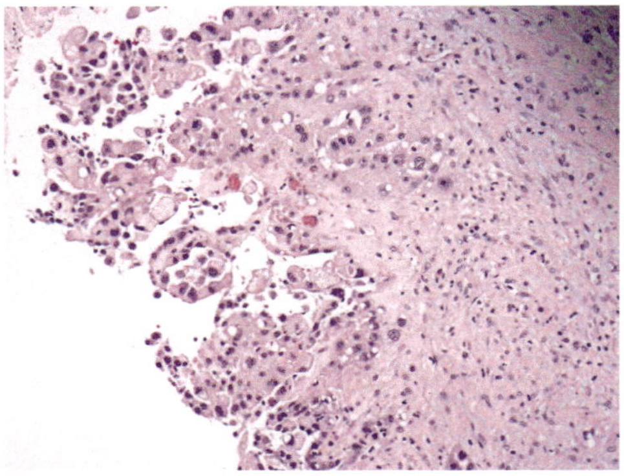

Fig. 1.86. Ox. Peritoneum. Mesothelioma. The mesothelioma is characterized histologically by clusters of pleomorphic cells with large hyperchromatic nuclei. The neoplastic cells form papilla projections and rest on a fibrovascular stroma. The histologic and immunohistochemical identification of mesothelioma and differentiation from carcinoma historically has always been challenging (H&E).

1.8 MISCELLANEOUS

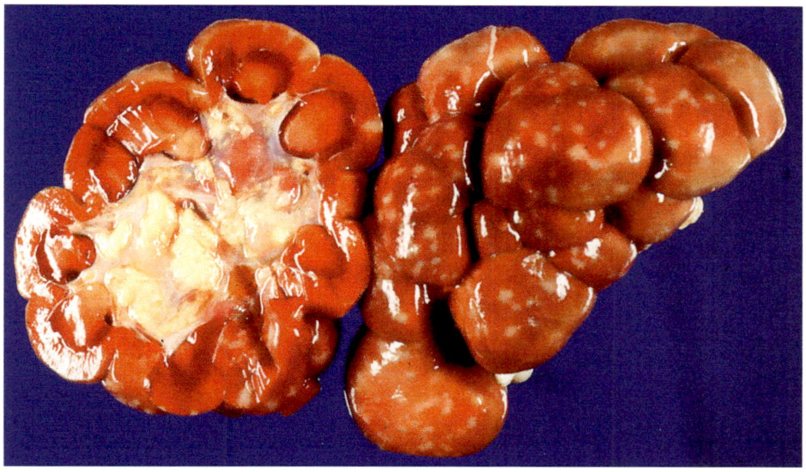

Fig. 1.87. Ox. Kidney. White spotted kidney (WSK). Thromboembolic glomerulonephritis. The cortical surface is studded by small white foci of inflammation. It is hypothesized that bacteria from a preceding enteric infection, especially *Escherichia coli*, hematogenously shower the glomeruli, inciting a purulent inflammation. When the primary inflammatory changes resolve, chronic interstitial nephritis develops (see Chapter 7: Diseases of the Urinary System).

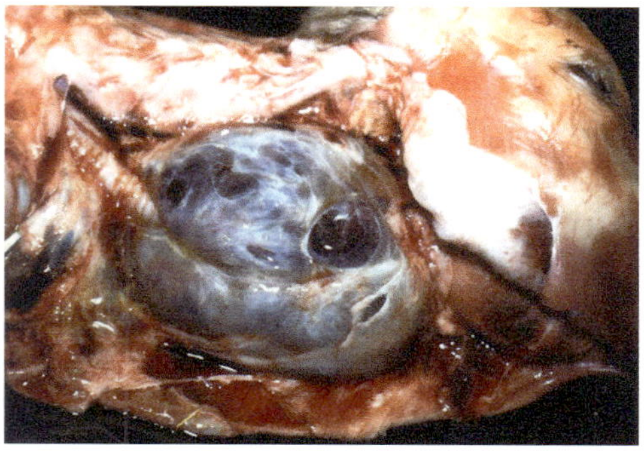

Fig. 1.88. Ox. Thyroid. Neonatal goiter. Hypotrichosis. Bilateral thyroid hypertrophy. The affected calves are born to iodine-deficient dams. In drought conditions with poor-quality feed, the thyroid glands should be collected for histologic examination, especially in stillborn and non-viable neonate calves. These will often show very little colloid production, but the cause for this condition is unknown. Vitamin E deficiency has been proposed. These affected animals grossly will not have goiter-type changes. For adult goiter, see Chapter 9: Diseases of the Endocrine System.

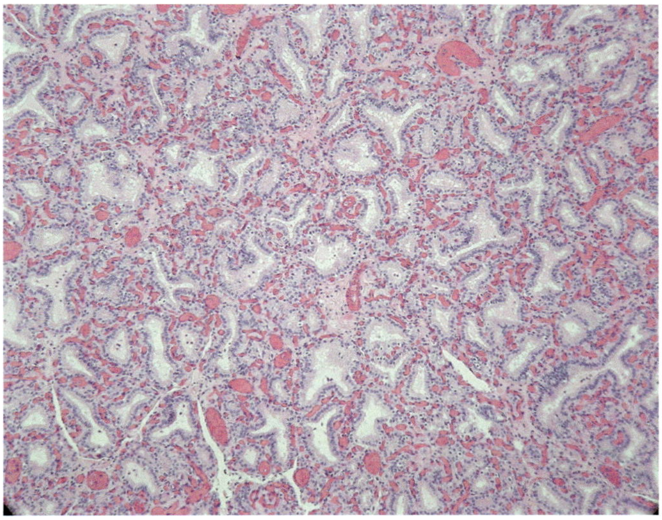

Fig. 1.89. Ox. Thyroid. Stillborn. Hyperplasia with little colloid (H&E).

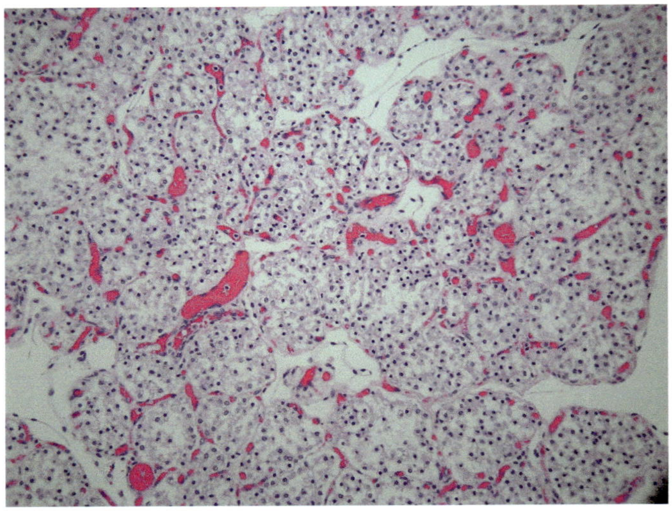

Fig. 1.90. Ox. Thyroid. Stillborn. Severe degeneration. No colloid (H&E).

1.8.1 Bovine neonatal pancytopenia (BNP)

Introduction. A hemorrhagic diathesis syndrome affecting neonatal calves emerged on the continent of Europe in 2008. The syndrome was characterized by pancytopenia and internal and external bleedings. The clinical signs were observed after the ingestion of colostrum. The history included that the dams of the affected calves received a killed vaccine against BVDV containing a novel adjuvant. Maternal alloantibodies produced against adjuvant antigen were secreted into the colostrum and, when ingested by calves, resulted in opsonization of leukocyte surface antigen, cytophagocytosis by macrophages, cytotoxicity to megakaryocytes and trilineage bone marrow hypoplasia.

Clinical signs. Dermal, nasal and rectal bleedings. Petechiae in visible mucous membranes.

Differential diagnoses. Bracken fern toxicity, nitrofurazone toxicity, infection with the thrombocytopenic strain of BVDV.

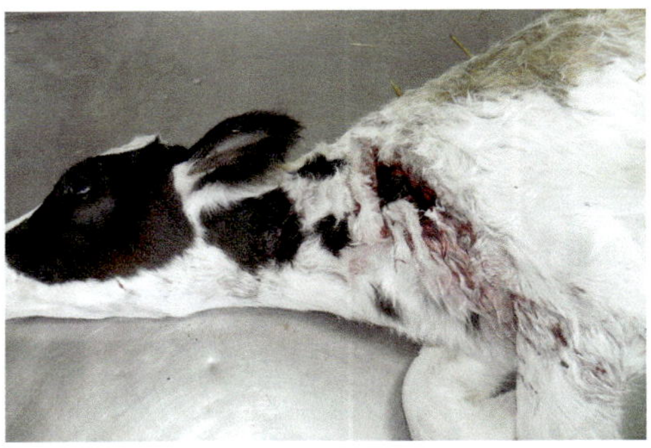

Fig. 1.91. Ox. Neck. Bovine neonatal pancytopenia (BNP). Dermal bleeding. Trauma to the cervical skin resulted in exudation of blood (unclotted). (Courtesy of Dr E. Lepri, University of Perugia, Italy.)

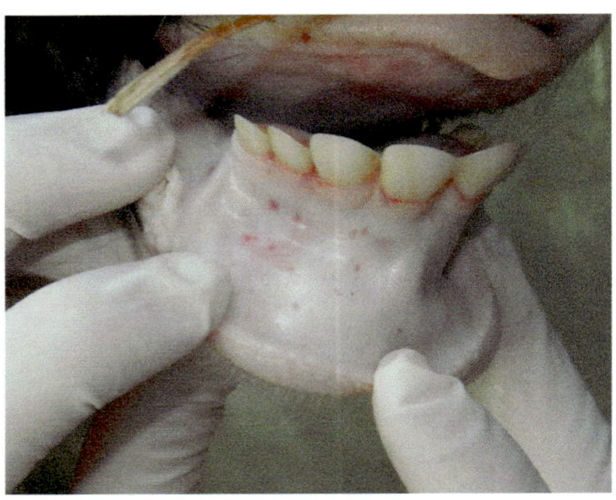

Fig. 1.92. Ox. Bovine neonatal pancytopenia (BNP). Oral mucous membranes. Hemorrhagic diathesis. Multiple petechiae are visible. Mucous membranes are pale. (Courtesy of Dr E. Lepri, University of Perugia, Italy.)

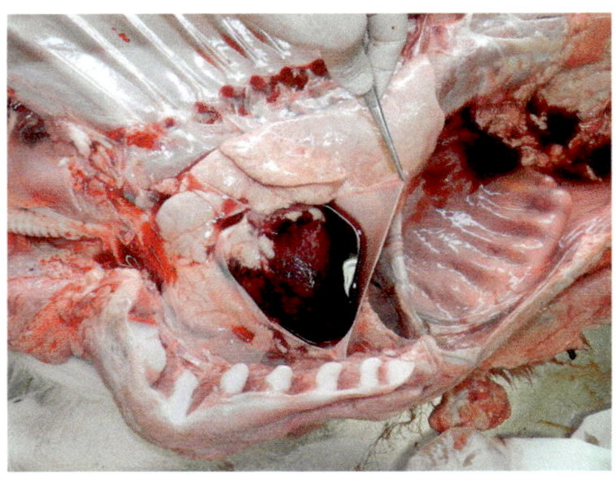

Fig. 1.93 Ox. Bovine neonatal pancytopenia (BNP). Epicardium. Effusive hemorrhage. The heart sac contains unclotted blood. The epicardial surface is tinged diffusely by blood. Tissue is pale. (Courtesy of Dr E. Lepri, University of Perugia, Italy.)

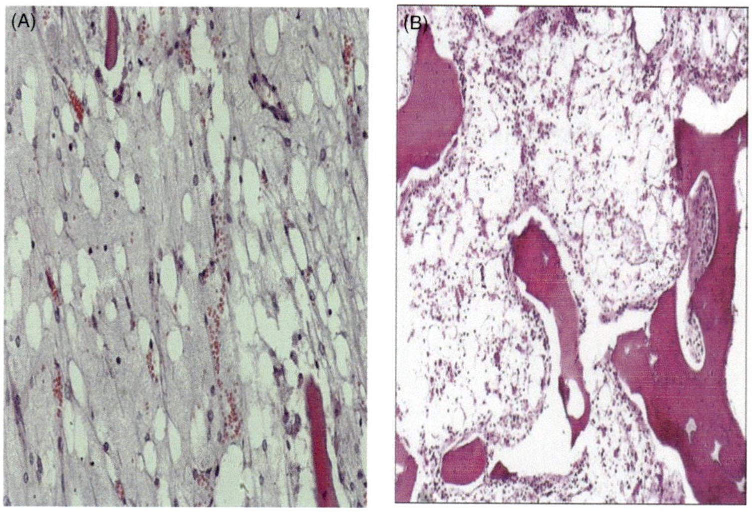

Fig. 1.94. Ox. Bovine neonatal pancytopenia (BNP). Bone marrow. Hypoplasia of hematopoietic cells. (A). All lineages are affected. (B) Normal bone marrow of unaffected animal (H&E). (Courtesy of Dr E. Lepri, University of Perugia, Italy.)

1.8.2 Floppy ear syndrome

Introduction. Infection of the middle ear and tympanic bullae in pre-weaned dairy calves fed waste milk from cows suffering from *Mycoplasma bovis* mastitis (see Chapter 15: Diseases of Eye and Ear).

Clinical signs. Drooping ear, head tilt, strabismus, stiff neck, opisthotonos, purulent aural discharge.

Differential diagnoses. Meningitis, cerebellar hypoplasia, ear mites (*Raillietia auris*).

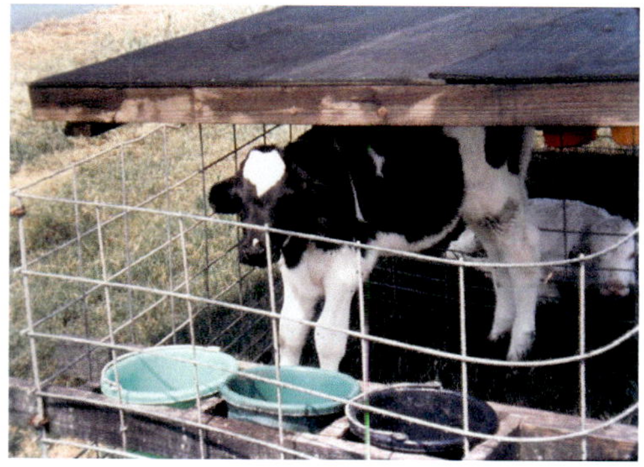

Fig. 1.95. Ox. Ears. Floppy ear syndrome. Calf with droopy ears.

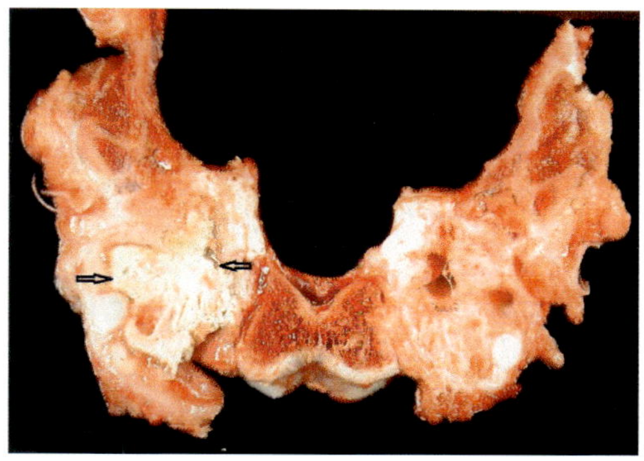

Fig. 1.96. Ox. Tympanic bulla. Floppy ear syndrome. Unilateral purulent otitis media. Arrow denotes purulent exudate in middle ear. *Mycoplasma bovis* is cultured from exudate.

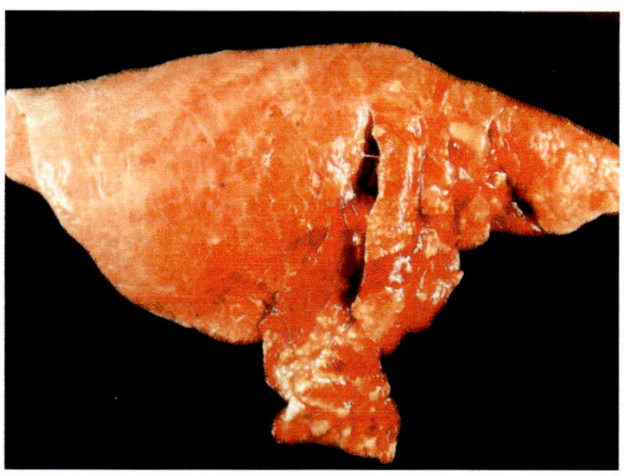

Fig. 1.98. Ox. Lung. Floppy ear syndrome. Cranioventral bronchopneumonia. Frequently, the floppy ear syndrome is associated with *Mycoplasma bovis* bronchopneumonia. It is postulated that exhaled tracheal exudate reaches the middle ear via the eustachian tube from the oral cavity. Oral ingestion of *Mycoplasma bovis* contaminated milk can also result in the colonization of tonsils and subsequent ascending infection to the middle ear.

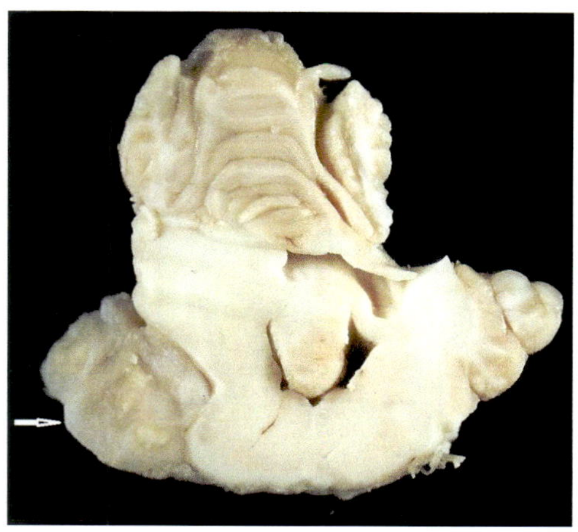

Fig. 1.97. Ox. Brainstem. Floppy ear syndrome. Purulent meningitis (arrow). The otitis media infection ascended to the meninges, producing an abscess.

SUGGESTED READING

Bastian, M., Holsteg, M., Hanke-Robinson, H., Duchow, K. and Cussler, K. (2011) Bovine neonatal pancytopenia: is this alloimmune syndrome caused by vaccine-induced alloreactive antibodies? *Vaccine* 29, 5267–5275.

Dittmer, K.E. and Thompson, K.G. (24 April 2015) Approach to Investigating Congenital Skeletal Abnormalities in Livestock. Doi: 10.1177/0300985815579999.

Edwards, G.T., Woddger, N.G., Barlow, A.M., Bell, S.J., Harwood, D.G., *et al.* (2008) Sarcina-like bacteria associated with bloat in young lambs and calves. *Veterinary Record* 163, 391–393.

Hoet, A.E., Nielsen, P.R., Hasoksuz, M., Thomas, C., Wittum, T.E. and Saif, L.J. (2003) Detection of bovine torovirus and other enteric pathogens in feces from diarrhea cases in cattle. *Journal of Veterinary Diagnostic Investigation* 15, 205–212.

Kirchhoff, J., Uhlenbruck, S., Goris, K., Keil, G.M. and Herler, G. (2014) Three viruses of the bovine respiratory disease complex apply different strategies to initiate infection. *Veterinary Record* 45, 20, doi: 10.1186/1297-9716-45-20.

Marshall, T.S. (2009) Abomasal ulceration and tympany in calves. *Veterinary Clinics North America Food Animal Practice* 25, 209–220.

Maunsell, F., Brown, M.B., Powe, J., Ivey, J., Wooland, M., *et al.* (2012) Oral inoculation of young dairy calves with *Mycoplasma bovis* results in colonization of tonsils, development of otitis media and local immunity. *PLoS One* 7(9): e44523, doi: 10.1371/journal.pone.0044523. Epub.

Santin, M., Trout, J.M. and Fever, R. (2008) A longitudinal study of cryptosporidiosis in dairy cattle from birth to 2 years of age. *Veterinary Pathology* 155, 15–23.

Songer, J.G. and Miskimins, D.W. (2005) Clostridial abomasitis in calves: case report and review of the literature. *Anaerobe* 11, 290–294.

CHAPTER 2

Diseases of the Nervous System

2.1 Removal of the Brain and Spinal Cord

2.2 Degeneration
- 2.2.1 Polioencephalomalacia (laminar cerebrocortical necrosis)
- 2.2.2 Acute lead poisoning (plumbism)
- 2.2.3 Salt intoxication (water deprivation)
- 2.2.4 Methyl and alkyl mercury poisoning
- 2.2.5 Organophosphate compounds poisoning
- 2.2.6 Vitamin A deficiency

2.3 Inflammation
- 2.3.1 Infectious prion protein (PrP)
  - 2.3.1.1 Bovine spongiform encephalopathy (BSE)
- 2.3.2 Viruses
  - 2.3.2.1 Rabies
  - 2.3.2.2 Bovine herpesvirus encephalomyelitis
  - 2.3.2.3 Malignant catarrhal fever (MCF)
  - 2.3.2.4 Neurotropic astrovirus
- 2.3.3 Bacteria
  - 2.3.3.1 Listeriosis
  - 2.3.3.2 Thrombotic meningoencephalomyelitis (TME)
  - 2.3.3.3 Sporadic bovine encephalomyelitis (SPE, transmissible serositis)
  - 2.3.3.4 Bovine cowdriosis (heartwater, bovine ehrlichiosis)
  - 2.3.3.5 Abscesses
  - 2.3.3.6 Meningitis
- 2.3.4 Fungi
  - 2.3.4.1 Cryptococcosis
- 2.3.5 Protozoa
  - 2.3.5.1 Cerebral babesiosis
  - 2.3.5.2 Cerebral theileriosis
  - 2.3.5.3 Cerebral amoebiasis
  - 2.3.5.4 Cerebral trypanosomiasis
- 2.3.6 Parasites
  - 2.3.6.1 Cerebral coenurosis

2.4 Trauma

2.5 Neoplasia

2.6 Miscellaneous
- 2.6.1 Breed-specific encephalomyelopathies
  - 2.6.1.1 Multifocal symmetrical encephalomyelopathy of juvenile Simmental cattle
  - 2.6.1.2 Bovine progressive degenerative myeloencephalopathy (BPDME)
  - 2.6.1.3 Spinal muscular atrophy
  - 2.6.1.4 Inherited progressive myelinopathy in Murray Grey cattle
  - 2.6.1.5 Progressive ataxia of Charolais cattle
  - 2.6.1.6 Bovine ceroid-lipofuscinosis in Devon cattle

INTRODUCTION

Nervous system diseases have multiple etiologies and necessitate a thorough clinical examination to rule out the participation of other systems such as the locomotor system. Some metabolic causes (hypocalcemia, hypomagnesemia) and infectious diseases (tetanus, botulism) are associated with marked clinical signs, but have no pathologic findings. Some disorders present a recumbent, but alert animal; some a disoriented, depressed, uncoordinated and abnormally behaving animal. It should be stressed that for thorough pathologic examination, the careful removal of a non-mutilated brain and spinal cord is paramount.

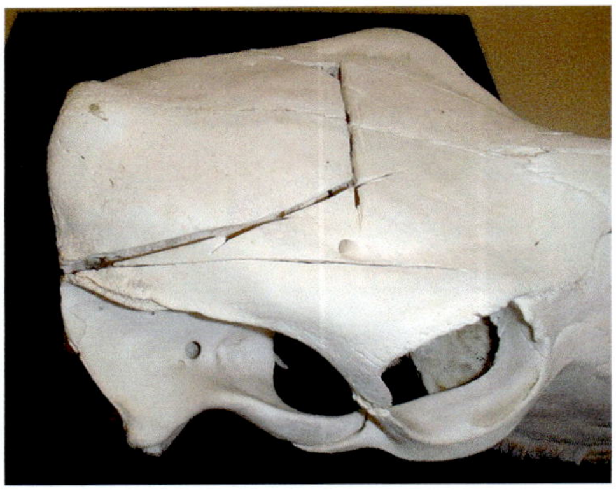

Fig. 2.1. Ox. Skull. Illustration of cut lines for the removal of the calvaria. It can be lifted off after these three cuts are made and the entire brain will be exposed for safe removal by cutting through the cerebral nerves.

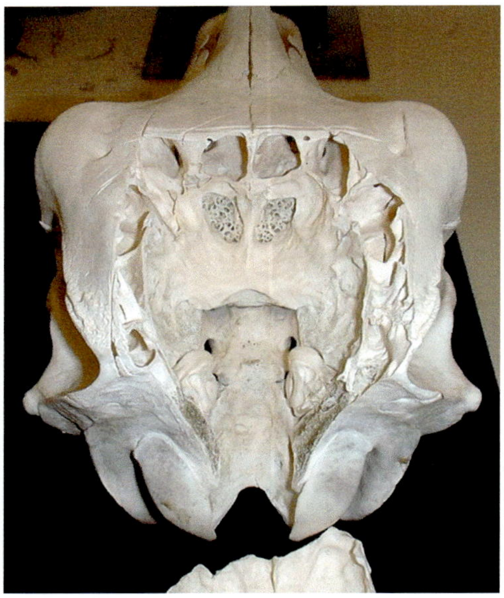

Fig. 2.2. Ox. Skull. After the removal of the skull, the exposed frontal sinuses extend caudally towards the occipital condyles. Note that the saw cuts will break through the frontal sinuses before reaching the cerebral cavity. The pituitary fossa is exposed. The pituitary needs to be removed from underneath the dura.

2.1 REMOVAL OF THE BRAIN AND SPINAL CORD

Both tissues are heavily protected by musculature and bone. The musculature has to be fleshed and the bone accessed with a handsaw or electric bandsaw where available. The goal is to maintain structural integrity and to avoid organ mutilation for pathologic examination. Before removing the head, cerebrospinal fluid can be collected by syringe from the atlanto-occipital cistern for analysis. The severed head is placed in a vise and held tightly, or placed on a solid surface against a rigid object such as a stone wall. The mandible can be removed at this time at the temporomandibular joints and across the pterygomandibular folds, for inspection of the deeper oral cavity or teeth.

For the removal of the calvaria and access to the brain, three cuts are made, as depicted in the following specimen of a bleached bovine skull (Figs 2.1 and 2.2): one transverse at the site of the zygomatic arch and two paramedian sagittal cuts, with the aim to saw caudally inside the sagittal cuts directed medially about 35 degrees inner angles of the occipital condyles at the site of the foramen magnum.

An alternative and simple method for brain removal is to perform a transverse sectioning via handsaw through the middle of the head caudal to the last molar tooth, toward the palatine bone and oral cavity, thus splitting the head into rostral and caudal parts. With the cranium open, both rostral and caudal portions of the bone can be removed with a gentle push. This technique is easier to perform if the mandible is removed to reduce the bulkiness of the bovine head.

Spinal cord removal can be achieved under field conditions, by dividing the vertebral column into three to four major segments (cervical, thoracic, lumbosacral) with a handsaw after fleshing the surrounding soft tissues. Depending on the anatomic location of the lesion(s), transverse cuts are made with a handsaw through the arches and vertebral bodies of the adjacent vertebrae on either side of the intervertebral articulations. The dura is lifted from one end of the vertebral canal with a pair of forceps. The spinal cord segment is then removed by cutting with scissors through the spinal cord nerves in the epidural space. The procedure can be repeated in as many vertebrae as necessary. Each section of the spinal cord is labelled separately and the dura is opened dorsally and longitudinally to facilitate thorough penetration of the fixative.

An alternative method is to saw the fleshed vertebral column into several sections, bag the segments in formalin and ship them expeditiously to a laboratory equipped with a bandsaw for removal of the spinal cord for histologic examination. The sections need to be small so that formalin can penetrate the cord.

Splitting the vertebral column sagittally with a meat cleaver may be a simpler method, but is discouraged because of possible mutilation and damage of the spinal cord for adequate histologic examination.

2.2 DEGENERATION

This chapter encompasses metabolic, toxic and nutritional brain diseases.

2.2.1 Polioencephalomalacia (laminar cerebrocortical necrosis)

Introduction. The most common predisposing factor observed in North America for this condition is excessive sulfur intake from diet or external sources such as alkaline water, plants or forage (>0.4% sulfur or >2% sulfate). Ruminal metabolism converts sulfur into hydrogen sulfide, which is a metabolic poison inhibiting cytochrome oxidase in the electron transport chain. Its action can be compared to cyanide poison. The disease has originally been associated with thiamine deficiency or with too much thiaminase activity of fermenting ruminal bacteria. Older calves and yearlings (6–18 months range) are mostly affected. In cattle, a second type of cerebrocortical necrosis can occur with feed rich in carbohydrates. This type occurs in all feedlot cattle kept high on carbohydrate diets.

Pathologic changes may be acute or chronic, and at the gross level are confined mainly to the cerebral cortex, featured as segmental laminar necrosis and cavitation. There is yellow discoloration of the depths and sides of sulci in the acute form, and the brain is yellow and shrunken in the chronic form. Basal nuclei, thalamic nuclei and colliculi may also be affected. In alkaline water containing high sulfur concentration, deep hemorrhage (thalamic/brainstem) due to vascular necrosis is common. Occasionally, cerebellar herniation may occur. Microscopic changes of the acute form include cortical edema and necrosis, neuronal necrosis, and microcavitation (subacute cases) with gitter cells in the chronic form. The necrotic tissue will fluoresce under UV light (Wood's lamp).

Clinical signs. Acute onset of ataxia, blindness, head pressing, recumbency, opisthotonos and convulsion.

Differential diagnoses. Toxicoses such as acute plumbism, alkaline water toxicosis, nervous ketosis, carbohydrate overload in diet, metabolic disorders such hypomagnesemia.

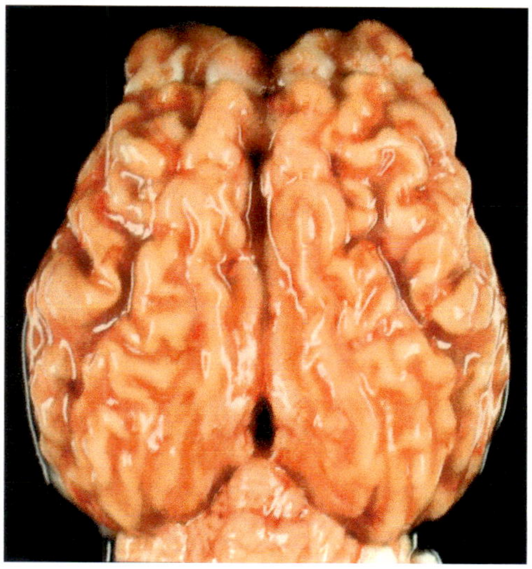

Fig. 2.3. Ox. Cerebrum. Polioencephalomalacia (PEM). Chronic form. The cerebral sulci are widened. The gyri look atrophic. There is diffuse yellow discoloration.

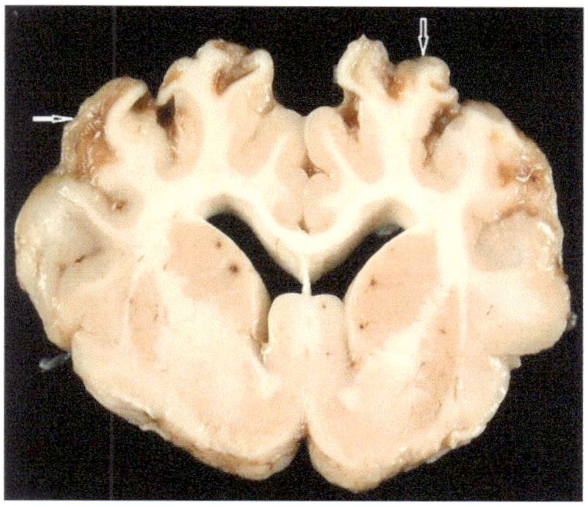

Fig. 2.4. Ox. Cerebrum. Polioencephalomalacia (PEM). Chronic form. A transverse section reveals segmental skipped lytic changes in several cerebral folia (arrows), but not in all. This morphologic feature is not observed in acute lead poisoning where generally all folia are involved.

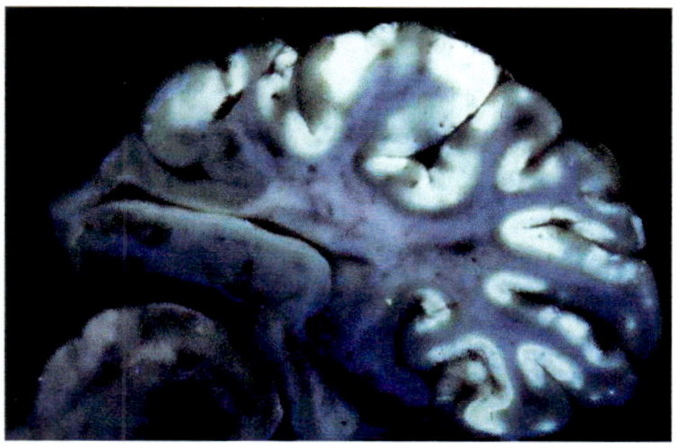

Fig. 2.5. Ox. Cerebrum. Polioencephalomalacia (PEM). UV light. Autofluorescence identifies the necrotic areas in the cortex and thalamus.

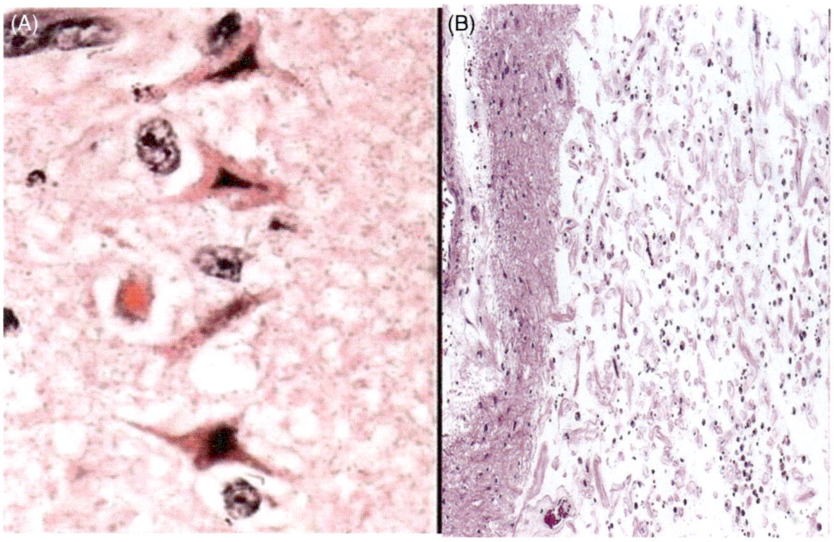

Fig. 2.6. Ox. Polioencephalomalacia (PEM). (A) Microscopic changes are characterized by edema, neuronal necrosis in the acute form; (B) spongiosis, microcavitation of the neuropil, isolation of prominent blood vessels, and small numbers of lymphocytes and macrophages in the chronic form (H&E).

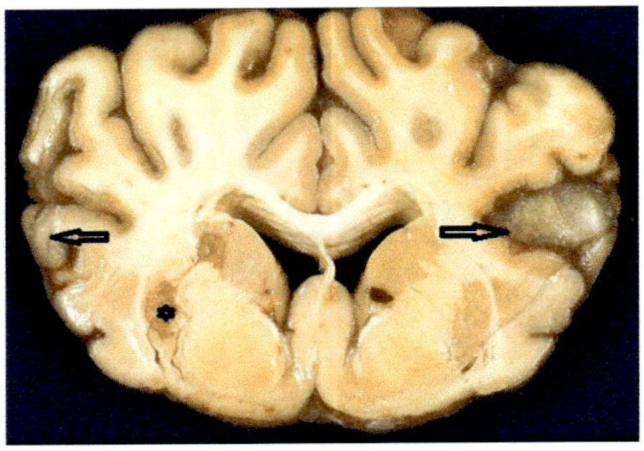

Fig. 2.7. Ox. Cerebrum. Polioencephalomalacia (PEM). High carbohydrate induced. Cortical necrosis (arrows) is present in some folia. Deep foci of necrosis in basal nuclei are indicated by asterisk.

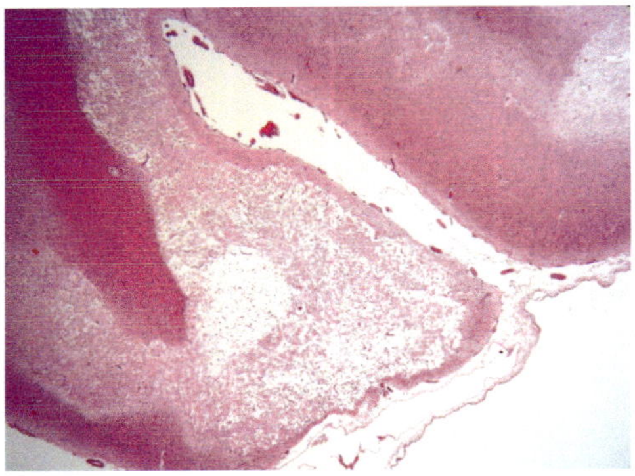

Fig. 2.8. Ox. Cerebrum. Polioencephalomalacia (PEM). High carbohydrate induced. Loss of gray matter substance is intense in cortex with microcavitation and little inflammation (H&E).

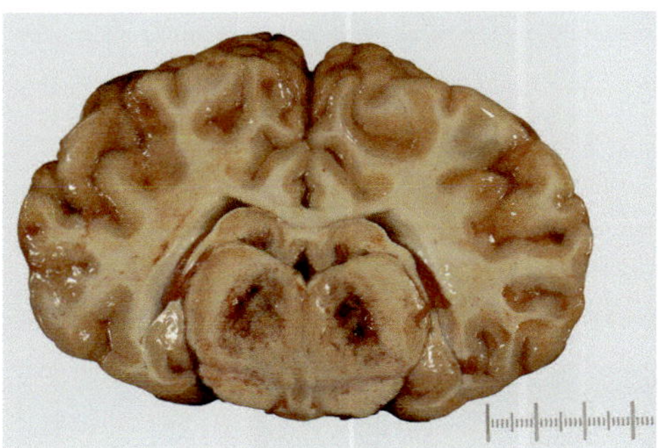

Fig. 2.9. Ox. Cerebrum. Polioencephalomalacia (PEM). Sulfur induced. A transverse section exhibits symmetrical foci of hemorrhage and malacia in the thalamus.

Fact Sheet: Polioencephalomalacia (PEM)

Definition
- Cerebrocortical necrosis caused by a variety of toxins, feed element excesses and deficiencies

Causes
- High dietary sulfur intake
- Altered thiamine status
- Increased ruminal thiaminase activity
- High carbohydrate intake
- Plants of family of *Brassicaceae*
- Coccidiostatic amprolium

Clinical features
- Blindness
- Head pressing
- Opisthotonos
- Coma

Gross findings
- Segmental laminar necrosis in cerebral cortex
- Cerebellar herniation

Microscopic findings
- Microcavitation of gray matter substance
- Neuronal necrosis
- Hemorrhage deep in brain

Differential diagnoses
- Acute plumbism
- Salt poisoning/water deprivation

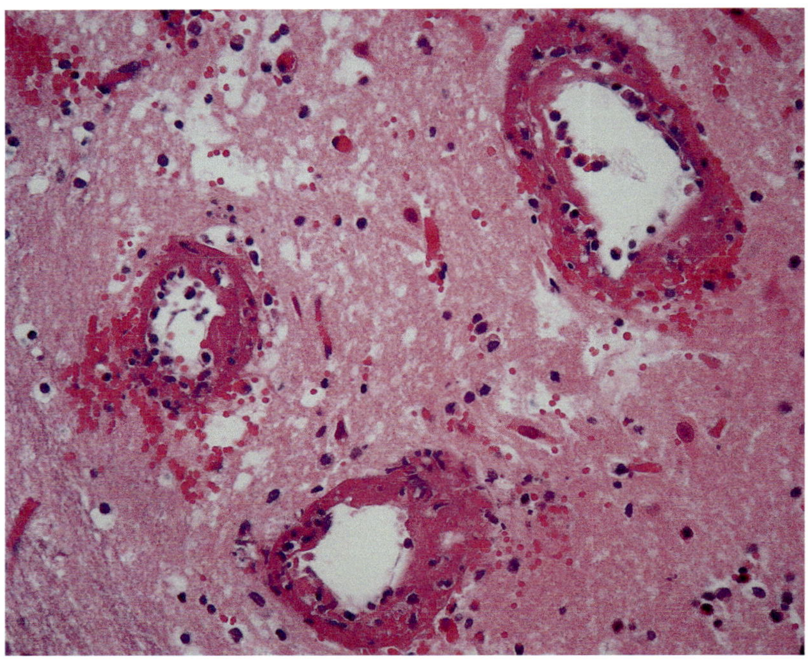

Fig. 2.10. Ox. Cerebrum. Polioencephalomalacia (PEM). Sulfur induced. Blood vessels are characterized by fibrinoid necrosis of the wall and perivascular extravasation. Hemorrhage is also present in the adjacent neuropil; so is vacuolation (H&E).

2.2.2 Acute lead poisoning (plumbism)

Introduction. Acute lead poisoning causes laminar cortical necrosis, mainly affecting the tips of the cerebral folia. The damage is mainly at the tips of the gyri. Lead has a direct toxic impact on neurons, astrocytes and endothelial cells. Astrocytes containing metallothionein are the principal target cells. The protein binds and sequesters metals, thus protecting the cells from injury. Direct injury to endothelial cells disrupts the blood–brain barrier, leading to edema and hemorrhage. It is important when suspecting plumbism not to rely on the brain lesions to make the diagnosis, but to perform lead analysis on organ tissues such as the kidney.
Clinical signs. Excessive salivation, muscle tremors, seizures, head pressing.
Differential diagnoses. PEM, rabies, meningoencephalitis, hepatic encephalopathy.

2.2.3 Salt intoxication (water deprivation)

Introduction. Feeding errors allowing excessive sodium chloride uptake or water deprivation cause hypernatremia. Both sodium and chloride levels are elevated in serum (>160 mEq/l) and central nervous system (CNS) fluid. Sodium analysis can also be performed on fresh brain tissue.
Clinical signs. Depression, weakness, seizures, diarrhea, blindness.
Differential diagnoses. Electrolyte abnormalities, meningitis, PEM, rabies.

Gross abnormalities other than increased moistness to the brain are absent. Histologic lesions are characterized by generalized edema.

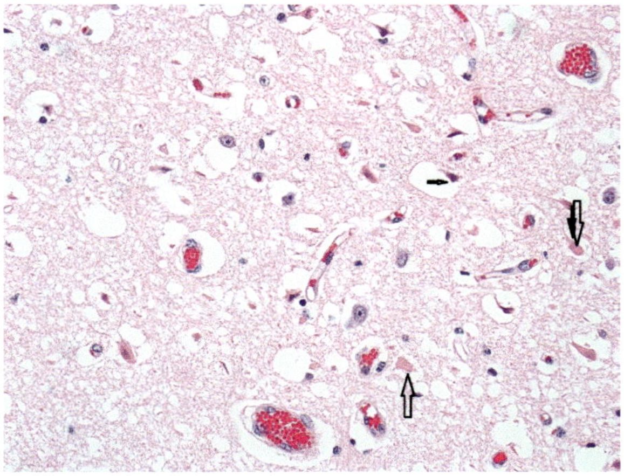

Fig. 2.11. Ox. Brain. Cerebral cortex. Salt intoxication. Vasogenic edema. The perivascular spaces are largely expanded and multiple clear spaces are present in the neuropil (closed arrow). Neurons (open arrows) are red and shrunken, indicating necrosis. Post-mortem changes can look similar if carcass is not fresh (H&E).

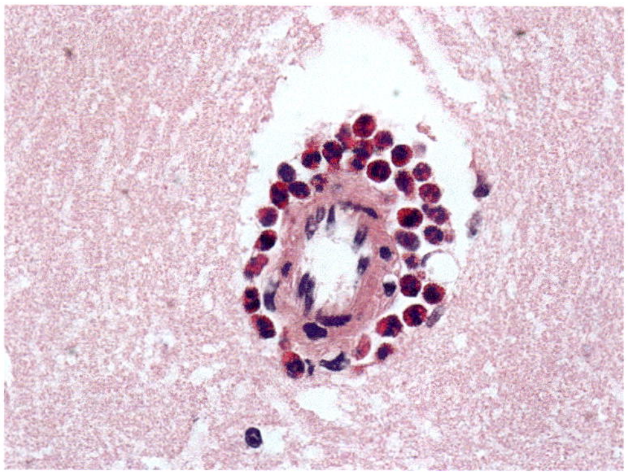

Fig. 2.12. Ox. Brain. Salt intoxication. Eosinophilic cuffing. Prominent perivascular eosinophilic cuffs are diagnostic in pigs for salt poisoning. In this bovine case with proven hypernatremia, it was also a feature, albeit rare (H&E).

2.2.4 Methyl and alkyl mercury poisoning

Used as fungicides and basically renal toxins like lead, they may cause granular cell necrosis in the bovine cerebellum.

Clinical sign. Ataxia.

Differential diagnoses. Autolysis. Granular cerebellar cells disappear fast after death.

2.2.5 Organophosphate compounds poisoning

Caused by organophosphate (OP) esters used as anticholinesterase (pesticides, herbicides, fungicides, rodenticides). Accumulating at synaptic junctions, persistent depolarization is the result. The acute form causes respiratory failure with no lesions. The chronic form is characterized by pathologic changes present in the brainstem and spinal cord. These include bilateral symmetrical axonal fragmentation and neuraxonal degeneration of distal axons (dying back neuropathy). Neuronal chromatolysis is an additional pathological feature. Distal axonal degeneration occurs in peripheral nerves. This condition can only be diagnosed with a good history and fresh brain cholinesterase analysis.

Clinical signs. Salivation, tremors, weakness.

Differential diagnoses. Rabies, plumbism, electrolyte abnormalities.

2.2.6 Vitamin A deficiency

Outbreaks are usually seen in young feedlot cattle.

Clinical signs. Blindness, seizures, circling, head elevation.

Differential diagnoses. Polioencephalomalacia, plumbism.

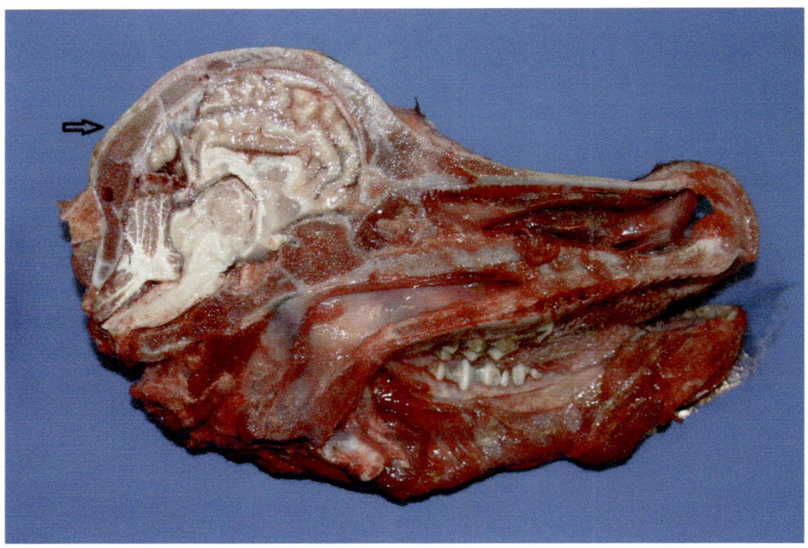

Fig. 2.13. Ox. Head. Vitamin A deficiency. Calvaria osteopetrosis and meningeal thickening. The bone plate of the calvaria is markedly thickened due to failure of bone resorption (arrow). The dura also is thickened due to fibroplasia. Both scenarios create compression on the adjacent brain, resulting in edema from increased cerebral system fluid (CSF) pressure. Blindness is caused by pressure on the optic nerve. It is important to dissect the optic nerve for histopathology and to examine the optic tract in the brain. (Courtesy of Dr F. Uzal, University of California, USA.)

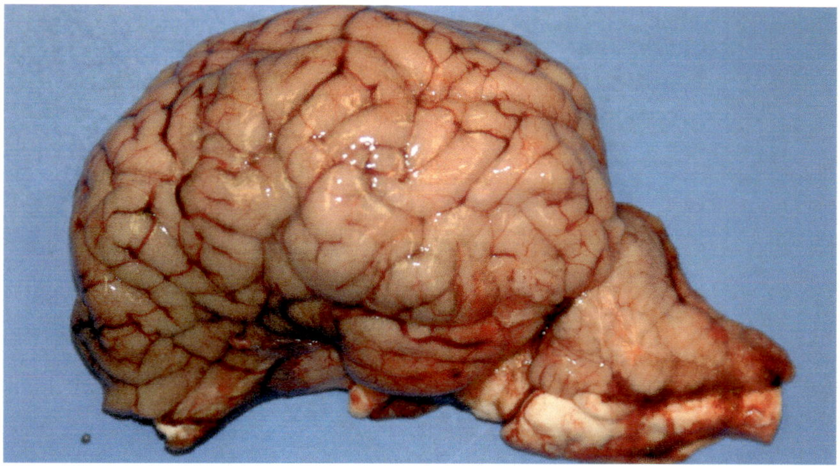

Fig. 2.14. Ox. Cerebellum. Vitamin A deficiency. Cerebellar coning. Increased pressure on the brain from the surrounding thickened meningeal tissue and bone plates leads to herniation of the cerebellar vermis through the foramen magnum (cerebellar coning). (Courtesy of Dr F. Uzal, University of California, USA.)

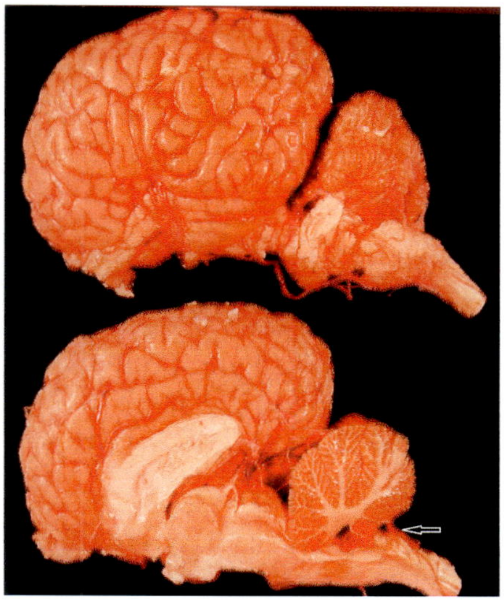

Fig. 2.15. Ox. Brain. Bovine spongiform encephalopathy (BSE). Arrow depicts anatomic location of obex at the level of the caudal aspect of the cerebellum as the preferred site for taking samples for BSE testing. In practice, the sample can be taken with a sharp spoon.

2.3 INFLAMMATION

2.3.1 Infectious prion protein (PrP)

2.3.1.1 Bovine spongiform encephalopathy (BSE)

Introduction. Also known as mad cow disease, this novel neurologic disorder started in Great Britain in 1986. It reached the potential of a zoonotic disease defined as variant Creutzfeldt–Jacob disease (vCJD), affecting mainly young human adults after consuming infected bovine meat. Neurologic and neuropathologic changes in cows are similar to those in sheep scrapie or mink encephalopathy. The agent known as infectious prion protein was introduced to cattle by feeding sheep products (bonemeal, meat) containing scrapie prions. BSE has been reported in over 30 countries worldwide. In the UK alone, roughly 20,000 cases of BSE have been confirmed. Of 50 million cattle screened in Europe, 7000 cases tested positive. Japan reported 35 confirmed bovine cases, Canada 20 and the USA 3, according to the World Organisation for Animal Health (OIE). The incidence of BSE has declined through avoiding ruminant-derived feed concentrates, quarantine and chemical digestion or other safe removal of positively diagnosed cows from the food chain. A total of 177 human cases have been reported in the UK as of 2014, and 49 in other countries.

The prion protein (PrP) is an infectious protein in a misfolded form and is very resistant to external influences. Ante-mortem diagnosis is difficult, but can be achieved via conjunctival and tonsillar biopsy submitted for immunohistochemistry of pathogenic PrP. Post-mortem diagnosis is performed via immunohistochemistry of brain tissue obtained from the obex by spoon scooping. Various molecular-based immunoblot kit tests are also in use.

Clinical signs. Gait abnormalities, muscle twitching, imbalance, recumbency, and occasional aggression.

Differential diagnoses. Rabies, listeriosis, metabolic and toxic disorders, locoweed toxicosis.

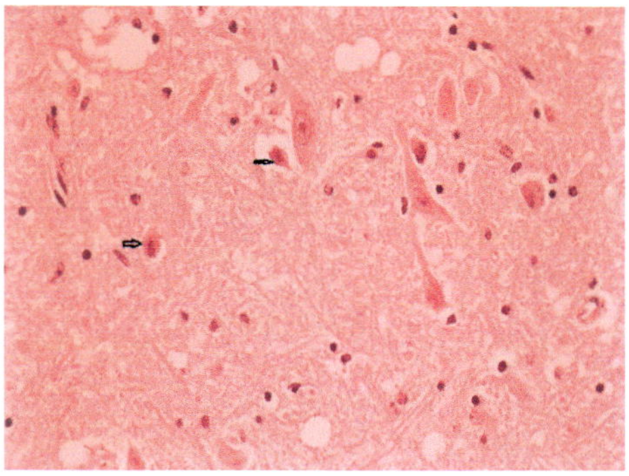

Fig. 2.16. Ox. Brain. Bovine spongiform encephalopathy (BSE). Neuropil vacuolation and neuronal necrosis. Red neurons (arrows) indicate neuronal necrosis. Neuronal cytoplasmic vacuolation can occur (H&E).

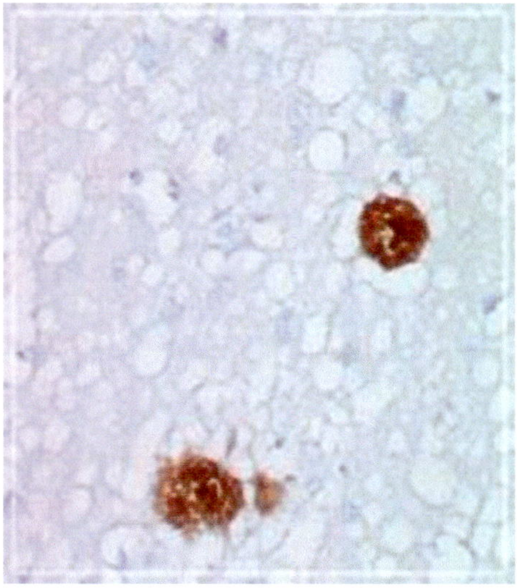

Fig. 2.17. Ox. Brain. Bovine spongiform encephalopathy (BSE). Immunohistochemical identification of aggregates of PrP in neuropil (IHC).

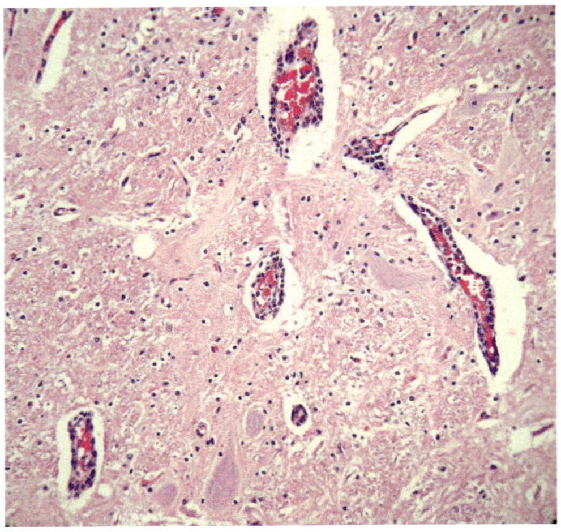

Fig. 2.18. Ox. Brain. Rabies. Lymphocytic polioencephalitis. Cuffs of lymphocytes surround blood vessels. By themselves they are non-diagnostic for rabies. A few perivascular macrophages, neuronal necrosis, glial nodules and neuronophagia can be present. Plasma cells can be present in ruminants. Microscopic changes can be expected in 100% of rabies cases in the spinal cord of cattle, with the brainstem and cerebellum next highest (H&E).

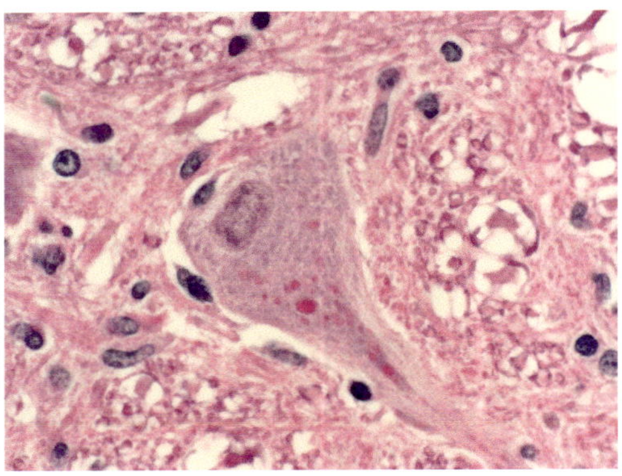

Fig. 2.19. Ox. Brain. Rabies. Negri inclusions. The presence of magenta intracytoplasmic Negri inclusion bodies in neurons is conclusive for the diagnosis of rabies. They are detected best in the spinal cord. They may be absent in some cases of rabies, necessitating other methods of diagnosis (H&E).

2.3.2 Viruses

2.3.2.1 Rabies

Introduction. Gross lesions in cows infected with this neurotropic rhabdovirus are usually absent in the brain, but the spinal cord may show multifocal hemorrhage in the gray matter, best encountered in the cervical segments. Clinical signs are variable and usually non-furious (dumb form). The urinary bladder may be dilated and the rectum may be impacted with feces. From the bite site, the virus reaches the central nervous tissue via retroaxonal transport. Brain, cerebral ganglia and spinal cord are affected. Microscopic changes are characterized by small to medium-sized lymphocytic perivascular cuffs with a few histiocytes. The brainstem is a good anatomic site to find these changes. The detection of intraneuronal intracytoplasmic inclusion bodies (Negri bodies) in hippocampus or cerebellar Purkinje cells helps to establish the etiologic diagnosis. Negri bodies can be absent. The abundant rabies antigen can be demonstrated with indirect immunohistochemistry in microscopic sections. The direct fluorescent antibody technique remains the official gold standard test. Strict protocols are established and should be followed when handling suspect rabies cases, as the virus is a dangerous zoonotic agent.

Clinical signs. Behavioral changes to salivation, bellowing, paralysis, and death. Uncontrolled aggression rarely occurs.

Differential diagnoses. Aujezky's disease, botulism, CNS bacterial infections, nervous ketosis.

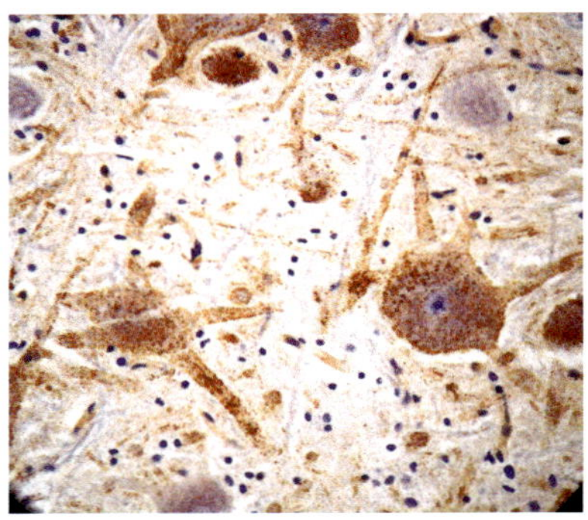

Fig. 2.20. Ox. Neocortex. Rabies. Abundant intracytoplasmic rhabdovirus antigen within neurons and fibers. Indirect immunohistochemistry proves a very effective tool in the etiologic diagnosis of rabies, but fluorescence antibody (FA) remains the primary official test (IHC).

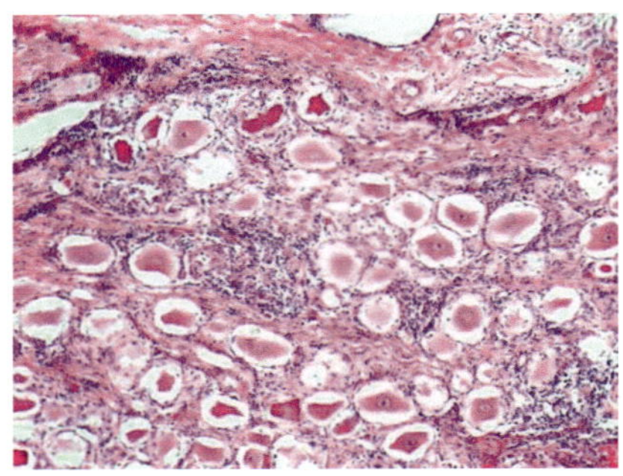

Fig. 2.21. Ox. Brain. Rabies. Lymphocytic ganglioneuritis. Aggregates of lymphocytes surround ganglionic neurons. There is neuronal necrosis. These changes can also be found in bovine herpesvirus encephalitis type 5 and bovine neurotropic astrovirus. It should be mentioned that the Gasserian ganglia in cattle often have some lymphocytes normally without any disease (H&E). (Courtesy of Dr D. Driemeier, Universidade Federal do Rio Grande do Sul, Brazil.)

2.3.2.2 *Bovine herpesvirus encephalomyelitis*

Introduction. The prototype of the bovine herpesviruses is bovine herpesvirus type 1 (BHV-1). It is the causative agent of infectious bovine rhinotracheitis (IBR), pustular vulvovaginitis, and abortion. In calves and aborted foetuses, it can sporadically induce a non-purulent meningoencephalomyelitis. It is dormant, presumably in ganglia, but lymphoid tissue has not been ruled out. A trigeminal ganglionitis can be the site of persistent infection and reactivation. The related BHV-5 is a neurotrophic agent and is within the subfamily of Alphaherpesvirinae. It occurs with some frequency in young cattle in Brazil.

Clinical signs. Fever, respiratory distress, and seizures without visual deficits.

Differential diagnoses. Infectious encephalitides, metabolic and toxic diseases.

Bovine lymphotropic herpesvirus type 6 (BHV-6) is a Gammaherpesvirus also known as caprine herpesvirus. Occurring sporadically, it causes a non-suppurative encephalitis with multilayered variously sized T- and B-lymphocyte vascular cuffing. A hemogram may exhibit persistent lymphocytosis.

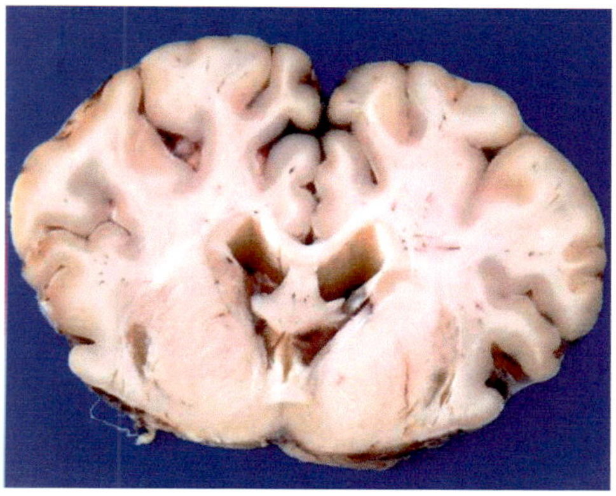

Fig. 2.22. Ox. Brain. Bovine herpesvirus type 5 (BHV-5). Malacia. There is very little gross pathology. The coronal section shows prominent vessels in the white matter substance and some softening of parenchyma. (Courtesy of Dr F. Riet-Correa, INIA, National Institute for Agricultural Research, Uruguay.)

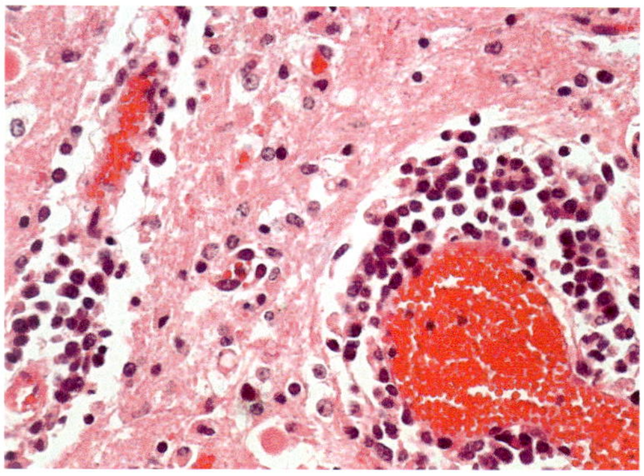

Fig. 2.23. Ox. Brain. Bovine herpesvirus type 5 (BHV-5). Lymphocytic encephalitis. There are distinct inflammatory cuffs composed of small and medium-sized lymphocytes (H&E).

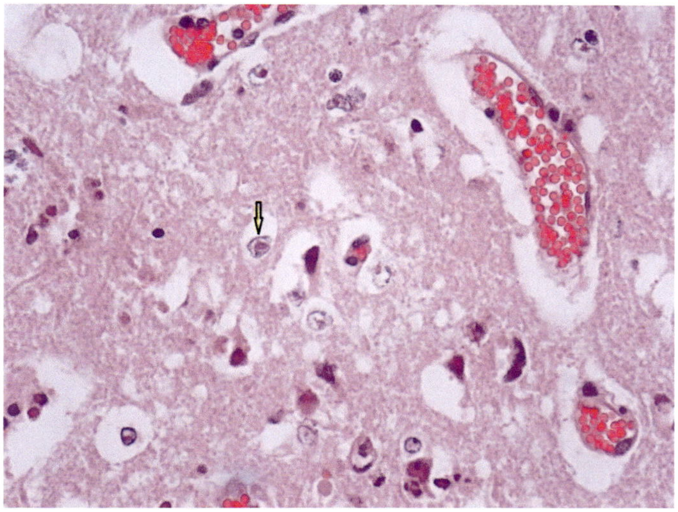

Fig. 2.24. Ox. Brain. Bovine herpesvirus type 5 (BHV-5). There is an occasional intranuclear herpesvirus inclusion (arrow) together with edema and neuronal necrosis (H&E).

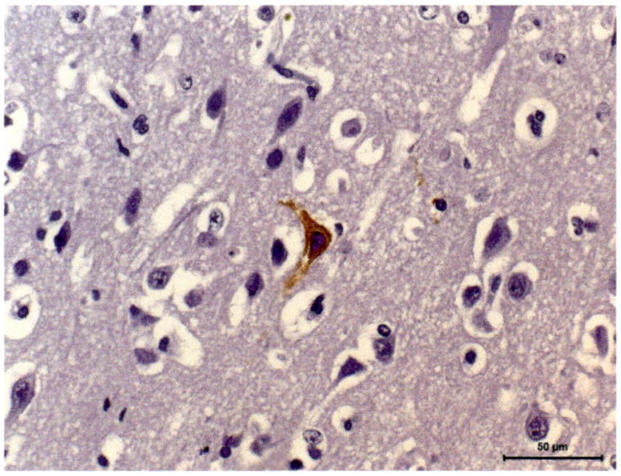

Fig. 2.25. Ox. Brain. Bovine herpesvirus type 5 (BHV-5). Demonstration of herpesviral antigen in the cytoplasm of a neuron (IHC). (Courtesy of Dr. D. Cagnini, Universidade Estradual Paulista, Brazil).

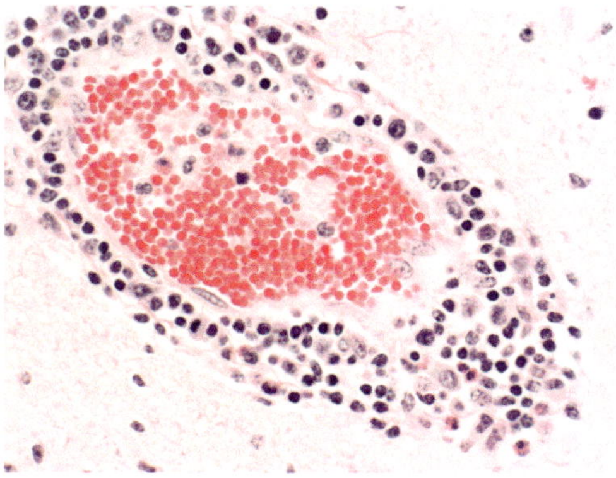

Fig. 2.26. Ox. Brain. Bovine herpesvirus type 6 (BHV-6). Thick perivascular cuffs are composed of small and large lymphocytes and macrophages. No inclusions are encountered (H&E).

Bovine Alphaherpesviruses – Strains and Targets

- BHV-1: IBR, IBV, abortion, infertility, encephalitis.
- BHV-2: bovine herpetic mammillitis, necrotizing dermatitis.
- BHV-4: mastitis. Detected in leukocytes, lymph nodes, nervous tissue, in aborted fetal tissues and aborted placentas. Post-partum metritis.
- BHV-5: meningoencephalitis in young cattle (South America).
- BHV-6: lymphotropic CNS caprine herpesvirus. CNS, respiratory tract, abortion.

2.3.2.3 *Malignant catarrhal fever (MCF)*

Introduction. Malignant catarrhal fever (MCF) is a fatal lymphoproliferative disease caused by a group of ruminant Gammaherpesviruses including *Alcelaphine Herpesvirus 1* and *2* (AlHV-1 and -2) and *Ovine Herpesvirus 2* (OvHV-2). The viruses cause inapparent infection in their reservoir hosts (sheep with OvHV-2 and wildebeest with AIHV-1), but are usually fatal in cattle and other ungulates such as deer, antelope, and bison.

MCF is an important disease reservoir and susceptible animal mix. There is a particular problem with Bali cattle in Indonesia, bison in North America and in pastoralist herds in eastern and southern Africa.

Outbreaks of MCF typically affect younger cattle. There are several clinical and morphologic forms of the disease: nervous, ocular, dermal, alimentary, and urinary. Microscopically, a ubiquitous necrotizing vasculitis affecting medium-sized arteries and veins is the hallmark lesion of MCF. Microscopic examination of the carotid rete mirabile for the

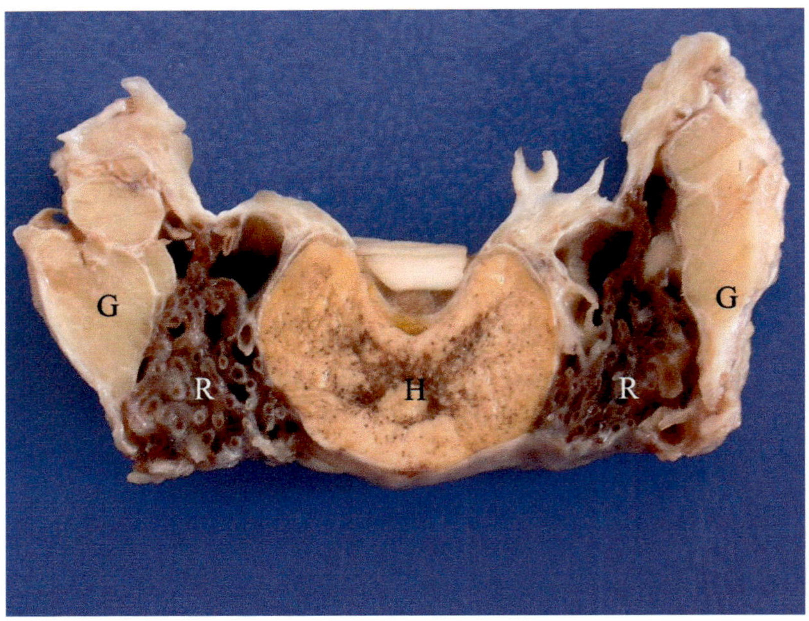

Fig. 2.27. Ox. Carotid rete mirabile. Normal tissue. The cross section depicts a pair of Gasserian ganglia (G) of the fifth cranial nerve, the carotid rete mirabile (R), and the hypophysis (H). The carotid rete mirabile tissue should be sampled for the diagnosis of malignant catarrhal fever (MCF). The ganglion should be examined for ganglionitis in the case of rabies or herpesvirus infection. (Courtesy of Dr C. Barros, Universidade Federal de Santa Maria, Brazil.)

demonstration of arteritis–phlebitis is recommended for the morphologic confirmation of bovine MCF. Additional pathologic aspects of bovine MCF will be presented in the specific organ systems involved.

Clinical signs (nervous form). Fever, depression, weakness.

Differential diagnoses. CNS viral and bacterial diseases.

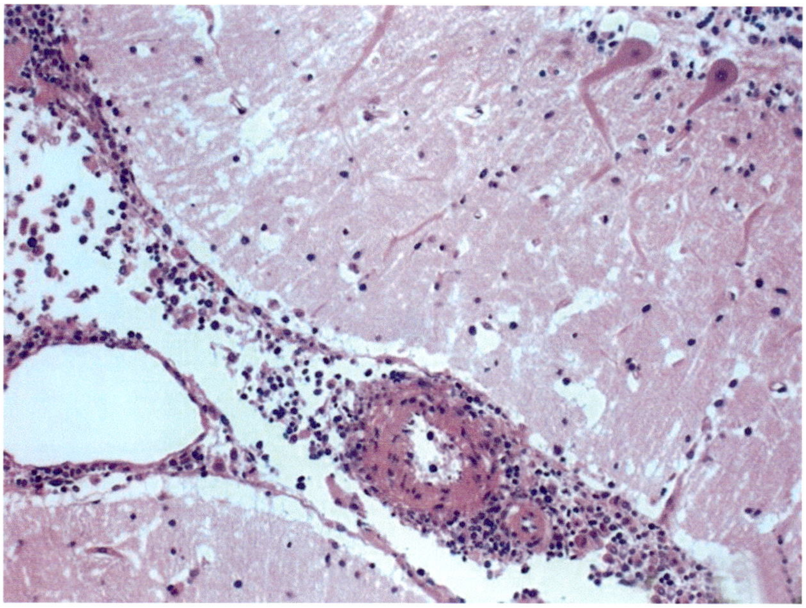

Fig. 2.28. Ox. Brain. malignant catarrhal fever (MCF). Lymphocytic meningoencephalitis. The pia mater is infiltrated with moderate numbers of lymphocytes, some of which are clustered around arteries showing fibrinoid necrosis of the tunica media (H&E). (Courtesy of Dr C. Barros, Universidade Federale de Santa Maria, Brazil.)

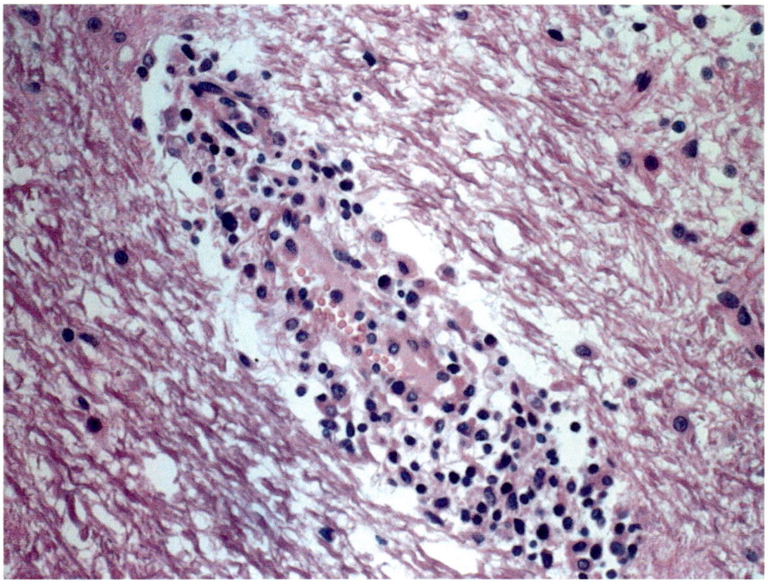

Fig. 2.29. Ox. Brain. malignant catarrhal fever (MCF). Lymphocytic vasculitis and perivasculitis. Moderate numbers of small and medium-sized lymphocytes with occasional plasma cells and macrophages have infiltrated the wall of an intraparenchymal blood vessel and are expanding the Virchow–Robin space (H&E). (Courtesy of Dr C. Barros, Universidade Federal de Santa Maria, Brazil.)

2.3.2.4 Neurotropic astrovirus

Introduction. Astroviruses are small, single-stranded RNA viruses infectious to mammals, including humans and birds. Being mainly enteric, they may infect young, elderly, and immunocompromised individuals. Transmission occurs via the fecal–oral route.

The novel neurotropic strain of bovine astrovirus (BoAstV-NeuroS1) induces a non-suppurative meningoencephalomyelitis, ganglioneuritis, and polyneuritis. Preferential anatomic sites are the cerebellar folia, mesencephalon, metencephalon, rhombencephalon, and spinal cord. It should be considered in the differential diagnosis of undiagnosed cases of bovine encephalitis.

Clinical signs. Weakness, paresis, paralysis, ataxia, recumbency.

Differential diagnoses. Rabies, bovine herpesvirus, BSE-prion, listeriosis, thromboembolic meningoencephalitis, babesiosis.

Diagram. Central nervous system (CNS). Anatomic distribution of bovine astrovirus. (Modified from *Emerging Infectious Diseases*, Vol 19, 2013, p. 1385.)

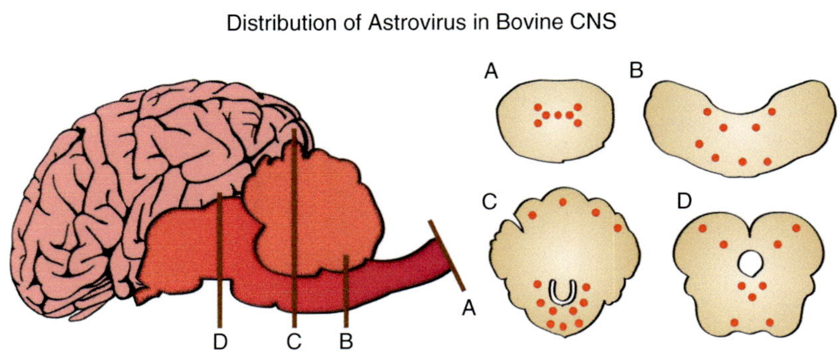

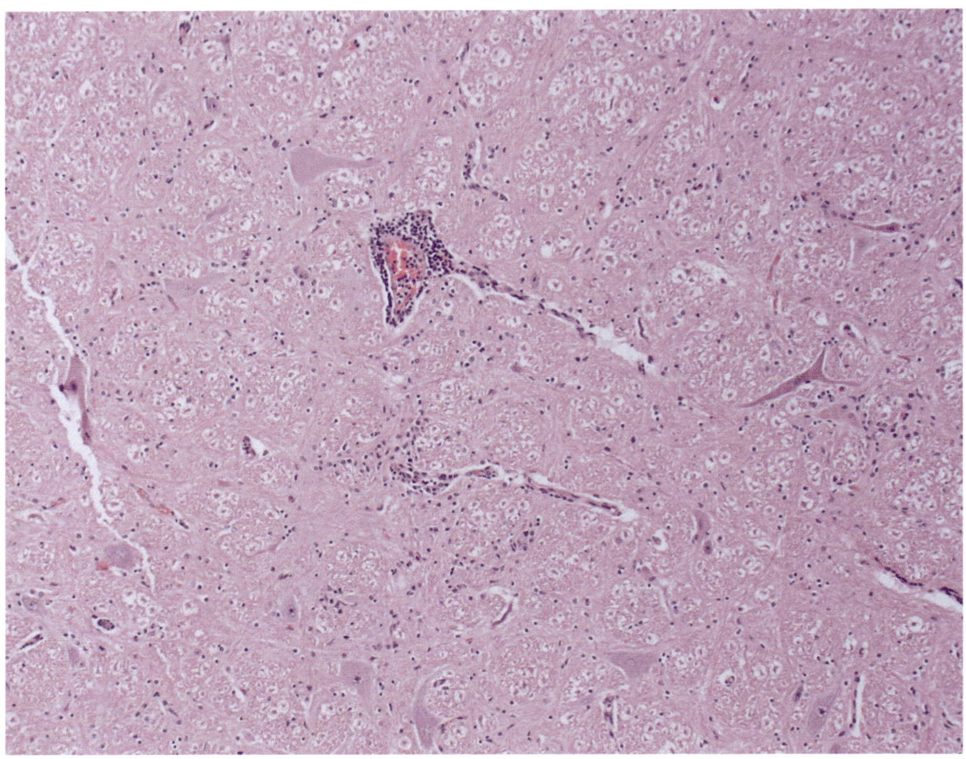

Fig. 2.30. Ox. Brain. Neurotropic astrovirus. Lymphocytic encephalitis. The gray matter substance is characterized by moderate perivascular lymphocytic cuffs, microgliosis, and neuronal degeneration. Swollen axons and spheroids may be additional findings. Viral inclusions are absent. Meningitis may be minimal (H&E). (Courtesy of Dr P. Pesavento, University of California, USA.)

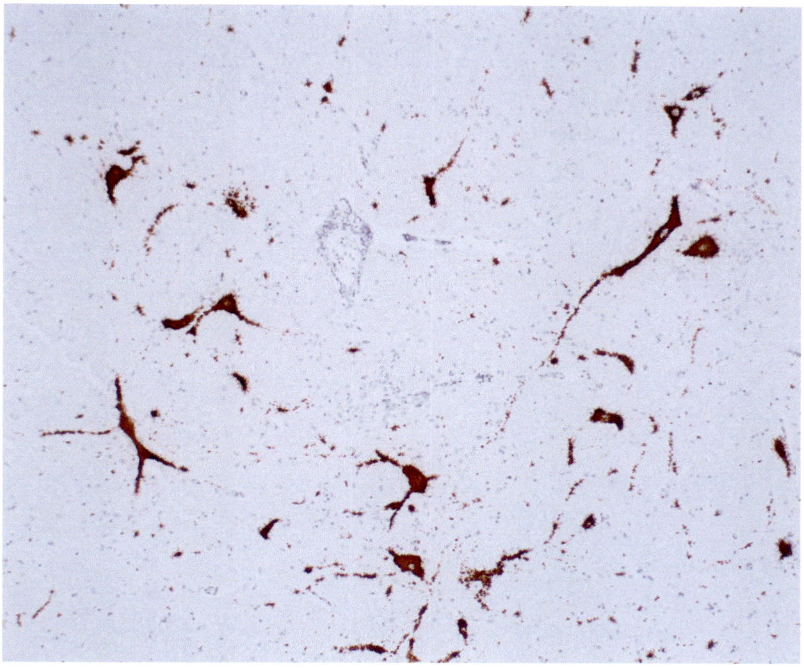

Fig. 2.31. Ox. Brain. Neurotropic astrovirus. Punctate or diffuse distribution of viral antigen in the cytoplasm of neurons and along neurofilaments (*in situ* hybridization). (Courtesy of Dr P. Pesavento, University of California, USA.)

2.3.3 Bacteria

2.3.3.1 Listeriosis

Introduction. Infectious disease with zoonotic potential caused by *Listeria monocytogenes* with nervous system and abortion components. Silage is the traditional reservoir for the agent. The route of entry is postulated from the oral cavity via cranial nerves to the medulla and brainstem. Here, the bacteria may cause multifocal hemorrhages at the gross level in some cases. The morphologic diagnosis is made by microscopic examination, with findings of microabscesses, and perivascular lymphocytic and plasmacytic cuffs. The organism is widespread and can be isolated from many organs in an infected ruminant. In the encephalon, lesions are restricted to the brainstem. Myelitis can also be observed.

Clinical signs. Circling and head pressing, facial nerve paralysis, tongue protrusion, ear drooping.

Differential diagnoses. Rabies, botulism, viral and bacterial meningoencephalitis, toxicoses.

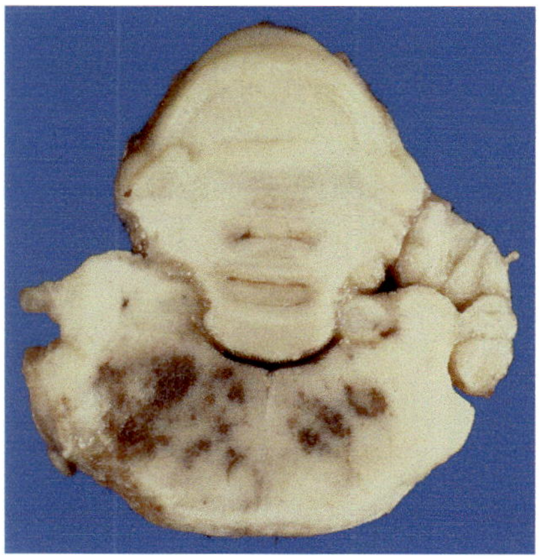

Fig. 2.32. Ox. Brainstem. Listeriosis. Hemorrhagic rhombencephalitis. Unilateral distribution of locally extensive foci of hemorrhage and malacia. These gross lesions are relatively infrequent in bovine listeriosis. (Courtesy of Dr P. Habecker, University of Pennsylvania, USA.)

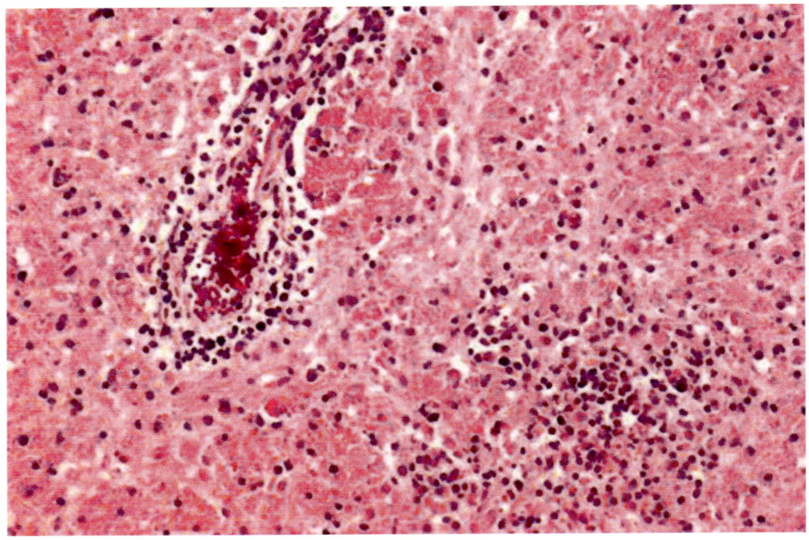

Fig. 2.33. Ox. Brainstem. Listeriosis. Lymphoplasmacytic meningoencephalitis with microabscesses. Perivascular cuffs and intraparenchymal mononuclear aggregates are composed of lymphocytes, a few plasma cells and macrophages, suggesting a chronic phase of the infection. There is some astrogliosis. Microabscesses composed of neutrophils are hallmark lesions of infection (H&E).

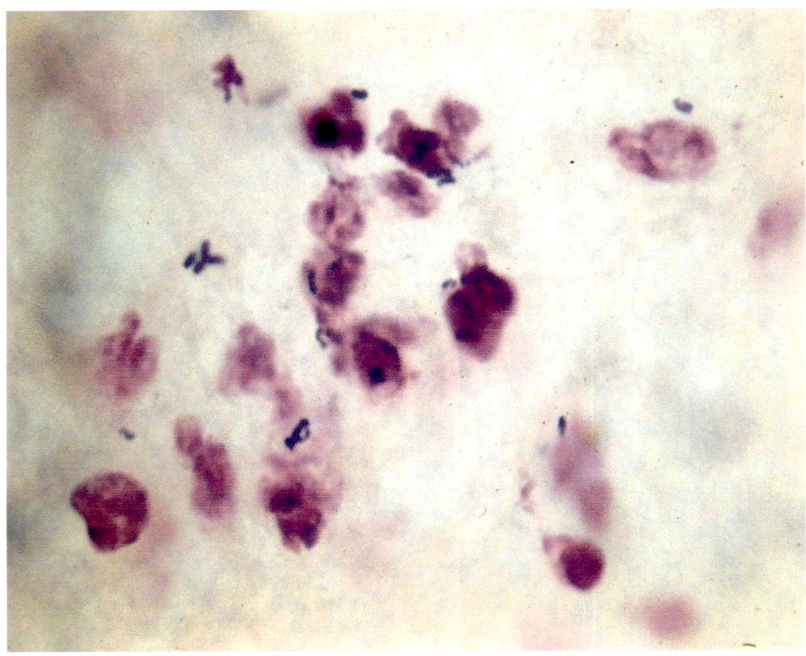

Fig. 2.34. Ox. Listeriosis. A cytologic spin from central nervous system (CNS) fluid stained with a Gram stain reveals intracytoplasmic and extracellular small gram-positive rods (Gram-stain).

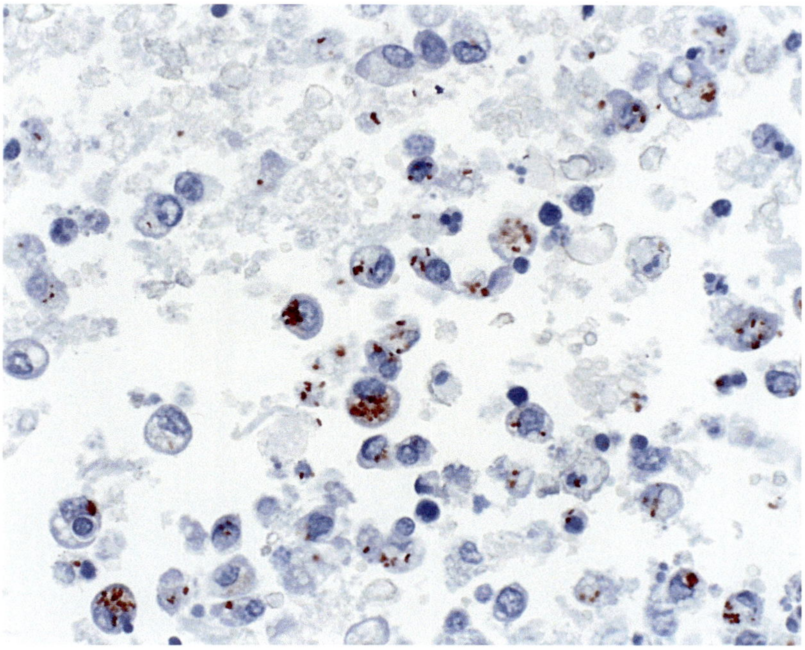

Fig. 2.35. Ox. Brain. Listeriosis. Indirect immunohistochemistry identifies the presence of small intracytoplasmic rods in gitter cells. Frequently, the bacteria can be identified in the cytoplasm of neutrophils (IHC).

2.3.3.2 Thrombotic meningoencephalomyelitis (TME)

Introduction. Originally described in feedlot operations to involve brain and spinal cord, the infection caused by *Histophilus somni*, a gram-negative, microthermophilic bacterium, has now been demonstrated to involve multiple other organs, such as tonsils, larynx, lung, pleura, heart, joints, muscle, the male and female reproductive tracts, udder, and eyes. As a disseminated infectious disease, it is frequently overlooked as such, both clinically and pathologically. In the CNS, it affects both brain and spinal cord, causing a thrombotic vasculitis (thrombophlebitis). *H. somni* infections in feedlot cattle are considered not to be associated with transient BVDV infections. In respiratory disease, *H. somni* is part of the bovine respiratory disease (BRD) complex.

Clinical signs. High fever, recumbency, sudden death.

Differential diagnoses. Viral and bacterial encephalitides, botulism, cerebral theileriosis, cerebral babesiosis, toxicoses.

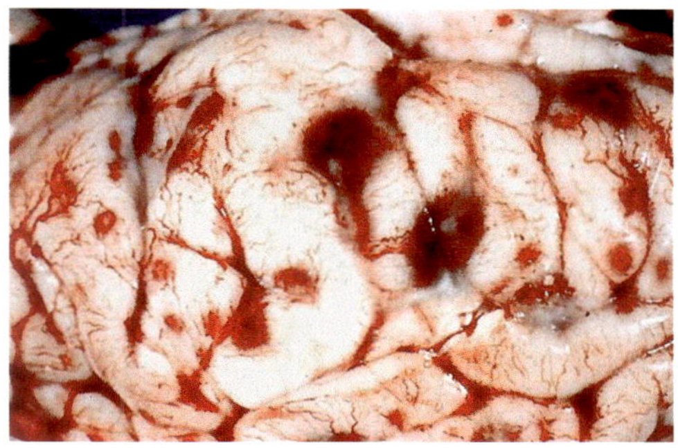

Fig. 2.36. Ox. Brain. Thrombotic meningoencephalitis (TME). There are multiple random foci of hemorrhage on the surface of the brain. These can also be visualized in the gray and white matter when performing coronal sections. They can occur in any part of the spinal cord. Antibiotic treatment can make the gross lesions less obvious to find only deeper in the brain.

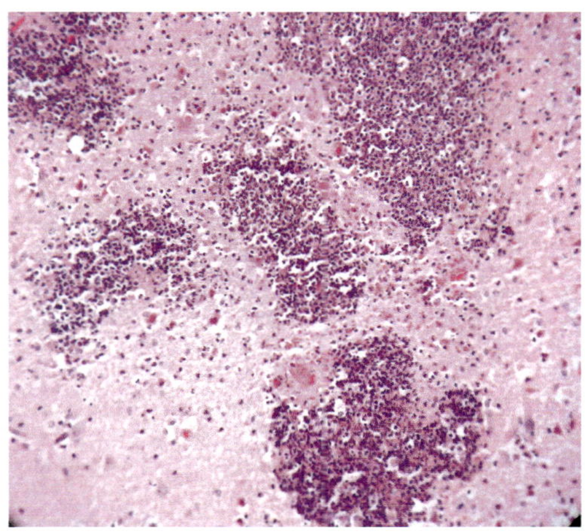

Fig. 2.37. Ox. Brain. Thrombotic meningoencephalitis (TME). Large areas of the neuropil are infiltrated by neutrophils, many of which are degenerate, and lymphocytes. (H&E).

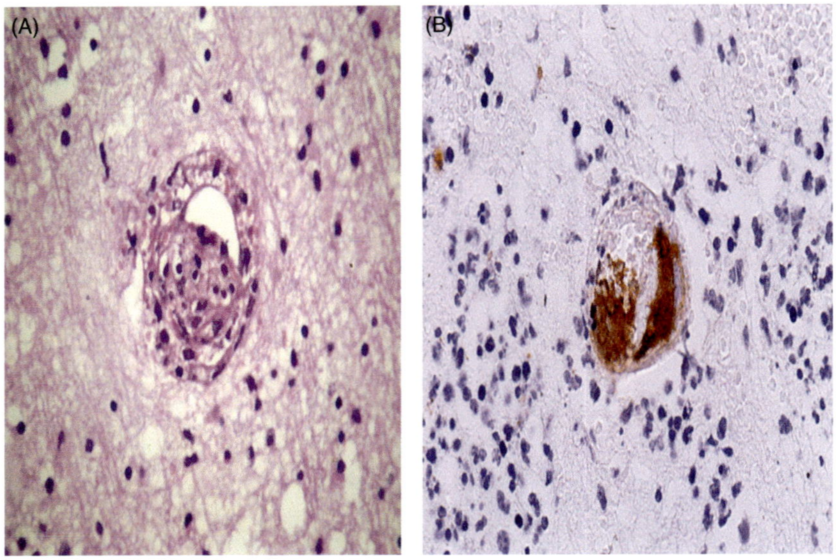

Fig. 2.38. Ox. Brain. Thrombotic meningoencephalitis (TME). Blood vessel. (A). A thrombus partially occludes a medium-sized artery with mural vacuolation, suggesting edema and necrosis. Vascular thrombosis and necrosis are the microscopic hallmark changes in TEM, and are responsible for infarcts. Apoptosis of endothelial cells and activated platelets may play a role in the pathogenesis of vascular damage (H&E). (B) (*Histophilus somni*) antigen is demonstrated with the thrombus (IHC).

Fact Sheet: Thrombotic Meningoencephalitis (TME) (Histophilus somni Disease Complex (HSDC)

Definition
- Central nervous system infection with septicemic spread to multiple organs caused by gram-negative microthermophilic bacterium, *Histophilus somni.*

Complications
- Septicemia and sequelae
- Myelitis; myocarditis/pericarditis; pleuritis; tonsillitis, laryngitis; bronchopneumonia; arthritis; nephritis; myositis; intestinal infarcts; ocular infection
- Reproductive losses
- Sporadic mastitis; abortion; vagino-cervicitis; endometritis; orchitis; balanoposthitis; seminal vesiculitis

Gross findings (CNS)
- Multiple, random foci of hemorrhage (infarcts)

Microscopic findings
- Thrombovasculitis and thrombolymphangitis (in case of pleuritis)

Differential diagnoses (CNS)
- Viral and bacterial encephalitides; polioencephalomalacia; septicemia; toxicoses

Other observations
- Not associated with transient BVDV infection
- Vaccines not consistently effective

2.3.3.3 Sporadic bovine encephalomyelitis (SBE, transmissible serositis)

Introduction. Also known as transmissible serositis, SBE is caused by *Chlamydophila pecorum*. The uncommon disease affects brain, pericardium, pleural and peritoneal surfaces, as well as the synovium of multiple joints, inducing a fibrinous exudative inflammation in each. Morbidity and mortality are low. Giemsa-stained impression smears are helpful for the diagnosis of SBE.

Gross lesions in the brain may include fibrin tags, congestion and edema. Histologic CNS lesions are featured by a non-suppurative meningoencephalomyelitis, particularly extensive in the cerebellum and expressed as lymphohistiocytic vasculitis and focal infiltration of the neuropil. Immunohistochemistry (IHC) staining can be used for demonstration of elementary bodies (EB)

Clinical signs. Fever, stiffness, incoordination, and depression.

Differential diagnoses. MCF, BHV, TME, listeriosis, salt intoxication.

2.3.3.4 Bovine cowdriosis (heartwater, bovine ehrlichiosis)

Introduction. A tick-transmitted disease, it is caused by *Ehrlichia ruminantium* (formerly *Cowdria ruminantium*). The vector tick, *Amblyomma* spp., is present in the Caribbean rim countries, and thus a threat to introducing the disease to the American mainland.

Brain swelling, edema with herniation through the foramen magnum and petechiation are gross findings. Microscopic changes are widened perivascular spaces, necrotic astrocytes, swollen axons, spongiosis and microcavitations, as well as a fibrinoid vasculitis with lymphocytes and macrophages.

E. ruminantium organisms can be demonstrated in the cytoplasm of endothelial cells of brain capillaries by Giemsa-stained tissue or smears.

Clinical signs. Respiratory distress, opisthotonos, leg peddling, recumbency, convulsions.

Differential diagnoses. MCF, cerebral babesiosis, cerebral theileriosis, viral and bacterial encephalitides.

2.3.3.5 Abscesses

Introduction. Multiple bacteria can cause brain and spinal cord abscesses. The more common organisms in cattle are *Trueperella pyogenes*, *Fusobacterium necrophorum*, *Pasteurella multocida* and *Pseudomonas aeruginosa*. The bacteria may reach the brain site hematogenously or from adjacent primary sites such as pituitary gland, ears, nasal cavity, or sinuses. Infected wounds from dehorning may be another portal of entry.

Clinical signs. These depend on the anatomic site. Blindness, ataxia, paresis, depression, recumbency may be some of them.

Differential diagnoses. Listeriosis, TME, lead poisoning, neoplasia, trauma.

2.3.3.6 Meningitis

Introduction. In adult cattle and encountered more frequently in juveniles associated with septicemia. Organism may include *Pasteurella* spp. or *Streptococcus* spp. and gram-negative bacteria. When bovine tuberculosis was widespread in Europe, granulomatous meningitis was a frequent event.

Clinical signs. Dullness, imbalance, recumbency, fever.

Differential diagnoses. Bacterial or viral encephalitides.

2.3.4 Fungi

2.3.4.1 Cryptococcosis

Introduction. Fungal encephalitis is a sporadic event occurring in immunocompromised animals. Systemic fungi reach the brain hematogenously

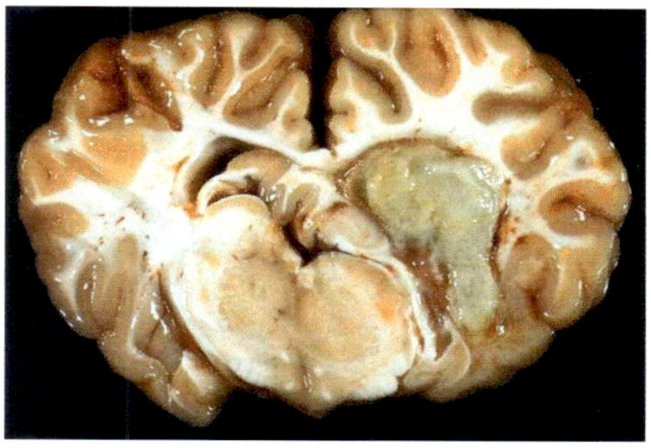

Fig. 2.39. Ox. Brain. Abscess. A purulent exudate occupies the brain parenchyma next to the lateral ventricle, which is compressed.

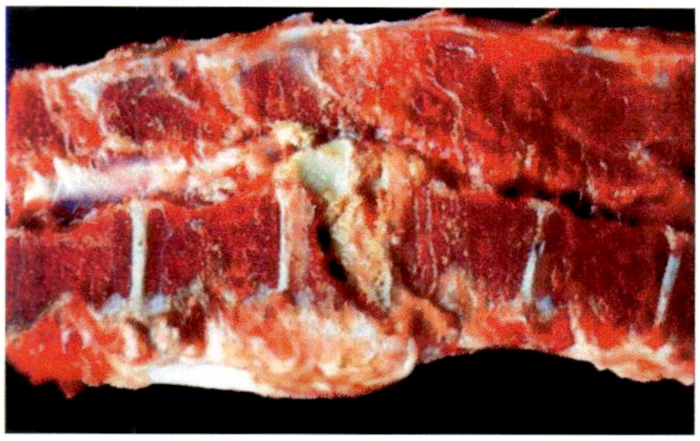

Fig. 2.40. Ox. Spinal cord. Abscess and discospondylitis. The vertebral body contains a purulent exudate expanding into the epidural space. Ventrally, there is evidence of discospondylitis.

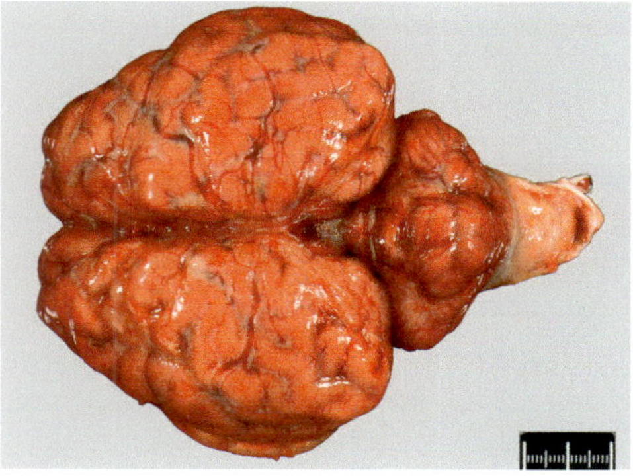

Fig. 2.41. Ox. Brain. Fibrinopurulent meningitis. A milky exudate is especially visible in the depths of sulci. (Courtesy of Department of Veterinary Pathology, WCVM, University of Saskatchewan, Saskatoon, Canada.)

from primary sites located somewhere else, generally forestomachs and abomasum. Occasionally, cows with mycotic abortions will get fungal embolic lesions in the brain. The identity of the organism can be established by culture or special tissue stains. Infections are usually caused by *Aspergillus*, *Candida*, *Mucor*, *Rhizopus*, *Absidia*, *Mortierella* spp.

Clinical signs. Behavioral changes similar to viral or bacterial encephalitides.

Differential diagnoses. Bacterial, viral encephalitis.

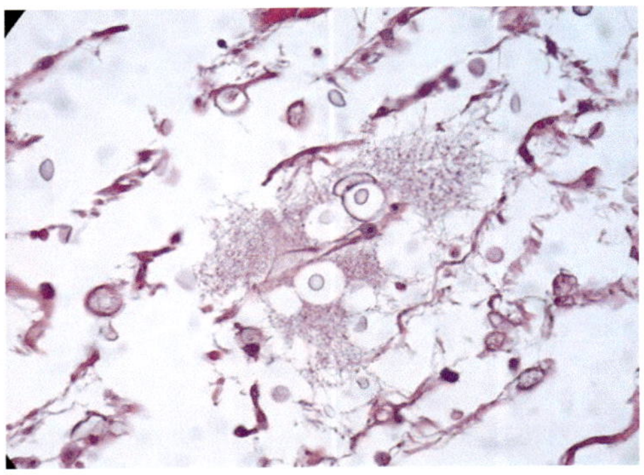

Fig. 2.43. Ox. Brain. Cryptococcosis. The finding of spherical yeasts with a thick, unstained capsule resulting in multiple clear spaces (halos) indicates cryptococcosis. The capsule can be stained with mucicarmine, other histochemical stains and identified via IHC. (Courtesy of Dr F. Riet-Correa, National Institute for Agricultural Research, Uruguay.)

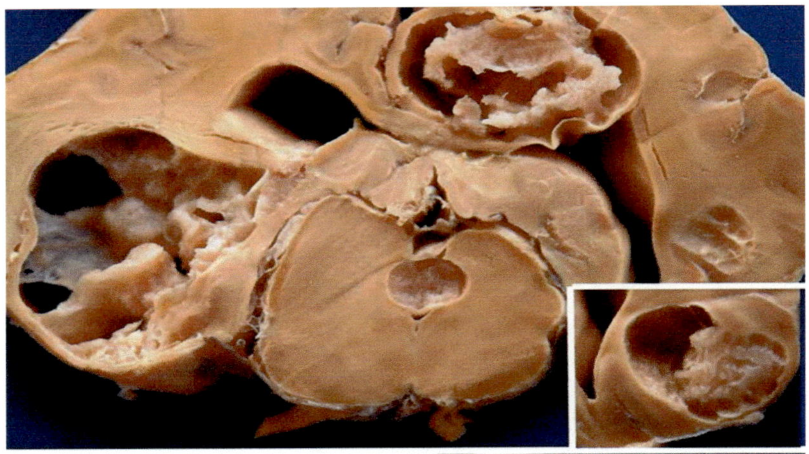

Fig. 2.42. Ox. Brain. Cryptococcosis. Multicavitary, mucinous, pyogranulomatous encephalitis. Multiple cavitations are scattered throughout the transverse section of the brain. Inset: cavitation is partially filled with glistening, mucinous, partially gelled capsular material typical for *Cryptococcus neoformans*. (Courtesy of Dr F. Riet-Correa, National Institute for Agricultural Research, Uruguay.)

2.3.5 Protozoa

2.3.5.1 Cerebral babesiosis

Introduction. Bovine babesiosis or redwater is a tick-borne disease caused by an intra-erythrocytic protozoon parasite, *Babesia*. *Babesia bovis* is one of four species of *Babesia*. Cerebral babesiosis develops in some infected animals and its outcome is mostly fatal (see Chapter 11: Diseases of the Hematopoietic and Hemolymphatic System).

Clinical signs. Hyperesthesia, nystagmus, circling, head pressing, convulsions, paralysis.

Differential diagnoses. Heartwater, cerebral theileriosis, bacterial meningoencephalitis.

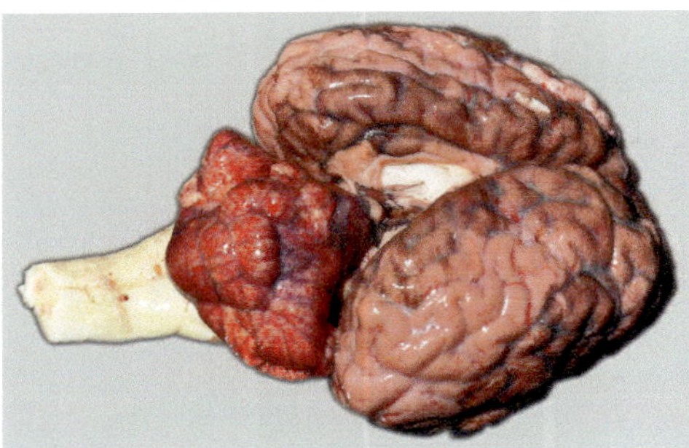

Fig. 2.44. Ox. Brain. Cerebral babesiosis. Meningeal congestion. The cerebellar meninges are dilated, highlighted by a cherry-pink color. (Courtesy of Dr D. Driemeier, Universidade Federal do Rio Grande do Sul, Brazil.)

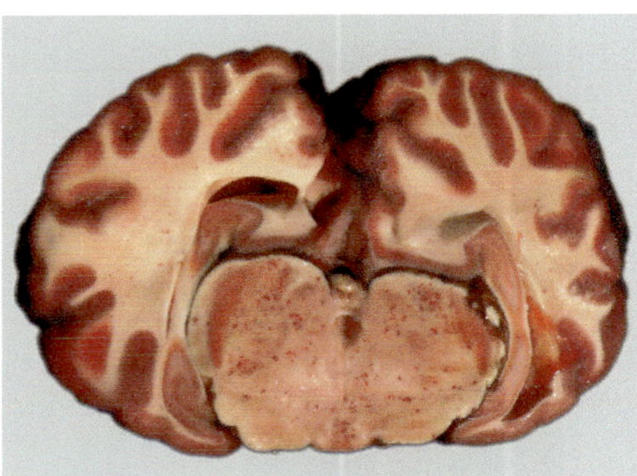

Fig. 2.45. Ox. Brain. Cerebral babesiosis. Congestion. Distinct red foci in the mesencephalon suggests vascular dilatation. (Courtesy of Dr D. Driemeier, Universidade Federal do Rio Grande do Sul, Brazil.)

2.3.5.2 Cerebral theileriosis

Introduction. Tick-borne, the protozoal parasite penetrates erythrocytes. It causes extravascular hemolysis, leading to anemia, jaundice, and abortions. The benign form of theileriosis, caused by *Theileria segmentalis* or *orientalis*, occurs in Latin America.

Grossly, meninges and brain are markedly congested (cherry-pink discoloration). Intense hemorrhage may occur in ventricles. Histological examination reveals obstruction of arterioles by large numbers of parasitized lymphoblasts, with thrombosis and necrosis of affected blood vessels. The brain parenchyma shows hemorrhage, and spongiosis with an infiltration of gitter cells, as well as glial cell proliferation.

Clinical signs. Circling, head pressing, blindness, ataxia, paralysis.

Differential diagnoses. Listeria, TEM, heartwater, rabies.

2.3.5.3 *Cerebral amoebiasis*

Introduction. *Naegleria fowleri* has been reported to cause sporadic meningoencephalitis in young cattle. It also affects the human central nervous system. The source of origin is stagnant water in hot climates. The protozoa tend to migrate into the encephalon from the nasal cavities via the lamina cribrosa of the ethmoid bone. Grossly multifocal areas of malacia tend to involve olfactory lobes and cerebellum. Histologically, there is a necrosuppurative meningoencephalitis with amoebic trophozoites in areas of malacia.

Clinical signs. Circling, seizures, nasal discharge.

Differential diagnoses. TME, PEM, cerebral abscess, bacterial meningitis, trauma.

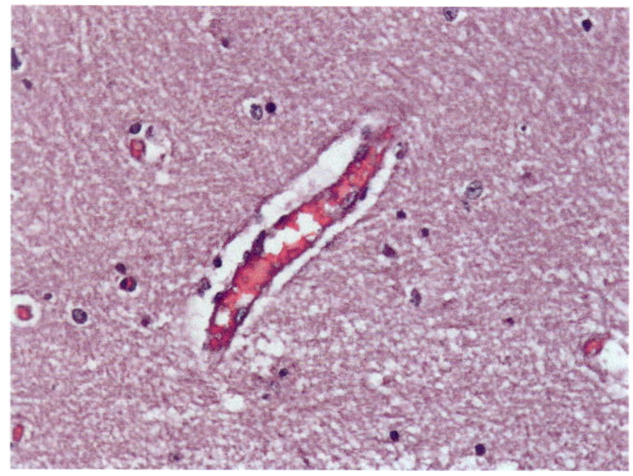

Fig. 2.46. Ox. Brain. Cerebral babesiosis. Red blood cell agglutination. Sludging of red blood cells can be seen in arterioles (and venules), but is non-specific (H&E). (Courtesy of Dr O. Illanes, Ross University, St Kitts.)

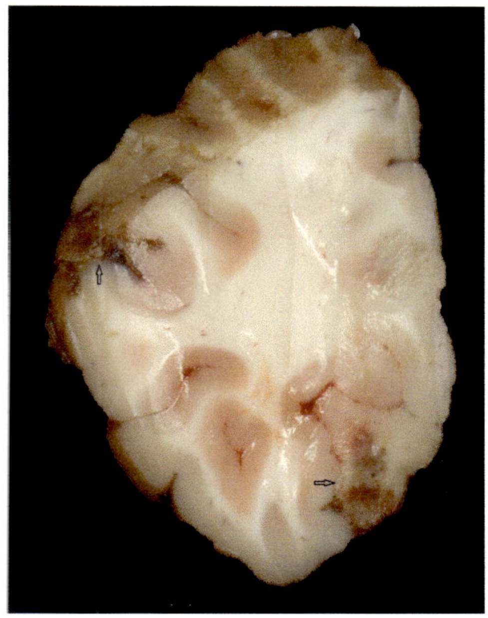

Fig. 2.47. Ox. Brain. Cerebral amoebiasis. Meningeal hemorrhage and foci of cerebral malacia. The meninges are focally red, brown, and a few areas of malacia are present in the neocortex (arrows). Olfactory lobes and cerebellum are mainly affected grossly with *Naegleria fowleri* infection. (Courtesy of Dr F. Uzal, University of California, USA.)

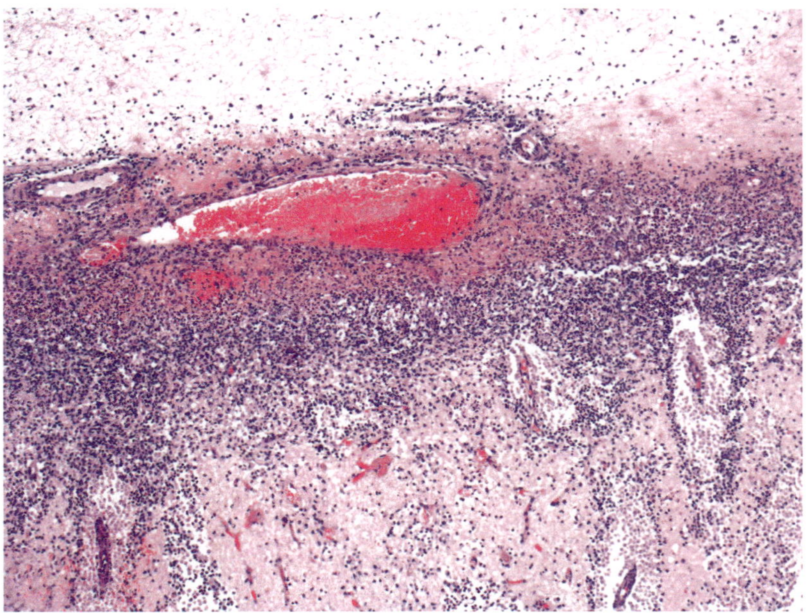

Fig. 2.48. Ox. Brain. Cerebral amoebiasis. Necrosuppurative meningoencephalitis. *Naegleria fowleri.* There is evidence of malacia, thrombosis, and infiltration by dense aggregates of neutrophils, many of them degenerate (H&E). (Courtesy of Dr F. Uzal, University of California, USA.)

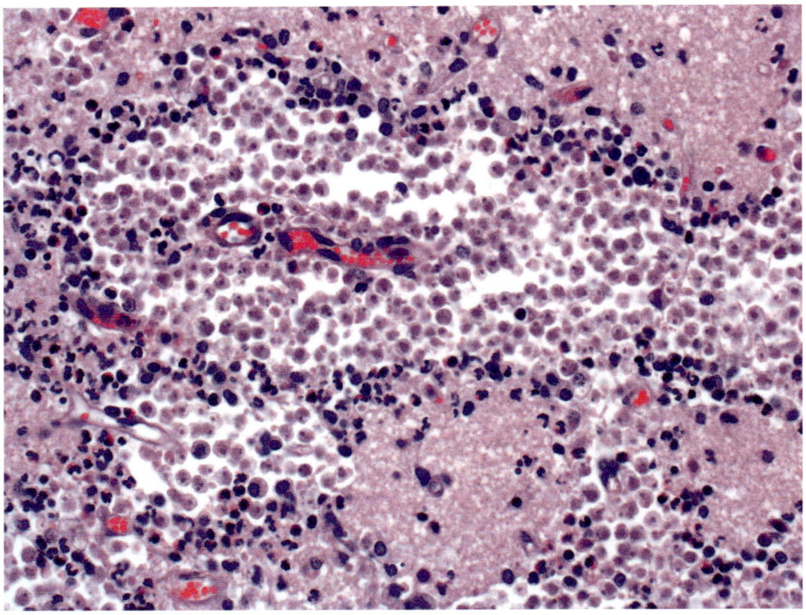

Fig. 2.49. Ox. Brain. Cerebral amoebiasis. Clusters of intralesional, weakly basophilic, round to ovoid amoebae are present in necrotic neuropil. (Courtesy of Dr F. Uzal, University of California, USA.)

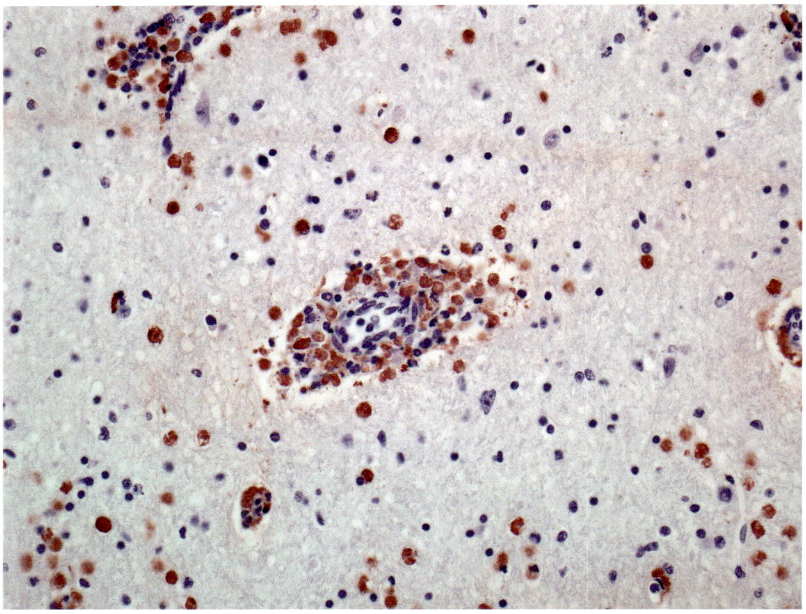

Fig. 2.50. Ox. Brain. Cerebral amoebiasis. Numerous brown staining (*Naegleria fowleri*) amoebae surround blood vessels. Individual organisms have invaded the neuropil (IHC). (Courtesy of Dr F. Uzal, University of California, USA.)

2.3.5.4 Cerebral trypanosomiasis

Caused by *Trypanosoma vivax*, the disease should be considered as differential diagnosis of non-suppurative menigoencephalitis in Latin American countries. The hemoprotozoon is transmitted by the horse fly belonging to the family *Tabanidae* (Diptera).

2.3.6 Parasites

2.3.6.1 Cerebral coenurosis

Introduction. Parasites are of infrequent occurrence in the bovine CNS.
Clinical sign. Circling.
Differential diagnosis. Listeriosis.

2.4 TRAUMA

Introduction. The brain and spinal cord are well protected by the musculature in cattle, and the compact, bony structures themselves are quite resistant to the impact of trauma. Injuries to the brain and spinal cord depend on three factors: severity, speed, and duration. Trauma to the skull may result in meningeal hemorrhage, subdural hematomas, or contra-coup hemorrhage. Trauma to the spinal column may lead to vertebral fractures or spinal cord hemorrhage, necrosis or laceration.
Clinical signs. Disorientation, convulsions, ataxia, paresis, paralysis, recumbency.
Differential diagnoses. Electrocution, lightning strike, fibro-cartilagenous embolic myelopathy (spinal cord), septicemia, bilateral poliomyelomalacia associated with selenium toxicosis, and prolonged anesthesia after dorsal recumbency.

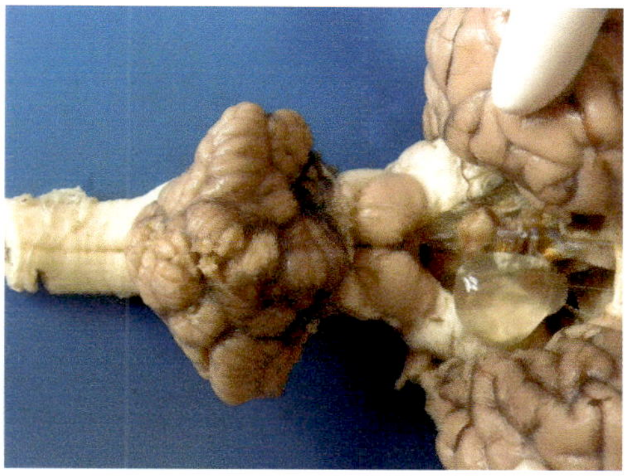

Fig. 2.51. Ox. Brain. Cerebral coenurosis. A fluid-filled cyst (white star) is located caudal to the occipital lobe. It contains the scolex of *Coenurus cerebralis*, metacestode of *Taenia multiceps* (*Multiceps multiceps*). (Courtesy of Dr C. Barros, Universidade Federal de Santa Maria, Brazil.)

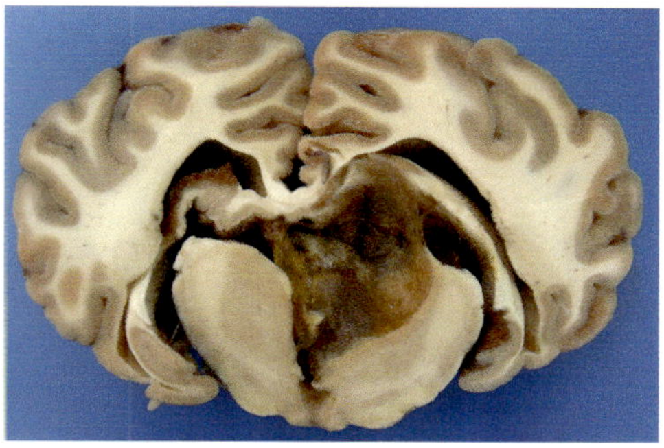

Fig. 2.52. Ox. Brain. Cerebral coenurosis. Cut section demonstrates anatomic location of cyst with contents compressing cerebral tissue. (Courtesy of Dr C. Barros, Universidade Federal de Santa Maria, Brazil.)

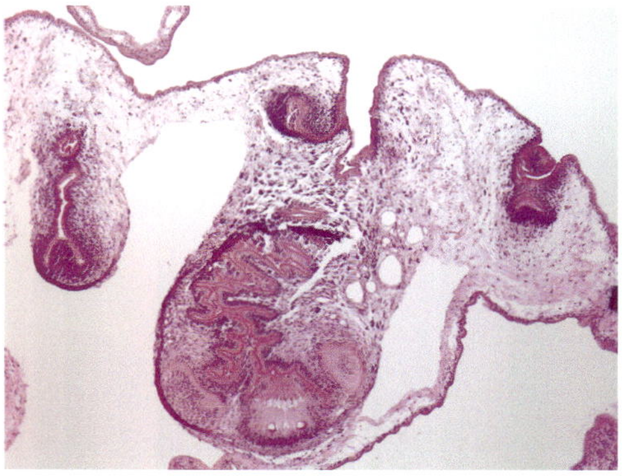

Fig. 2.53. Ox. Brain. Cerebral coenurosis. Histologic demonstration of metacestode within cyst (H&E). (Courtesy of Dr C. Barros, Universidade Federal de Santa Maria, Brazil.)

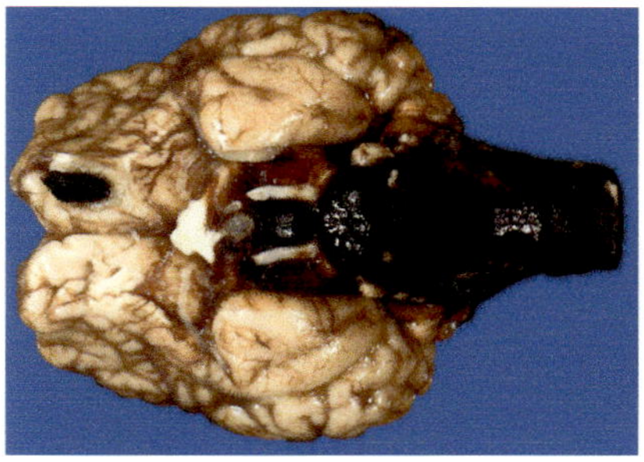

Fig. 2.54. Ox. Brain. Hemorrhage. The ventral surface of the brainstem is covered by blood. If not the result of trauma, the hemorrhage could have been caused by coliform septicemia or an attempt to collect central nervous system (CNS) fluid.

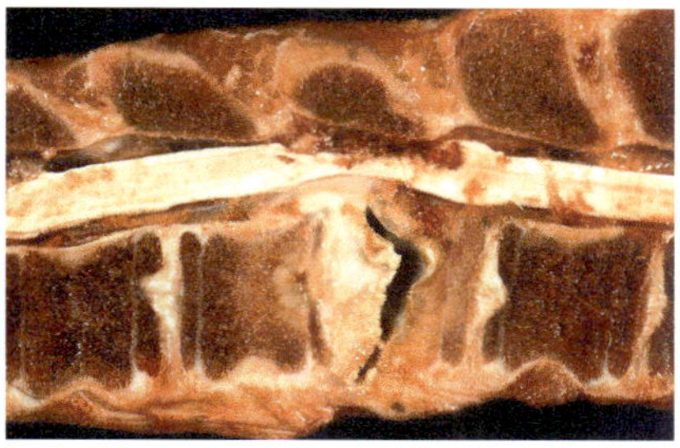

Fig. 2.55. Ox. Vertebral column. Abscess and fracture. Vertebral abscess resulted in secondary fracture, with dislodged bone segments traumatizing adjacent cord by impingement.

2.5 NEOPLASIA

Introduction. Primary CNS neoplasms originating from specific cells of the histological neuroanatomy are unusual in the bovine, perhaps due to a short lifespan. Medulloblastoma as an example is listed in the chapter on calves (see Chapter 1: Diseases of Neonates and Calves). Likewise, metastatic neoplasia is uncommon.

Clinical signs. Neuroanatomic location of the tumor determines the expression of clinical signs. Compressing neoplasms in the epidural space of the spinal cord creates an alert downer cow. Preceding signs can range from paresis to ataxia.

Differential diagnoses. Trauma, fracture, abscesses.

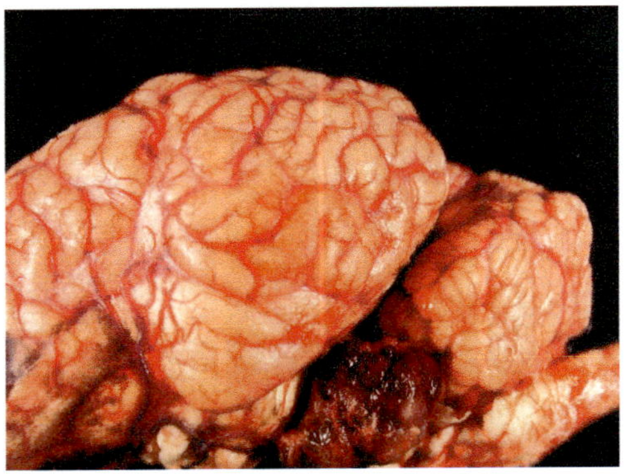

Fig. 2.56. Ox. Central nervous system (CNS). Benign peripheral nerve sheath tumor (schwannoma). A unilateral, cauliflower-like growth is present laterally between the cerebrum and cerebellum. The tumor arose from a cranial nerve root. The animal exhibited a head tilt clinically and some aggressive behavior, and was euthanized with a presumptive diagnosis of rabies.

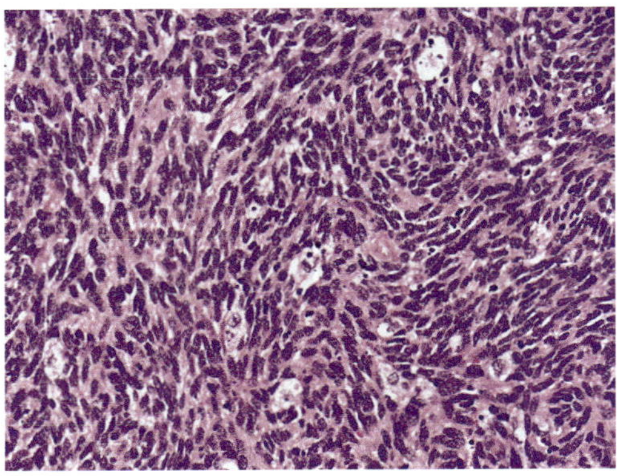

Fig. 2.57. Ox. Central nervous system (CNS). Benign peripheral nerve sheath tumor (schwannoma). Histological features reveal spindle-shaped tumor cells with elongated nuclei and a pattern of interwoven, whirling bundles (H&E).

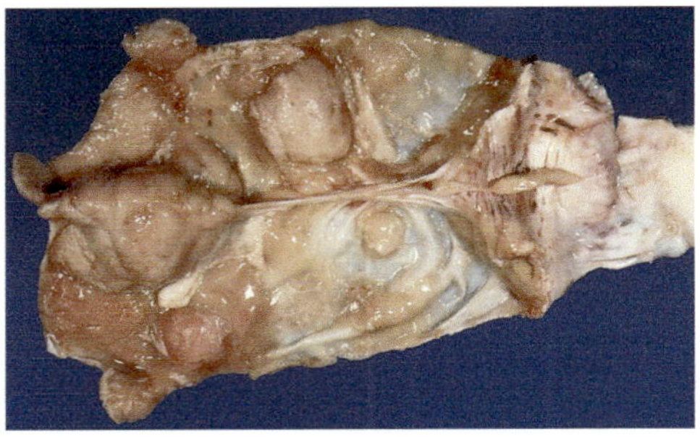

Fig. 2.58. Ox. Cerebral dura mater. Meningeal lymphoma. Multiple sessile, soft nodules are attached tightly to the dura. Central nervous system (CNS) lymphomas can occur as primary or metastatic tumors. Fibroblastic meningioma is a rare tumor that should be considered in the differential diagnosis.

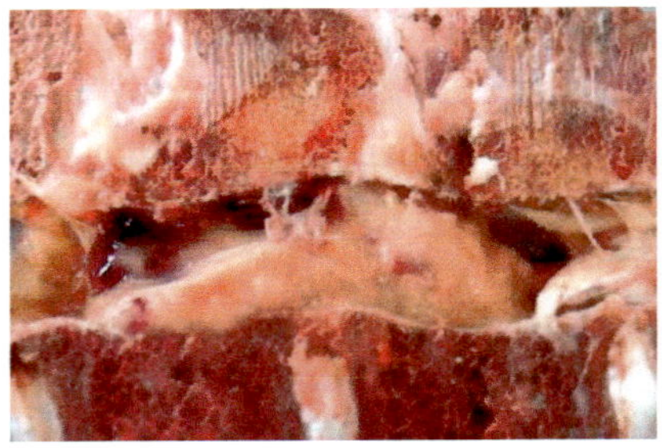

Fig. 2.59. Ox. Spinal cord. Epidural lymphoma. A fleshy, monotonous, soft mass focally occupies the epidural space in a cow with ataxia. It was diagnosed as lymphoma.

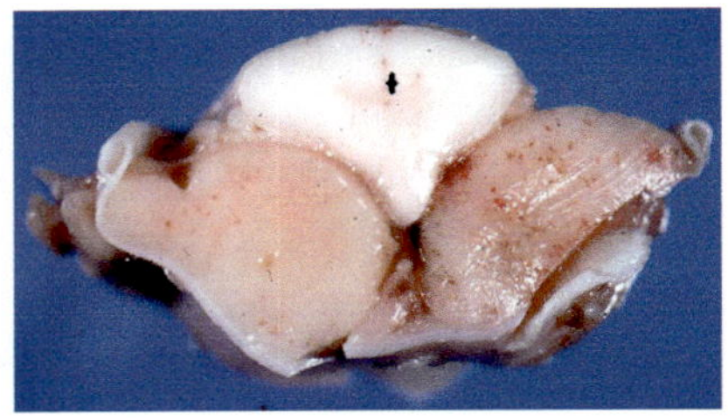

Fig. 2.60. Ox. Spinal cord. Epidural lymphoma. The compressive effect of an epidural space-occupying mass on the adjacent spinal cord is depicted on cut section. (Courtesy of Dr J.M. King and Section of Anatomic Pathology, Cornell University, USA.)

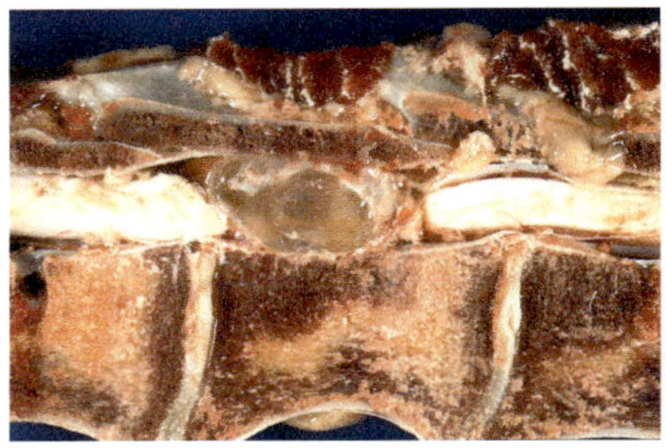

Fig. 2.61. Ox. Spinal cord. Epidural nerve sheath tumor (schwannoma). A focal, brown, gelatinous growth has invaded a segment of the spinal cord, compressing it.

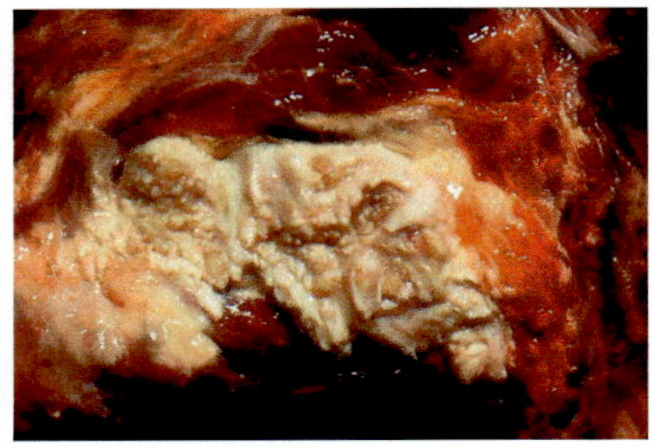

Fig. 2.62. Ox. Brachial plexus. Neurofibromatosis. A thickened, multinodular, firm growth is expanding within the medial part of the shoulder. The condition is considered a multi-site type of schwannoma.

2.6 MISCELLANEOUS

This chapter contains a short text and some images on familial myelopathies affecting certain bovine breeds.

2.6.1 Breed-specific encephalomyelopathies

Introduction. Occurrence within one breed in multiple geographic areas suggests inherited factors contributing to the development of the disorders. A few selective hereditary and familial myelopathies are presented with the following.

2.6.1.1 Multifocal symmetrical encephalomyelopathy of juvenile Simmental cattle

Also seen in the Limousin breed and in cross-animals of both breeds. Pathologic features are neuronal degeneration and demyelination. Grossly, bilateral and symmetric malacic, depressed, cavitating foci are present in the brainstem of affected animals. The caudal olivary nucleus is also a consistent target. Foci of malacia are also seen in the thoracic spinal cord.

Clinical signs. Ataxia and hindlimb paresis.

Differential diagnoses. Fracture, spinal cord compression, deficiency diseases affecting locomotor system.

2.6.1.2 Bovine progressive degenerative myeloencephalopathy (BPDME)

Also known as Weaver syndrome, occurring in Brown Swiss cattle, Braunvieh, and crosses. A familial pattern of distribution suggests hereditary pathogenesis.

Gross changes are not common. Microscopic lesions affecting the white matter substance of the spinal cord are most prominent in the thoracic segment and consist of axonal degeneration, leading to the formation of spheroids, loss of axons and myelin. Cerebellar lesions are characterized by degeneration or loss of Purkinje cells; brainstem nuclei show occasional axonal swelling. Degenerative changes appear to be a primary axonopathy.

Clinical signs. Posterior ataxia, atrophy of pelvic limb muscles.

Differential diagnoses. Trauma, spinal cord compression. Deficiency diseases affecting locomotor system.

2.6.1.3 Spinal muscular atrophy

Seen in young Brown Swiss, Red Danish dairy breeds and occasional Holstein–Friesians, the diagnosis is based on histological findings of degenerative and necrotic and loss of spinal motor neurons the ventral horns with neuronophagia, neurofilament accumulations and astrocytosis, leading to secondary neurogenic muscular atrophy. Again, a familial pattern traced to breeding bulls suggests a hereditary condition. An autosomal recessive gene has been located at chromosome 24.

Clinical signs. Progressive symmetric weakness, quadriparesis, sternal recumbency, atrophy of appendicular muscles.

Differential diagnoses. Trauma, deficiency diseases affecting locomotor system.

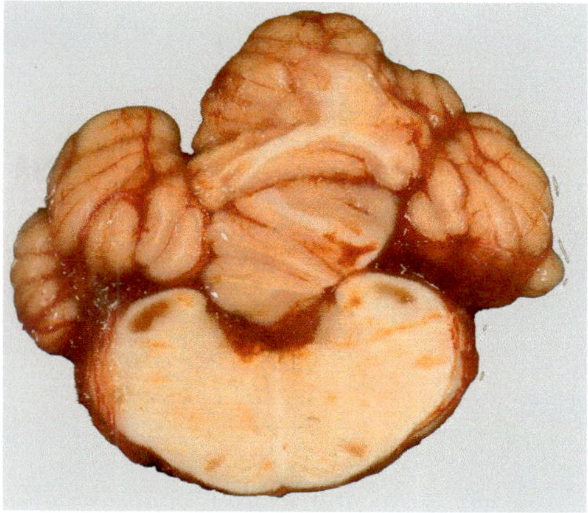

Fig. 2.63. Ox. Brainstem. Symmetrical encephalomyelopathy of Simmental cattle. Bilateral symmetrical hemorrhage, malacia and cavitations are evident. (Courtesy of Dr E. Waters, Prairie Diagnostic Services, Saskatoon, Saskatchewan, Canada.)

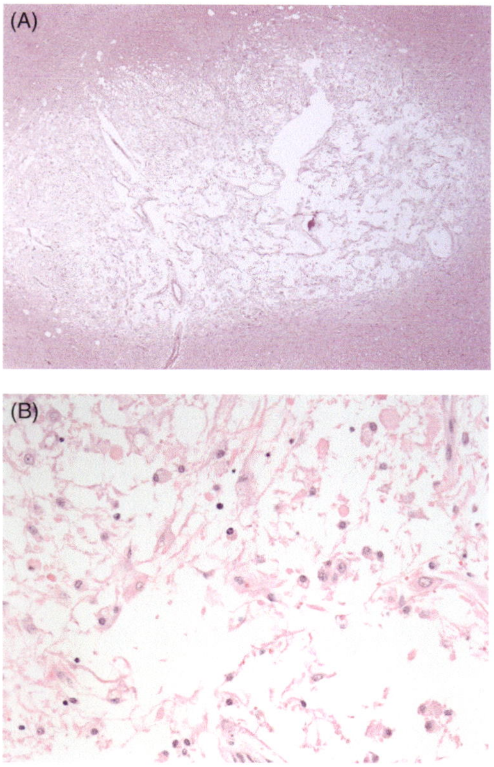

Fig. 2.64. Ox. Brainstem. Symmetrical encephalomyelopathy of Simmental cattle. Malacia. (A) Microscopic features are rarefaction of neuropil, neuronal degeneration, and demyelination (H&E). (B) Higher magnification of lesions (H&E). (Courtesy of Dr G. McGregor, Department of Pathology, WCVM, University of Saskatchewan, Saskatoon, Canada.)

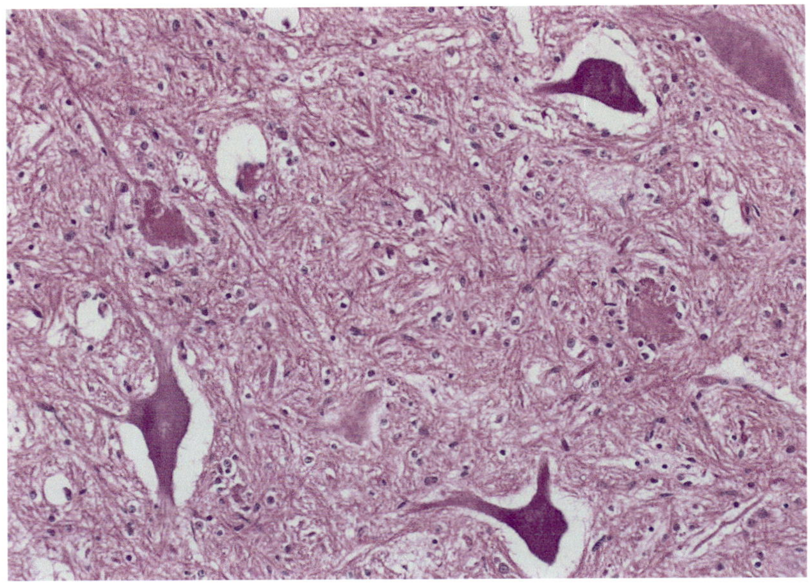

Fig. 2.65. Ox. Spinal cord. Spinal muscular atrophy. Lower motor neuron disease (LMND). Shrunken (fading ghosts), degenerate, eosinophilic neurons are present. Occasional somatic motor neurons are swollen (H&E). (Courtesy of Dr B. Summers, Cornell University, USA.)

2.6.1.4 Inherited progressive myelinopathy in Murray Grey cattle

This autosomal recessive disorder is characterized by brain and spinal cord neuronal degeneration and demyelination. Affected sites are primarily spinal cord white matter and gray matter, medulla oblongata, and cerebellum.

Clinical sign. Ataxia.

Differential diagnoses. Trauma, deficiency diseases affecting locomotor systems.

2.6.1.5 Progressive ataxia of Charolais cattle

The disease is diagnosed by histologic findings of areas of myelin loss in the white matter of the central nervous system and of multifocal, acellular, pale, eosinophilic plagues throughout the cerebellum and spinal cord. The condition is thought to be an oligodendroglial dysplasia, resulting in leukodystrophy.

Clinical signs. Ataxia, weakness, paralysis.

Differential diagnoses. Trauma, deficiency diseases affecting locomotor system.

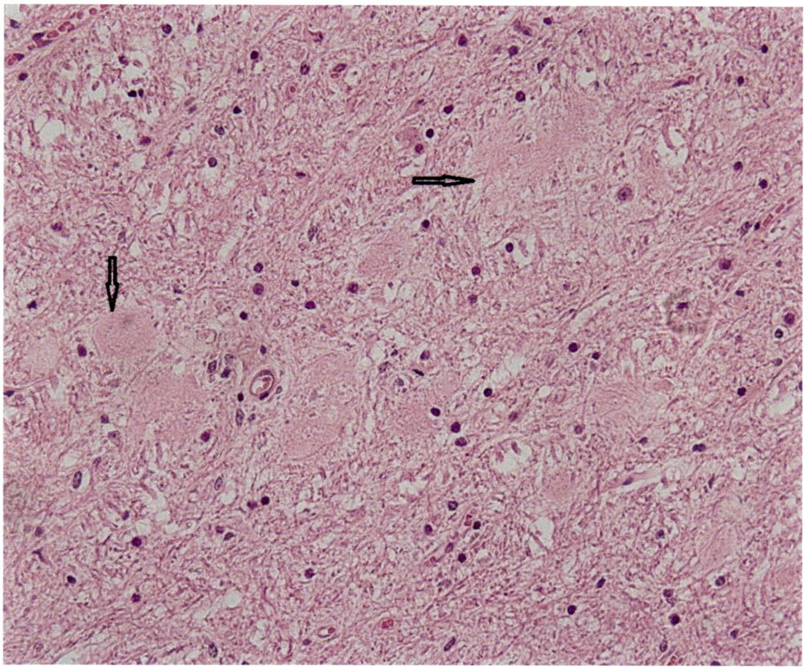

Fig. 2.66. Ox. Brain. Progressive ataxia of Charolais cattle. Leukodystrophy. Multiple eosinophilic plaques (arrows) are present in the white matter substance (H&E). (Courtesy of Dr S. Greenwood, Department of Pathology, WCVM, University of Saskatchewan, Saskatoon, Canada.)

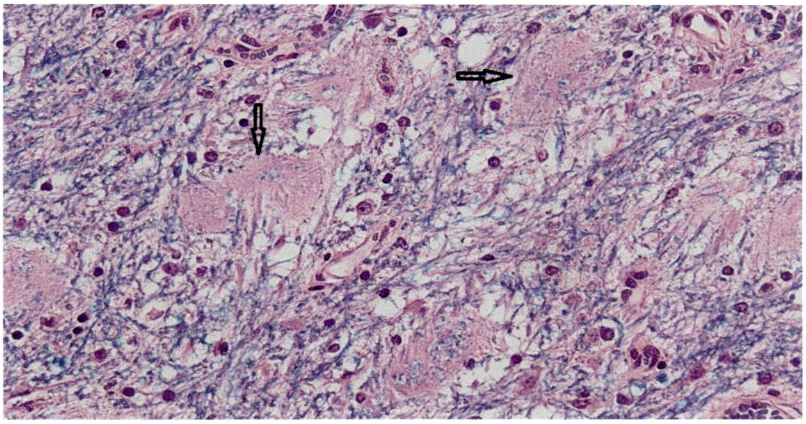

Fig. 2.67. Ox. Brain. Progressive ataxia of Charolais cattle. Dysmyelination. Plaques (arrows) are interfering with distribution of myelin (Luxol Fast Blue Cresyl Violet). (Courtesy of Dr S. Greenwood, Department of Pathology, WCVM, University of Saskatchewan, Saskatoon, Canada.)

2.6.1.6 Bovine ceroid-lipofuscinosis in Devon cattle

Characterized grossly by severe cerebellar atrophy, the disease microscopically exhibits accumulation of fluorescent lipopigment granules in neurons of the central nervous system, in retinal ganglionic cells, and in major visceral organs. Inheritance suggests an autosomal recessive trait.
Clinical signs. Blindness, ataxia.
Differential diagnoses. BVD, inflammations.

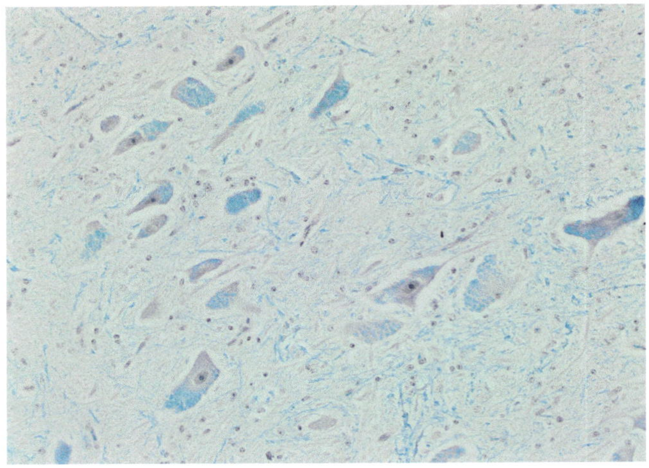

Fig. 2.68. Ox. Brain. Ceroid-lipofuscinosis. Several neurons are involved in the deposition of lipopigment (Luxol Fast Blue stain). (Courtesy of Dr B. Summers, Cornell University, USA.)

SUGGESTED READING

Bassuino, D.M., Konradt, G., Cruz, R.A.S., Silva, G.S., Gomes, D.C., *et al.* (2016) Characterization of spinal cord lesions in cattle and horses with rabies: the importance of correct sampling to the diagnosis. *Journal of Veterinary Diagnostic Investigation*, doi: 10.1177/1040638716647992.

Corbeil, L.B. (2007) *Histophilus somni* host relationship. *Animal Health Research Review* 8, 151–160.

Cordoso, T.C., Ferrari, H.F., Garcia, A.F., Bregano, L.C., Andrade A.L. and Nogueira, A.H. (2010) Immunohistochemical approach to the pathogenesis of clinical cases of bovine Herpesvirus type 5 infections. *Diagnostic Pathology* 10, 57–63.

Daft, B.M., Visvesvara, G.S., Read, D.H., Kinde, H., Uzal, F.A. and Manzer, M.D. (2005) Seasonal meningoencephalitis in Holstein cattle caused by *Naegleria fowleri*. *Journal of Veterinary Diagnostic Investigation* 17, 605–609.

Linlin, L., Diab, S., McGraw, S., Barr, B., Traslavina, R., *et al.* (2013) Divergent astrovirus associated with neurologic disease in cattle. *Emerging Infectious Diseases* 19, 1385–1392.

Nandi, S., Kumar, M., Manohar, M. and Chauhan, R.S. (2009) Bovine herpesvirus infection in cattle. *Animal Health Research Review* 10, 85–98.

O'Toole, D. and Sondgeroth, K.S. (2015) Histophilosis as a natural disease. *Current Topics in Microbiology and Immunology*, doi: 10.1007/82_2015_5008.

Rachid, M.A., Filho, E.F., Carvalho, A.U., Vasconcelos, A.C. and Ferreira, P.M. (2011) Polioencephalomalacia in cattle. *Asian Journal of Animal and Veterinary Advances* 6, 126–131.

Schock, A., Gray, D. and Howie, F.E. (2008) Multifocal symmetrical necrotizing encephalopathy in Simmental cross cattle in Scotland. *Veterinary Record* 162, 694–695.

Vandevelde, M., Higgens, R.J. and Oevermann, A. (2012) *Veterinary Neuropathology*, 1st edn. Wiley-Blackwell, Oxford, UK.

CHAPTER 3

Diseases of the Respiratory System

3.1 Upper Respiratory Tract
- 3.1.1 Nostrils
  - 3.1.1.1 Inflammation
- 3.1.2 Sinonasal compartment
  - 3.1.2.1 Cysts
  - 3.1.2.2 Inflammation
  - 3.1.2.3 Neoplasia
- 3.1.3 Larynx
  - 3.1.3.1 Inflammation

3.2 Lower Respiratory Tract
- 3.2.1 Trachea
  - 3.2.1.1 Inflammation
  - 3.2.1.2 Honker's syndrome
- 3.2.2 Lung
  - 3.2.2.1 Inflammation
  - 3.2.2.2 Neoplasia
  - 3.2.2.3 Miscellaneous

3.3 Pleura
- 3.3.1 Effusion
- 3.3.2 Inflammation

INTRODUCTION

The respiratory tract can be divided anatomically and functionally into upper and lower respiratory tract, with the lung playing a critical role in bovine respiratory disease (BRD). Many predisposing factors determine the scope and outcome of BRD. Predisposing factors include physical stressors, environmental disturbances, and viruses (BVDV) compromising the system's defense mechanisms to allow pulmonary colonization and destructive inflammation by bacteria, many of which are normal residents of the upper respiratory tract.

The respiratory defense mechanism is a complex process involving the mucociliary apparatus as the first line of defense, followed by the bronchus-associated lymphoid tissue (BALT), bronchoalveolar lining fluid and lining cells, alveolar macrophages, and bactericidal alveolar neutrophils. Viral and bacterial pathogens overpowering the respiratory defense system exert virulent, suppressive, or toxic effects on the various elements of the respiratory defense mechanism.

3.1 UPPER RESPIRATORY TRACT

3.1.1 Nostrils

3.1.1.1 Inflammation

Introduction. The structure is an important anatomic site to recognize clinical signs of respiratory infectious diseases externally, particularly viral diseases such as vesicular and erosive viruses and viruses with internal dissemination.

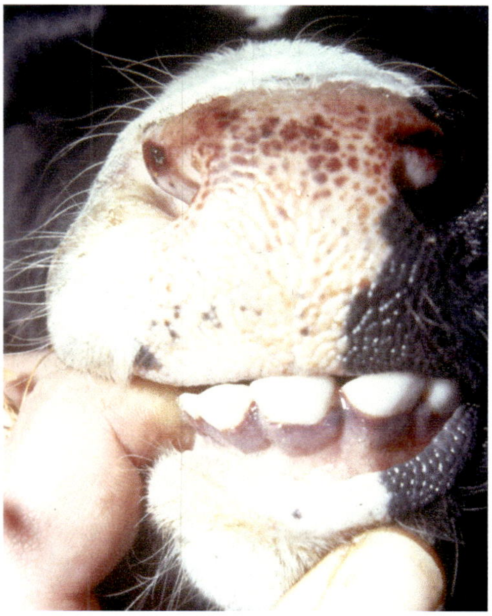

Fig. 3.1. Ox. Planum nasale. Infectious bovine rhinotracheitis (IBR; bovine herpesvirus type 1 (BHV-1)). Hemorrhagic, ulcerative dermatitis. The hairless skin is locally extensively red ('red nose'), an external indicator of IBR. (Courtesy of Dr R. Whitlock, University of Pennsylvania, USA.)

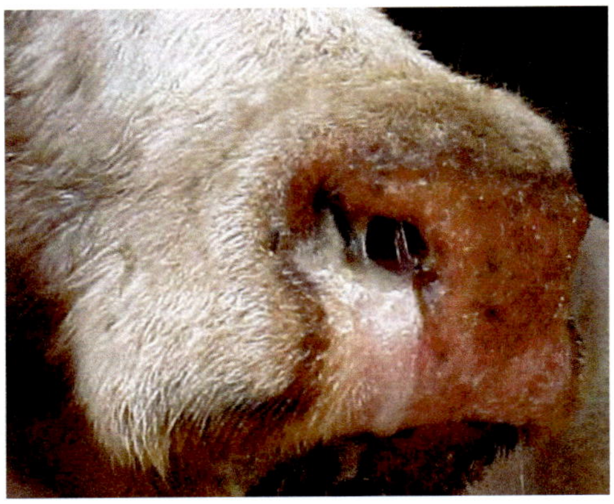

Fig. 3.2. Ox. Planum nasale. Malignant catarrhal fever (MCF), ovine herpesvirus-2 (OHV-2). Fibrinonecrotic, hemorrhagic dermatitis with catarrhal rhinitis. (Courtesy of Dr C. Barros, Universidade de Santa Maria, Brazil.)

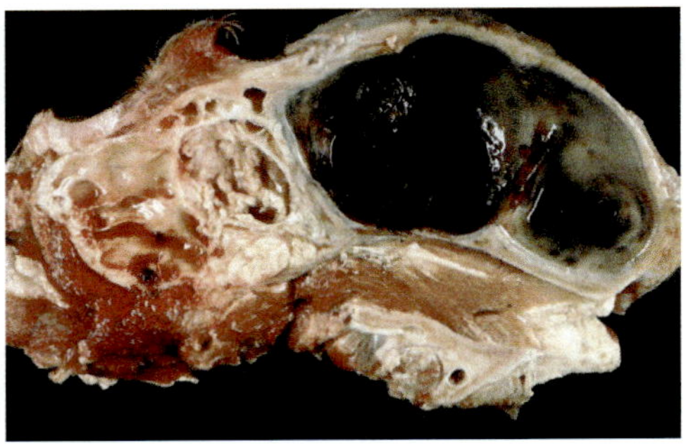

Fig. 3.4. Ox. Frontal sinus. Gangrenous sinusitis. A green discoloration suggests tissue putrefaction from gangrenous bacteria.

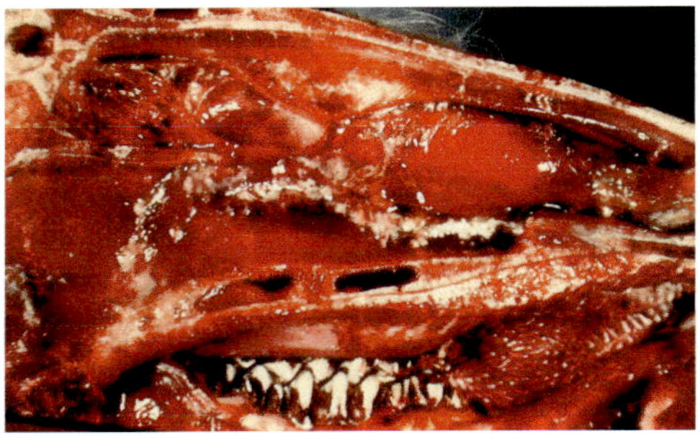

Fig. 3.5. Ox. Nasal septum. Diffuse hemorrhagic rhinitis. Turbinates and palatine sinus are covered by blood. The etiology ranges from epistaxis, congestion, blood disorders, to trauma and infection, such as infectious bovine rhinotracheitis (IBR).

3.1.2 Sinonasal compartment

3.1.2.1 Cysts

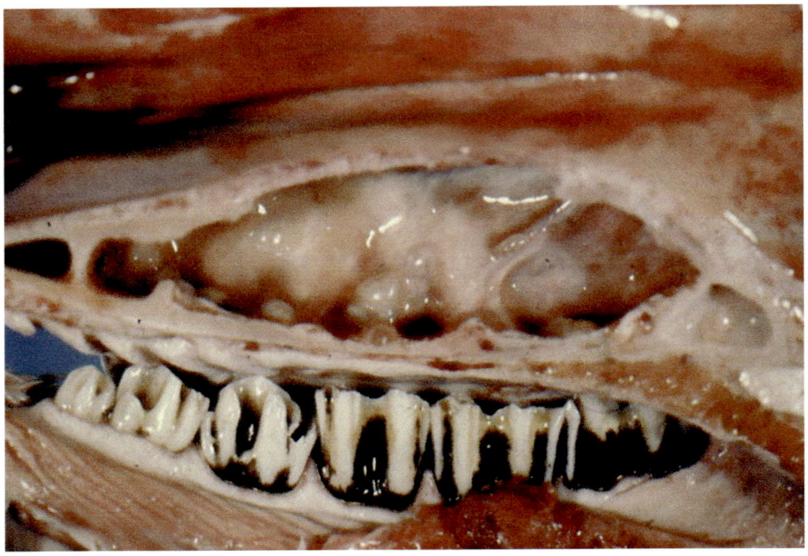

Fig. 3.3. Ox. Palatine sinus. Cysts. Multiple fluid-filled cysts protrude from the mucosal glands. These cysts can also develop within the frontal sinuses.

3.1.2.2 Inflammation

Introduction. Inflammation affects multiple structures of the nasal passages, including frontal sinuses. A mucinous to purulent exudate of mainly bacterial etiology accumulates.

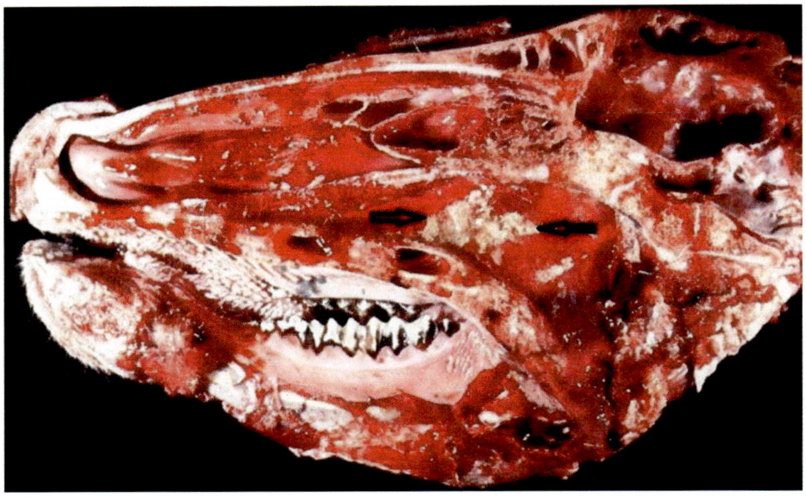

Fig. 3.6. Ox. Nasal septum. Infectious bovine rhinotracheitis (IBR). Fibrinonecrotic rhinitis. The mucosa of the nasal septum is diffusely red. The palatine sinus is partially covered by yellow fibrin (arrows). (Courtesy of Dr J.M. King and Section of Anatomic Pathology, Cornell University, USA.)

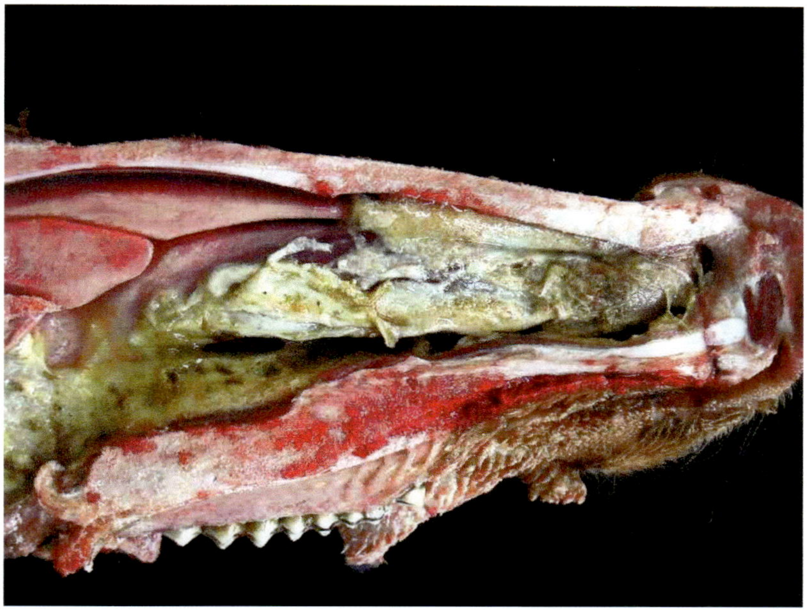

Fig. 3.7. Ox. Nasal septum. Malignant catarrhal fever (MCF). Fibrinonecrotic rhinitis and aspiration. The nasal passages are covered by a dense sheath of fibrin intermixed with digesta.

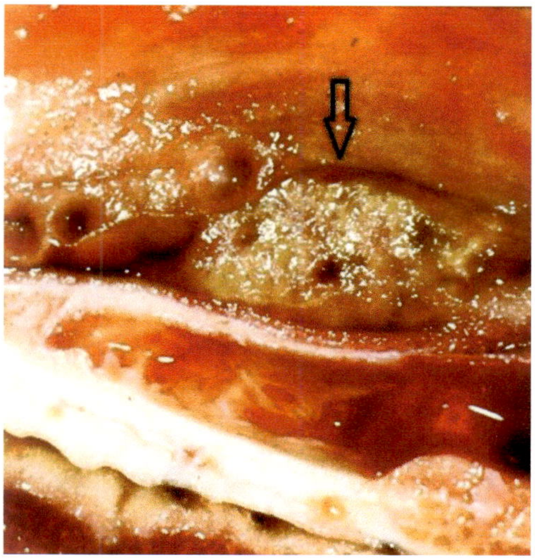

Fig. 3.8. Ox. Nose. Focal granulomatous rhinitis. A bronze focal growth (arrow) is the result of bovine eosinophilic nasal granuloma formation. Its etiology ranges from immediate type of hypersensitivity (bovine atopic rhinitis) to environmental allergens and to various bacteria and fungi. Nasal neoplasia should be considered as a differential diagnosis.

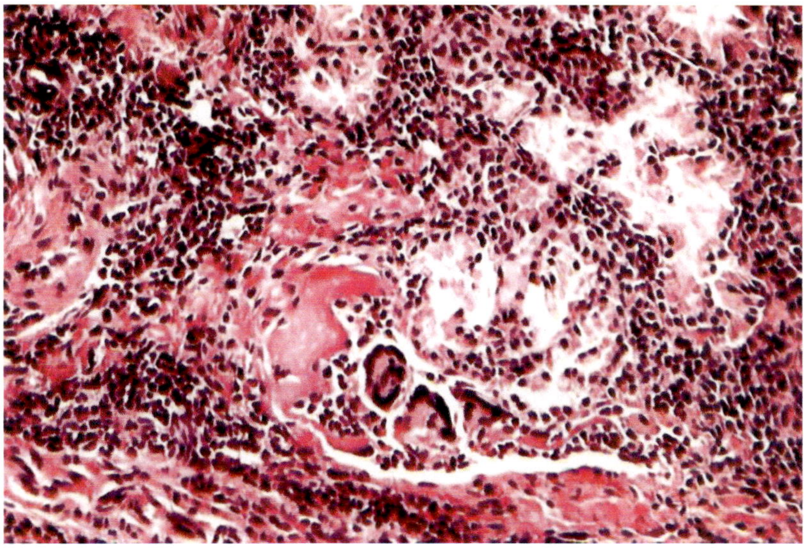

Fig. 3.9. Ox. Nasal granuloma. Granulomatous rhinitis. Microscopically, there are macrophages, lymphocytes and multinucleated imflammatory giant cells. Splendore–Hoeppli material and the deposition of acellular eosinophilic material suggestive of amyloid can also be encountered (H&E).

3.1.2.3 *Neoplasia*

Primary nasal neoplasia is rare in cattle. Squamous cell tumors have been encountered in older cows.

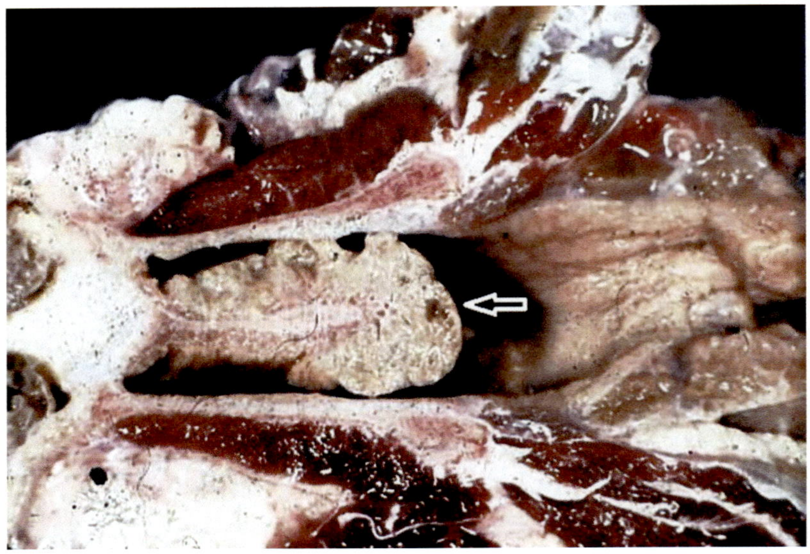

Fig. 3.10. Ox. Nose. Nasal carcinoma. A cauliflower, solid growth is expanding within the nasal cavity (arrow). Endemic carcinoma-sarcomas originating from the cribriform plate have been described in the literature.

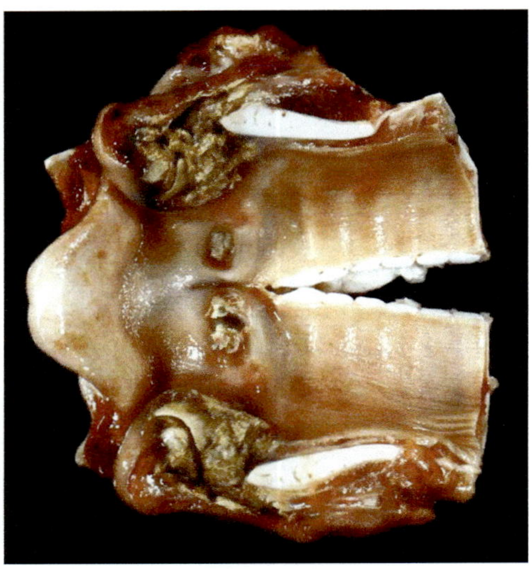

Fig. 3.11. Ox. Larynx. Ulcerative, necrotizing laryngo-tracheitis. The larynx and foci of cranial tracheal tissue are covered by necrotic material. Differential diagnoses and agents should include IBR, MCF, *Fusobacterium necrophorum* and fungi.

3.1.3 Larynx

3.1.3.1 *Inflammation*

Inflammation of the larynx is usually the result of viral (IBR, MCF) or bacterial invasion. In feedlots, many of these cases will develop aspiration pneumonia.

3.2 LOWER RESPIRATORY TRACT

3.2.1 Trachea

Introduction. The trachea remains relatively unaffected by disease processes. It is the target organ for infectious bovine rhinotracheitis, however, with its key lesion of fibrinonecrotic inflammation. Regurgitation and aspiration may resemble IBR-induced tracheitis.

3.2.1.1 *Inflammation*

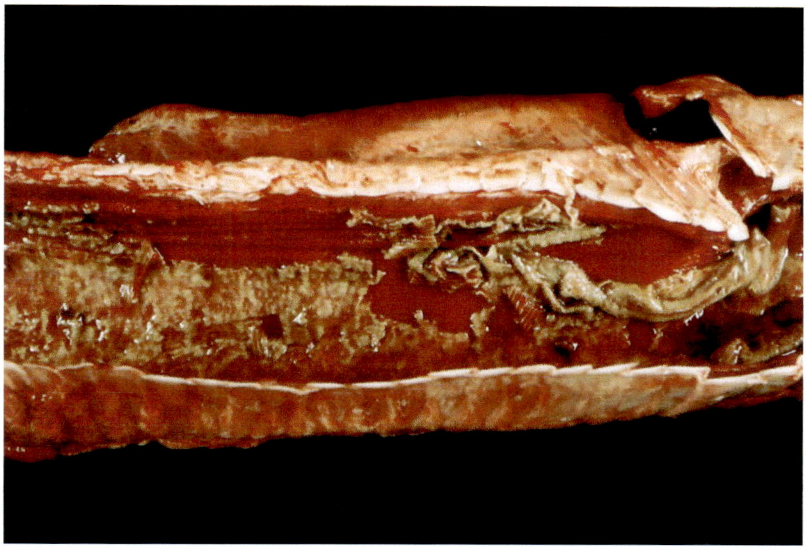

Fig. 3.12. Ox. Trachea. Infectious bovine rhinotracheitis (IBR). Necrotizing, fibrinous, hemorrhagic tracheitis. Sheaths of fibrin cover a denuded red tracheal surface. Being the principal target organ in the upper respiratory tract for bovine herpesvirus type 1 (BHV-1) infection, multiple other organs are involved in infection with this virus.

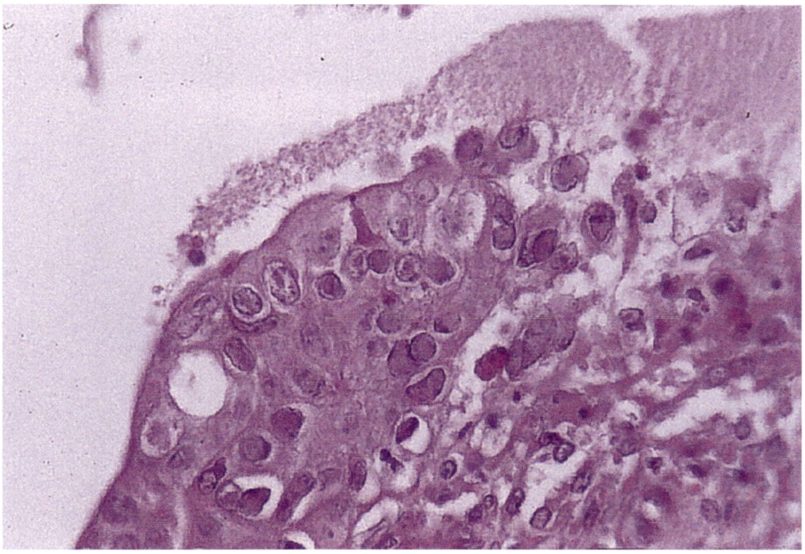

Fig. 3.13. Ox. Trachea. Infectious bovine rhinotracheitis (IBR). Fibrinous tracheitis. There is microscopic evidence of multiple intranuclear herpesvirus inclusions in respiratory epithelial cells. These are best seen at the junction between necrotic and intact epithelium. Fibrin covers the respiratory epithelial layer (H&E).

Fact Sheet: Infectious Bovine Rhinotracheitis (IBR)

Definition
- Infectious multi-organ viral disease caused by bovine herpesvirus 1 (BHV-1)

Virus subtypes

BHV-1.1	Respiratory subtype
BHV-1.2	Genital subtype
BHV-1.3 (BHV-5)	Encephalitic subtype

Organs involved
- Conjunctiva
- Nostrils
- Nose
- Larynx
- Trachea
- Lung
- Mouth
- Esophagus
- Rumen
- Brain
- Placenta
- Fetus
- Adrenal glands
- Abomasum

Specific gross findings in respiratory form
- White mucosal plaques on nasal septum, tongue, conjunctiva
- Fibrinonecrotic tracheitis, laryngitis, rhinitis

Clinical signs
- Hyperthermia
- Anorexia
- Hyperventilation
- Nasal discharge

Complications
- Secondary bacterial bronchopneumonia
- Abortions

Differential diagnoses
- BVD
- MCF
- BT

3.2.1.2 Honker's syndrome

Introduction. Occurs in cattle nearing market weight, and no predisposing causes are known. No associated significant lung pathology.

Clinical signs. Acute onset of respiratory distress with stertorous respiration or sudden death in respiratory distress.

Differential diagnosis. Inhaled clotted blood from bleeding in neighboring organs, smoke inhalation.

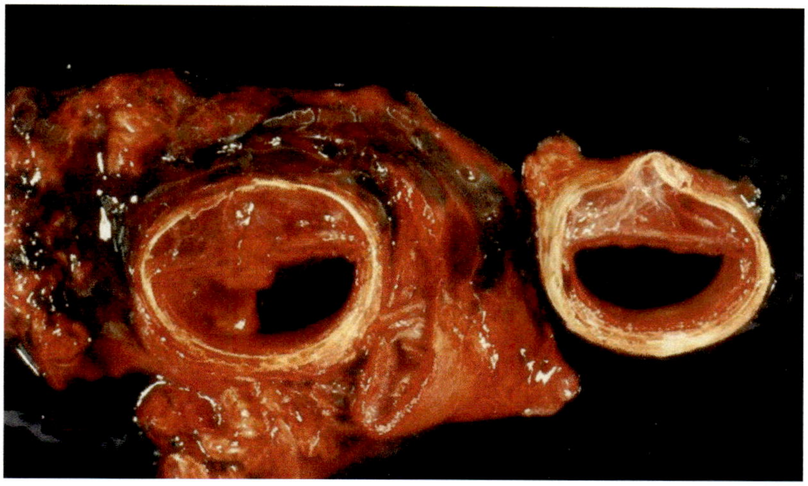

Fig. 3.14. Ox. Trachea. Honker's syndrome. Submucosal hemorrhage and edema. The tracheal lumen is significantly occluded by clotted blood being partially organized. Peritracheal tissue is edematous and hemorrhagic. Some cases have an inflammatory component, and squamous cell metaplasia of the tracheal epithelium is occasionally seen with undetermined cause.

3.2.2 Lung

The lung is the largest organ of the chest. Anatomically, especially in cattle, the lung is arranged in compartments, meaning that different pathologic processes are ongoing in adjacent lobes and lobules. Physiologically, the bovine lung has a limited cardiovascular reserve, making cattle highly susceptible to infectious respiratory disease. The lung's main function is gas exchange. For this, it depends on continuous ventilation and large intact surface areas. When the lung's defense mechanism breaks down, disease develops to invoke inflammation.

Many lung infections are due to aspiration from laryngitis or pharyngitis.

The lungs of feedlot cattle are especially susceptible to infectious processes. When cattle from different farms are housed together with different histories of vaccination and exposure to many new infectious agents, and arriving under severe stress, it is not surprising that respiratory diseases are so common.

At the gross level, pattern recognition and distribution of inflammation helps to categorize types of pathologic changes and etiologies (see the diagram on pneumonia pattern recognition). An important aspect for the diagnosis of lung disorders, in addition to visualization, is systematic palpation of lung parenchyma. If the lung does not feel firm, pneumonia can usually be excluded from the diagnosis. It should be emphasized that the collection of sterile samples for microbial culture and viral isolation is a prerequisite before palpation. Suspicious sites should be collected for ancillary tests and for histologic examination. Serial sectioning of the lung parenchyma should be attempted and larger airways and major vessels should be opened.

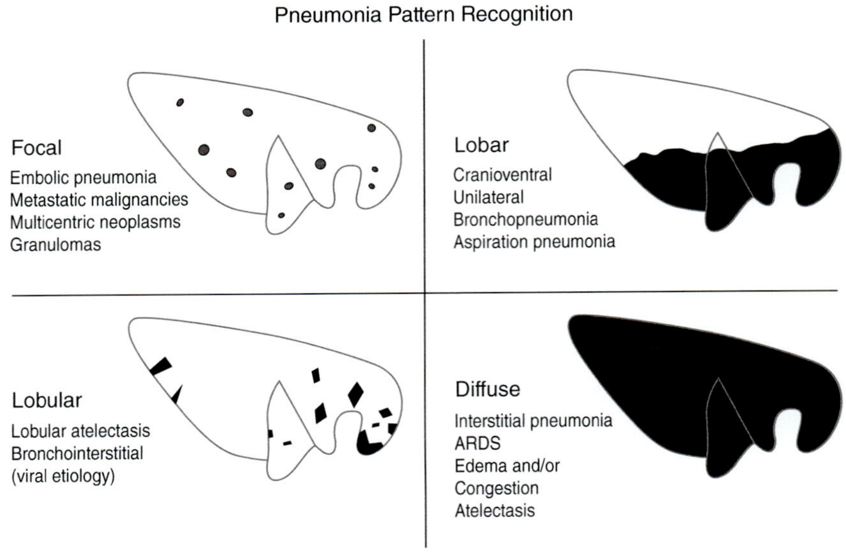

3.2.2.1 *Inflammation*

Introduction. Bovine respiratory disease (BRD) is a complex condition inflicting heavy economic losses to the cattle industry. The colonization of the lung by bacterial and/or viral and parasitic pathogens often invokes a severe inflammatory response, resulting in significant pulmonary damage. Much attention has been paid to the viral–bacterial synergism in BRD. Preceding viral infection causing bronchiolitis inhibits the pulmonary defense mechanisms, with bacteria taking advantage through colonization. Lack of regular deworming creates a condition of multiple lungworm cases in a herd. The role of fungi in bovine pulmonary disease is of lesser economic significance as only individual animals are affected.

The main pathogens contributing to bovine shipping fever pneumonia are *Mannheimia haemolytica*, *Histophilus somni* and/or *Pasteurella multocida*.

VIRUSES

Infectious bovine rhinotracheitis (IBR)

Introduction. Caused by bovine herpesvirus 1 (BHV-1), the virus infects multiple organs. The virus has its reservoir for latency in the trigeminal ganglion. It is largely controlled by vaccination. None the less, IBR abortions still occur in the field.

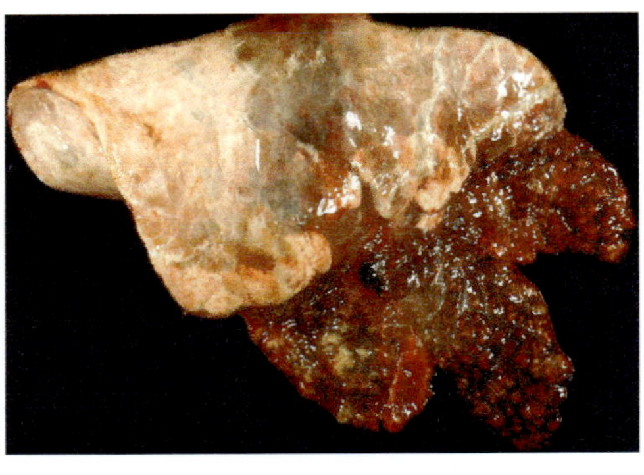

Fig. 3.15. Ox. Infectious bovine rhinotracheitis (IBR). Bronchiolitis and bronchiectasis. The cranial lung lobe is afflicted and exhibits multiple gray-yellow nodules in indurated lobules. These are markedly distended bronchioles filled with purulent exudate. The dorsal aspects of the diaphragmatic lobe has an area of brown consolidation. This is a very chronic case with secondary bacterial infection resulting in bronchiectasis.

Differential diagnosis. Cranioventral bronchopneumonia with pulmonary abscesses.

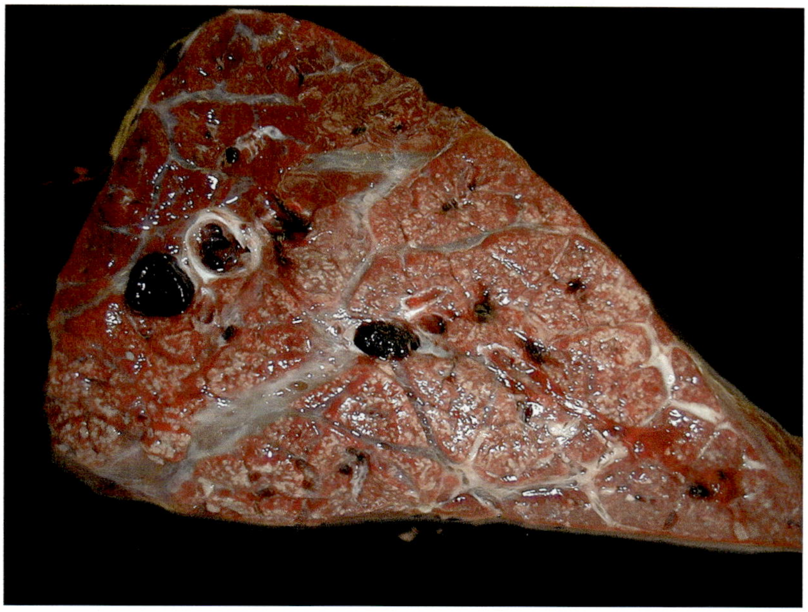

Fig. 3.16. Ox. Infectious bovine rhinotracheitis (IBR). Necrotizing bronchiolitis. On cut section, the lung is characterized by multiple gray, partially bulging foci. There is evidence of marked interstitial edema and emphysema.

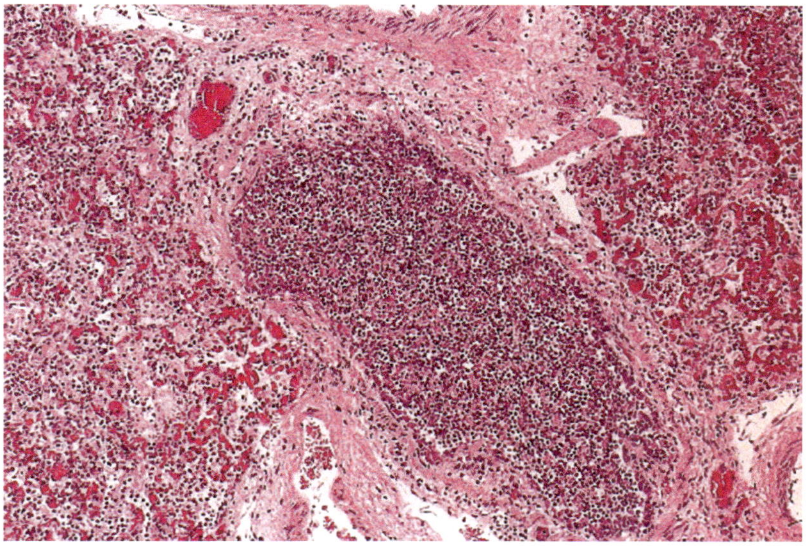

Fig. 3.17. Ox. Lung. Infectious bovine rhinotracheitis (IBR). Necrotizing, purulent bronchitis. The epithelial lining is mostly effaced, and the lumen of the bronchiole is markedly filled with mixed inflammatory cells and fibrin. The adjacent alveoli are distended by fibrin and by a moderate inflammatory infiltrate, all of these being indicators of a secondary bacterial colonization. Interstitial capillaries are congested (H&E).

Bovine respiratory syncytial virus (BRSV)

Introduction. This pneumovirus within the paramyxovirus family is endemic in cow-calf operations. It is a cause of enzootic pneumonia in dairy calves. It causes fatal bronchointerstitial pneumonia in feedlot cattle. The virus causes bronchial epithelial cell necrosis and interferes with pulmonary alveolar macrophage function. In some herds, exposure to the virus exceeds 50%. It predisposes to bacterial bronchopneumonia.

The disease in some herds may occur in two phases or scenarios. Phase I inflicts a syncytial cell bronchiolitis, and most animals recover. Phase II often occurs up to 1 month later, and animals die suddenly or after a few hours of severe respiratory distress. This stage is also known as reinfection syndrome, but only an occasional isolated case appears, for reasons not understood. The affected lungs grossly look like atypical interstitial pneumonia (AIP), not implying that all cases of AIP should be considered to be caused by BRSV. Some are, if specifically sampled and studied.

Clinical signs. Hyperthermia, dyspnea, cough, salivation, nasal discharge, milk reduction, subcutaneous emphysema. Sudden death in phase II cases is a most common outcome.

Differential diagnoses. Atypical interstitial pneumonia (AIP), bacterial bronchopneumonia.

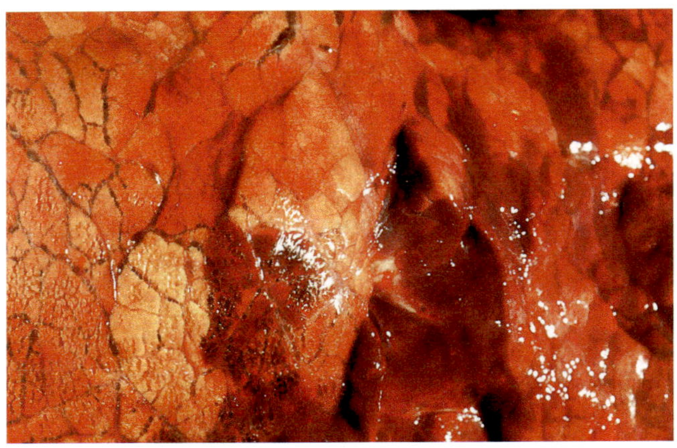

Fig. 3.18. Ox. Lung. Bovine respiratory syncytial virus (BRSV). Cranioventral bronchopneumonia. Phase I. There is evidence of moderate brown consolidation with a lobular pattern.

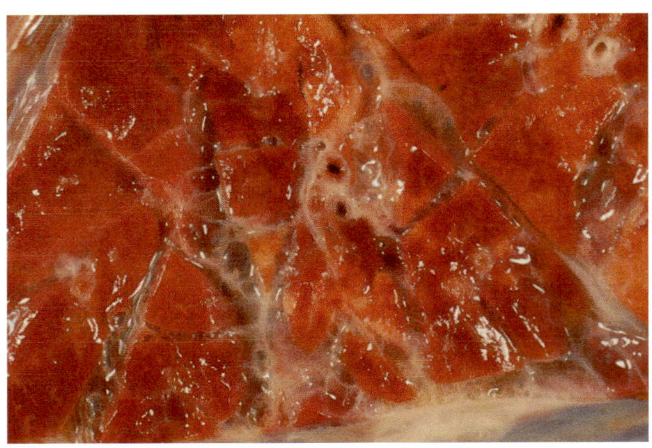

Fig. 3.19. Ox. Lung. Bovine respiratory syncytial virus (BRSV). Interlobular edema and emphysema. In addition to lobular consolidation, marked distension of the interlobular interstitium by edematous fluid and air pockets is present.

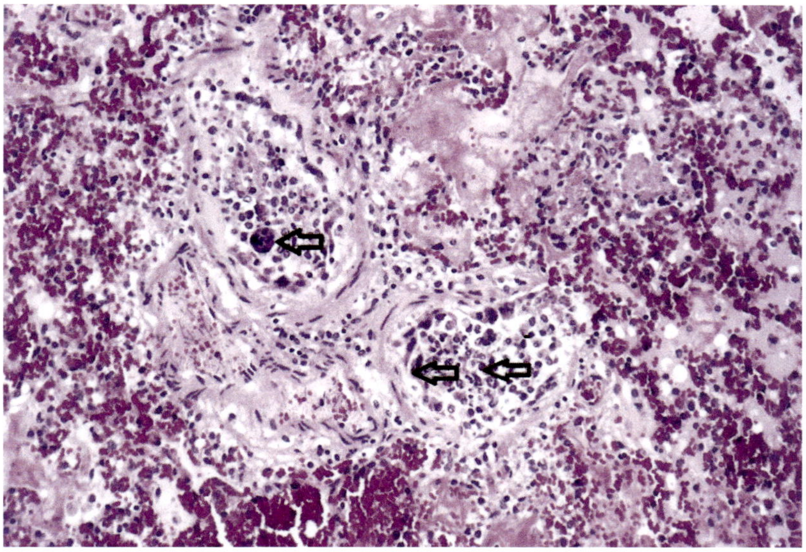

Fig. 3.20. Ox. Lung. Bovine respiratory syncytial virus (BRSV). Necrotizing bronchiolitis with intralesional syncytial cells. The bronchial epithelial cells exhibit necrosis. The lumen of the bronchioles is filled with mixed inflammatory cells and several syncytial cells (arrows). Adjacent alveoli contain fibrin, red blood cells, and moderate amounts of inflammatory cells (H&E).

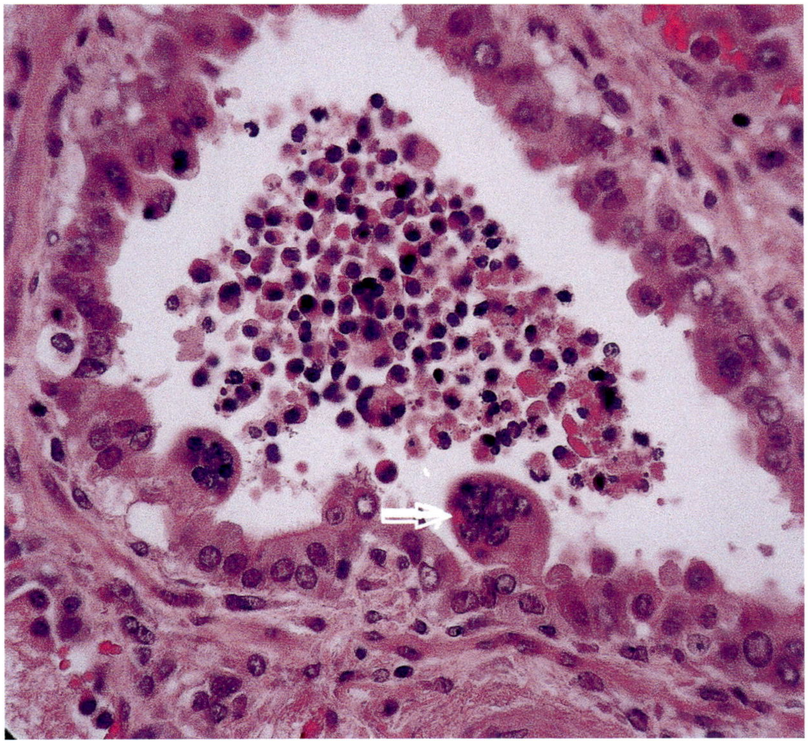

Fig. 3.21. Ox. Lung. Bovine respiratory syncytial virus (BRSV). Bronchiole. Formation of syncytial cells. Multinucleated cells form from the lining epithelial cells (arrow) (H&E).

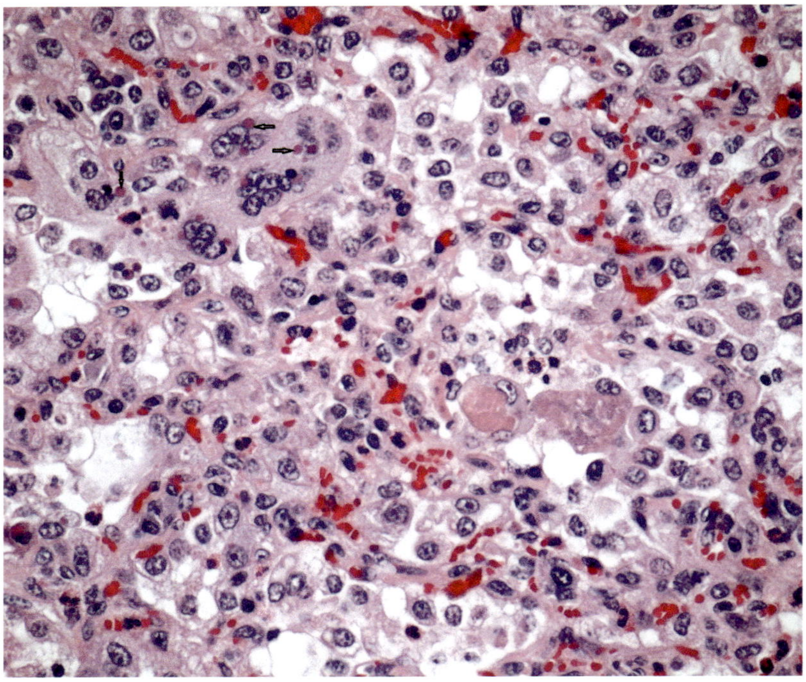

Fig. 3.22. Ox. Lung. Bovine respiratory syncytial virus (BRSV). Interstitial-type pneumonia with eosinophilic cytoplasmic inclusions. Some syncytial cells contain eosinophilic intracytoplasmic inclusions, exhibiting the size of a red blood cell (arrows) (H&E).

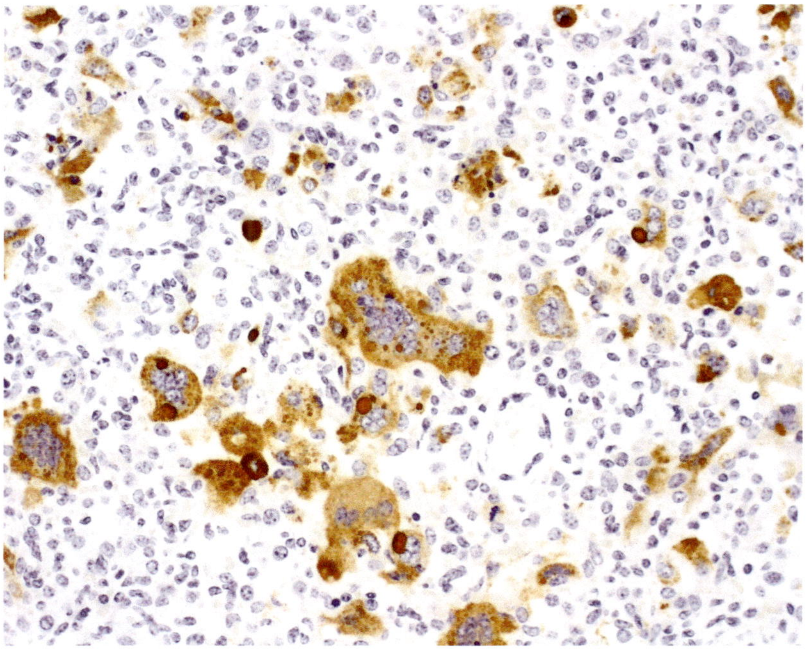

Fig. 3.23. Ox. Lung. Bovine respiratory syncytial virus (BRSV). Localization of viral antigen. As viral replication takes place in the respiratory epithelium and in syncytial cells, viral antigen can be demonstrated in the cytoplasm of these cells. The image depicts a heavy diffuse distribution of viral antigen in the cytoplasm of syncytial cells (IHC).

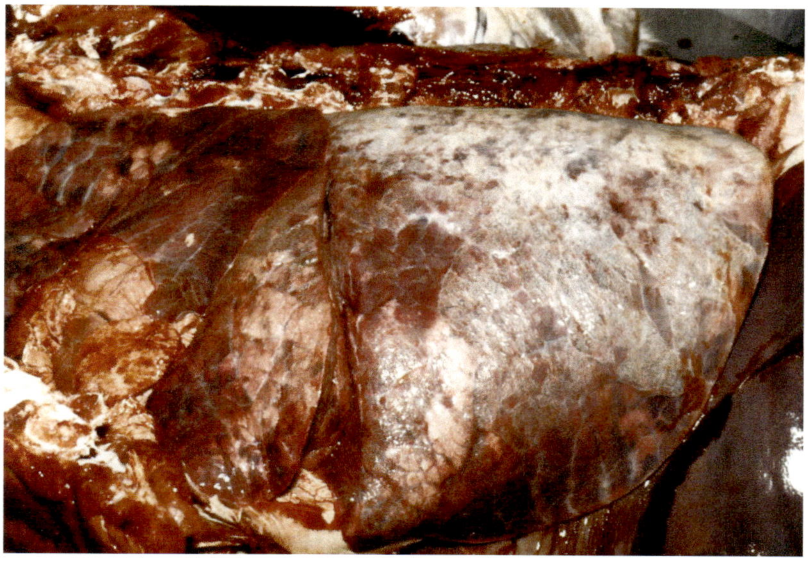

Fig. 3.24. Ox. Lung. Bovine respiratory syncytial virus (BRSV). Diffuse bronchointerstitial pneumonia. Phase II. The lung is poorly collapsed, with consolidation affecting all lobes. Phase II lesions are grossly essentially the same as interstitial pneumonia of feedlot cattle. Affected lung feels firm on palpation. For the specific diagnosis of BRSV infection, it is crucial that sections for histology are taken from the cranial portions of the lung to look for syncytial cells, inclusion bodies, and viral antigen by IHC or other diagnostic techniques.

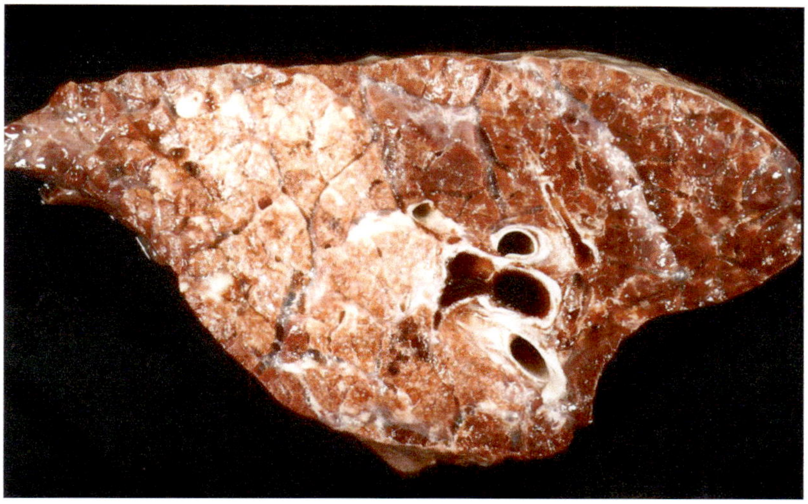

Fig. 3.25. Ox. Lung. Bovine respiratory syncytial virus (BRSV). Diffuse interstitial pneumonia. On cut section, mottling of meaty lobules is apparent. There is evidence of variable edema and emphysema. Such lung has little airspace left for aeration and is responsible for the clinical signs of respiratory distress.

Bovine viral diarrhea virus (BVDV). Though primarily targeting the gastrointestinal tract, this pestivirus plays a significant predisposing role in the development of BRD through its immunosuppressive effect on pulmonary defense mechanisms. Persistently BVDV infected animals (PI) are much more prone to develop serious BRD than uninfected animals. Immunosuppression also occurs in transient infections.

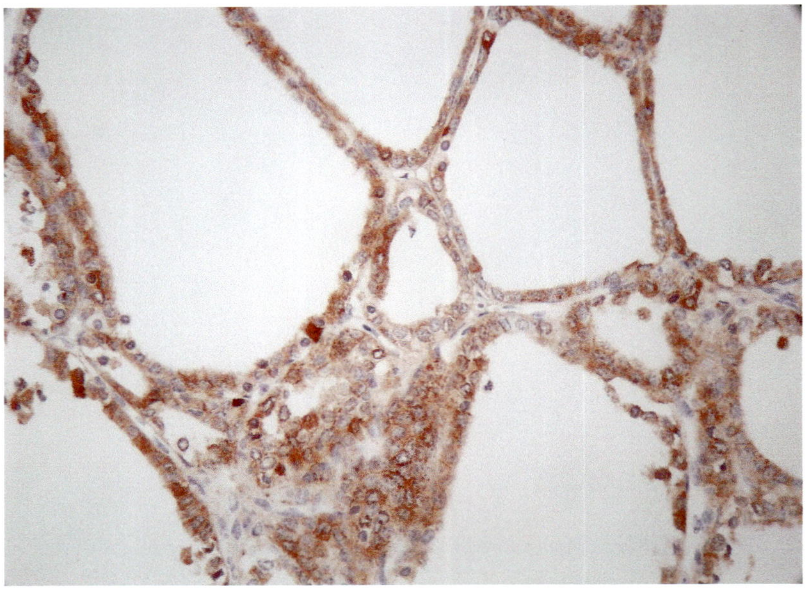

Fig. 3.26. Ox. Lung. Bovine viral diarrhea virus (BVDV). Evidence of a large amount of BVDV antigen location in the cytoplasm of alveolar cells, typically encountered in persistently infected animals (IHC).

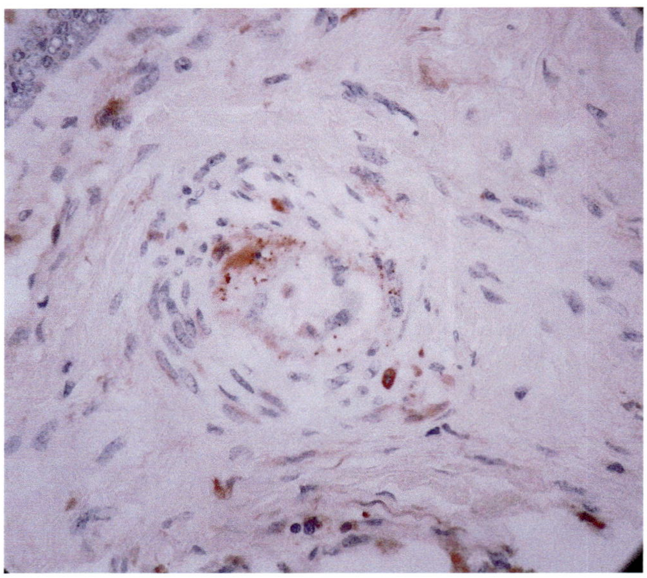

Fig. 3.27. Ox. Lung. Bovine viral diarrhea virus (BVDV). Pulmonary artery. Evidence of BVD viral antigen location in the cytoplasm and nucleus of monocytes. This feature is more typical of transiently infected animals, as is IHC positive staining in the walls of myocardial vessels (IHC).

Other viruses contributing to the BRD complex are bovine parainfluenza-3 virus (PI-3), and bovine respiratory coronavirus (BRCV). These viral diseases are covered in Chapter 1: Diseases of Neonates and Calves.

BACTERIA

Mannheimia haemolytica

Introduction. *Mannheimia haemolytica* is a gram-negative bacterium, residing in the nasopharynx and tonsils, and an important primary pathogen for lung disease, especially in feedlot cattle. There are 12 serotypes. Virulent strains of *M. haemolytica* are responsible for the severe pathologic changes induced in the lung. The major virulent constituent of the bacterium is leukotoxin, an exotoxin, produced by the capsule, inhibiting phagocytosis by alveolar macrophages, causing lysis of neutrophils and generating cytokine production. Other virulence factors are endotoxin, causing vascular injury, lipopolysaccharide, and iron-binding proteins. Stress (transport, crowding) is a primary risk factor for *M. haemolytica* infection ('shipping fever').

Clinical signs. Fever, cough, nasal discharge, increased respiration, decreased milk production.

Differential diagnoses. *Mycoplasma bovis*, *H. somni*, *Trueperella pyogenes*, *Bibersteinia trehalosi*, BRSV infection, contagious bovine pleuropneumonia (CBPP).

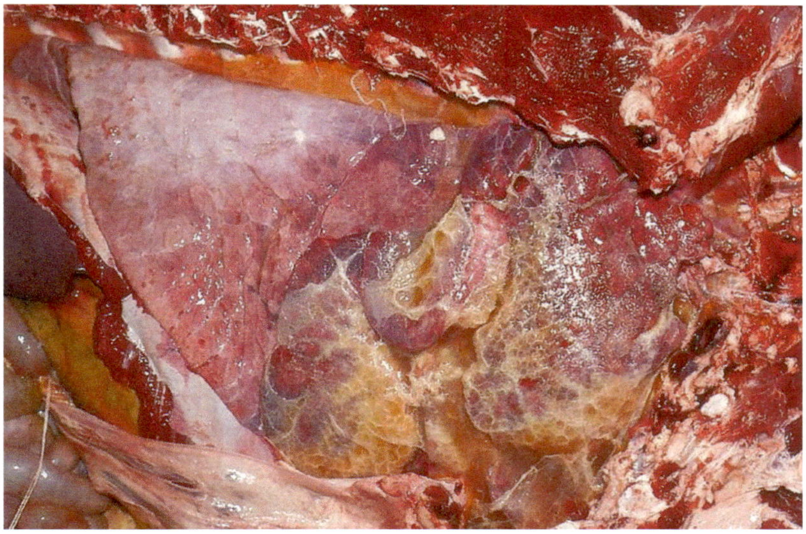

Fig. 3.28. Ox. Lung. *Mannheimia haemolytica*. Fibrinous cranioventral bronchopneumonia with fibrinous pleuritis. Multiple lobes of the cranioventral lung are consolidated. The pleura is covered by tan, yellow fibrin. The condition occurs bilaterally. Pleural adhesions are common.

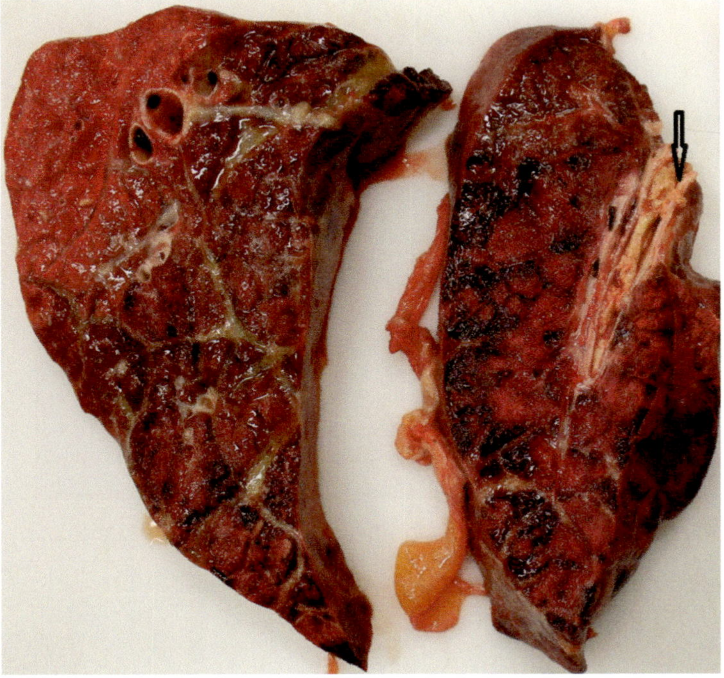

Fig. 3.29. Ox. Lung. *Mannheimia haemolytica*. Hemorrhagic, necrotizing bronchopneumonia. On cut section, red foci of lobular hemorrhage and necrosis are present. The interstitium is widened and filled with fibrin. Note the fibrin in large airways (arrow).

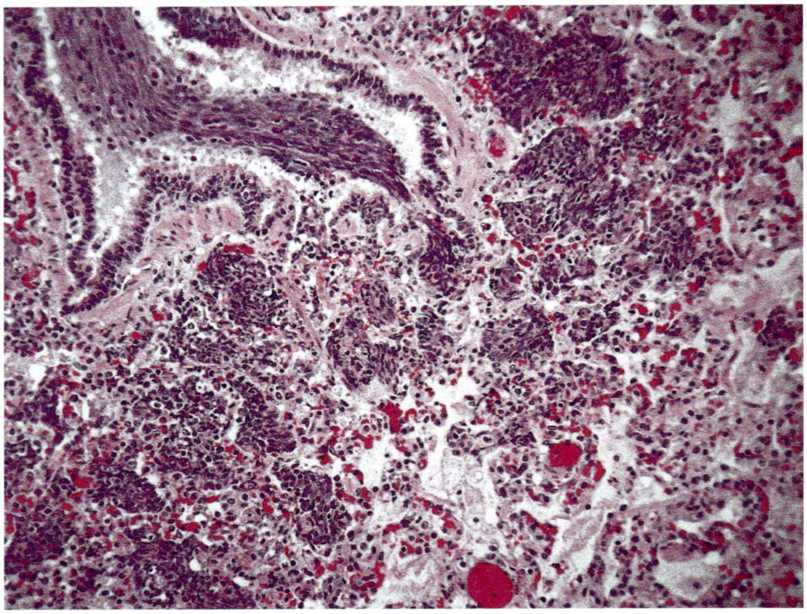

Fig. 3.30. Ox. Lung. *Mannheimia haemolytica*. Suppurative bronchopneumonia. Bronchiole and adjacent alveoli are densely filled with necrotic neutrophils and some mononuclear cells. Inflammatory cells in bronchiole have a streaming appearance of basophilic chromatin ('oat cells') (H&E).

Pasteurella multocida

Introduction. The bacterium infects both calves and adult dairy cows opportunistically as a frequent pathogen in BRD. A normal inhabitant of the upper respiratory system, when reaching the lung, it depresses the antibacterial defense mechanism. The bacterium produces vascular injury by toxin generation, resulting in fibrin exudation and lymphatic thrombosis.

Clinical signs. Increased respiration, cough, and fever.

Differential diagnoses. Primary bacterial and viral bronchopneumonia.

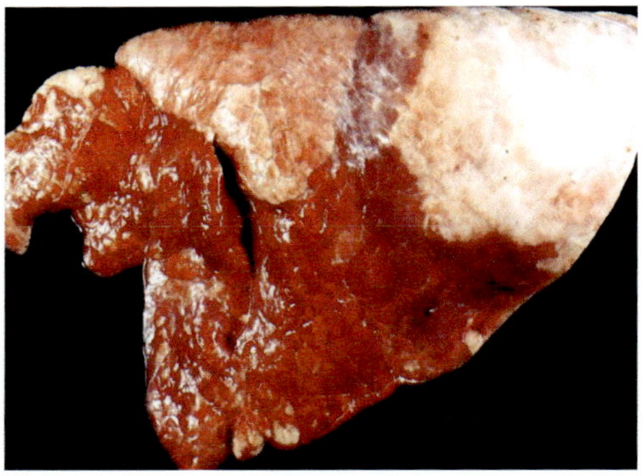

Fig. 3.31. Ox. Lung. *Pasteurella multocida*. Cranioventral bronchopneumonia. Brown lobar consolidation is apparent. The visceral pleura is not affected in this case. Fibrinous pleuritis, however, may occur. Bronchiectasis and microabscesses may be additional findings. Gross changes tend to be bilateral.

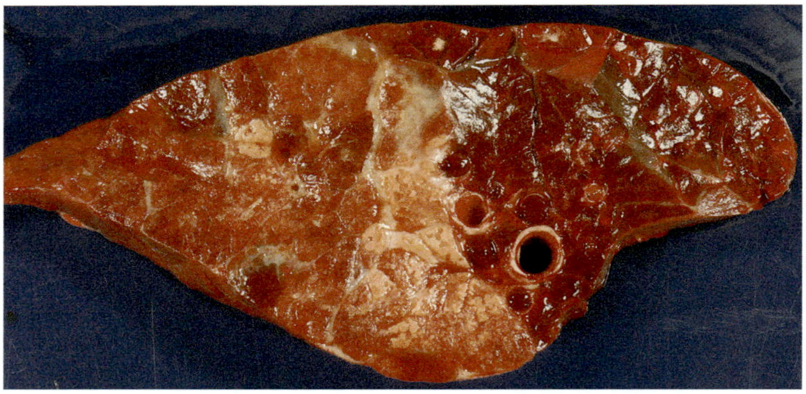

Fig. 3.32. Ox. Lung. *Pasteurella multocida*. On cut section, various stages of inflammation are characterized by a marbling pattern.

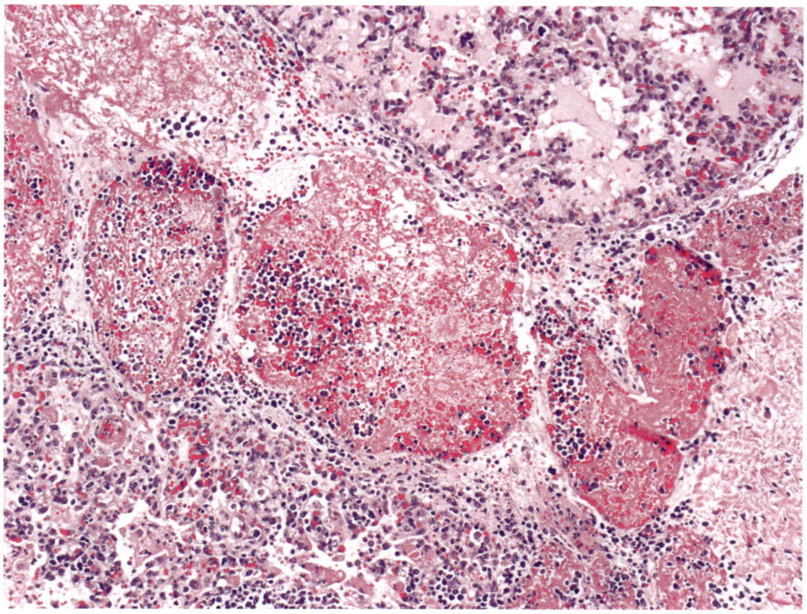

Fig. 3.33. Ox. Lung. *Pasteurella multocida*. Fibrinosuppurative bronchopneumonia. Microscopic lesions consist of severe alveolar fibrinous exudation and neutrophilic inflammation, with edematous widening of the interstitium and fibrin thrombi in interstitial lymphatics. Differential etiology. *Histophilus somni* (H&E).

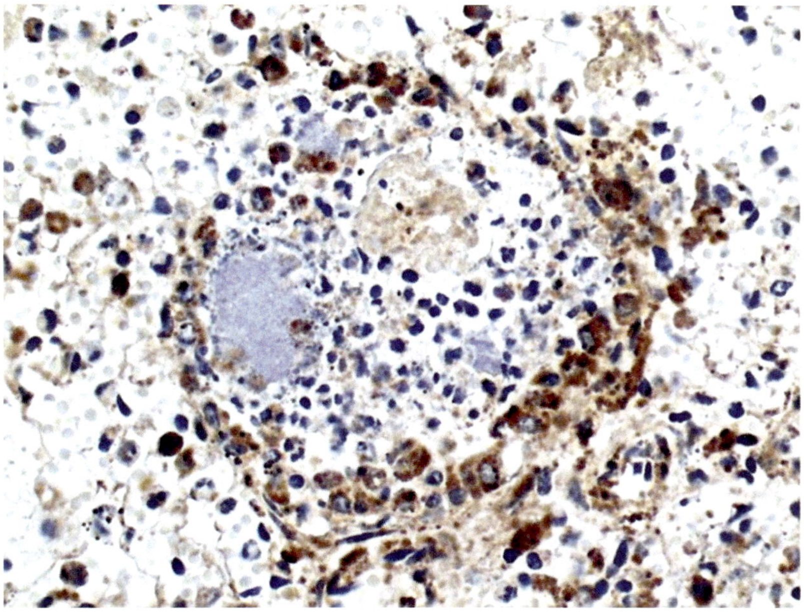

Fig. 3.34. Ox. Lung. *Pasteurella multocida* pneumonia. Bovine viral diarrhea virus (BVDV) viral synergism. BVDV viral antigen is demonstrated in the cytoplasm of alveolar macrophages and of type 2 pneumocytes. BVDV infection is immunosuppressive, facilitating susceptibility to bovine respiratory disease (BRD) pathogens (IHC).

Histophilus somni

Introduction. The thermophilic, gram-negative bacterium is the most important pathogen in BRD of feedlot cattle. It causes severe bronchopneumonia or pleuritis. The bacterium is involved in surviving alveolar macrophage phagocytosis, apoptosis of endothelial cells, platelet aggregation and the production of chemotactic factors that act as inflammatory mediators.

Clinical signs. Increased respiration, cough, and purulent discharge, similar to previous pulmonary pathogens. Sudden death is common in cases of acute fibrinous pleuritis with pleural effusion.

Differential diagnoses. Mannheimiosis, pulmonary mycoplasmosis, contagious bovine pleuropneumonia.

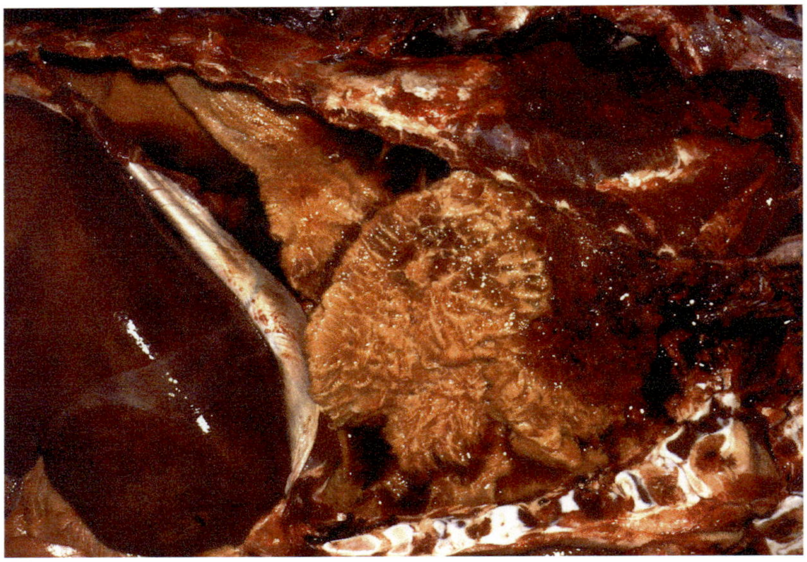

Fig. 3.35. Ox. Lung. *Histophilus somni*. Fibrinous pleuritis with pleural effusion. Tan fibrin covers the visceral pleura and visible parietal pleura. The entire lung is consolidated due to atelectasis from fibrin compression.

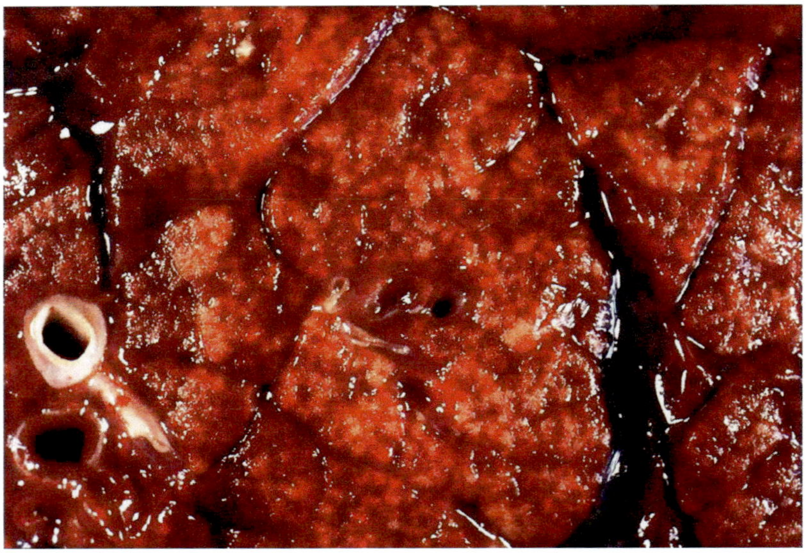

Fig. 3.36. Ox. Lung. *Histophilus somni*. Bronchopneumonia with microabscesses. On cut section, white protruding nodules imply airway involvement and are intermixed with brown areas of consolidation. The interstitium is wet, hemorrhagic, and widened.

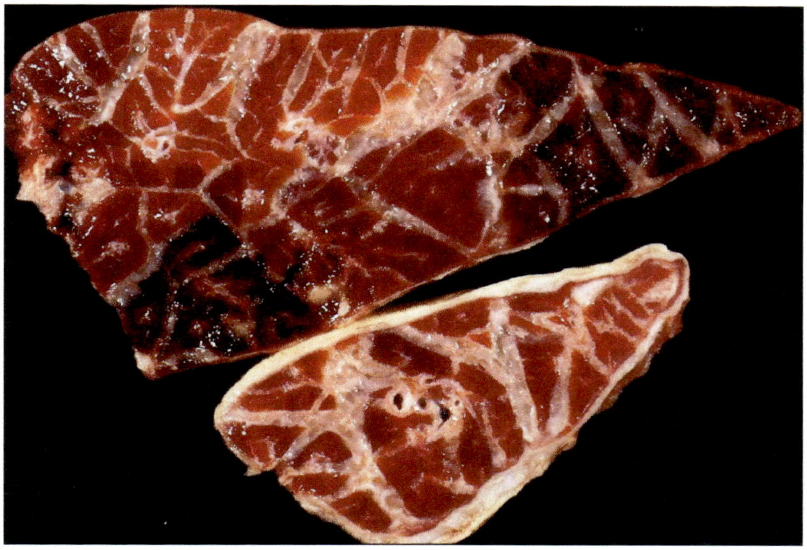

Fig. 3.37. Ox. Lung. *Histophilus somni*. Fibrinous pleuritis with extension of fibrin into interlobular spaces. Mottling on cut section suggests compression of alveolar parenchyma, causing atelectasis. Should not be misinterpreted as Mannheimiosis.

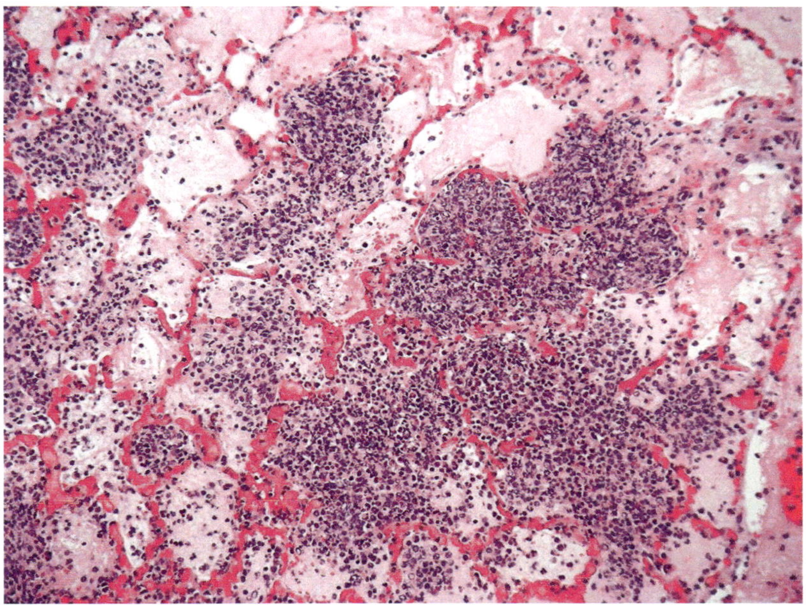

Fig. 3.38. Ox. Lung. *Histophilus somni*. Necrotizing, fibrinous, suppurative alveolitis. The alveolar septa are effaced, and alveoli are distended by the presence of neutrophils and fibrin. Alveolar capillaries are congested (H&E).

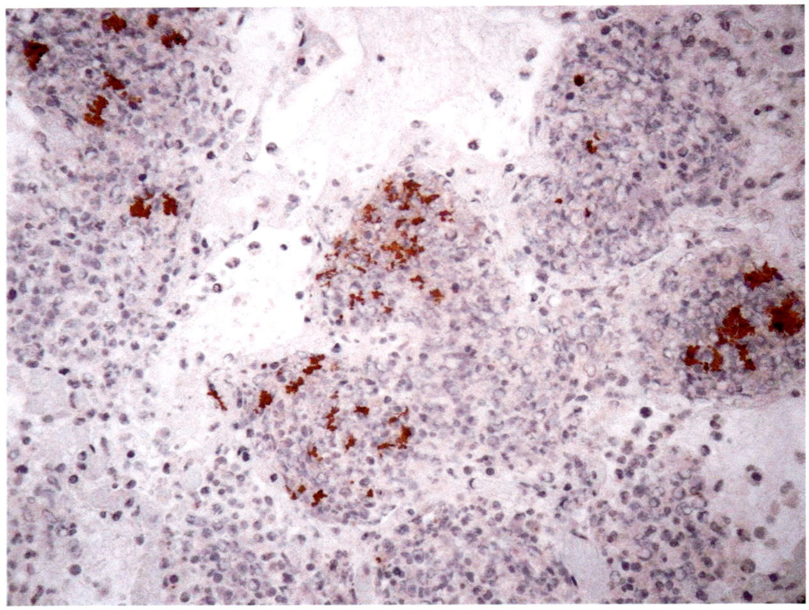

Fig. 3.39. Ox. Lung. *Histophilus somni*. The presence of aggregated colonies of *H. somni* are recognized within suppurative foci of inflammation (IHC).

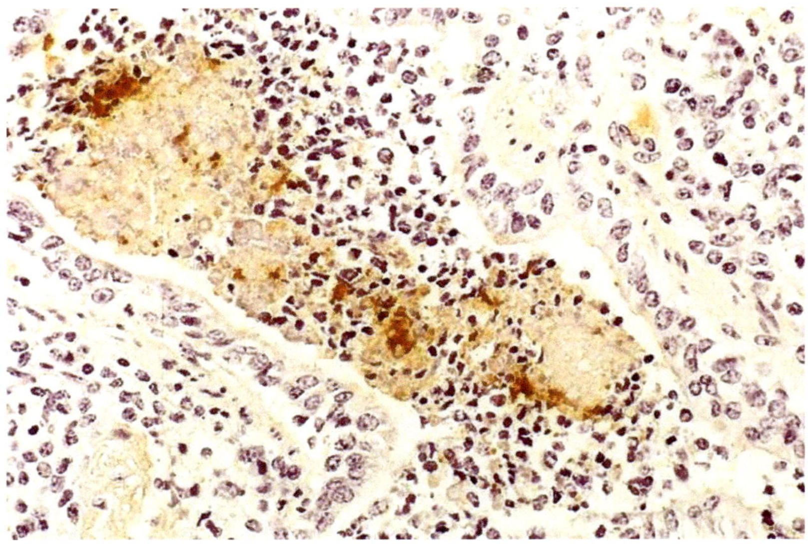

Fig. 3.40. Ox. Lung. *Histophilus somni*. Extracellular *H. somni* antigen aggregates are demonstrated in airway (IHC).

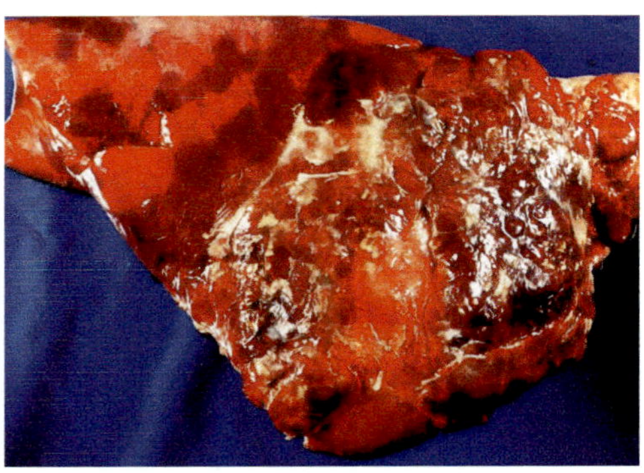

Fig. 3.41. Ox. Lung. *Trueperella pyogenes*. Fibrinous pleuritis and bronchopneumonia. Multifocal lobules exhibit consolidation. There is evidence of locally extensive, moderate fibrinosuppurative pleuritis. *Bibersteinia trehalosi* should be considered in the differential etiology.

Trueperella pyogenes

Introduction. This gram-positive, ubiquitous bacterium invades the lung of individual animals, both calves and adult cows. The organism is common on all mucous membranes. A break in mucous membranes is usually needed to allow invasion to occur. The most common scenario of infection is secondary lung invasion, when ulcerative or erosive laryngitis, tracheitis or pharyngitis are present. Infection can also be preceded by immunosuppression such as persistent or transient BVDV and bovine leukocyte adhesion deficiency (BLAD).

Mycoplasma bovis

Introduction. *Mycoplasma bovis* is a major pathogen in chronic BRD of feedlot cattle. In about 10% of the cases, concurrent single or multiple arthritis and tenosynovitis exist. This combination led to the introduction of the term: chronic pneumonia and polyarthritis syndrome (CPPS). In addition to pneumonia and arthritis, *M. bovis* also can induce mastitis in dairy cattle and otitis media in calves (see Chapter 1: Diseases of Calves and Neonates. Chapter 14: Diseases of the Udder and Teats, and Chapter 15: Diseases of Eye and Ear). The lung lesions in feedlot cattle are quite severe, with *M. bovis* starting to develop inflammation in bronchi and bronchioles and then to coalesce into large areas of yellow, caseous necrosis, with invasion and spread via interlobular lymphatics or direct extension into adjacent viable parenchyma. Concurrent fibrinous pleuritis is common. Mycoplasmosis accounts for joint problems and sometimes other organ involvement. Lung lesions can combine with other bacterial or viral infectious agents, especially *M. haemolytica*. When examined by indirect immunohistochemistry, transient BVDV infection is commonly found. As *M. bovis* is antibiotic resistant, extensive antibiotic therapy promotes *M. bovis* growth, enhancing the resulting pneumonia. *M. bovis* can be isolated from most feedlot lungs, thus cultures alone do not confirm the diagnosis of mycoplasmosis, nor does polymerase chain reaction (PCR). The test of choice is IHC of formalin-fixed tissue to associate the lesions with *M. bovis* antigens.

Other types of mycoplasma pathogens include *Mycoplasma dispar* and *Mycoplasma bovirhinus*.

Clinical signs. Cough, nasal discharge, lameness.

Differential diagnoses. Bacterial bronchopneumonia, mycobacterosis, and contagious bovine pleuropneumonia. The latter disease has been eradicated from North America but the gross lesions and clinical disease are very similar.

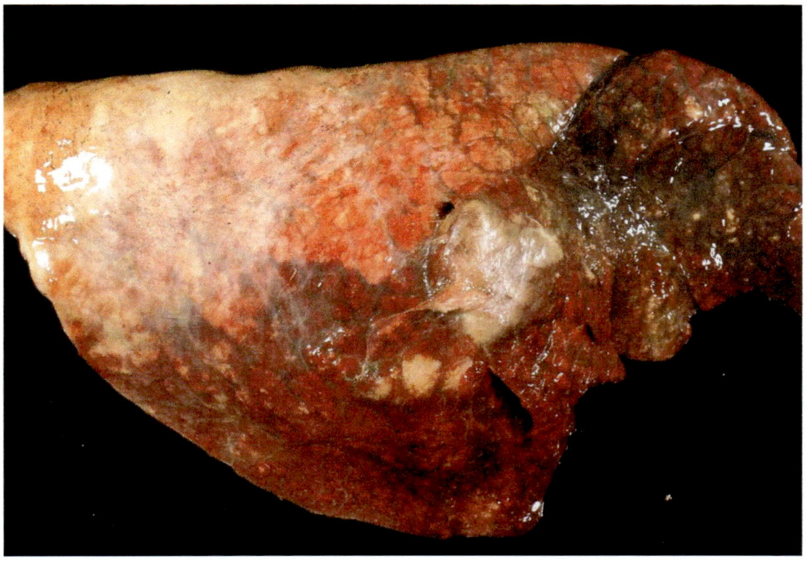

Fig. 3.42. Ox. Lung. *Mycoplasma bovis*. Cranioventral bronchopneumonia with foci of caseous necrosis. These are not true abscesses. There is evidence of extensive cranioventral distribution of pneumonia with scattered caseous to inspissated foci of necrosis of varying size. Typical lesions project above the pleural surface. Tuberculosis always has to be considered in the differential diagnosis when these gross lesions are seen.

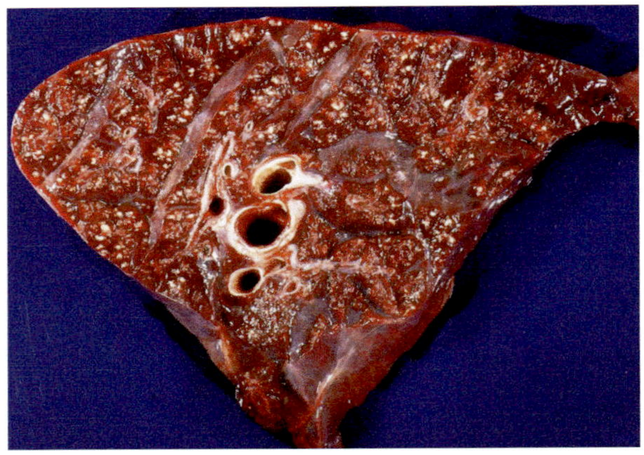

Fig. 3.43. Ox. Lung. *Mycoplasma bovis*. Caseous necrotizing bronchitis and/or bronchiolitis. Airways are filled and extended by caseous necrotic material, rendering a miliary pattern of inflammation to the lung parenchyma. This is an early case involving bronchiolar lumina only.

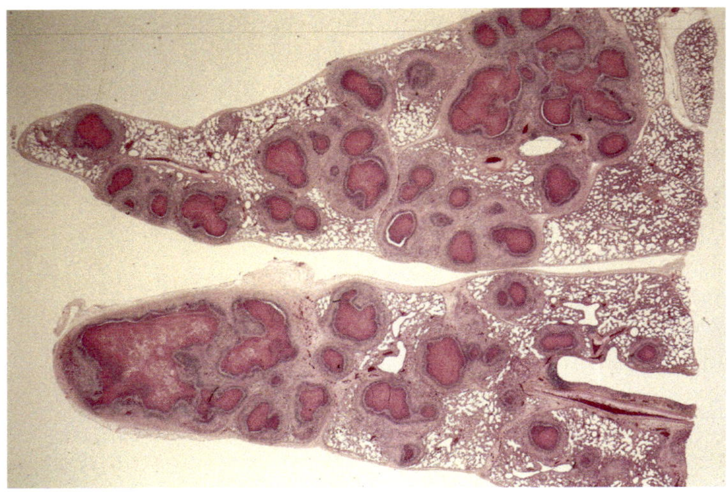

Fig. 3.44. Ox. Lung. *Mycoplasma bovis*. Bronchiectasis with peribronchiolitis. The eosinophilic center is the result of caseous necrosis with a pale blue ring reflecting inflammation in adjacent alveoli. Some of these foci are coalescing. Another microscopic feature of *M. bovis* infection is peribronchiolar lymphoid aggregation (H&E).

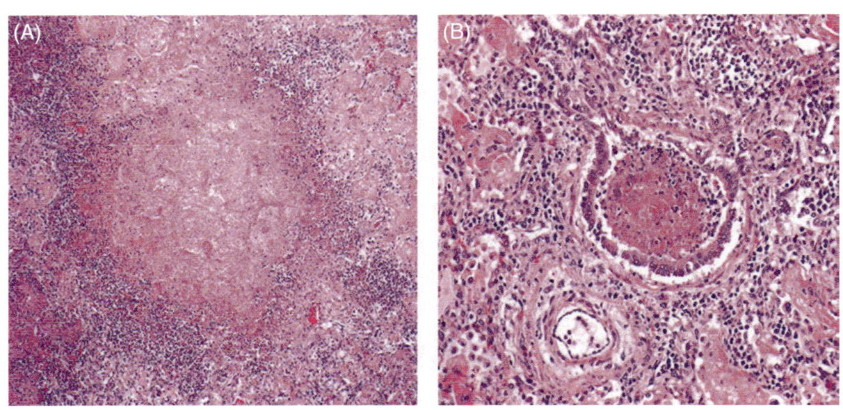

Fig. 3.45. Ox. Lung. *Mycoplasma bovis*. Early inflammation. (A) Fibrinonecrotic pneumonia. Central eosinophilic material indicates coagulative necrosis of large alveolar areas. The necrotic focus is surrounded by degenerating inflammatory cells. (B) Fibrinous bronchiolitis with lymphocytic alveolitis and perivasculitis. A bronchiole is filled with fibrin and some necrotic cells. The surrounding alveoli contain dense aggregates of inflammatory cells with some fibrin intermingled (H&E).

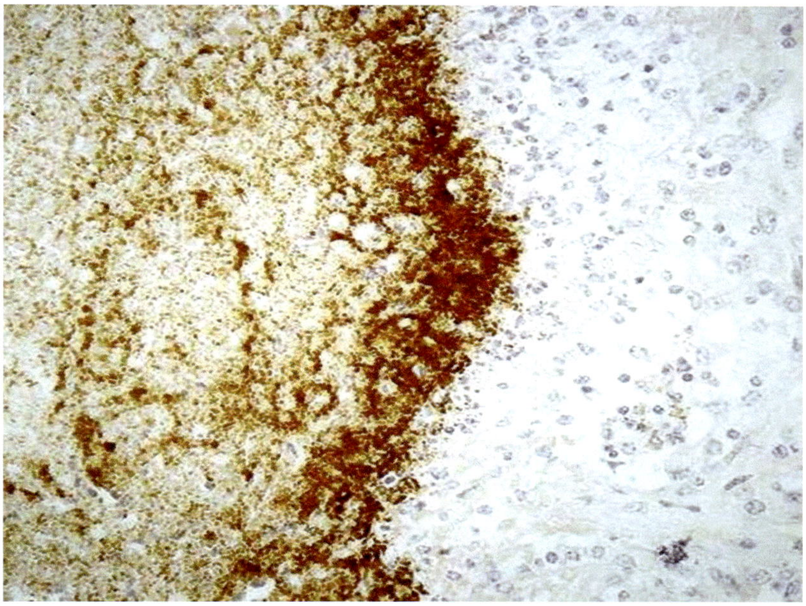

Fig. 3.46. Ox. Formalin-fixed tissue. *Mycoplasma bovis*. Demonstration of dense distribution of *M. bovis* antigen by indirect immunohistochemistry. Bacteria are usually not visible on H&E stained sections, unless in densely populated areas as basophilic granular material, but this is not specific for the organism. Silver stains such as Warthin Starry or Warthin Faulkner stain the organism when densely populated and help rule out other bacterial populations by morphology (IHC).

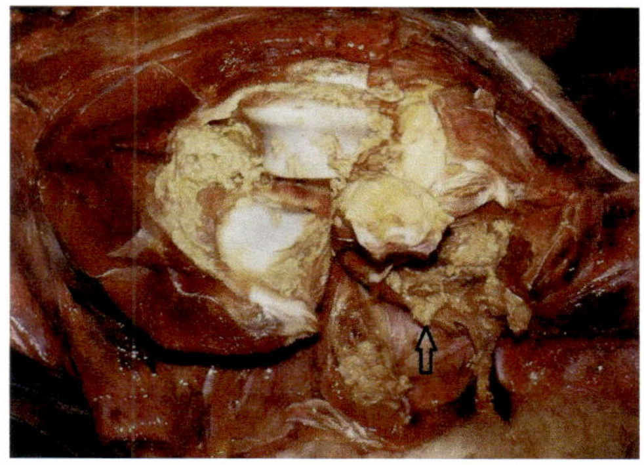

Fig. 3.47. Ox. *Mycoplasma bovis*. Stifle joint. Purulent arthritis. Arthritic component of chronic pneumonia and polyarthritis syndrome (CPPS) infection. There is also evidence of muscle necrosis (arrow) of the peroneus tertius muscle and its tendon. In joint infections, surrounding soft tissue involvement is common.

Fact Sheet: Contributors to Bovine Respiratory Disease (BRD)

(Adopted from World Buiatrics Conference 2014, Cairns, Australia)

Risk factors
- Feeding (22%)
- Colostrum (28%)
- Climate (67%)
- Housing (79%)

Infectious agents
- IBR virus (4%)
- PI-3 virus ?
- BRS virus (18%)
- Mycoplasma (14%)
- *Mannheimia* (67%)
- Other
  - *Pasteurella multocida*
  - *Histophilus somni*
  - *Trueperella pyogenes*

Immunosuppression
- BVD virus (18%)
- Adverse weather conditions

Mycoplasma mycoides subsp. *mycoides* (small colony type)

Introduction. The organism is the cause of contagious bovine pleuropneumonia (CBPP) and is foreign to the northern American continent. Sporadic outbreaks of CBPP were reported from some countries in Europe in the late 1980s. The hallmark gross pathologic feature is that of a fibrinous pleuropneumonia, often unilateral, characterized by marbling, edematous interlobular septa and trachebronchial lymphadenitis. Pulmonary sequestra containing a brown exudate can be observed. The extensive severe natural cases are difficult to reproduce via experimental infection. Sometimes, renal infarcts are also observed in cattle with CBPP. As the organism shares this morphologic feature with other pulmonary pathogens, *M. bovis* for example, it is important to consider *Mycoplasma mycoides* subsp. *mycoides* in the differential diagnosis to recognize and help to prevent the pathogen entering disease-free geographic areas.

Clinical signs. Respiratory distress, cough, high fever, nasal discharge.

Differential diagnoses. Mannheimiosis, histophilosis, *P. multocida*, *T. pyogenes, M. bovis* and/or other mycoplasmas.

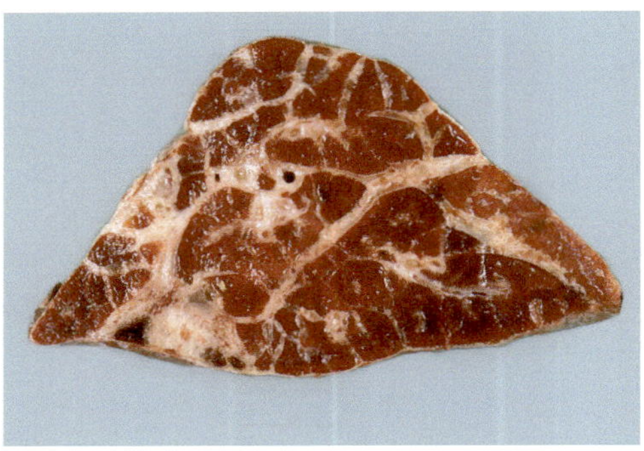

Fig. 3.49. Ox. Lung. Contagious bovine pleuropneumonia (CBPP). Fibrinous pneumonia. On cut section, a marbling effect is the result of varying stages of inflammation in the lobular compartment. There is marked widening of the interlobular septa by fibrin, edema, and lymphatic thrombosis. Lobules are indurated. In chronic cases, tissue sequestration may occur. The same cut surface appearance can occur in *Histophilus somni* pleuritis.

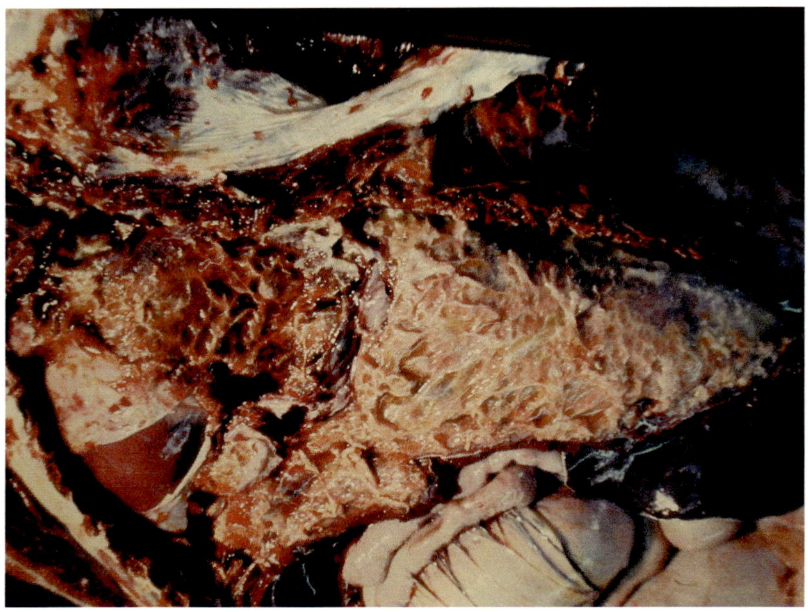

Fig. 3.48. Ox. Lung. Contagious bovine pleuropneumonia (CBPP). Fibrinous pleuropneumonia. Yellow fibrin covering of the pleura is dense and diffuse, with a ruffled surface appearance.

Bibersteinia trehalosi

Introduction. This pathogen is emerging in BRD. Some strains produce leukotoxins, others not. Dairy calves and adult cattle are more affected, but the infection can also occur in beef operations. Outbreaks jump from small ruminants (sheep). Gross lesions often resemble those of *M. haemolytica*, though are less severe.

Clinical signs. Similar to pathogens previously discussed.

Differential diagnoses. Similar to other members of BRD.

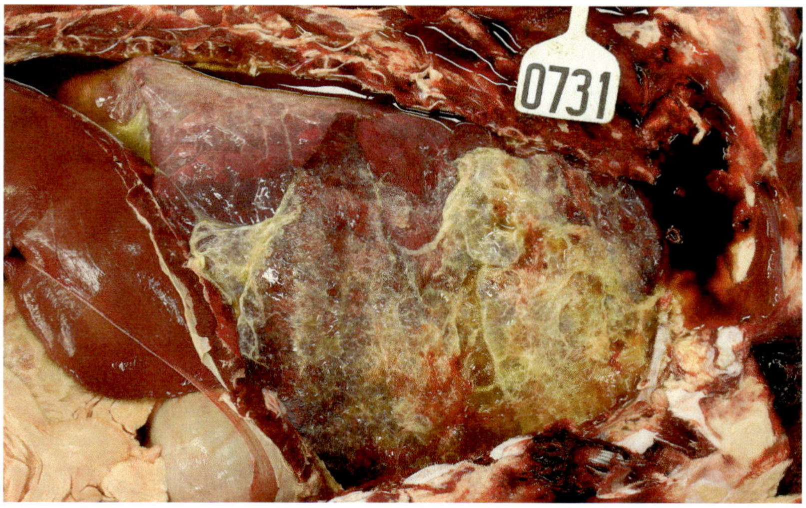

Fig. 3.50. Ox. Lung. Fibrinous pleuropneumonia. Major portions of the cranial lung are characterized by consolidation, and the visceral pleura is covered by strands and sheets of yellow fibrin. *Mannheimia haemolytica* was isolated from this case, but *Bibersteinia trehalosi* can induce similar lesions.

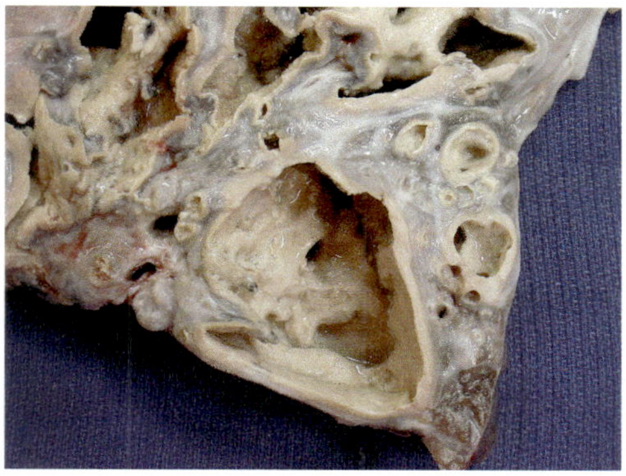

Fig. 3.51. Ox. Lung. Chronic suppurative bronchopneumonia with bronchiectasis. *Trueperella pyogenes* as well as *Escherichia coli* and *Mycoplasma bovis* were isolated. The gross lesions are extensive, distorting pulmonary architecture. Sometimes, *M. bovis* is not the only pathogen isolated in outbreaks of BRD; others including *Histophilus somni* and *Pasteurella multocida* are also isolated in combination.

Mycobacterium bovis

Introduction. *Mycobacterium bovis* is part of the *Mycobacterium tuberculosis* complex responsible for tuberculosis in humans and animals. The disease has been eliminated from many countries, but lurks in others. Wildlife (farmed deer, badgers, opossums) serves as a reservoir for the bacillus in some countries and interferes with eradication.

Clinical signs. Cough, dyspnea, emaciation.

Differential diagnoses. Mycoplasmosis, *T. pyogenes* abscesses, lymphoma (tracheal lymph nodes).

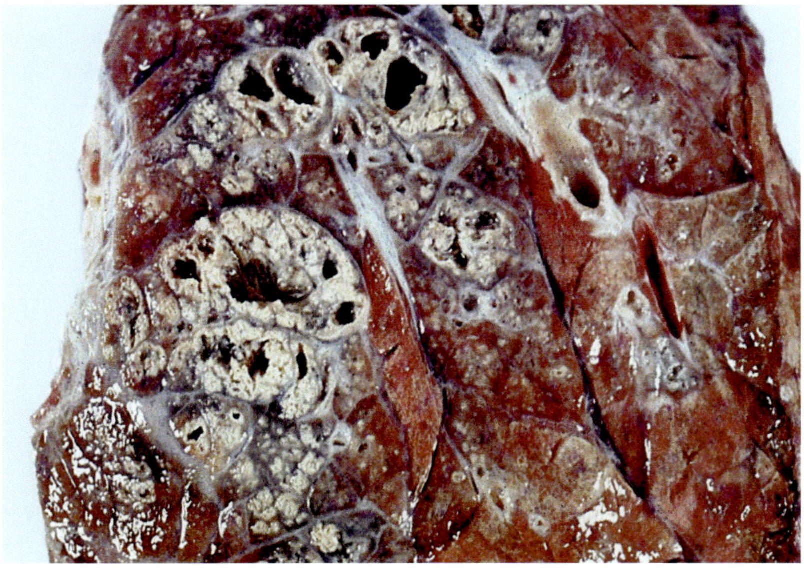

Fig. 3.52. Ox. Lung. Bovine tuberculosis. Caseous bronchiectasis and granulomatous pneumonia. On cut section, multiple bronchi are filled and distended by a caseous exudate. Multiple miliary nodules with a caseous exudate are disseminated next to the extended bronchi. (Courtesy of Prof E. Scanziani, University of Milan, Italy.)

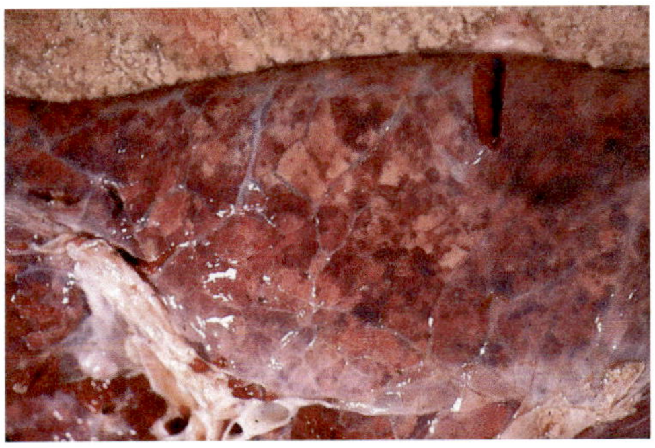

Fig. 3.53. Ox. Lung. Mycotic pneumonia. Multiple, red-brown, somewhat regular-sized foci seed, suggesting hematogenous spread.

Fungi

Introduction. Deep fungi (*Aspergillus* spp.; *Zygomycetes* spp.) reach the lung from a nidus of infection somewhere else (rumen, abomasum, udder, liver, or focal ulcerative enteritis). Usually, individual animals in a herd are affected.

Clinical signs. Rales, cough, sporadic epistaxis.

Differential diagnosis. Disseminated bacterial abscesses.

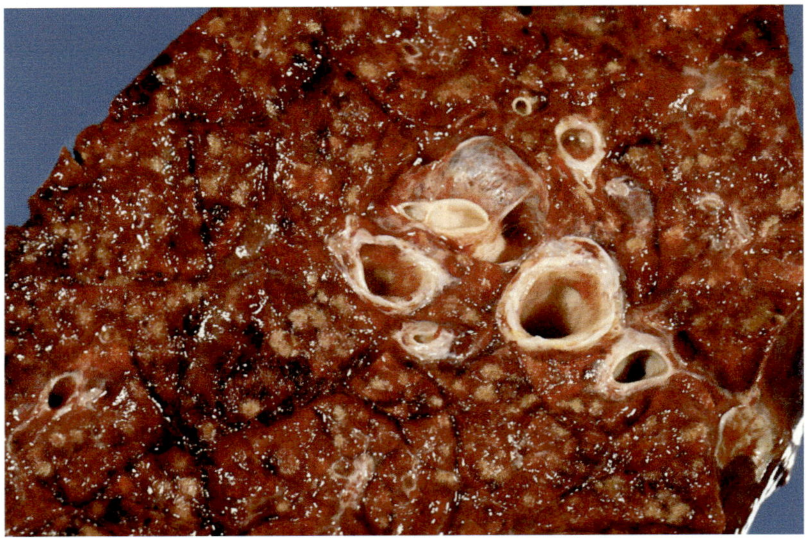

Fig. 3.54. Ox. Lung. Mycotic pneumonia. Cut section exhibits monotonous distribution of multiple tan nodules throughout lung parenchyma. Differential diagnoses should consider bacterial granulomas, metastatic neoplasia.

Parasites

Introduction. *Dictyocaulus viviparus* is the lungworm in cattle causing verminous pneumonia. It has a direct life cycle. Maturing larvae and adults occupy trachea and bronchi.

Clinical signs. Dyspnea, moist cough ('husk'), emaciation.

Differential diagnoses. Aspiration pneumonia, atypical interstitial pneumonia, bacterial pneumonias.

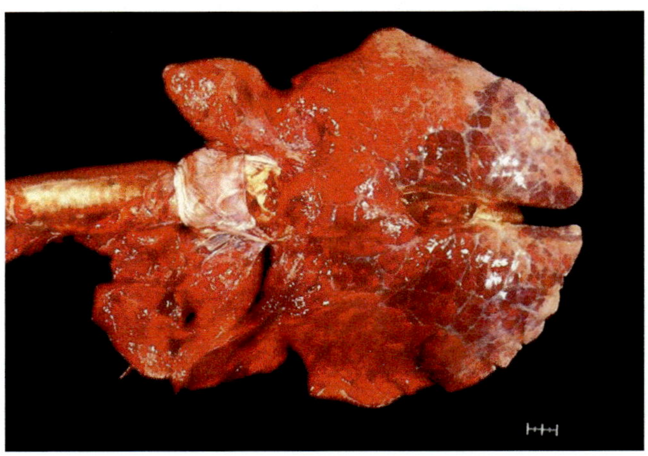

Fig. 3.55. Ox. Lung. *Dictyocaulus viviparus*. Verminous pneumonia. Locally extensive consolidation of dorsal lung lobes. One should look for lungworms by opening the right dorsal bronchus, which extends to the caudal aspect of the caudal lung lobe.

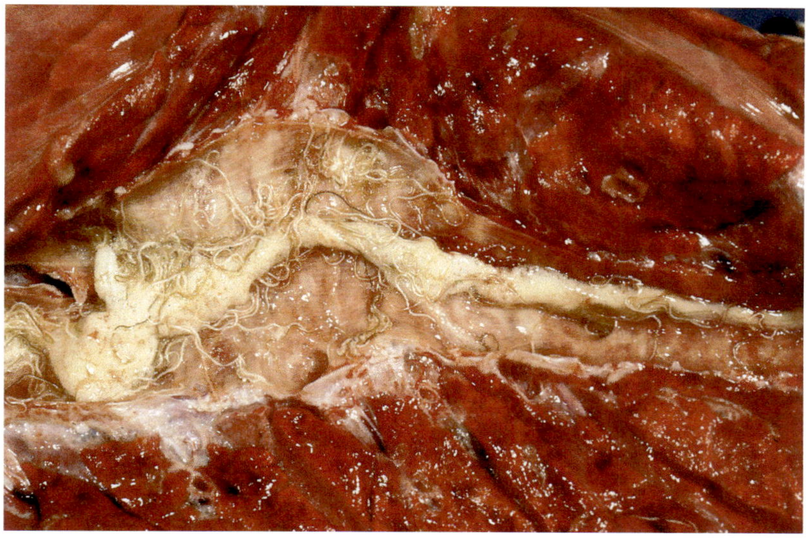

Fig. 3.56. Ox. Lung. *Dictyocaulus viviparus*. Verminous bronchitis. Opened bronchus contains nematode worms embedded in fibrin.

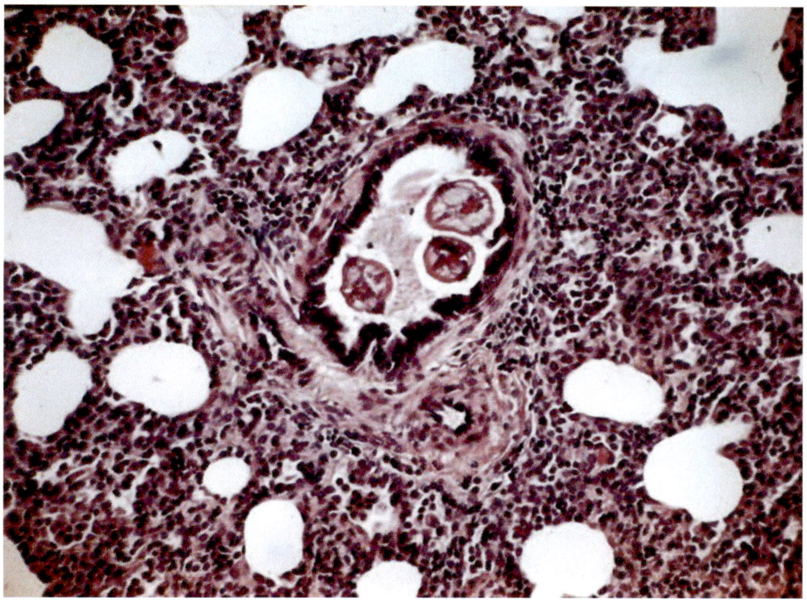

Fig. 3.57. Lung. *Dictyocaulus viviparus*. Verminous bronchiolitis. The lumen of a bronchiole contains several larvae. The lining epithelium has sloughed, and dense inflammation is present in the lumen and peribronchiolar and adjacent alveolar tissues.

3.2.2.2 Neoplasia

Primary neoplasms such as adenoma or adenocarcinoma have occasionally been reported in older cows. Metastasizing neoplasms are often of uterine origin.

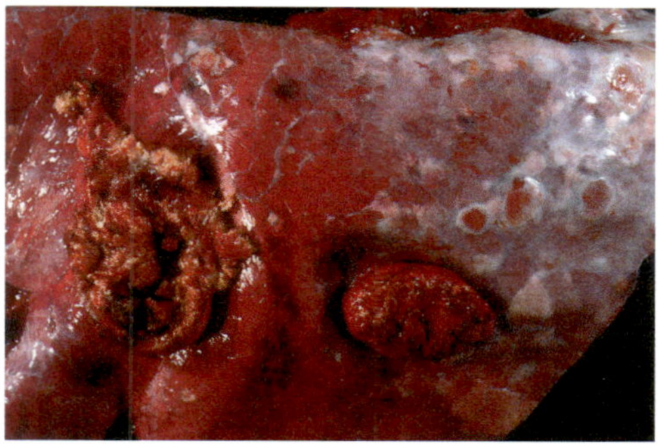

Fig. 3.58. Ox. Lung. Metastasis of mammary gland carcinoma. Multiple round, partially elevated and necrotic nodules occupy the lung parenchyma. (Image courtesy of the Government of Alberta, Canada.)

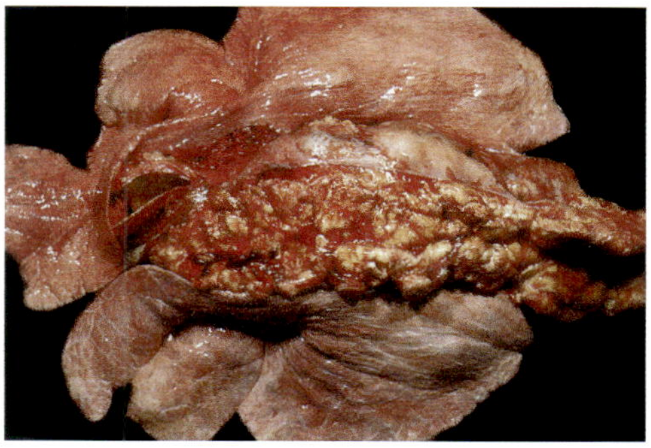

Fig. 3.59. Ox. Lung. Mediastinal lymphosarcoma (lymphoma). Multiple coalescing gray nodules have infiltrated the dorsal mediastinum. Bovine tuberculosis should be considered in differential diagnosis.

3.2.2.3 Miscellaneous

Introduction. This subsection deals with individual pulmonary categories difficult to integrate with the previous disease entities presented.

Aspiration pneumonia

Introduction. Foreign material reaching the lung through inhalation causes septic or gangrenous cranioventral pneumonia. Causes are multiple, ranging from regurgitation of ruminal contents, neurologic or metabolic disorders, to iatrogenic manipulations such as balling gun application or stomach tubing. The far most common cause is aspiration from stomatitis, pharyngitis and especially laryngitis. These tissues and sites always need to be examined thoroughly.
Clinical signs. Repeated coughing, nasal discharge, rapid respiration, septicemia.
Differential diagnosis. Bacterial cranioventral bronchopneumonia.

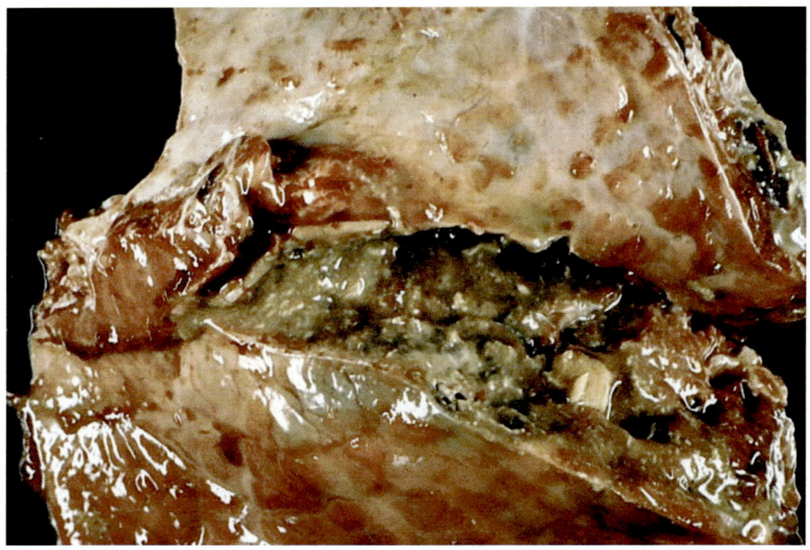

Fig. 3.60. Ox. Lung. Aspiration. Gangrenous pneumonia. Ruminal contents are present within airways, causing necrosis of surrounding lung parenchyma. The pleura is studded with multiple gray to red nodules, suggesting fibrosis.

Atypical interstitial pneumonia (AIP)

Introduction. This non-infectious disorder of cattle is multifactorial. The terminology for the condition varies from acute bovine pulmonary emphysema and edema complex, used by clinicians, and proliferative pneumonia, preferred by some pathologists. The condition is commonly seen in feedlot cattle and, to a lesser degree, in dairy cattle. AIP is a poorly understood entity and should be considered a syndrome. Factors confirmed to be involved are pneumotoxic 3-methylindole, a metabolite of L-tryptophan, hypersensitivity reactions from moldy feed, milk allergy or repeated exposure to lungworm larvae, plant pneumotoxins such as 4-ipomoenol from moldy sweet potatoes (*Ipomoea batatas*), perilla ketones from purple mint (*Perilla frutescens*), nitrogen gases (silo filler's disease), lush pastures, fog conditions. Lush pasture-associated AIP occurs in adult cattle, and feedlot-associated AIP in younger ages.

Clinical signs. Dyspnea, open-mouth breathing, respiratory distress, subcutaneous emphysema.

Differential diagnosis. Bacterial pneumonias with diffuse anatomic pattern, congestion and edema, anaphylaxis, atelectasis.

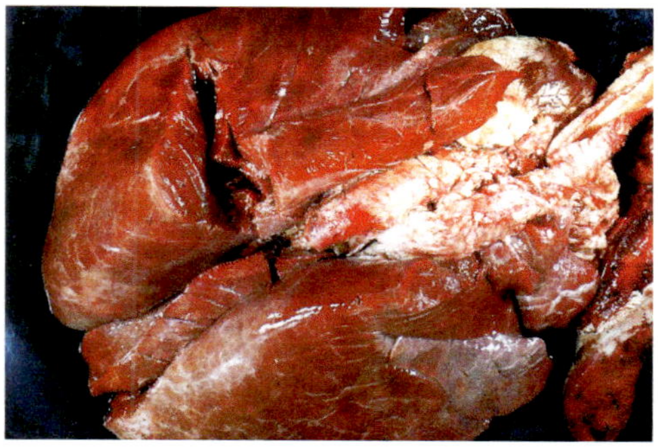

Fig. 3.61. Ox. Lung. Atypical interstitial pneumonia (AIP). Adult cow with lush pasture-associated AIP. The main gross feature of AIP is a heavy, non-collapsed lung, with firm, rubbery texture (meaty), brown discoloration, and diffuse pattern of distribution. These features are expressed best and most consistently in the caudal lobes.

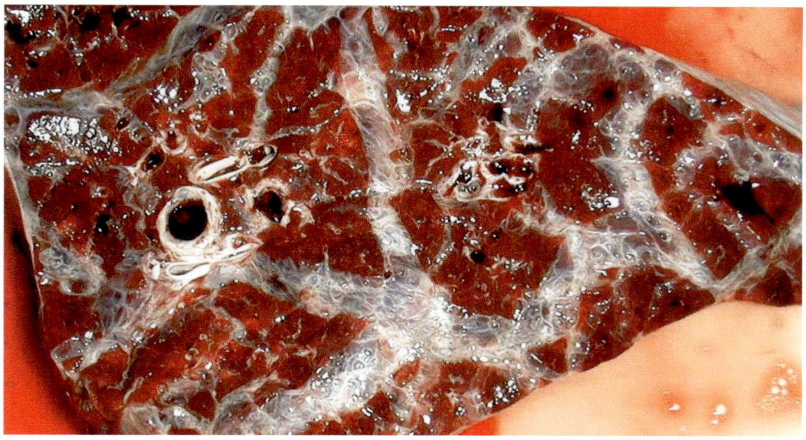

Fig. 3.62. Ox. Lung. Atypical interstitial pneumonia (AIP). Interlobular edema and emphysema. Excessive breathing in acute respiratory distress and damage to the integrity of alveolar structures lead to alveolar rupture and escape of residual air and fluid into the interlobular interstitium. The extent of edema and emphysema varies from case to case, and even in different parts of the lung.

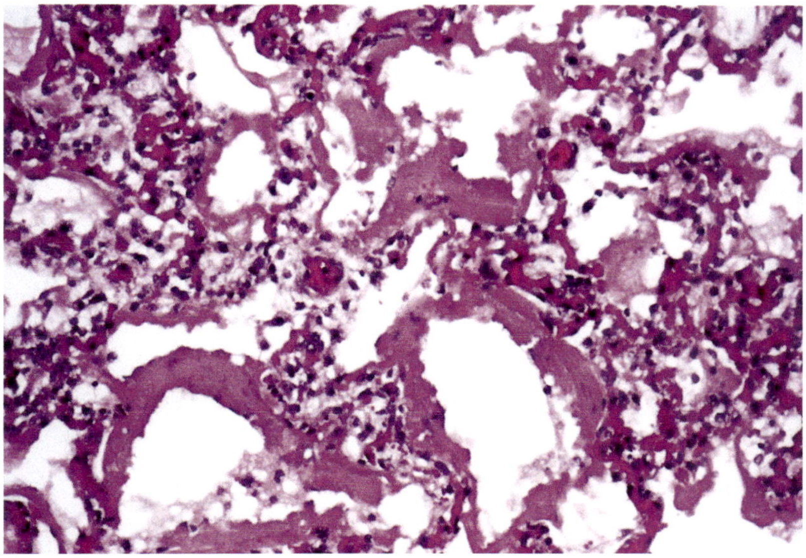

Fig. 3.63. Ox. Lung. Atypical interstitial pneumonia (AIP). Membranous alveolitis. The alveolar-interstitial unit is damaged in the acute phase of AIP, leading to the formation of hyaline membranes covering the spillage. Alveolar septa are disrupted. During the process, type 1 pneumocytes and Clara cells undergo necrosis (periodic acid–Schiff).

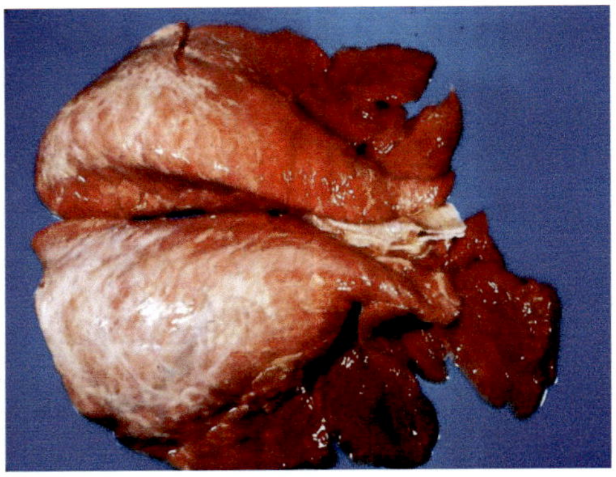

Fig. 3.65. Ox. Lung. Secondary atypical interstitial pneumonia (AIP). Cranioventral bronchopneumonia with secondary proliferative pneumonia. In young animals, a sequential bacterial cranioventral bronchopneumonia, usually due to *Pasteurella multocida* or *Mannheimia haemolytica*, and subsequent acute caudal proliferative pneumonia has been recognized. It is hypothesized that the proliferating pneumonia is a delayed hypersensitivity reaction to bacterial components of a resolving bronchopneumonia. The image exhibits brown consolidation of the cranial lung and a non-collapsed, firm lung in the caudal portion. Sometimes, careful histologic examination of cranial lung lobes will reveal remaining bovine respiratory syncytial virus (BRSV) antigen by IHC. (Courtesy of Dr J.M. King and Section of Anatomic Pathology, Cornell University, USA.)

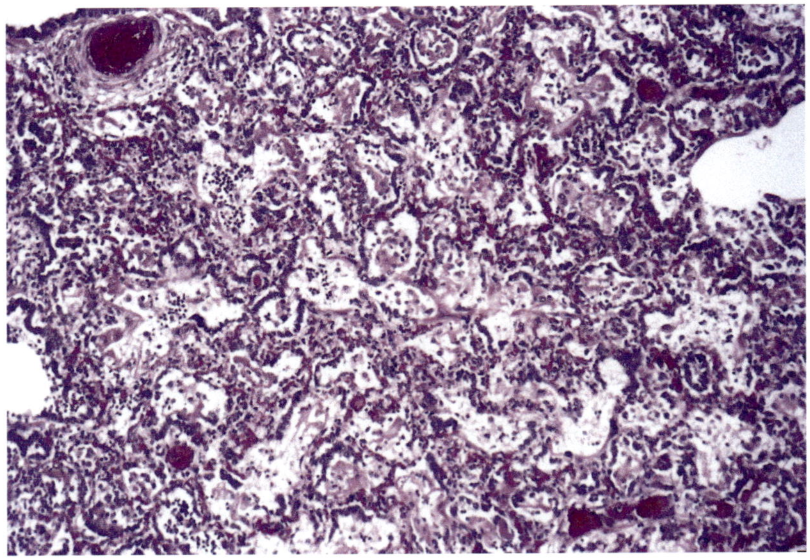

Fig. 3.64. Ox. Lung. Atypical interstitial pneumonia (AIP). Type 2 pneumocyte hyperplasia. Epithelialization of the alveolar lining by proliferating type 2 pneumocytes characterizes the chronic phase of AIP. The alveolar lumen is filled by necrotic cells and alveolar macrophages. It is the cellular proliferation, protein content of the hyaline membranes and interstitial edema that make the lung heavy and meaty (H&E).

Fact Sheet: Atypical Interstitial Pneumonia (AIP)

Definition
- Acute respiratory disease syndrome of multifactorial origin resulting in alveolar damage, type 2 pneumocyte hyperplasia, and interstitial emphysema and edema

Clinical signs
- Open-mouth breathing
- Coughing
- Head extension
- Tongue protrusion

Differential diagnoses
- Bovine respiratory disease (BRD)
- Heart failure
- Hypersensitivity/allergy

Gross findings
- Diffuse meaty, wet, heavy lung
- Severe interstitial emphysema and edema

Microscopic findings
- Alveolar hyaline membranes
- Type 2 pneumocyte proliferation
- Alveolar macrophages

Causes
- Pneumotoxins
  - 3-methylindole
  - Ketones from perilla (purple) mint
  - Ipomoenol from moldy sweet potatoes

- Infectious agents
  - BRSV
  - Pulmonary bacterial pathogens
- Parasites
  - Reinfection with *Dictyocaulus viviparus*
- Environmental factors
  - Dust
  - Toxic gases (nitrogen dioxide)
  - Allergens
  - Lush pastures

Pulmonary abscess

Introduction. When solitary, aerogenous in origin; when multiple, likely hematogenous.

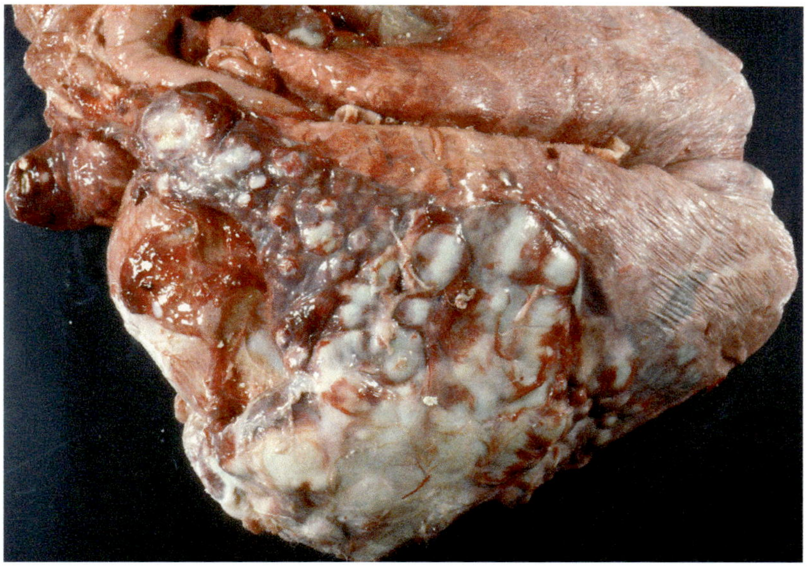

Fig. 3.66. Ox. Lung. A large abscess of bacterial origin occupies the cranioventral lung and has extended caudally. When rupturing, it releases its contents into the thorax to induce exudative pleuritis. Bronchiectasis is a secondary finding.

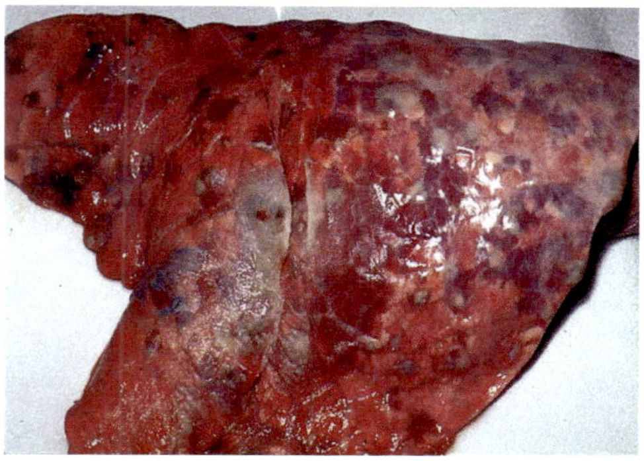

Fig. 3.67. Ox. Lung. Multifocal, suppurative embolic pneumonia with focal fibrinous pleuritis. Multiple, circumscribed foci, some of them confluent, are disseminated throughout the lung. The foci have a two-color pattern of central gray and brown peripheral coloration. Origin of the embolic shower might have been septic foci in the liver, feet, or joints. There is evidence of focal fibrinous pleuritis. The most common cause in feedlot cattle is posterior vena cava syndrome and therefore it is important to examine the vessel just caudal to the diaphragm at the dorsal aspect of the liver when embolic pneumonia is diagnosed (see Chapter 6: Diseases of the Hepatobiliary System and Pancreas). (Courtesy of Dr J.M. King and Section of Anatomic Pathology, Cornell University, USA.)

Embolic pneumonia

Introduction. The condition occurs when septic emboli hematogenously shower the lung from primary inflammatory foci somewhere else. Septic pathogens may be of bacterial or mycotic origin. Multifocal, even-sized foci are distributed randomly within lung lobes grossly. Microscopically, the inflammatory response is typically oriented around pulmonary blood vessels (angiocentric).

Pulmonary emphysema

Introduction. Excessive air may accumulate grossly as interlobular bullae, interlobular emphysema, and subpleural emphysema. A fourth form is alveolar emphysema, seen in chronic obstructive pulmonary disease and diagnosed mainly by microscopy. Emphysema alone does not constitute a primary diagnosis as it is often secondary to some other lung pathologic process.

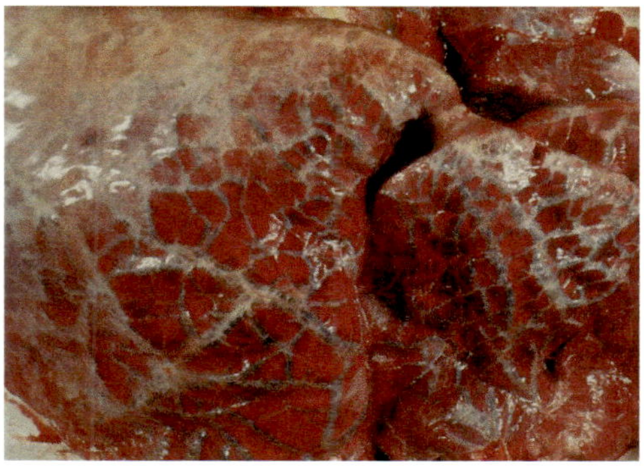

Fig. 3.68. Ox. Lung. Subpleural and interlobular emphysema. Small air pockets are extending the visceral pleura and are widening the interlobular interstitium. Non-transparent appearance of parietal pleura of dorsal caudal lung lobe is normal in the adult bovine lung.

Pulmonary edema, congestion, and anaphylaxis

Introduction. Excessive fluid accumulation in the trachea, airways, and interlobular septa leads to froth in airways when intermixed with air and respiratory labor. Causes of excessive fluid in the lung range from chronic heart failure, acute septic bacterial pneumonia, acute hypersensitivity reactions to exogenous causes such as vaccines or drugs, and endogenous causes such as milk proteins.

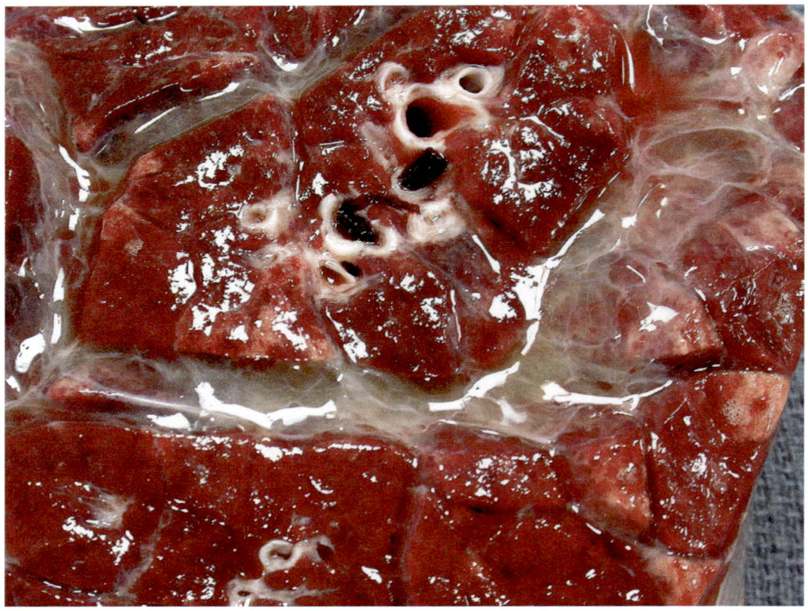

Fig. 3.69. Ox. Lung. Interlobular edema. Interlobular septa are flooded by watery, mucinous fluid. Surrounded lobules are consolidated.

Bronchiectasis

Introduction. Distension of bronchi occurs following bronchitis and accumulation of dense purulent exudate in the lumen. During this process of inflammation, the wall of bronchi disintegrates.

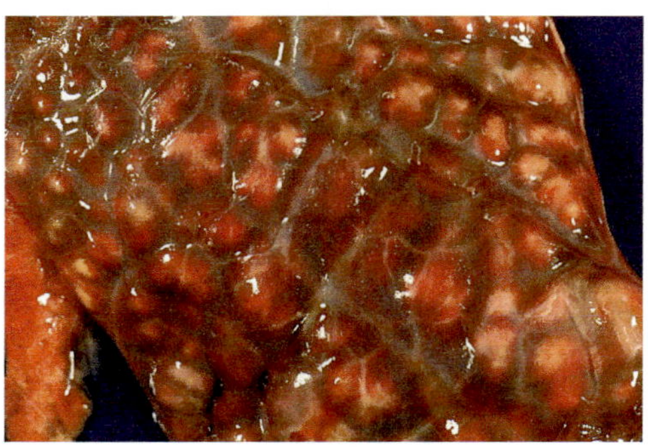

Fig. 3.70. Ox. Lung. Bronchiectasis. The lung lobe contains distended bronchi. Adjacent parenchyma is characterized by atelectasis.

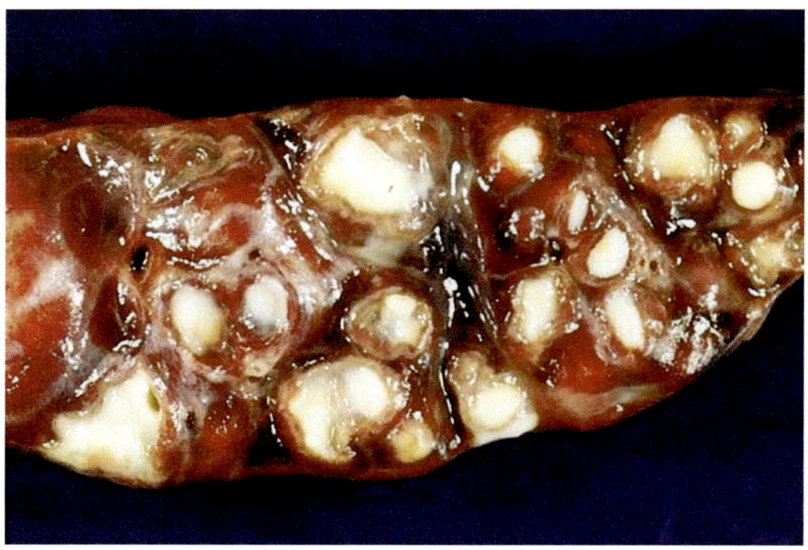

Fig. 3.71. Ox. Lung. Bronchiectasis. On cut section, distended bronchi are filled by purulent exudate. These should be differentiated from pulmonary abscesses.

Bronchiolitis obliterans

Introduction. Defined as fibrosing inflammatory reaction to bronchiolar injury. Certain pulmonary viruses (BRSV, PI-3) or toxic gases may cause necrosis to the bronchiolar lining cells, damage to the basement membrane, and fibrin influx. When necrotic debris is not removed from the lumen, fibroblasts invade and transform into fibrovascular luminal projections.

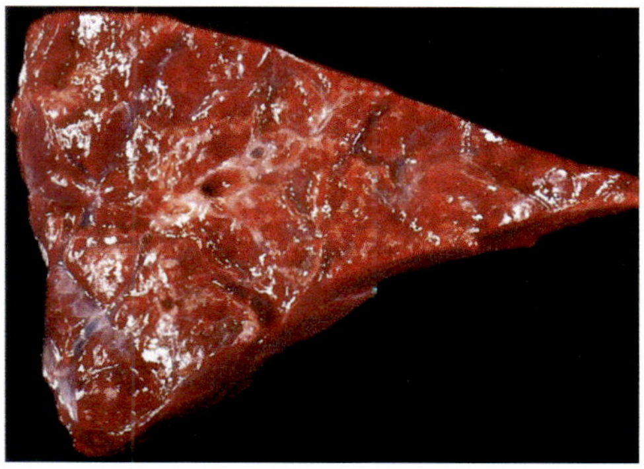

Fig. 3.72. Ox. Lung. Bronchiolitis obliterans. On cut section, lobules are under-aerated and solid. There is evidence of interstitial emphysema and edema. The gross changes do not differ from atypical interstitial pneumonia (AIP) and bacterial bronchopneumonia, and require microscopic examination to verify the diagnosis of bronchiolitis obliterans.

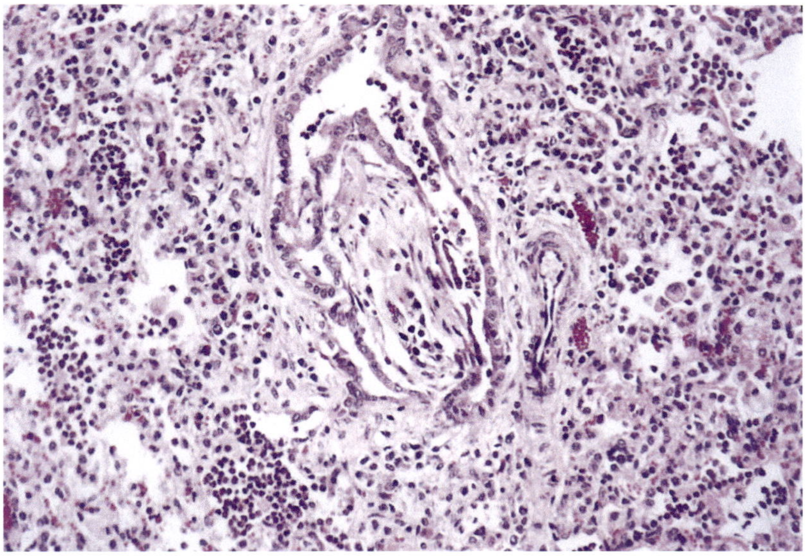

Fig. 3.73. Ox. Lung. Bronchiolitis obliterans. On microscopic examination, a bronchiole is obliterated by a finger-like projection of fibrovascular tissue lined by respiratory epithelium. The projection originated from one focus in the bronchiole where the lining cells were lost. There is evidence of clusters of inflammatory cells within and outside the bronchiolar projection. The surrounding alveoli are densely filled with inflammatory cells and poorly aerated (H&E).

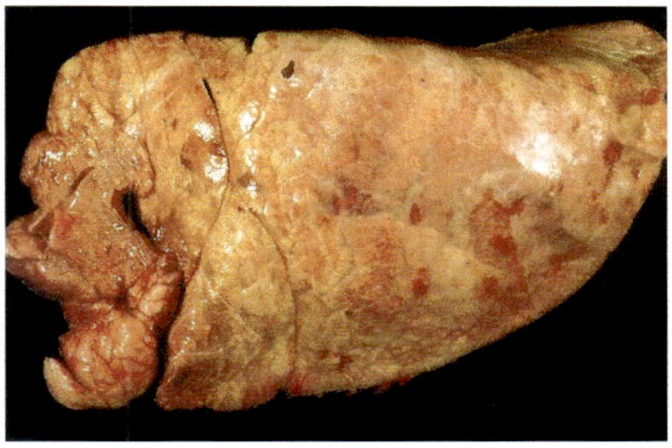

Fig. 3.74. Ox. Lung. Pulmonary fibrosis. The lung is not collapsed and lobules are pale. Such a lung feels firm on palpation.

Pulmonary fibrosis

Introduction. Chronic response to presumable pneumotoxins such as metabolites, gases, or toxic plants. The likely target structure in the lung is the alveolar-interstitial unit with structural repair characterized by type 2 pneumocyte hyperplasia and alveolar fibrosis. These cases usually terminate in cor pulmonale, or right-sided heart failure.

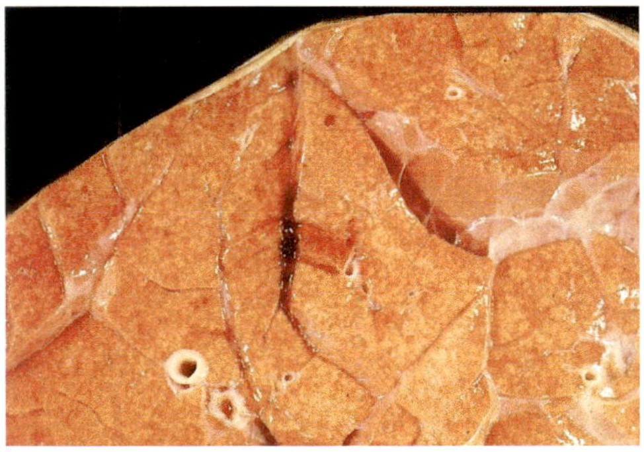

Fig. 3.75. Ox. Lung. Pulmonary fibrosis. Lung lobules are uniformly pale and dense, suggesting a lack of aeration and vascularization. Microscopic examination is needed to verify the gross diagnosis.

Caudal vena cava thrombosis (CVC)

Introduction. The condition is a syndrome often leading to sudden death by nasal–oral exsanguination. It is a common problem in feedlot cattle, and severe embolic pneumonia along with emphysema is the outcome. The pathogenesis of CVC begins in the rumen, often from rumenitis due to grain overload and secondary bacterial inflammation (*Fusobacterium necrophorum*, *Trueperella pyogenes*). Bacterial seeding into the liver and the development of hepatic abscesses ensue. Some of the abscesses migrate towards and erode into the adjacent overriding caudal vein. Caudal venous thrombosis develops. Septic emboli shower the lung and build up in the pulmonary vasculature. Aneurysms and vasculo-bronchial fistulas form in the lung. Severe pulmonary hemorrhage is the fatal consequence (see Chapter 6: Diseases of the Hepatobiliary System and Pancreas).

Clinical signs. Hemoptysis, recurrent epistaxis, melena in dairy cattle; respiratory distress and/or sudden death in feedlot cattle.

Differential diagnoses. Nasal disease, chronic bronchopneumonia, abomasal ulcers, vegetative valvulitis, nasal tubing.

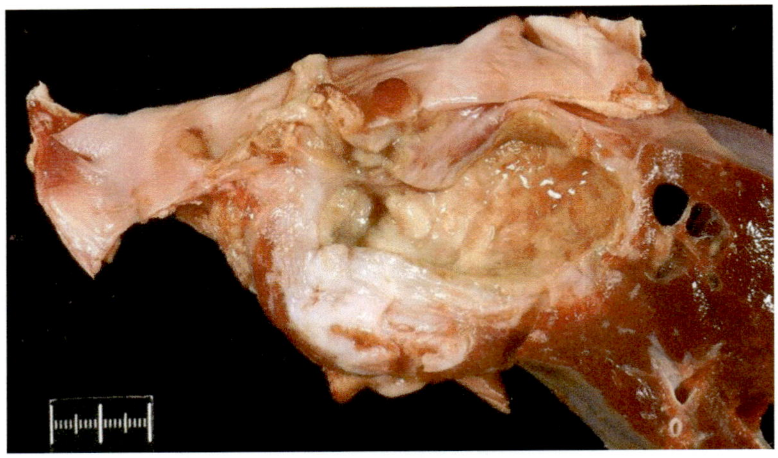

Fig. 3.76. Ox. Caudal vein. Abscess. A large liver abscess has eroded the overriding vena cava.

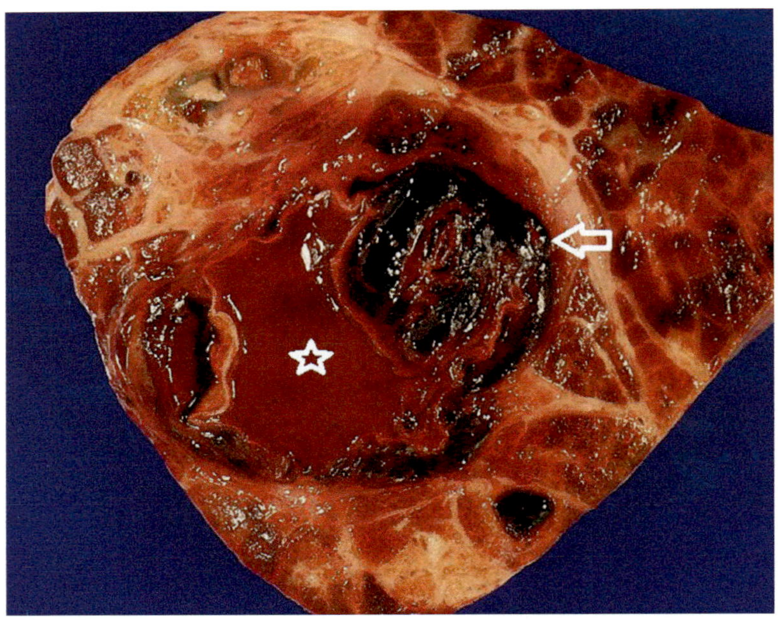

Fig. 3.77. Ox. Lung. Thromboembolism. A septic embolus (arrow) has been dislodged from the caudal vein into a larger lung vessel and a vasculo-bronchial fistula has resulted in massive hemorrhage within the airway (asterisk), being responsible for the fatal epistaxis seen clinically.

3.3 PLEURA

3.3.1 Effusion

Pleural effusions of non-inflammatory origin may result in hydrothorax or hemothorax.

3.3.2 Inflammation

Introduction. Inflammation of the pleura (pleuritis) usually occurs secondary to pneumonia, often as a result of a ruptured lung abscess or as part of a primary pleuropneumonia such as Mycoplasmosis or Mannheimiosis. Thoracic puncture or foreign body (traumatic reticulopericarditis) may be another source of pleuritis. Pleuritis may be acute or chronic, unilateral or bilateral. It is classified according to the nature of the exudate accumulating in the pleural cavity. In chronic pleuritic, fibrosis and adhesions may occur.

Clinical signs. Labored breathing, fever, head extension.

Differential diagnosis. Pleuropneumonia from *Mannheimia haemolytica* or *Mycoplasma bovis*.

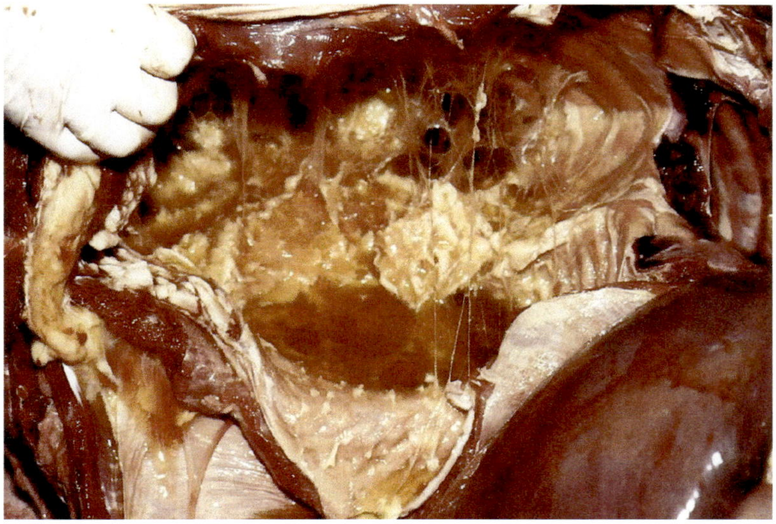

Fig. 3.78. Ox. Pleura. Fibrinous pleuritis. The thorax is filled with a serofibrinous exudate, and both the visceral and parietal pleurae are covered by dense layers of fibrin. Fibrinous adhesions and fibrous villosities are present. *Histophilus somni* was isolated. *H. somni* pleuritis usually occurs without concurrent pneumonia.

SUGGESTED READING

Caswell, J.L. (2014) Failure of respiratory defenses in the pathogenesis of bacterial pneumonia in cattle. *Veterinary Pathology* 51, 393–409.

Caswell, J.L., Bateman, K.G., Cai, H.Y. and Castillo-Alcala, F. (2010) *Mycoplasma bovis* in respiratory diseases of feedlot cattle. *Veterinary Clinics of Food Animals* 26, 365–369.

Doster, A.R. (2010) Bovine atypical interstitial pneumonia. *Veterinary Clinics of Food Animals* 26, 395–407.

Griffin, D. (2010) Bovine pasteurellosis and other bacterial infections of the respiratory tract. *Veterinary Clinics of Food Animals* 26, 57–71.

Panciera, R.J. and Confer, A.W. (2010) Pathogenesis and pathology of bovine pneumonia. *Veterinary Clinics of Food Animals* 26, 191–214.

Sacco, R.E., McGill, J.L., Pillatzki, A.E., Palmer, V. and Ackermann, M.R. (2014) Respiratory syncytial virus infection in cattle. *Veterinary Pathology* 51, 427–436.

Singh, K., Ritchey, J.W. and Confer, A.W. (2011) *Mannheimia haemolytica*: bacterial–host interactions in bovine pneumonia. *Veterinary Pathology* 48, 338–348.

CHAPTER 4

Diseases of the Cardiovascular System

4.1 Dissection and Examination of the Heart

4.2 Heart

- 4.2.1 Congenital cardiovascular anomalies
- 4.2.2 Pericardial diseases
  - 4.2.2.1 Effusion
  - 4.2.2.2 Inflammation
- 4.2.3 Myocardial diseases
  - 4.2.3.1 Necrosis/degeneration/fibrosis
  - 4.2.3.2 Inflammation
- 4.2.4 Endocardial disorders
  - 4.2.4.1 Fibrosis and calcification
  - 4.2.4.2 Valvular cysts
  - 4.2.4.3 Endocarditis
- 4.2.5 Congestive heart failure
  - 4.2.5.1 Brisket (high-altitude) disease
- 4.2.6 Neoplasia

4.3 Vessels

- 4.3.1 Arteries
  - 4.3.1.1 Marfan syndrome
- 4.3.2 Veins
- 4.3.3 Lymphatics
- 4.3.4 Neoplasia

INTRODUCTION

The healthy bovine heart fulfills three physiologic functions: (i) as a muscular pump it supplies oxygenated blood to the organs of the body and returns venous blood to the lung for oxygenation; (ii) specialized cardiocytes (Purkinje fibers) in the ventricles receive and respond to electric stimuli from the intracardiac conduction system; and (iii) as an endocrine organ it synthesizes and secretes a peptide known as atrial natriuretic factor (ANF).

4.1 DISSECTION AND EXAMINATION OF THE HEART

A methodical dissection of the heart is paramount to avoid mutilation of anatomic structures and to destroy diagnostic pathologic processes. Various procedures have been proposed and can be looked up elsewhere. Excess blood within ventricles should be removed, and the heart should be rinsed softly with water for visualization of lesions, photography, recording of weight and measurements, and procurement of samples for histologic examination.

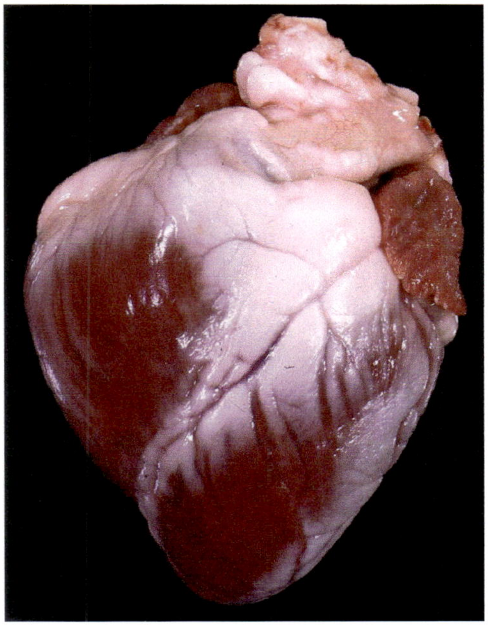

Fig. 4.1. Ox. Normal heart. The apex defines the left ventricle. The coronary groove is covered by adipose tissue. Atrial appendages and major vessels are located at the base of the heart.

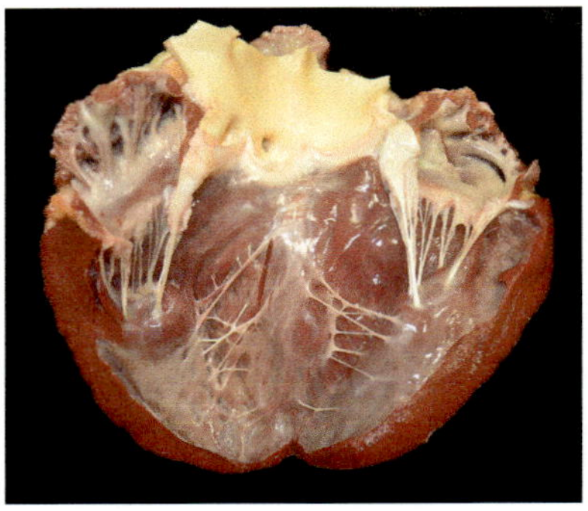

Fig. 4.2. Ox. Opened left heart. Ventricle, atrium, endocardium, ascending aorta, mitral valve leaflets, and chordae tendineae attachments are exposed. (Courtesy of Dr N. Crossland, Louisiana State University, USA.)

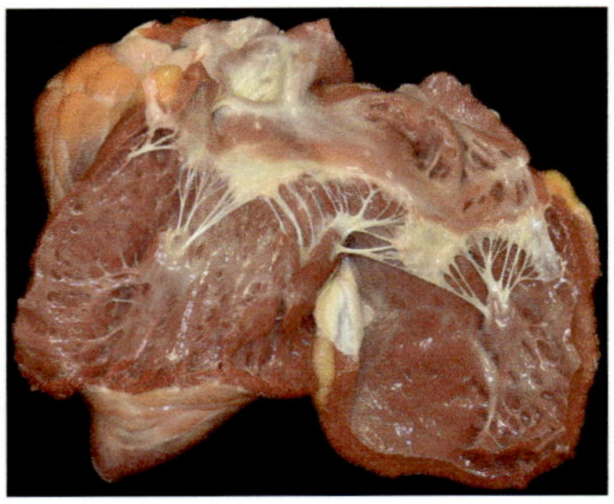

Fig. 4.3. Ox. Opened right heart. The same structures as in Fig. 4.2 are visible. Notice the right ventricle is not part of the apex. (Courtesy of Dr N. Crossland, Louisiana State University, USA.)

4.2 HEART

4.2.1 Congenital cardiovascular anomalies

Introduction. The most frequent bovine anomaly is a ventricular septal defect (VSD). An example of VSD is presented in Chapter 1: Diseases of Neonates and Calves. Other, less frequent anomalies occasionally encountered are atrial septal defect, transposition of greater vessels, tetralogy of Fallot, and ectopia cordis.
Clinical signs. Cyanosis, exercise intolerance, stunted growth.
Differential diagnoses. Pneumonia, intestinal diseases.

4.2.2 Pericardial diseases

4.2.2.1 Effusion

Introduction. Excessive fluid accumulation in the heart sac leads to hydropericardium or hemopericardium (cardiac tamponade).

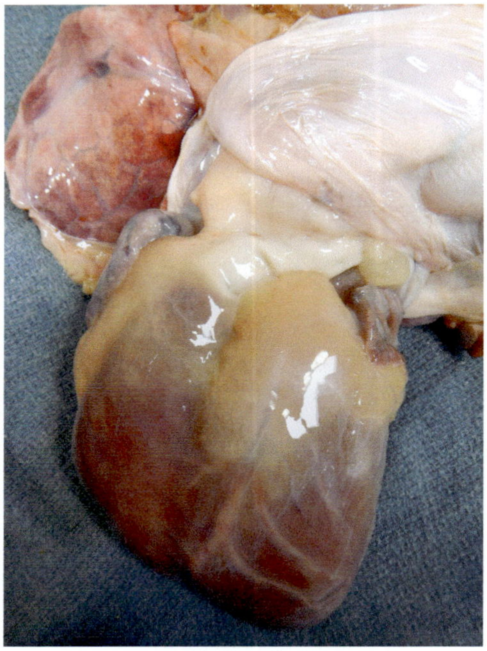

Fig. 4.5. Ox. Heart. Coronary groove. Serous atrophy of fat. A gelatinous fluid has replaced the adipose tissue in the coronary groove. This transformation is a reflection of poor nutritional history or long-lasting disease. A small amount of serous fluid will be within the pericardium normally to serve as a lubricant.

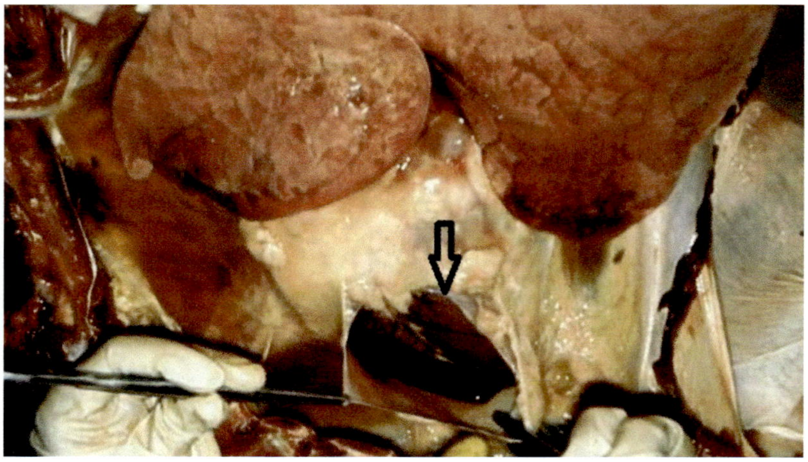

Fig. 4.4. Ox. Pericardium. Hydropericardium. Serous fluid surrounds the opened pericardium, with some fluid left within the heart sac (arrow). Causes are congestive heart failure, clostridial disease, and cowdriosis (heartwater). Notice the severe edema in the lung, with severe widening of the interlobular interstitium by fluid.

4.2.2.2 *Inflammation*

Septic pericarditis

Introduction. Septic (bacterial) spread to the pericardium invokes fibrinous pericarditis with adhesions to the epicardium, which is also inflamed. The best-known example in cattle is traumatic reticulopericarditis, or hardware disease. Hematogenous spread of bacteria to the bovine pericardium or local extension of pneumonia are additional routes of transmission.

Clinical signs. Pain over ventral chest on percussion, ventral edema, jugular vein distension.

Differential diagnoses. Cardiac lymphosarcoma, non-septic pericarditis.

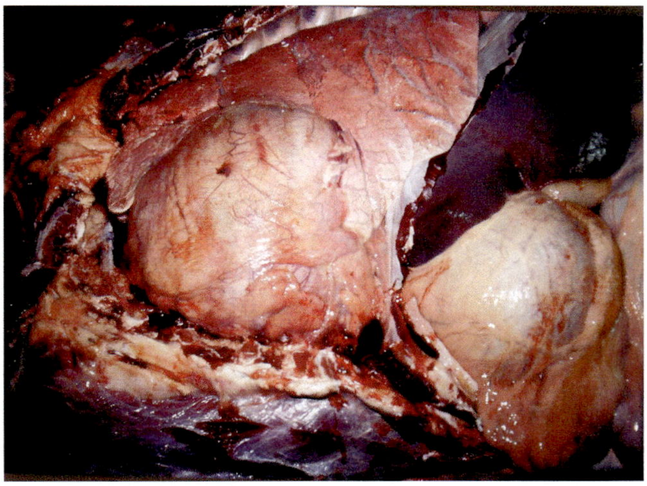

Fig. 4.6. Ox. Pericardium. Septic pericarditis. The heart sac is distended markedly, compressing the cranial lung lobe. Pericardial distension can also be seen with cardiomegaly.

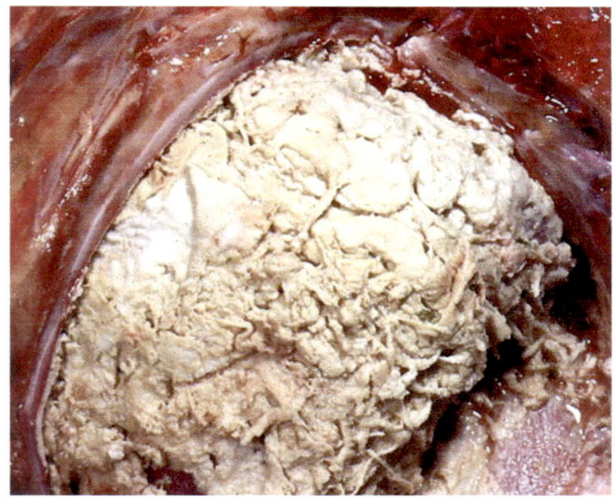

Fig. 4.7. Ox. Pericardium. Chronic fibrinopurulent (septic) pericarditis. The pericardium is thickened and contains fibrin and inspissated, purulent material which covers the entire surface of the epicardium. (Courtesy of Dr J.M. King and Section of Anatomic Pathology, Cornell University, USA.)

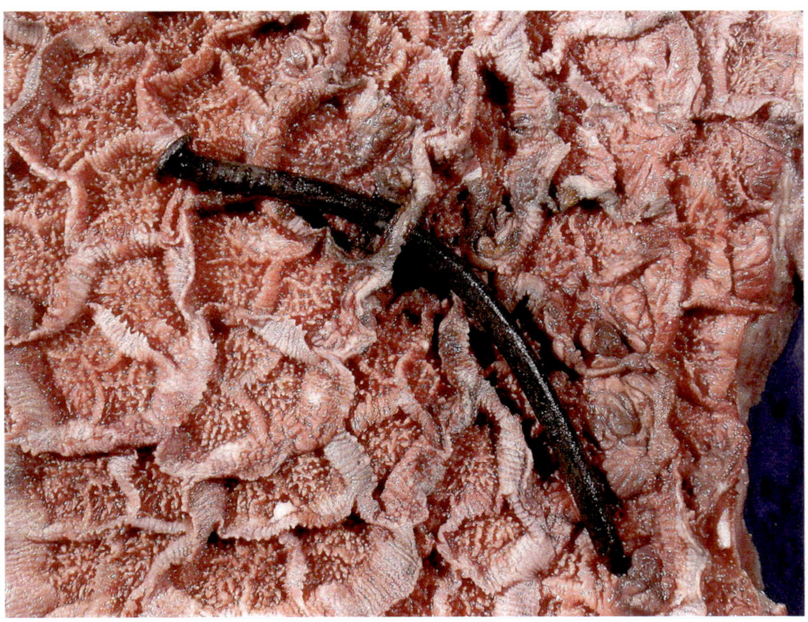

Fig. 4.9. Ox. Reticulum. Hardware disease. A penetrating nail and its migration in cranial direction through the diaphragm into the pericardium contaminates the pericardium with a plethora of bacteria, setting up the severe pericarditis and epicarditis.

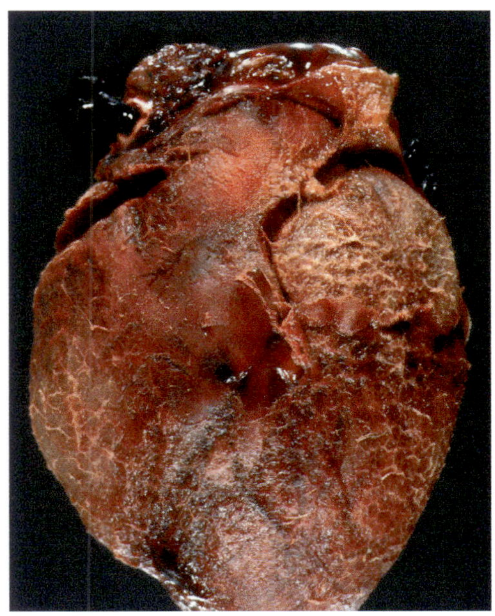

Fig. 4.8. Ox. Epicardium. Fibrinopurulent epicarditis. 'Bread and butter' or 'scrambled egg' appearance of fibrinopurulent exudate covering epicardium.

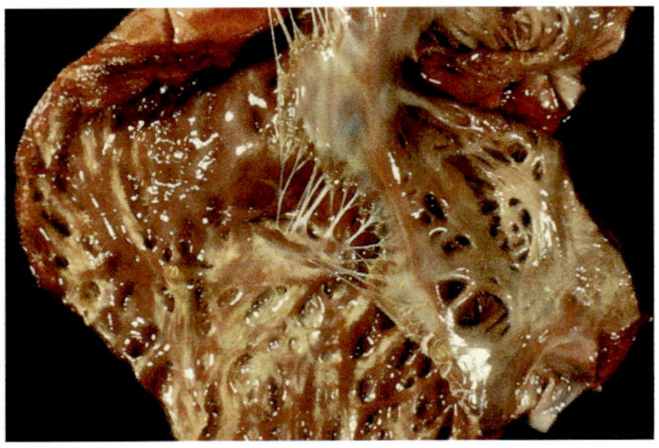

Fig. 4.10. Ox. Heart. Myocardium. Myodegeneration and necrosis. The myocardium of the left ventricle shows severe, multifocal and focally extensive white discoloration. The cause is undetermined. The ventricle is mildly dilated.

4.2.3 Myocardial diseases

4.2.3.1 Necrosis/degeneration/fibrosis

Introduction. Nutritional deficits (vitamin E/selenium), plant-associated selenium toxicosis (*Symphotrichium ascendens*), toxic plants (*Cassia occidentalis*), ionophore antimicrobials (monensin, salinomycin, maduramicin), oleander cardenolids (*Nerium oleander*), gossypol, locoweed, and mycotoxins are potential causes of primary myodegeneration. Many of these initiating causes also affect skeletal muscles.

Clinical signs. Congestive heart failure, sudden death.

Differential diagnosis. Severe myocarditis.

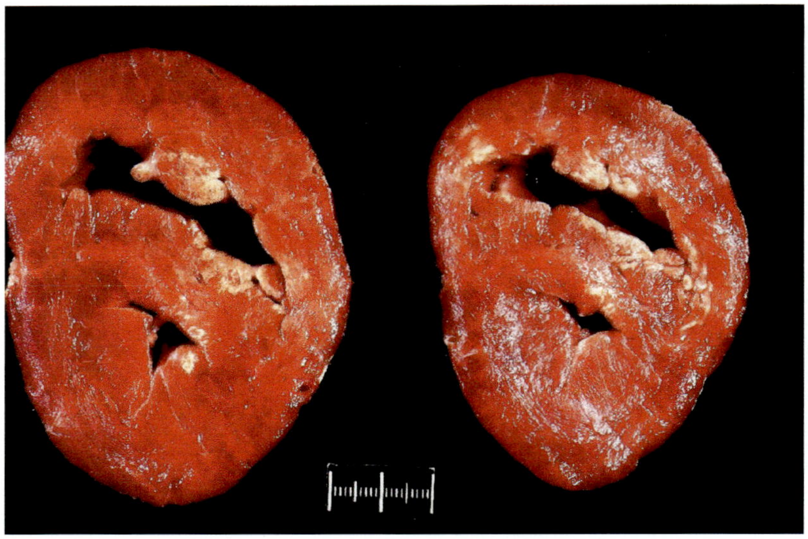

Fig. 4.11. Ox. Heart. Myocardium. Multifocal nutritional myopathy (white muscle disease). The subendocardial myocardium is affected by multiple foci of necrosis. The remaining myocardium exhibits diffuse pallor.

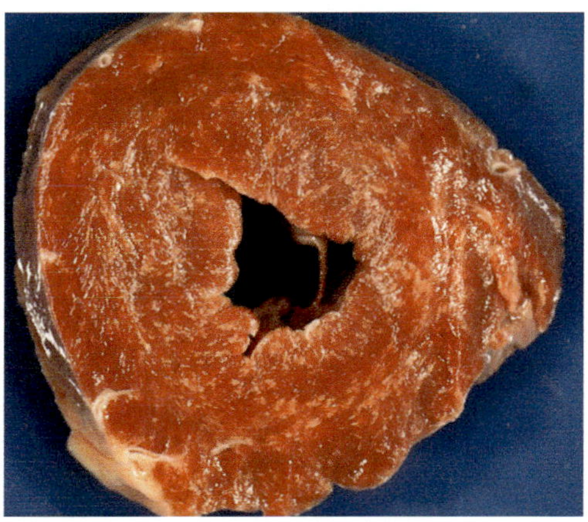

Fig. 4.13. Ox. Heart. Myocardium. Severe necrosis, calcification, and fibrosis. The entire myocardial plane has been replaced by multifocal fibrotic tissue, signalizing chronicity. Such chronic condition prevents recognition of the original etiology.

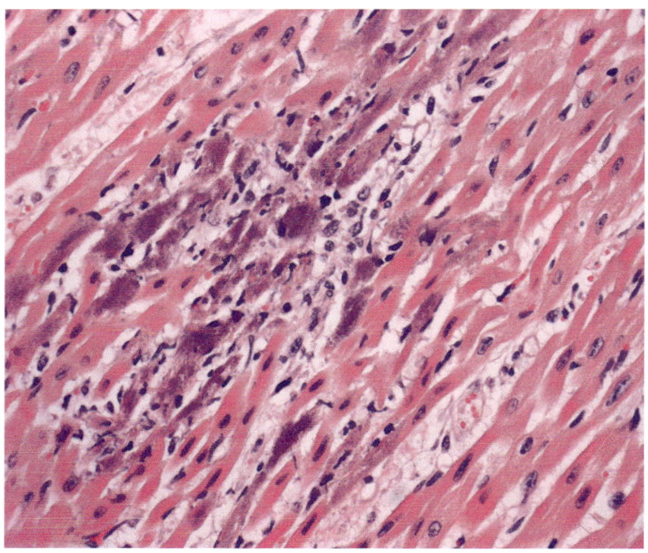

Fig. 4.12. Ox. Heart. Myocardium. Multifocal nutritional myodegeneration (white muscle disease). Cardiocytes are fragmented, necrotic, and mineralized. Many have lost their nucleus (H&E).

4.2.3.2 Inflammation

Introduction. Myocarditis is commonly caused by hematogenously spread bacteria, causing a wide spectrum of inflammatory response ranging from necrotizing, hemorrhagic, suppurative, lymphocytic to granulomatous. Affected animals have a pre-existing infection somewhere else in the body to produce episodes of bacteremia. To a lesser degree, fungi, protozoa or parasites may be involved. Two viral agents are capable of causing myocarditis, transient bovine viral diarrhea virus (BVDV) and malignant catarrhal fever (MCF). In BVDV cases, both lymphocytic myocarditis and vasculitis are expressed, but can only be diagnosed as such histologically and via IHC. Microscopic vasculitis is present in MCF.

Clinical signs. Congestive heart failure, septicemia, sudden death.

Differential diagnoses. Myodegeneration, neoplasia.

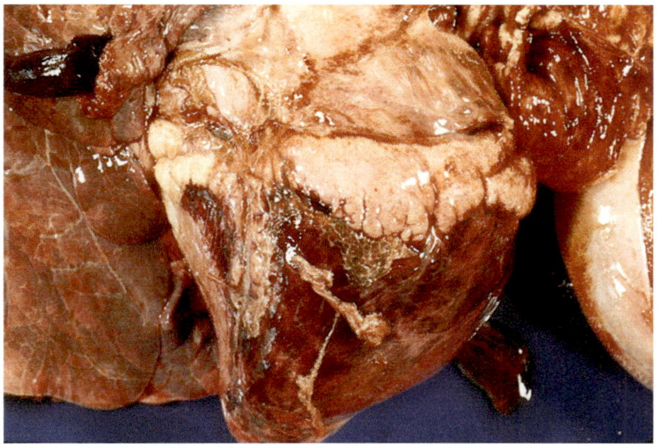

Fig. 4.14. Ox. Myocardium. Blackleg. Necrohemorrhagic myocarditis. The myocardium beneath the coronary groove is markedly hemorrhagic. Some fibrin strands cover the epicardium. The pericardium may also be covered by fibrin. The inflammation is the result of infection with *Clostridium chauvoei*. *Fusobacterium necrophorum* or *Actinomyces* spp. can occasionally be isolated from such lesions.

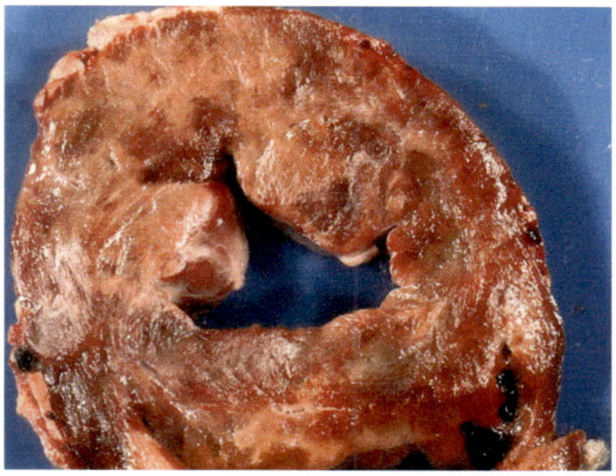

Fig. 4.15. Ox. Myocardium. Blackleg. Necrohemorrhagic myocarditis. *Clostridium chauvoei* is the causative agent. The severity of myocardial damage is reflected on the cut section.

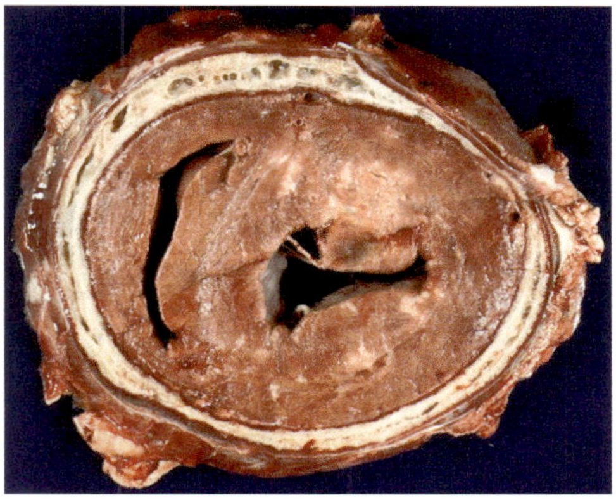

Fig. 4.16. Ox. Heart. Histophilosis. Diffuse fibrino-suppurative pericarditis and multifocal necrotizing myocarditis. *Histophilus somni* infection causes significant inflammatory damage to the myocardium. *H. somni* is considered the principal pathogen causing myocarditis in feedlot cattle. Lesions specifically involve papillary muscles of the left ventricle. Vasculitis is a concurrent microscopic finding in these sites.

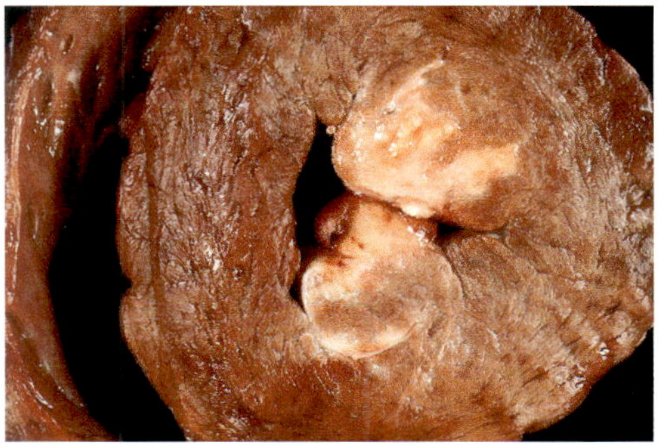

Fig. 4.17. Ox. Heart. Histophilosis. Infarcts. These are typically located in the papillary muscles of the left ventricle.

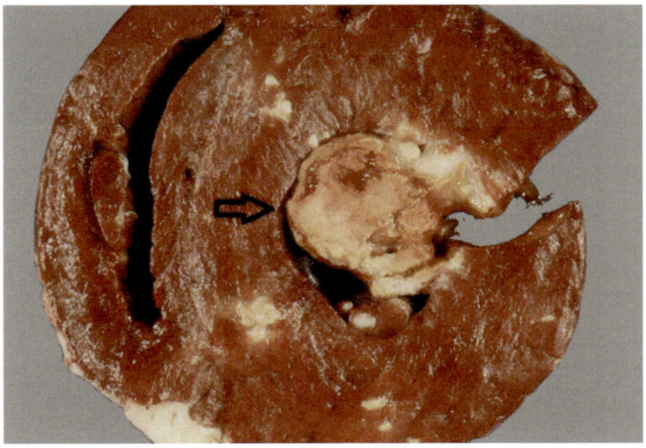

Fig. 4.18. Ox. Heart. Histophilosis. Sequestration of papillary muscle infarct. In addition to the multiple foci of myocardial inflammation, an infarct of the papillary muscle (arrow) has sequestered into the left ventricle. Rupture of such sequestrum may lead to sudden death. To re-emphasize, *Histophilus somni* in feedlot cattle appears to have a preference to affect the papillary muscle in the left ventricle most consistently.

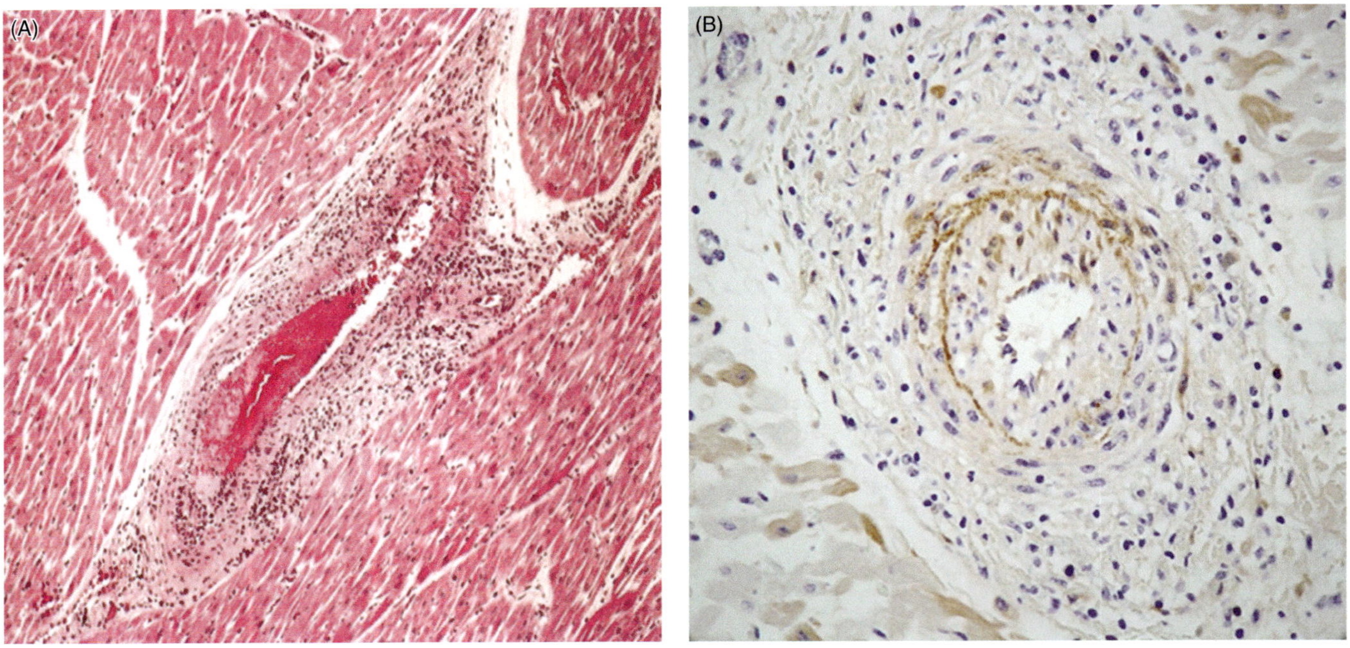

Fig. 4.19. Ox. Myocardium. Bovine viral diarrhea virus (BVDV)-induced arteritis. (A) An intracardiac artery is infiltrated and surrounded by moderate numbers of lymphocytes (H&E). (B) BVDV antigen is contained within the cytoplasm of media myocytes, and occasionally in the cytoplasm of histiocytes. This is a hallmark feature of some transient BVDV infection cases, but not of persistently infected (PI) animals (IHC).

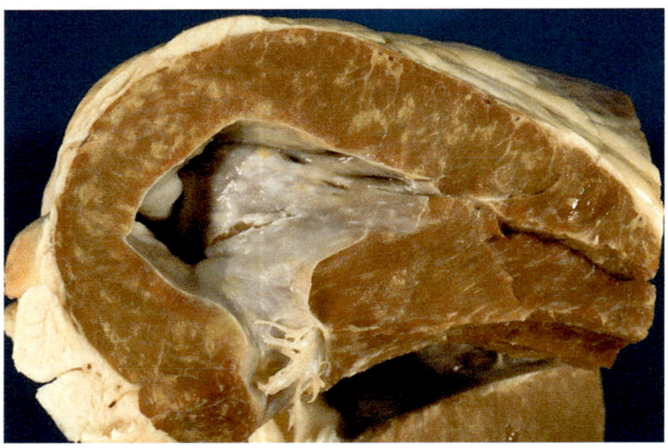

Fig. 4.21. Ox. Myocardium. Sarcocystosis. Granulomatous myocarditis. Multiple tan and slightly green-tinged foci occupy most of the myocardium. The green tinge results from the microscopic presence of eosinophils intermingled in the inflammation. It is hypothesized that the eosinophilic inflammation is an unusual host–parasite interaction to the presence of large numbers of bovine *Sarcocystis* spp. in the myocardium. Rarely, clinical signs ensue. The infection is diagnosed mostly as an incidental finding at slaughter. The protozoon has at least three host life cycles, with canids (*Sarcocystis bovicanis*), felids (*Sarcocystis bovifelis*) and primates (*Sarcocystis bovihominis*) as the definitive host and ruminants as an intermediate host.

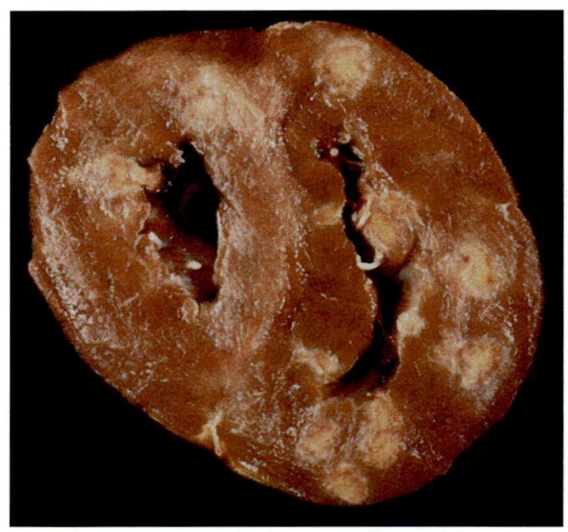

Fig. 4.20. Ox. Myocardium. Mycotic infarcts. On the cut section, multiple circumscribed and locally extensive angiocentric pale areas have resulted from mycotic thrombi in the coronary vasculature.

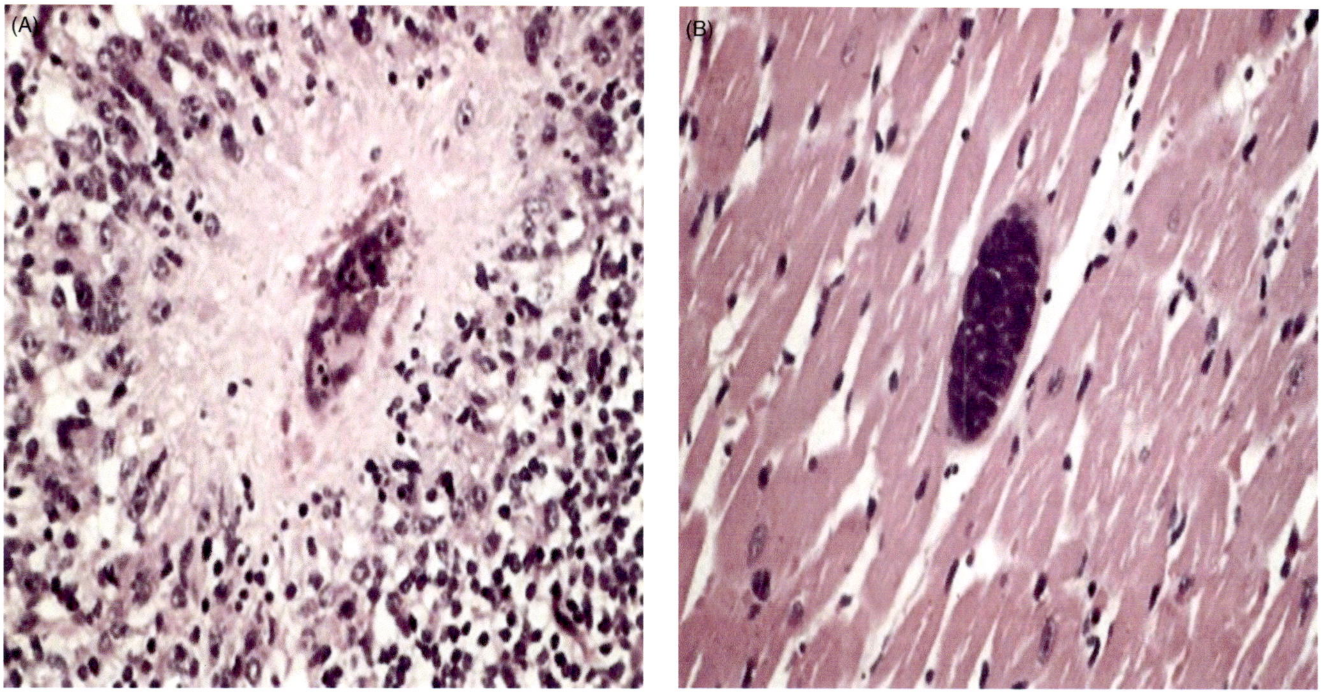

Fig. 4.22. Ox. Myocardium. Sarcocystosis. (A) Histologically, the inflammatory reaction to dead protozoa (center) in the myocardium is composed of histiocytes and lymphocytes, with eosinophils intermixed in earlier phases (H&E). (B) Very commonly in the bovine myocardium, one can detect intramyofiber *Sarcocystis* spp. cysts in cardiocytes without accompanying inflammation (H&E).

4.2.4 Endocardial disorders

4.2.4.1 Fibrosis and calcification

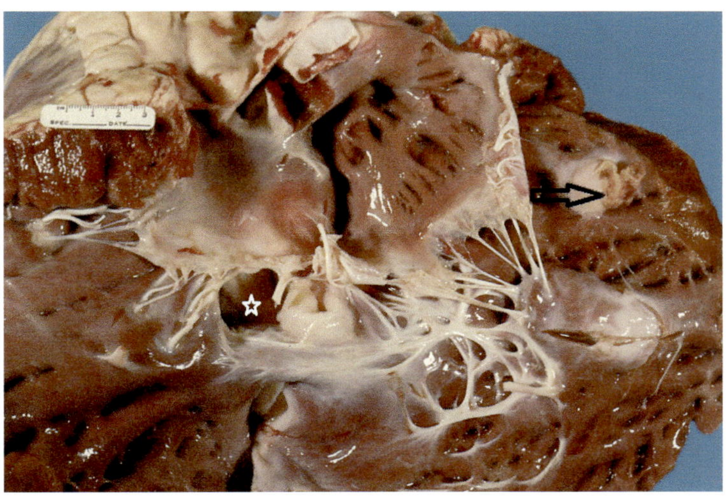

Fig. 4.24. Ox. Heart. Ventricular septal defect. Secondary endocardial fibrosis and myocardial abscess. The septal defect (asterisk) is fairly large, likely resulting in local laminar flow disturbances causing friction fibrosis in the surrounding endocardium. The myocardial abscess (arrow) is unrelated and likely of hematogenous origin.

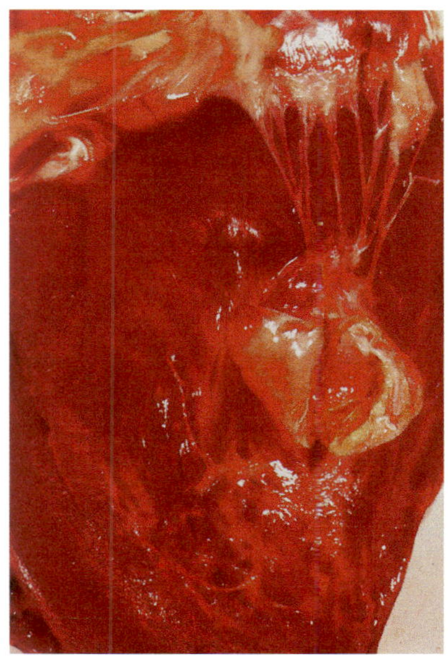

Fig. 4.23. Ox. Myocardium. Echinococcosis. Parasitic myocarditis. A solitary cyst of *Echinococcus granulosus* is lodged in the wall of the myocardium. The parasite mostly affects ruminant liver and lung. Livestock is the intermediate host. Domestic dogs play a key role in the transmission of this zoonotic tapeworm. *Cysticercus bovis* larvae also cause inflammatory changes in the myocardium. (Courtesy of the Department of Veterinary Pathology, WCVM, University of Saskatchewan, Saskatoon, Canada.)

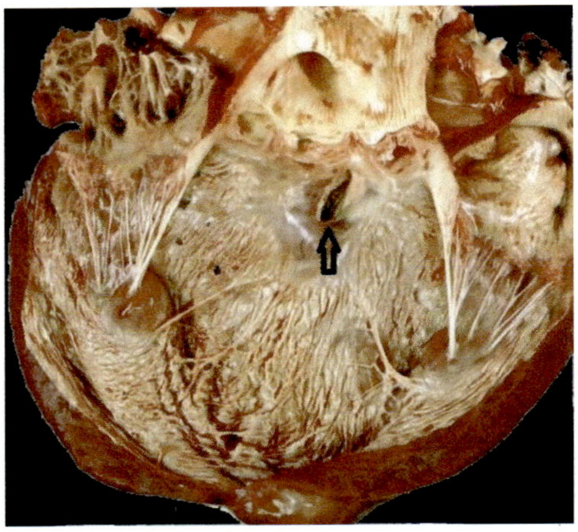

Fig. 4.25. Ox. Heart. Left atrium, ventricle, and ascending aorta. Endocardial and aortic calcification. Metastatic endocardial and intimal calcification develop from plant consumption such as *Cestrum diurnum*, *Solanum malacoxylon*, *Solanum glaucophylum*, or *Trisetum flavescens*, the latter being involved in the syndrome of enzootic calcinosis, since these plants contain calcinogenic glycosides. The lesions are also seen in vitamin D toxicosis resulting from a mixing error in the feed or excess vitamin D injections prepartum to prevent milk fever. They occasionally occur in bovine paratuberculosis (Johne's disease) as a by-product of activated macrophages (1,25-dihydroxcalciferol). Ventricular septal defect (arrow) is a second, unrelated diagnosis in this heart.

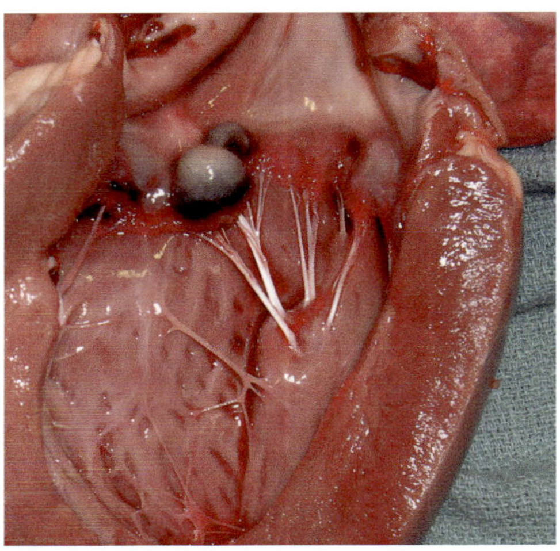

Fig. 4.26. Ox. Heart. Atrioventricular valve. Hematocyst. The red focal elevation within the mitral valve leaflet constitutes a blood-containing cyst often seen in neonate calves and increasing in number with age. (Courtesy of Dr P. Habecker, University of Pennsylvania, USA.)

4.2.4.2 Valvular cysts

Introduction: Hematocysts and lymphatic cysts are thought to be the result of segmental closure of blood or lymphatic vessels. Another suggestion implies that the cysts develop during the transition of fetal circulation to post-natal circulation following a sudden pressure change in the left ventricle. The cysts are of no clinical significance.

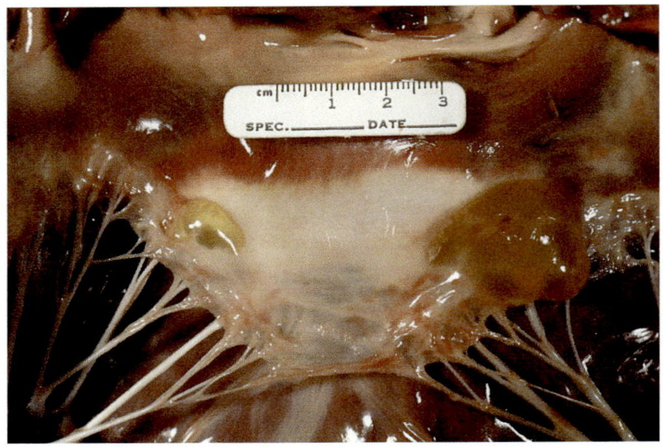

Fig. 4.27. Ox. Heart. Atrioventricular valve. Serous (lymphatic) cysts. Yellow fluid-containing cysts are located within the mitral valve leaflet. The serous fluid is biochemically similar to lymph.

4.2.4.3 Endocarditis

Introduction. Inflammation of the endocardium occurs at the valve and ventricular (mural) or atrial level. Valve involvement is more frequent and usually of bacterial etiology. Endocardial bacterial colonization follows a primary nidus of infection somewhere else in the body (mastitis, metritis, foot rot), with episodes of bacteremia being responsible for endocardial damage and inflammation.

Clinical signs. Fever, heart murmur, signs of heart failure, pain over ventral chest, drop of milk production.

Differential diagnosis. Traumatic reticulopericarditis.

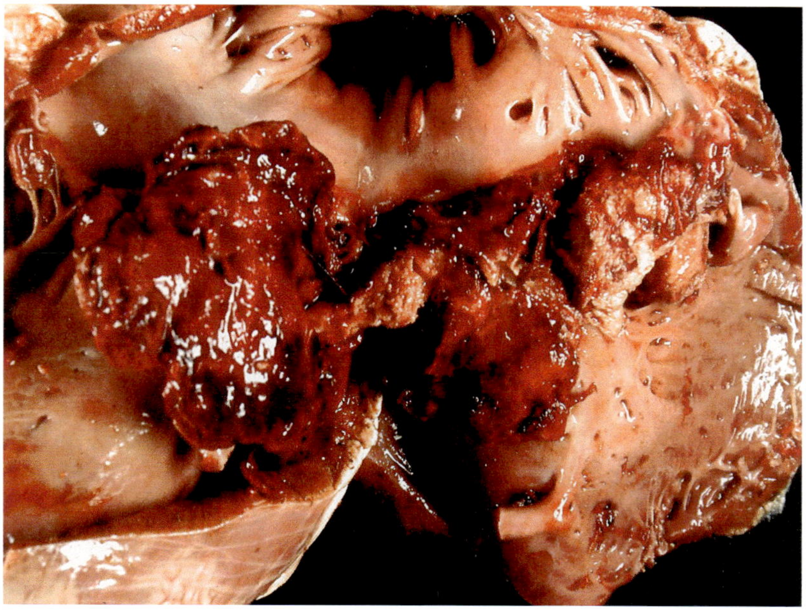

Fig. 4.28. Ox. Tricuspid valves. Bacterial valvular vegetative endocarditis. A cauliflower-like, friable red growth occupies the leaflets. The right anteroventral (AV) valve is the most affected in cattle, followed by the mitral valve. Emboli may shower into the circulation and, depending on the anatomic site of the valvulitis, infarcts may occur in the lung, spleen and kidney, usually with no clinical significance. Bacteria isolated from the endocardial lesion are *Trueperella pyogenes*, *Streptococcus* spp., *Staphylococcus* spp. and gram-negative organisms.

4.2.5 Congestive heart failure

Introduction. A healthy myocardium initially responds to damage with an increased compensatory workload, and thus stimulates myocardial hypertrophy. The ventricular walls become thicker. Hypertrophy of the left ventricle gives the heart a larger appearance. Right ventricular hypertrophy results in a rounded appearance of the heart and in double apex. When the limits of cardiac reserve are exhausted, cardiac decompensation, reduced cardiac output, and congestive heart failure occur. The consequences of a failing heart are best seen in the pulmonary and systemic vascular (venous) systems. These vascular changes induce the clinical syndrome of congestive heart failure.

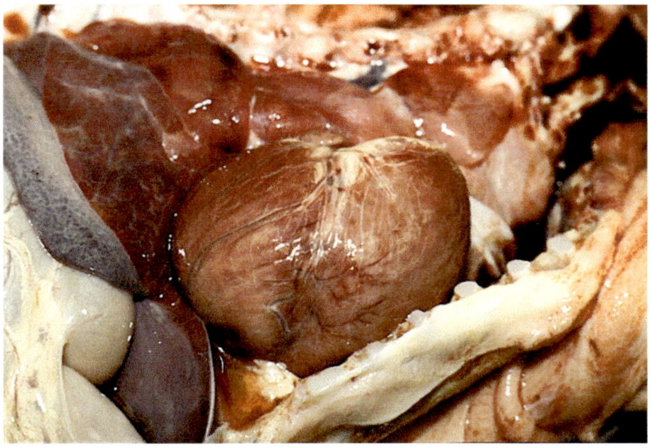

Fig. 4.29. Ox. Heart. Cardiomegaly. The enlarged heart exhibits a rounded appearance and has a double apex. The animal was diagnosed with goiter.

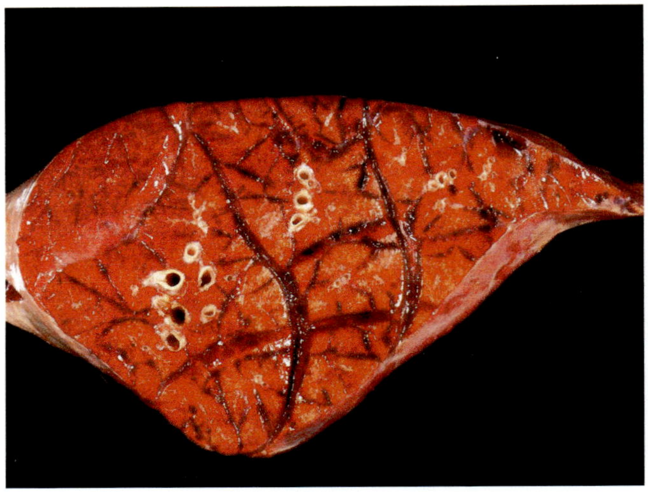

Fig. 4.30. Ox. Lung. Left-sided heart failure. Pulmonary edema mixed with red blood cells in interlobular spaces. The interlobular interstitium is widened markedly by fluid. The pulmonary cut section is moist.

4.2.5.1 Brisket (high-altitude) disease

The initial cause for brisket disease is pulmonary hypertension resulting from alveolar hypoxia. It leads to right-sided congestive heart failure.

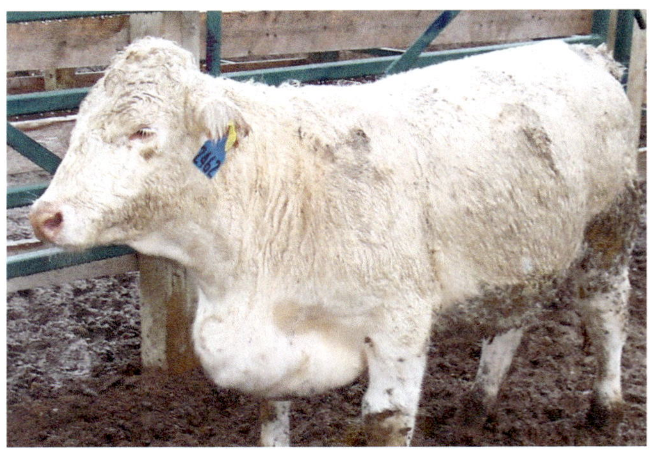

Fig. 4.31. Ox. Body. Brisket. Brisket disease. The skin over the brisket is distended due to subcutaneous edema.

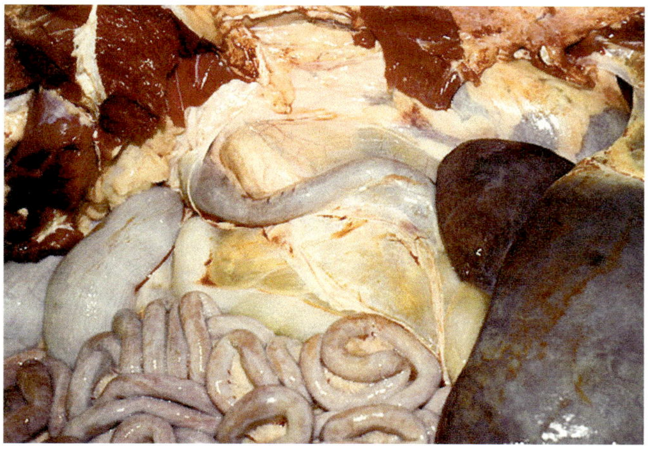

Fig. 4.32. Ox. Abdomen. Right-sided heart failure. Mesocolonic edema. Serous effusion. A straw-color fluid has accumulated in the abdominal cavity due to venous congestion. The liver is enlarged from congestion.

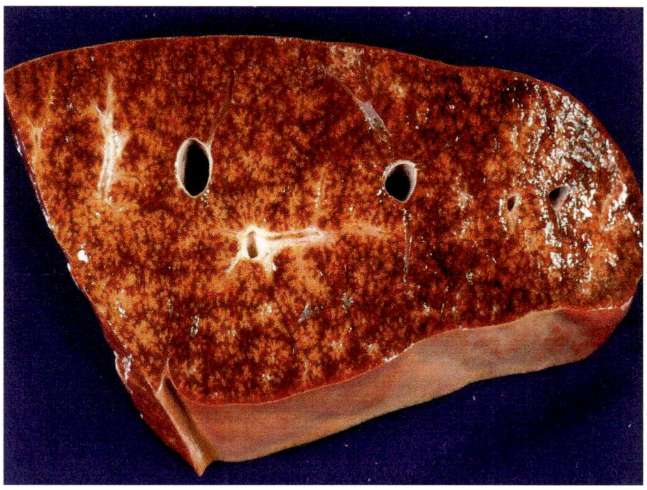

Fig. 4.33. Ox. Liver. Right-sided heart failure. Chronic passive congestion. The cut surface of the liver exhibits a 'nutmeg pattern' of periacinar necrosis and damage, but intact periportal, pale parenchyma, signalizing passive venous congestion.

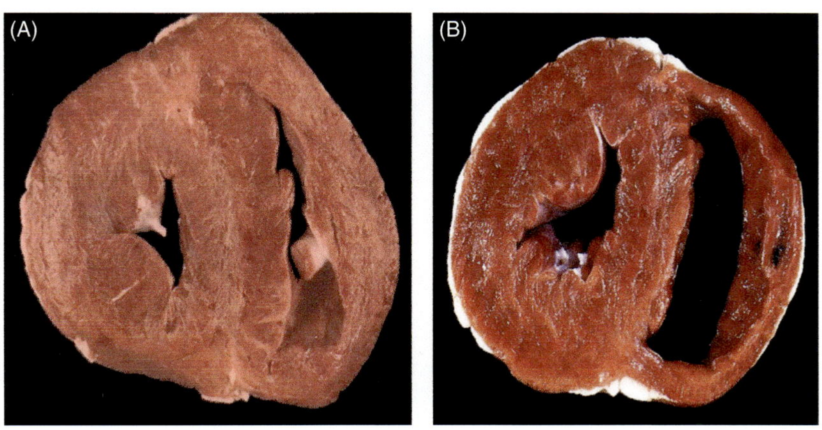

Fig. 4.34. Ox. Heart. Right ventricular hypertrophy (cor pulmonale) versus normal ventricular dimension. (A) The right ventricle is uniformly thickened, with narrowing of its lumen when compared with a normal heart. Note the moderator band hypertrophy on the left as well. (B) The normal ratio between left and right ventricular width is considered to be 3:1.

Fact Sheet: Cardiac Failure

- Left-sided failure (myocarditis, myocardial necrosis, cardiomyopathy, mitral/aortic valve disease, congenital heart diseases).
  - Acute = pulmonary congestion, edema.
  - Chronic = chronic lung congestion, chronic edema, heart failure cells in alveoli, fibrosis.
  - Chronic form often results in both left- and right-side failure due to pulmonary hypertension.
- Right-sided failure (pulmonary hypertension, cardiomyopathy, tricuspid and pulmonary valve disease, congenital heart disease).
  - Acute = enlargement and congestion of spleen and liver, sometimes mesocolonic edema.
  - Chronic = nutmeg liver, edema, ascites.
- Cor pulmonale – right-sided heart failure resulting from severe lung disease, causing pulmonary hypertension and right ventricular hypertrophy. Its prevalence has increased in North American feedlot cattle. Brisket disease is an example.

4.2.6 Neoplasia

Introduction. Primary tumors of the heart (rhabdomyoma, rhabomyosarcoma) are rare in ruminants. Multicentric lymphosarcoma is the most important secondary tumor affecting the heart of adult cattle. Peripheral nerve sheath tumors (schwannomas) originating from cardiac nerves are rare, and usually an incidental finding.

Clinical signs. Arrhythmia, cardiac failure, jugular venous distension, sudden death.

Differential diagnosis. Excessive adipose tissue.

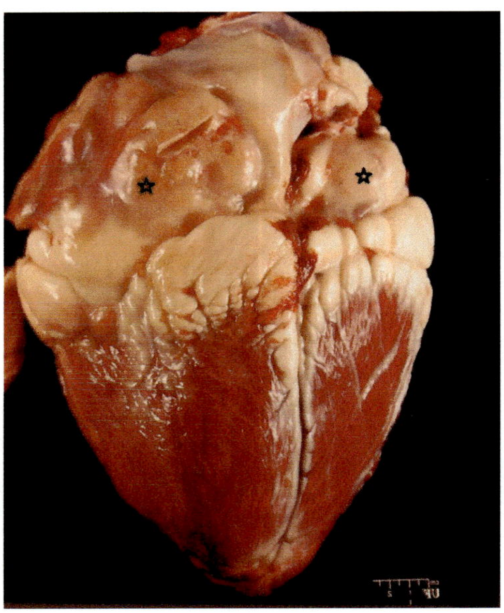

Fig. 4.35. Ox. Heart. Lymphosarcoma. Gray-yellow glistening, bulging tissue (asterisks) is eminent in both atria and blend into the adipose tissue below in the coronary groove. A common site for this tumor is the right atrium.

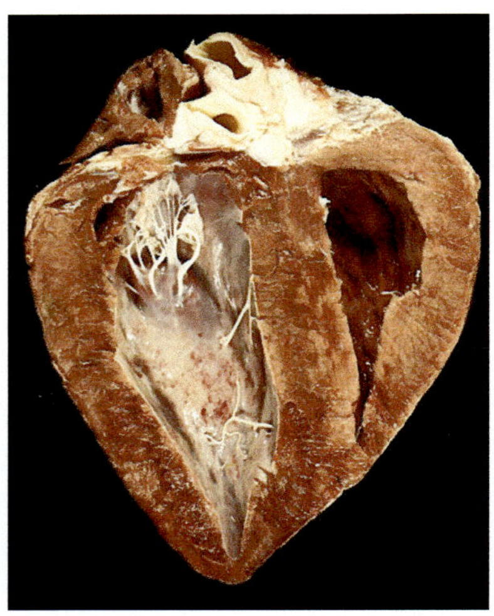

Fig. 4.36. Ox. Heart. Lymphosarcoma. Gray-yellow tissue has disseminated into myocardium of left atrium and both ventricles. The endocardium of the left ventricle bulges from gray tissue in subendocardial myocardium. Consider chronic inflammation in the differential diagnosis.

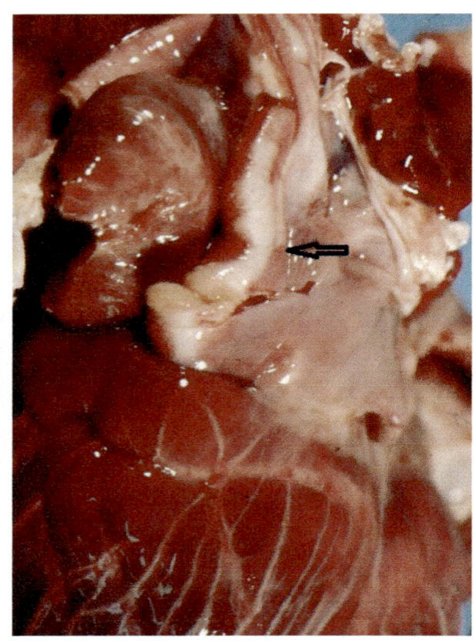

Fig. 4.37. Ox. Heart. Neurofibromatosis (multicentric schwannoma). A tubular, segmented growth (arrow) extends between the right auricle and pulmonary outflow tract at the base of the heart.

4.3 VESSELS

Introduction. Inflammatory disorders (vasculitis) of vessels can be divided into infectious and non-infectious causes and are classified as arteritis, phlebitis, and lymphangitis when specifically involving any one of the three categories of vessels. Non-infectious causes for distal extremity vasculopathy are toxic principles such as ergotism and fescue grass toxicosis. Infectious causes for vasculitis are viruses such as BVDV, MCF, and bluetongue. The non-thrombosing lymphocytic vasculitis that occurs in transient BVDV infections is seen most commonly in the myocardium, but also in the lung, ileum, and kidney. Vasculitis in PI cattle is rare. Bacteria such as *Histophilus somni*, *Salmonella* spp., *Mycobacterium avium* subsp. *paratuberculosis* (lymphangitis), rickettsia such as *E. ruminantium*, and chlamydophila such as in sporadic bovine encephalomyocarditis (SBE) have to be considered as etiologic agents. Some examples are presented in the respective disease chapters.

Fact Sheet: Bovine Infectious Diseases Causing Vasculitis

Viral	■ Bovine malignant catarrhal fever
	■ Bluetongue
	■ Bovine viral diarrhea
Bacterial	■ Histophilosis
	■ Salmonellosis
	■ Paratuberculosis
Rickettsial	■ Heartwater
Chlamydophila	■ Sporadic bovine encephalomyocarditis

4.3.1 Arteries

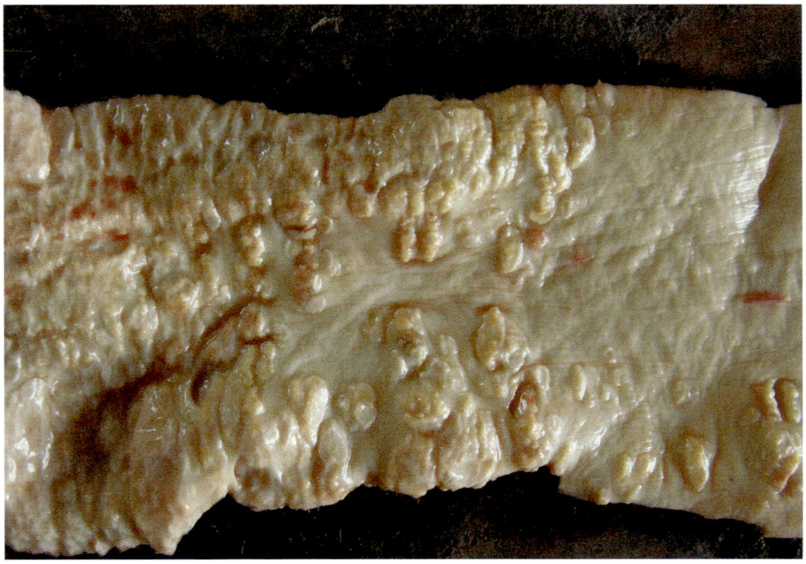

Fig. 4.38. Ox. Aorta. *Solanum malacoxylon*. Calcification. Several gritty plaques are located within the subintima. In Latin America, the condition is known as enteque seco. Additionally, tendons and joints are affected, causing lameness. (Courtesy of Prof L. Minatel, University of Buenos Aires, Argentina.)

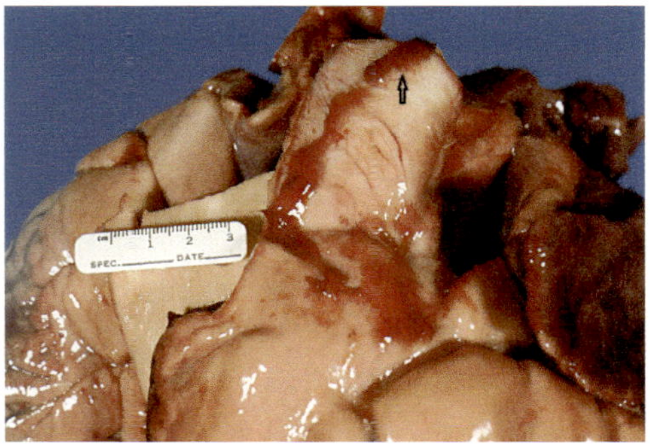

Fig. 4.39. Ox. Base of heart. Aorta. Granulation tissue. Fleshy elevations (arrow) are present in the adventitia of the ascending aorta at the base of the heart. The condition is a common incidental finding and likely induced by friction of the moving aorta.

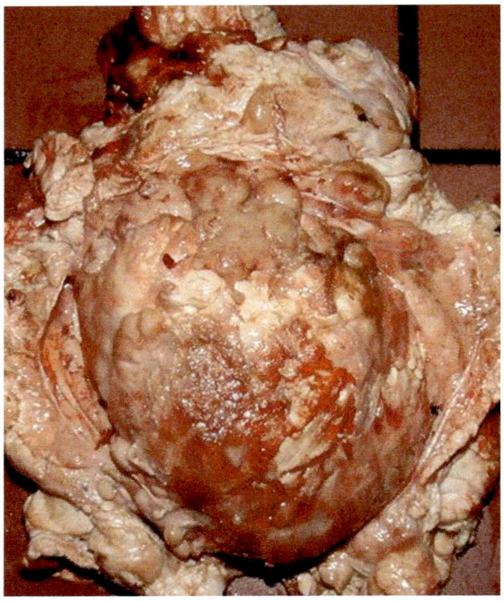

Fig. 4.41. Ox. Heart. Fibrovascular epicarditis and pericarditis. This case composed of extensive sterile fibrovascular tissue resulting in congestive heart failure. Differential diagnoses: traumatic reticulopericarditis; lymphosarcoma.

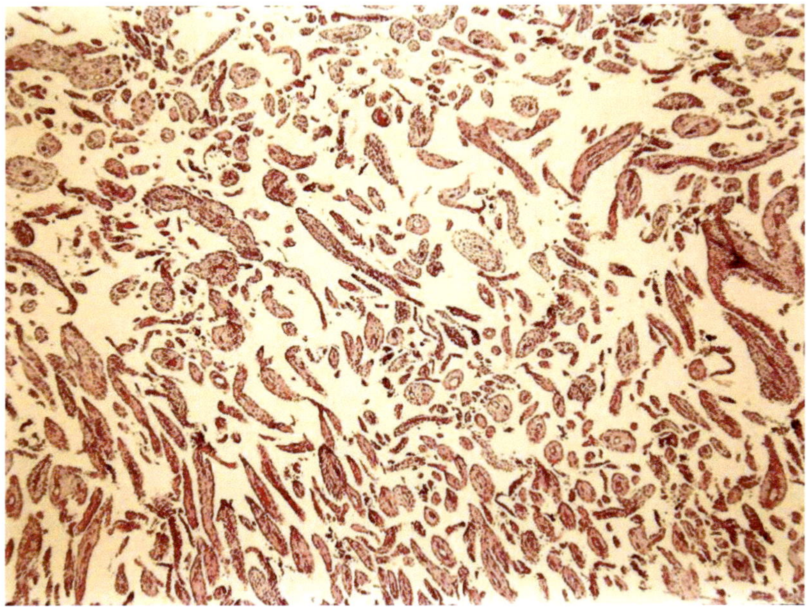

Fig. 4.40. Ox. Aorta. Granulation tissue. The microscopic appearance is characterized by fibrovascular proliferation with minimal inflammation (H&E).

4.3.1.1 Marfan syndrome

Aortic rupture and dissecting aneurysm of the major cardiac vessels in cattle have been described as pathologic manifestations of Marfan syndrome, a mutation of the gene of connective tissue fibrillin-1 that also occurs in humans.

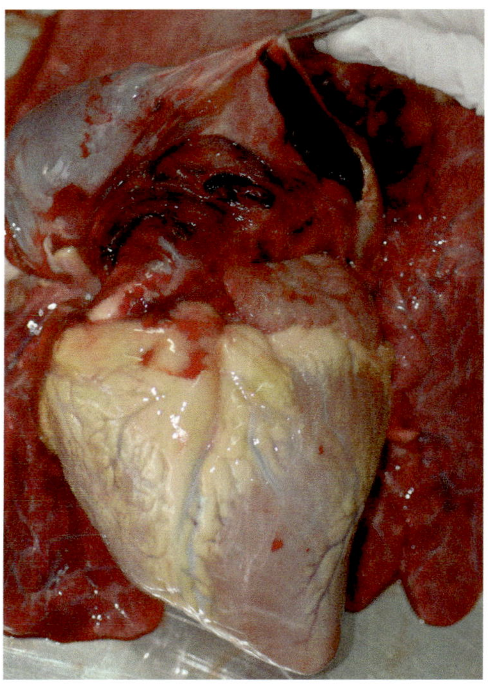

Fig. 4.42. Ox. Base of heart. Marfan syndrome. Pulmonary artery. Aneurysm and rupture. The pulmonary artery is dilated. Hemorrhage is present in the adventitia and pericardial sac (cardiac tamponade). (Courtesy of Dr E. Lepri, University of Perugia, Italy.)

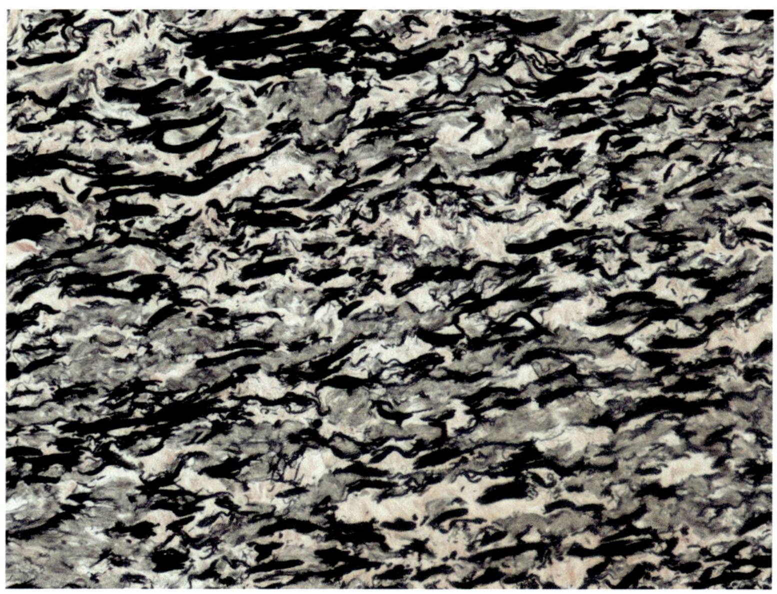

Fig. 4.43. Ox. Marfan syndrome. Artery. Elastic fibers in the media are fragmented, and are without parallel orientation. They are short and thick. Verhoeff–van Gieson silver impregnation. (Courtesy of Dr K. Potter, Washington State University, USA.)

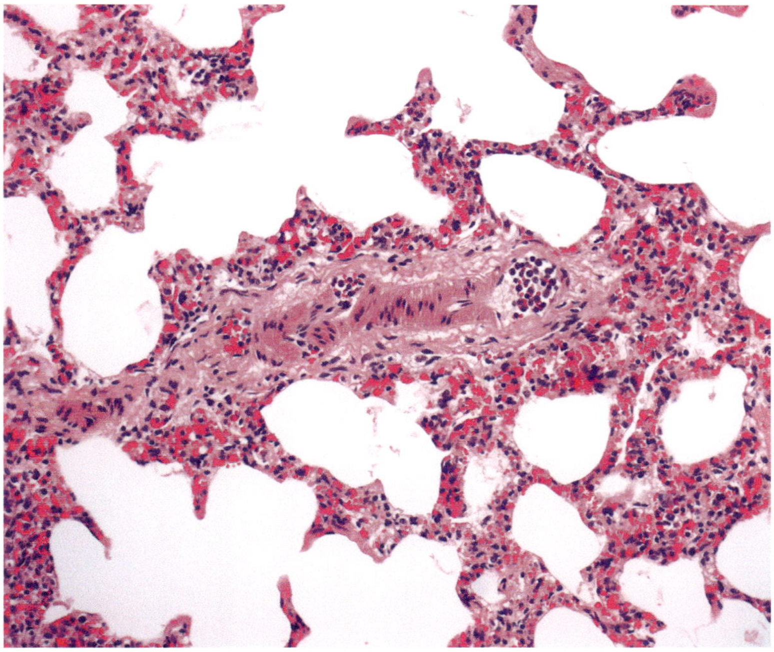

Fig. 4.44. Ox. Pulmonary arteriole. Normal spiral muscle. The blebs show up as hypercontracted state in chronic alveolar hypoxia or stress conditions. Specific examples are acute frothy bloat and atypical interstitial pneumonia (AIP) (H&E).

4.3.2 Veins

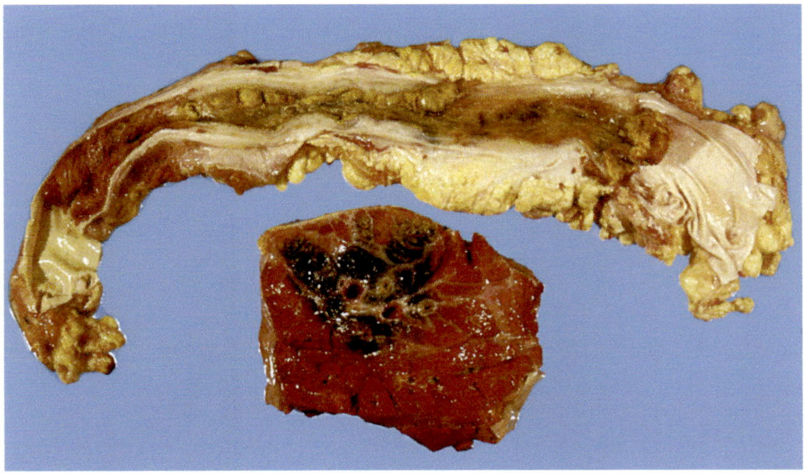

Fig. 4.45. Ox. Jugular vein. Septic thrombosis. Venipuncture is the main cause for septic thrombosis leading to lung embolism, with usually no clinical consequences. Sometimes, abscesses and gangrenous pneumonia (as seen in this image) ensue. Omphalophlebitis in neonates and its clinical consequences are discussed in Chapter 1: Diseases of Neonates and Calves. Vena cava thrombosis is discussed in Chapter 3: Diseases of the Respiratory System.

4.3.3 Lymphatics

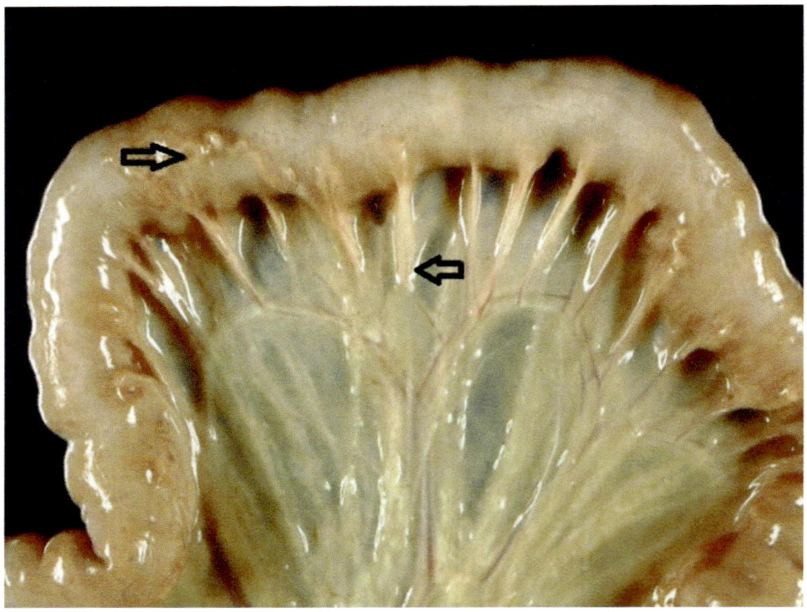

Fig. 4.46. Ox. Mesenteric lymphatics. Bovine paratuberculosis (Johne's disease). Granulomatous lymphangitis. Infection with *Mycobacterium avium* subsp. *paratuberculosis* primarily targets the small intestinal tract. From there, the macrophage-phagocytized mycobacteria are drained via the lymphatics to the regional mesenteric lymph nodes, causing a granulomatous reaction in mesenteric lymphatics and mesenteric lymph nodes. Gross evidence of mycobacterial inflammation is present, both in the intestinal subserosa (arrow) and by a beaded appearance of the thickened streaming lymphatics in the mesentery (arrow).

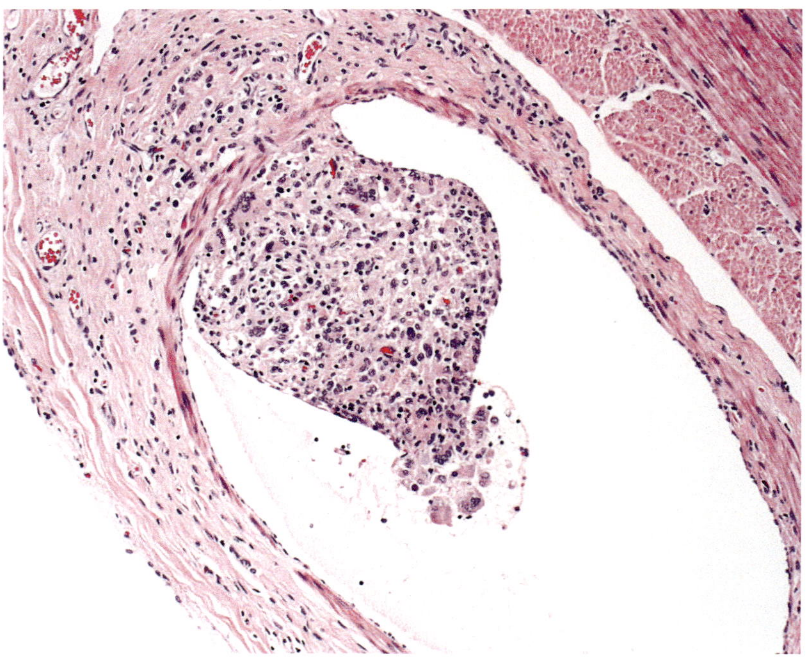

Fig. 4.47. Ox. Lymphatic vessel. Bovine paratuberculosis (Johne's disease). Granulomatous lymphangitis. An intravascular granuloma composed of macrophages, giant cells, and lymphocytes is attached to the lymphatic wall. There is mild perilymphatic lymphocytic inflammation (H&E).

4.3.4 Neoplasia

Introduction. Hemangioma/hemangiosarcoma are examples of vascular tumors. They are of endothelial origin. Such tumors can occur at any anatomic site containing blood vessels. They are very sporadic in cattle, perhaps due to lack of longevity.

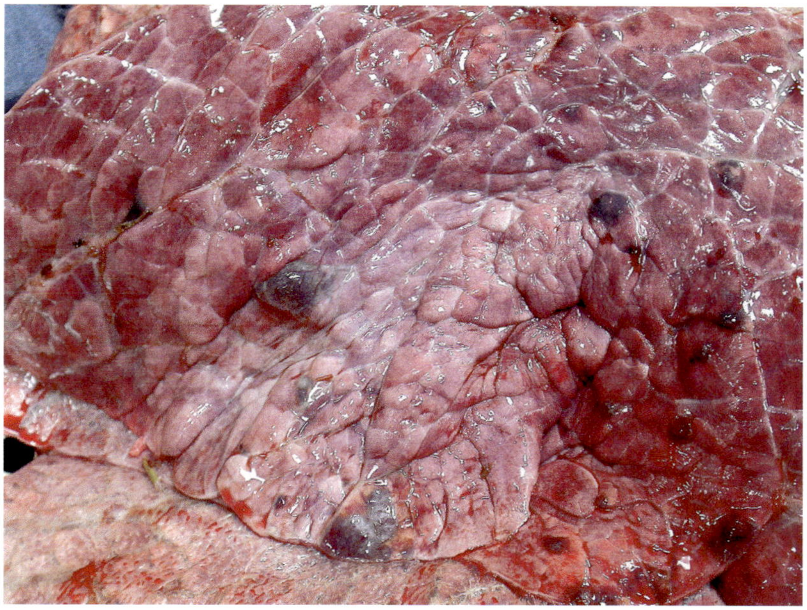

Fig. 4.49. Ox. Lung. Metastatic hemangiosarcoma. Several red-blue nodules are scattered within the lung parenchyma. The primary site is unknown.

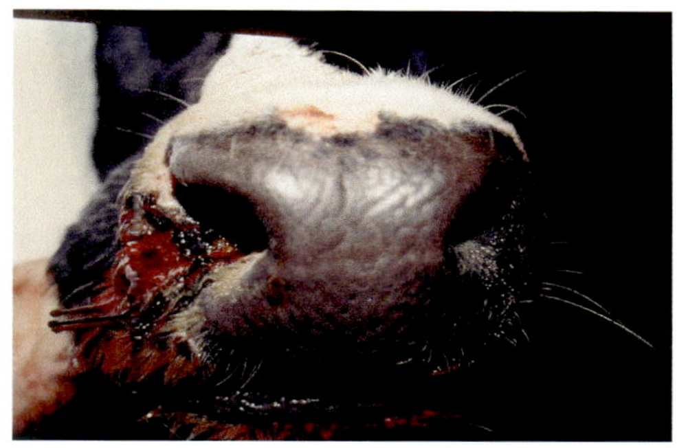

Fig. 4.48. Ox. Nostril. Dermal hemangiosarcoma. A focal red, ulcerated, poorly delineated growth protrudes from the nostril.

SUGGESTED READING

Bastianelo, S.S., McGregor, H., Penrith, M.L. and Fourie, N. (1996) A chronic cardiomyopathy in feedlot cattle attributed to toxic levels of salinomycin in the feed. *Journal of South African Veterinary Association* 67, 38–41.

Braun, U., Diener, M., Hibe, B., Busch, M., Bischoff, M. and Brosi, G. (2000) Enzootic calcinosis in 16 cows from 6 dairy farms in Unterengadin. *Schweizer Archiv fuer Tierheilkunde* 142, 333–338.

Davis, T.Z., Stegelmeier, B.L., Panter, K.E., Cook, D., Gardner, D.R. and Hall, J.O. (2012) Toxicokinetics and pathology of plant-associated acute selenium toxicosis in steers. *Journal of Veterinary Diagnostic Investigation* 24, 319–327.

Haines, D.M., Moline, K.M., Sargent, R.A., Campbell, J.R., Myers, D.J. and Doig, P.A. (2004) Immunohistochemical study of *Hemophilus somnus*, *Mycoplasma bovis*, *Mannheimia haemolytica* and bovine viral diarrhea virus in death losses due to myocarditis in feedlot cattle. *Canadian Veterinary Journal* 45, 231–234.

Harris, F.W. and Janzen, E.D. (1989) The *Haemophilus somnus* disease complex (Histophilosis): a review. *Canadian Veterinary Journal* 30, 816–822.

Marcatto, P.S., Benazzi, C., Bettini, G., Masi, M., Della Salda, L., *et al.* (1996) Blood and serous cysts in the atrioventricular valves of the bovine heart. *Veterinary Pathology* 33, 14–21.

Neary, J.M., Booker, C.W., Wildman, B.K. and Morley, P.S. (2016) Right-sided congestive heart failure in North American feedlot cattle. *Journal of Veterinary Internal Medicine* 30, 26–334.

O'Toole, D., Alien, T., Hunter, R. and Corbeil, L.B. (2009) Diagnostic exercise: myocarditis due to *Histophilus somni* in feedlot and background cattle. *Veterinary Pathology* 46, 1015–1017.

Penumatsa, K.C., Toksoz, D., Warburton, R.R., Hilmer, A.J., Liu, T., *et al.* (2014) Role of hypoxia-induced transglutaminase 2 in pulmonary artery smooth muscle proliferation. *American Journal of Lung Cell Molecular Physiology* 307, 576–585.

Potter, K.A. and Besser, T.E. (1994) Cardiovascular lesions in bovine Marfan syndrome. *Veterinary Pathology* 31, 501–509.

Potter, K.A., Hoffman, Y., Sakai, L.Y., Byers, P.H., Besser, T.E. and Milewicz, D.M. (1993) Abnormal fibrillin metabolism in bovine Marfan syndrome. *American Journal of Pathology* 142, 803–810.

Uzal, F.A., Paramidani, M., Assis, R., Morris, W. and Miyakawa, M.F. (2003) Outbreak of clostridial myocarditis in calves. *Veterinary Record* 152, 143–146.

CHAPTER 5

Diseases of the Gastrointestinal Tract

5.1 Diseases of the Oral Cavity
- 5.1.1 Anomalies
- 5.1.2 Inflammation
  - 5.1.2.1 Viral
  - 5.1.2.2 Bacterial
- 5.1.3 Dental diseases
- 5.1.4 Neoplasia

5.2 Diseases of the Esophagus
- 5.2.1 Obstruction (choke)
- 5.2.2 Trauma
- 5.2.3 Inflammation
- 5.2.4 Endoparasites
- 5.2.5 Neoplasia

5.3 Diseases of the Forestomachs
- 5.3.1 Metabolic disorders
  - 5.3.1.1 Rumen lactic acidosis
  - 5.3.1.2 Tympany (bloat)
  - 5.3.1.3 Urea toxicity (ammonia toxicosis)
  - 5.3.1.4 Ruminal papillary hypertrophy/ hyperplasia
- 5.3.2 Obstruction
  - 5.3.2.1 Ruminal indigestion
- 5.3.3 Inflammation
  - 5.3.3.1 Traumatic reticulitis
  - 5.3.3.2 Opportunistic pathogens secondary to lactic acidosis
  - 5.3.3.3 Rumen infected with BVDV
- 5.3.4 Endoparasites
- 5.3.5 Neoplasia
- 5.3.6 Miscellaneous disorders

5.4 Diseases of the Abomasum
- 5.4.1 Changes in position
  - 5.4.1.1 Abomasal displacement
  - 5.4.1.2 Abomasal torsion/volvulus
- 5.4.2 Obstruction
  - 5.4.2.1 Impaction
  - 5.4.2.2 Vagal indigestion (Hoflund syndrome)
- 5.4.3 Erosions and ulcers
- 5.4.4 Inflammation
- 5.4.5 Endoparasites
  - 5.4.5.1 Haemonchosis
  - 5.4.5.2 Ostertagiosis
  - 5.4.5.3 Trichostrongylus axei
- 5.4.6 Neoplasia

5.5 Diseases of the Intestinal Tract
- 5.5.1 Anomalies
- 5.5.2 Displacements and obstruction
- 5.5.3 Inflammation
  - 5.5.3.1 Catarrhal enteritis
  - 5.5.3.2 Hemorrhagic enteritis
  - 5.5.3.3 Fibrinonecrotic enteritis
  - 5.5.3.4 Erosive-ulcerative-necrotic enteritis
  - 5.5.3.5 Granulomatous enteritis
- 5.5.4 Intestinal endoparasites
  - 5.5.4.1 Nematodes
  - 5.5.4.2 Ascarids
  - 5.5.4.3 Cestodes
  - 5.5.4.4 Protozoa
- 5.5.5 Neoplasia
- 5.5.6 Miscellaneous
  - 5.5.6.1 Hemorrhagic bowel syndrome (HBS)
  - 5.5.6.2 Rectal perforation
  - 5.5.6.3 Diaphragmatic hernia
  - 5.5.6.4 Intestinal droplets

5.6 Diseases of the Peritoneum
- 5.6.1 Fat necrosis
- 5.6.2 Inflammation

INTRODUCTION

Great economic losses are inflicted to the cattle industry from disorders of the gastrointestinal tract that occur individually or as herd outbreaks on a larger scale. It is paramount to identify the cause(s) of enteric diseases quickly through targeted clinical investigation and thorough necropsy examination, to prevent spread and devastating losses. The gastrointestinal tract of ruminants is voluminous and occupies most of the abdominal cavity. For an organized approach for diagnosis at necropsy, segments of the gastrointestinal tract are divided in this chapter into upper gastrointestinal tract to include the oral cavity, esophagus, forestomachs and abomasum, and lower gastrointestinal tract, to include small and large intestines. Decomposition of the gastrointestinal tract occurs quickly after death, and the goal is to perform the necropsy as fresh as possible to avoid distortion of lesions and misinterpretation of changes from the normal appearance.

5.1 DISEASES OF THE ORAL CAVITY

5.1.1 Anomalies

The development of an anatomic normal oral cavity depends largely on the organized growth of a number of embryologic processes. Failure of integration and of fusion may lead to a variety of malformations, the most frequent being facial fissures and palatoschisis, which is illustrated in Chapter 1: Diseases of Neonates and Calves.

5.1.2 Inflammation

The recognition of morphologic types of inflammation may be extremely informative for the presence of specific etiologic factors. The following forms of inflammation can be distinguished in the oral cavity: catarrhal, vesicular, erosive-ulcerative, fibrinous, papular, pyogranulomatous.

5.1.2.1 Viral

VESICULAR – EROSIVE – ULCERATIVE

Bovine viral diarrhea (BVD)

Introduction. Bovine viral diarrhea (BVD) and mucosal disease (animals affected between 6 and 18 months of age) are two disease entities caused by the bovine viral diarrhea virus (BVDV), a highly mutable RNA virus and a member of the *Pestivirus* genus of the family *Flaviviridae*. Since its discovery in 1946, the virus has been one of the most challenging, most complex and crucial bovine infectious agents of our times, inflicting severe economic losses. It is characterized by a variety of epidemiologic manifestations. Although detectable through various diagnostic methods, the virus escapes effective treatment via vaccination and control modalities. In addition to the gastrointestinal tract, the virus has tropism for multiple other organ systems and tissues, including lymphoid, nervous, vascular, epithelial and reproductive system. Case examples will be presented with the respective organ systems.

Two isolates of the virus are recognized on cell culture: the non-cytopathic (ncp) and cytopathic (cp) biotypes. Unrelated to the biotype, two genotypes (BVDV-1 and BVDV-2) with subgenotypes (1a–1u) and (2a–2c) are identified through genetic sequencing. These have different genetic and antigenic properties. Genotype 2 is more virulent and causes disease.

Two forms of clinical BVDV are recognized in cattle: mucosal disease and severe acute BVD, associated with a non-cytopathic, virulent BVDV-2. In Europe, an atypical pestivirus, designated as BVDV-3 or HoBi-like virus, has emerged.

Mucosal disease (MD) occurs when an animal persistently infected with a non-cytopathic biotype post-natally is exposed (superinfected) to a second cytopathic strain that might have mutated from a non-cytopathic strain. Outbreaks of severe hemorrhagic diathesis are caused by an ncp thrombocytopenic strain of BVDV.

Vertical and horizontal transmissions of the virus occur. *In utero* transmission between days 30 and 120 of gestation leads to a persistently infected (PI) animal (non-cytopathic strain). These animals are lifelong carriers of the ncp BVDV and persistent shedders, making control of the virus in a herd extremely difficult. BVDV distribution in these animals is omnipresent in multiple organ systems of the body, with the virus being the initiator for the development of other infectious diseases via immunosuppression.

For the pathologist, virus antigen distribution can be demonstrated best with the help of indirect immunohistochemistry in infected tissues. Persistent infection is characterized by abundant virus antigen in numerous tissues, including the skin and brain. Transient infections are not. The present method of choice is the ear notch test, with the skin sample subjected to indirect immunohistochemistry (IHC) (see BVDV Fact Sheet below and also the discussion in Chapters 3, 4, and 12).

In feedlot cattle, it should always be determined first if the BVDV infection is the PI form or a transient infection. If the latter prevails, one should look for a vasculitis/perivasculitis or myocarditis histologically. If there is a severe or unusual manifestation of another infectious disease, it should be kept in mind that a transient BVD infection may be involved.

Clinical signs. (oral cavity). Sialorrhea, reduced food uptake.

Differential diagnoses. (oral vesicles/erosions). Foot and mouth disease (FMD), vesicular stomatitis (VS), bovine papular stomatitis (BPS), malignant catarrhal fever (MCF), bluetongue virus (BT), infectious bovine rhinotracheitis (IBR), rinderpest (officially eradicated).

Fact Sheet: Bovine Viral Diarrhea Virus (BVDV)

■ Virus:	genus Pestivirus; family Flaviviridae
■ Classification:	biotypes pathogenic (cp) and non-pathogenic (ncp) genotypes type 1 with 11 subgenotypes and type 2 with 2 subgenotypes
■ Infection forms:	acute transient persistently infected (PI) mucosal disease (MD)
■ Virus tropism:	pancytotropic (lymphoid, CNS, reproductive, digestive, megakaryocyte (thrombocytopenic strain)
■ Transmission:	secretions – excretions semen
■ Diagnosis:	virus isolation qRT-PCR IHC (skin or any other tissue) serology (antigen capture ELISA)
■ DDX:	MCF, IBR, bluetongue, salmonellosis
■ Control:	eradication of PI vaccination
■ Gross pathology:	gastrointestinal linear erosions Peyer's patch necrosis coronitis serosal hemorrhages (thrombocytopenic strain) cerebellar (pulmonary, renal) hypoplasia abortions
■ Hallmark histology:	multicentric (multi-organ) arteritis

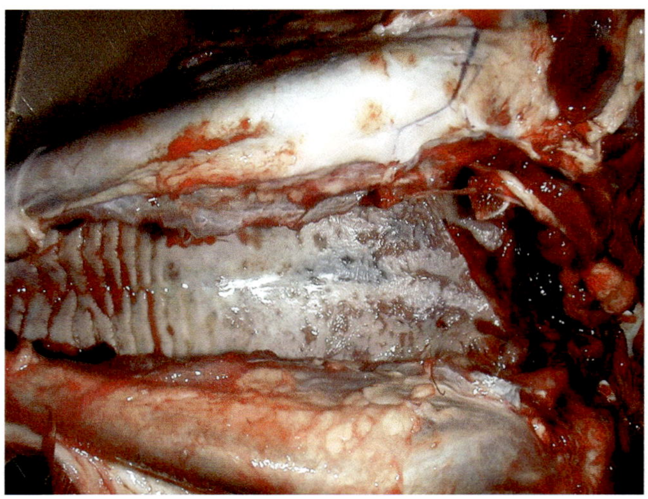

Fig. 5.1. Ox. Hard palate. Bovine viral diarrhea virus (BVDV). Erosive-ulcerative palatine stomatitis. Multiple shallow erosions are present. Additional BVDV changes in the oral cavity include erosive-ulcerative cheilitis and stomatitis, as well as blunting of oral papillae.

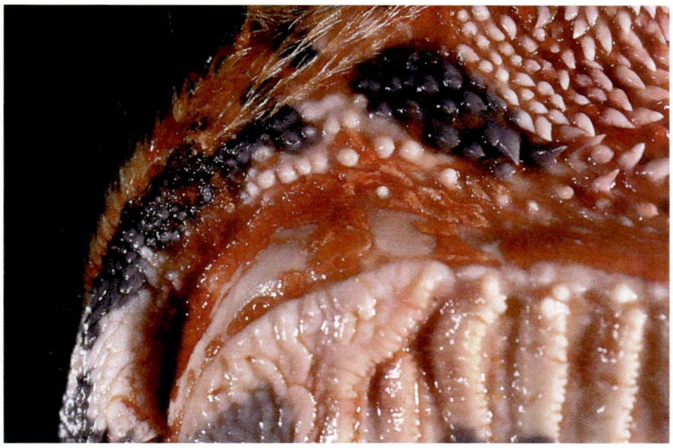

Fig. 5.2. Ox. Oral vestibule. Bovine viral diarrhea (BVDV). Erosive and ulcerative gingivitis. Gingiva is mottled and disrupted with islands of normal oral mucosa left below papillae.

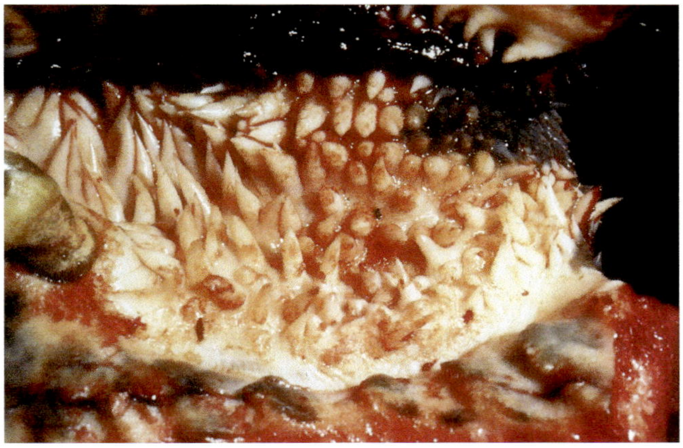

Fig. 5.3. Ox. Oral cavity. Bovine viral diarrhea (BVDV). Papillae blunting. Oral papillae vary in height, with some of them being reduced to blebs. (Courtesy of Dr R. Whitlock, University of Pennsylvania, USA.)

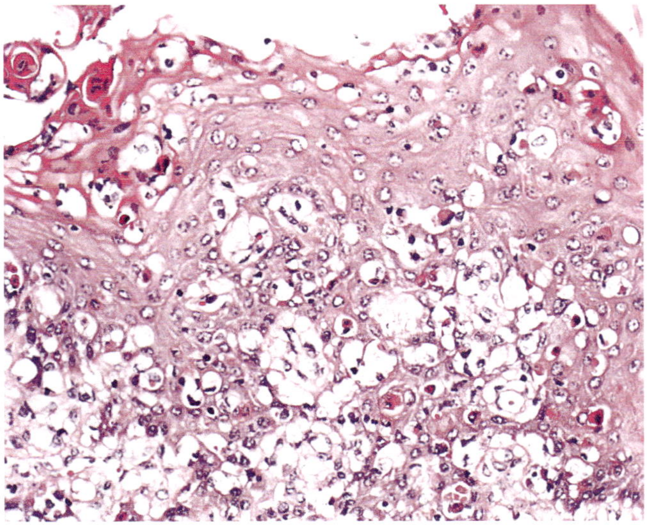

Fig. 5.4. Ox. Oral mucosa. Bovine viral diarrhea (BVDV). Erosive stomatitis. Vacuolar degeneration, dissociation and spongiosis of epithelial cells. Single cell death is a cytopathic effect but not diagnostic for BVDV (H&E).

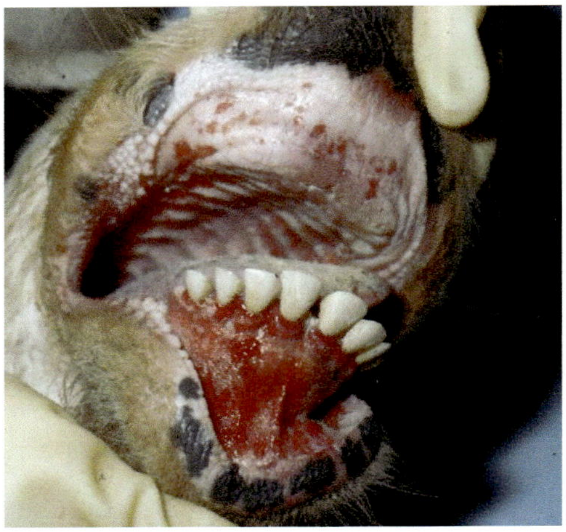

Fig. 5.5. Ox. Mouth. Bluetongue. Erosive, hemorrhagic gingivitis. Gums contain erosions and multifocal hemorrhage.

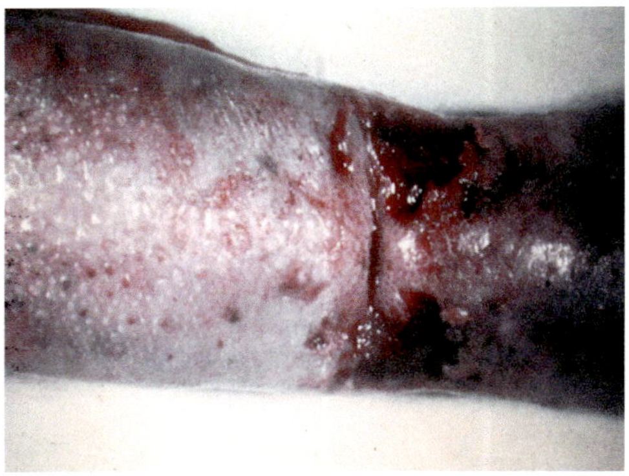

Fig. 5.6. Ox. Tongue. Bluetongue. Cyanosis and multifocal hemorrhagic ulcerative glossitis. The blue color of the lingual mucosa inspired the name of the disease. Glossal ulcers at the lingual fossa are covered by blood.

Bovine bluetongue (BT)

Introduction. This *Orbivirus* is transmitted by *Culicoides* spp. and infects domestic and wild ruminants, mainly sheep. The cyanotic appearance of the tongue mucosa is responsible for the name of the disease. There are many (at least 24) serotypes. The virus has a strong tropism for vascular endothelial cells. Hyperemia, edema and vascular permeability disturbances (hemorrhage), erosions, crusting, and excoriations occur in the oral cavity, face, neck, ears, feet (coronet perioplic band), and teat. Clinical and morphologic parameters overlap with other viral domestic and foreign diseases.

Clinical signs. Up to 95% of infected animals are asymptomatic. Transient fever, salivation, lachrymation, lameness in remaining animals.

Differential diagnoses. BVDV, FMD, MCF, IBR, EHDV (epizootic hemorrhagic disease virus).

Bovine malignant catarrhal fever (MCF)

Introduction. The ruminant Gammaherpesvirus, in particular the OvHV-2 strain, causes multisystemic disease in cattle. Individual morphologic changes have been discussed in Chapter 2: Diseases of the Nervous System and Chapter 3: Diseases of the Respiratory System. As far as the alimentary form of MCF is concerned, various segments of the upper and lower gastrointestinal tracts are involved. In the oral cavity, erosions and hemorrhage develop beneath the tongue, hard palate, gums, and tips of the buccal papillae.

Clinical signs. Fever, nasal exudate, excessive salivation, photosensitization.

Differential diagnoses. Vesicular, erosive, nodular viruses, IBR.

Fact Sheet: Bovine Malignant Catarrhal Fever (MCF)

- Virus: subfamily Gammaherpesvirus
- Members: alcelaphine herpesvirus 1 (AlHV-1)
ovine herpesvirus 2 (OvHV-2)
eight others
- Reservoir host: wildebeest (AlHV-1). Susceptible hosts: domestic cattle
domestic sheep (OvHV-2). Susceptible hosts: domestic cattle, cervids, American and European bison
- Clinical forms: nervous, ocular, dermal, digestive, urinary tract (American bison)
- DDX: mucosal disease, IBR, bluetongue, VS, FMD, photosensitization
- Gross pathology: keratitis, oral and esophageal ulcers, rhinitis, lymphadenopathy, dermatitis
- Hallmark histology: multicentric arteritis-phlebitis (carotid rete mirabilis
lymphoid proliferation

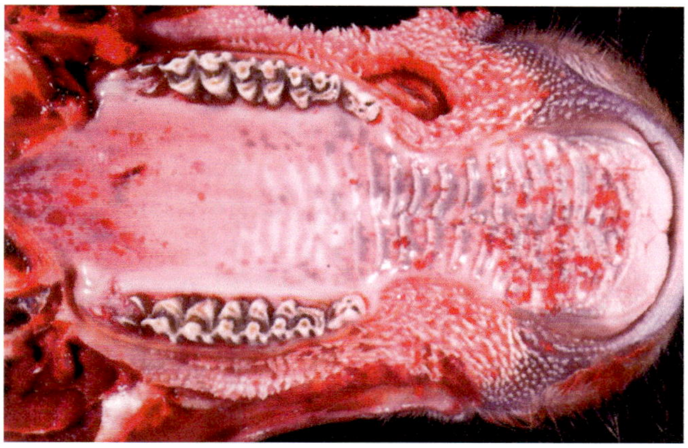

Fig. 5.7. Ox. Hard palate. Malignant catarrhal fever. Erosive, hemorrhagic palatine stomatitis. The mucosa of the hard palate contains erosions, petechiae, ecchymoses, and foci of hyperemia. Similar lesions can be found in the cranial part of the esophagus, forestomachs, and abomasum.

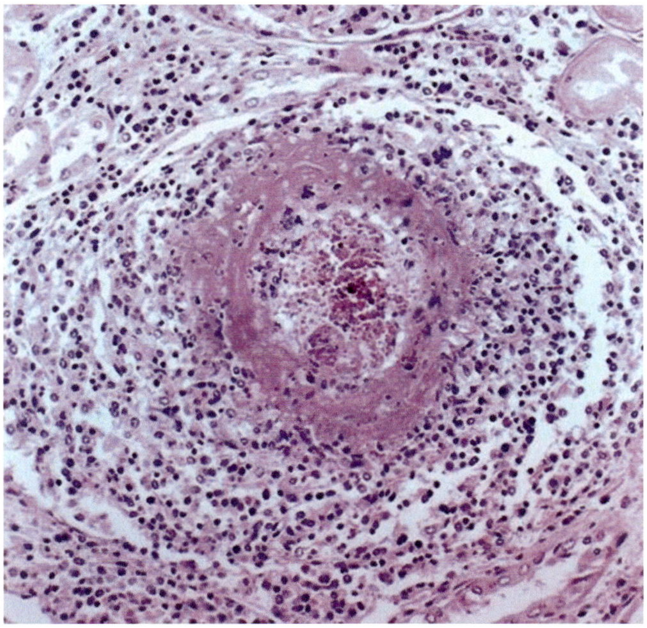

Fig. 5.8. Ox. Malignant catarrhal fever. Necrotizing panvasculitis. The microscopic hallmark lesion for the diagnosis of malignant catarrhal fever (MCF) is a necrotizing vasculitis affecting arteries and veins. The entire vessel wall is characterized by fibrinoid necrosis, with an influx of a few lymphocytes. Massive numbers of lymphocytes surround the blood vessel. Again, the microscopic vascular changes can be found in many organs, and best in the carotid rete (rete mirabile) (H&E). (Courtesy of Dr C. Barros, Universidade Federal de Santa Maria, Brazil.) (See the fact sheet on bovine malignant catarrhal fever.)

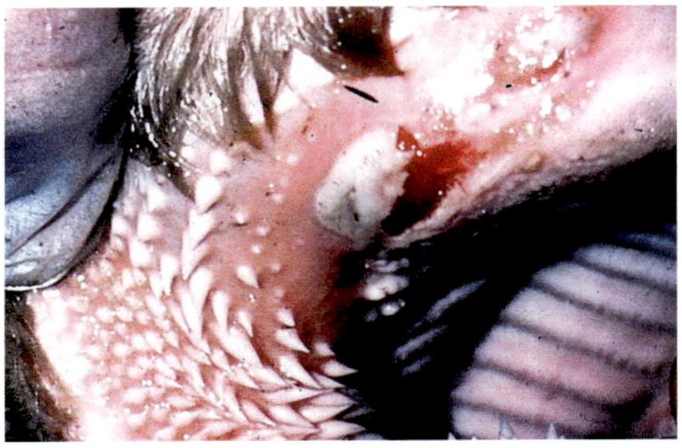

Fig. 5.9. Ox. Oral cavity. Vesicular stomatitis (VS). Ulcerative-vesicular gingivitis. Gums contain vesicles and a focal ulcer covered by blood. Vesicles also develop in tongue, lips, and muzzle. Other organs involved in VS are teats, interdigital spaces and coronary band. Oral lesions develop in 69% of the cases, teat lesions in 23%, oral and teat lesions in 6%, and foot lesions in 2% of the cases. (Courtesy of Dr J.M. King and Anatomic Pathology Section, Cornell University, USA.)

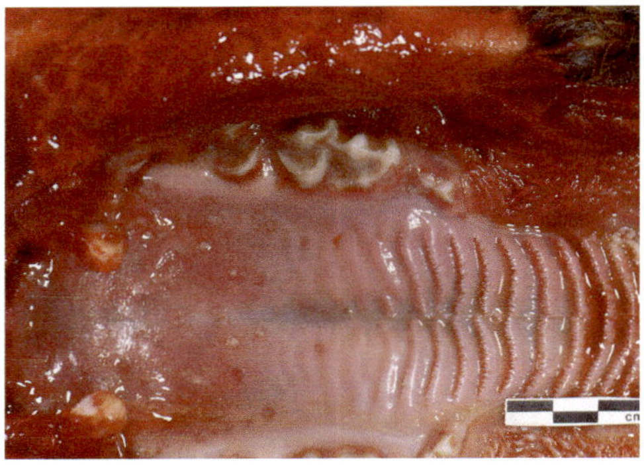

Fig. 5.10. Ox. Soft palate. Infectious bovine rhinotracheitis (IBR). Necrotic palatine stomatitis. Multifocal lesions need to be differentiated from malignant catarrhal fever (MCF), bovine viral diarrhea virus (BVDV), bluetongue (BT).

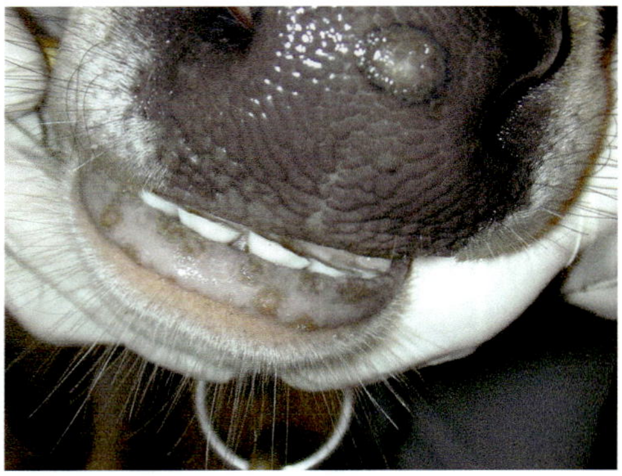

Fig. 5.11. Ox. Muzzle and gingiva. Papular stomatitis. A raised nodule is localized on the muzzle and several discrete, gray-green circular elevations on the gums. The papular lesions may become erosive and crusty. (Courtesy of Dr P. Habecker, University of Pennsylvania, USA.)

Bovine vesicular stomatitis (BVS)

Introduction. Vesicular stomatitis is caused by a group of distinct viruses belonging to the family of *Rhabdoviridae*. The disease is sporadic in cattle, but none the less alarming because of the close resemblance to foot and mouth disease (FMD), a feared livestock disease. Mosquitos and biting flies may be involved in the transmission. The virus is transmissible to humans.

Clinical signs. Salivation, lameness, secondary bacterial infections.

Differential diagnoses. FMD, other erosive, vesicular viruses, BPS, rinderpest (officially eradicated).

Infectious bovine rhinotracheitis (IBR)

Introduction. Though principally inflicting pathologic changes in the respiratory and reproductive systems, the virus has tropism for the alimentary system to induce ulcerative lesions in the oral cavity and raised lesions in the esophagus and abomasum.

PAPULAR

Bovine papular stomatitis (BPS)

Introduction. Caused by a *Parapoxvirus*, the causative virus invokes discrete raised nodules on the muzzle and oral gingiva. The virus is closely related to the *Pseudopoxvirus* and virus of ovine contagious ecthyma (ORF). It is transmissible to humans. Often seen in primary or transient BVDV infections.

Clinical signs. Usually mild sialorrhea. Lesions may regress.

Differential diagnoses. Various etiologies of stomatitis, oral gingival salmonellosis.

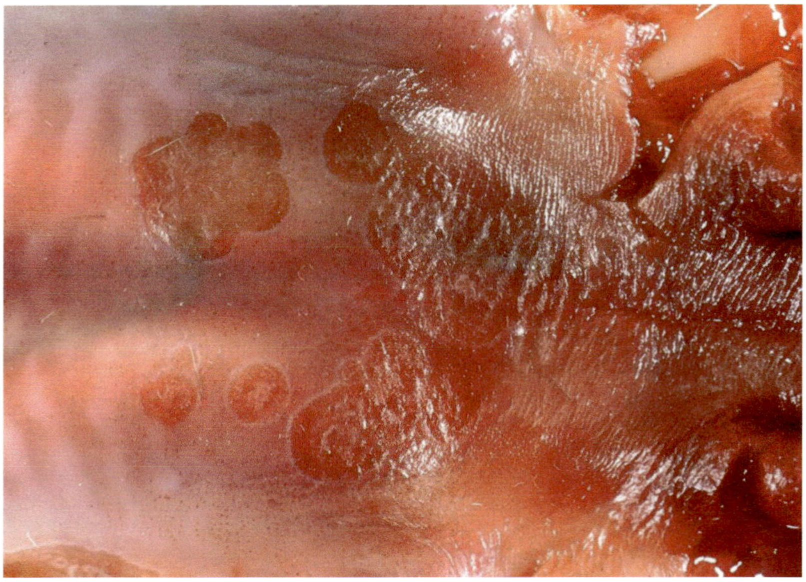

Fig. 5.12. Ox. Palate. Papular stomatitis. Tan, red circular plaques occupy the mucosa of the hard palate.

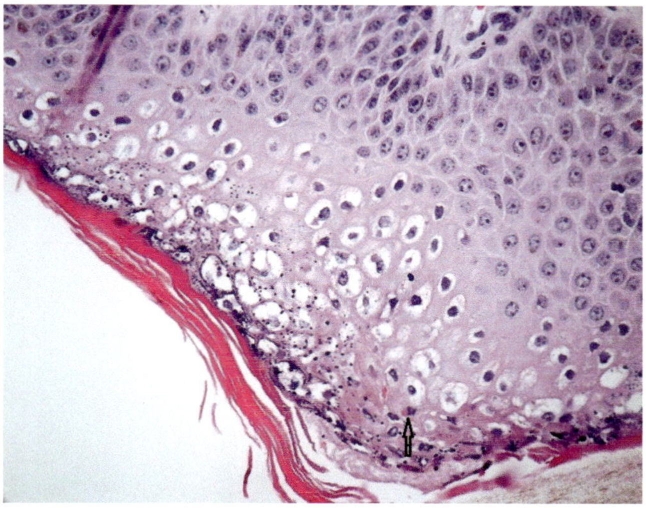

Fig. 5.13. Ox. Gingiva. Papular stomatitis. Mucosal cells are vacuolated. Occasional mucosal cells contain small eosinophilic inclusions in their cytoplasm (arrow) (H&E).

5.1.2.2 Bacterial

Introduction. The tongue is frequently involved in bacterial infections, usually preceded by traumatic events or dental disease. Actinobacillosis (*Actinobacillus lignieresii*) and actinomycosis (*Actinomyces bovis*) are the most notable infectious agents invading the tongue or adjacent tissue in the mouth. Other bacterial pathogens may be *Salmonella enterica* or *Clostridium chauvoei*.

Clinical signs. Salivation, tongue protrusion.

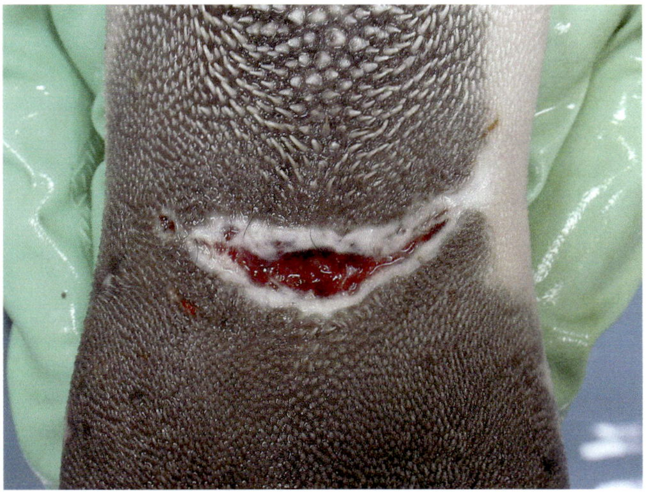

Fig. 5.14. Ox. Tongue. Lingual fossa ulcer. This site is susceptible to trauma and secondary invasion by *Actinobacillus lignieresii*, other bacteria and fungi (silage, hay).

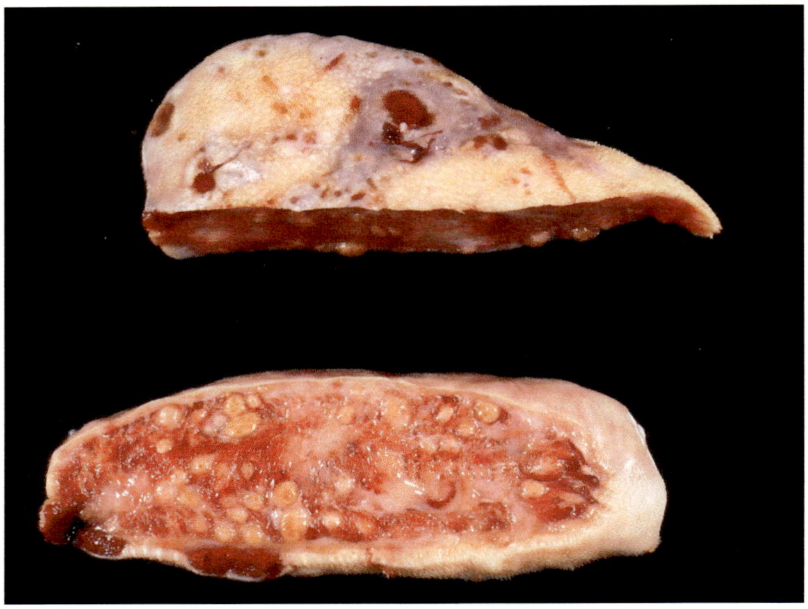

Fig. 5.15. Ox. Tongue. Actinobacillosis ('wooden tongue'). Pyogranulomatous glossitis. The tongue's surface (upper) exhibits areas of mucosal ulceration and thickening. The cut section has multiple foci of pyogranulomas (sulfur granules). Organisms are inoculated within lingual fossa by forage.

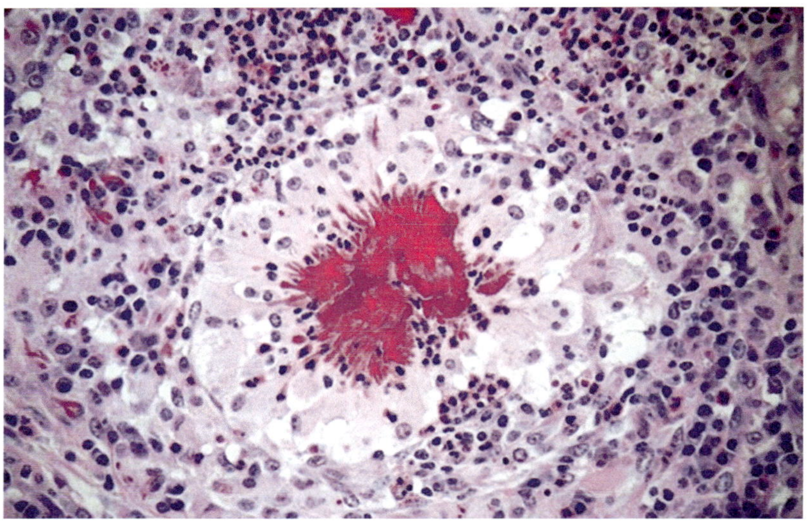

Fig. 5.16. Ox. Tongue. Actinobacillosis. Granuloma with Splendore–Hoeppli material. Starburst-type lesion is the typical club colony seen grossly as sulfur granules. The material is surrounded by macrophages, neutrophils, lymphocytes, and plasma cells (H&E).

For actinomycosis ('lumpy jaw') caused by *A. bovis*, refer to Chapter 8: Diseases of the Musculoskeletal System and Chapter 12: Diseases of the Integument.

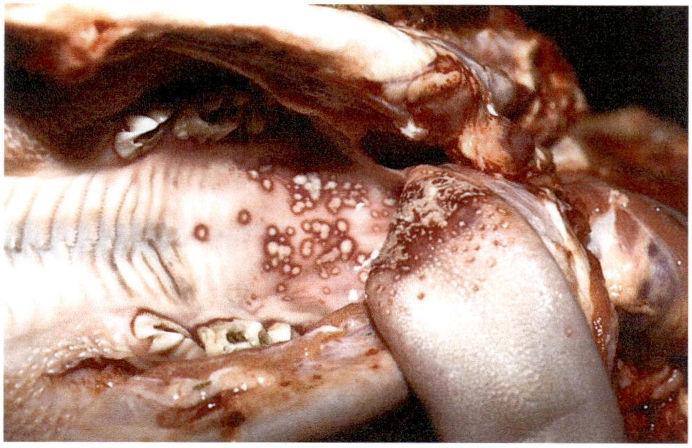

Fig. 5.17. Ox. Oral cavity. Salmonellosis. Nodular and necrotizing stomatitis and glossitis. Multiple discrete and confluent gray elevations are seeding the soft palate and the back of the tongue. *Salmonella enterica* was identified as the cause.

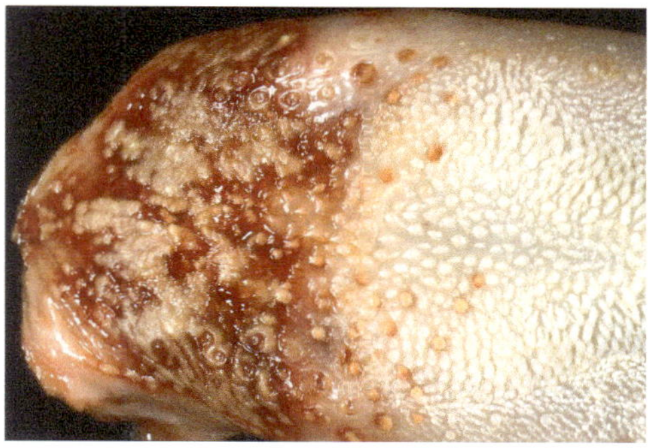

Fig. 5.18. Ox. Tongue. Salmonellosis. Multifocal nodular glossitis. Multiple uniform gray-yellow nodular elevations are present at the tip of the tongue. *Salmonella enterica* was isolated.

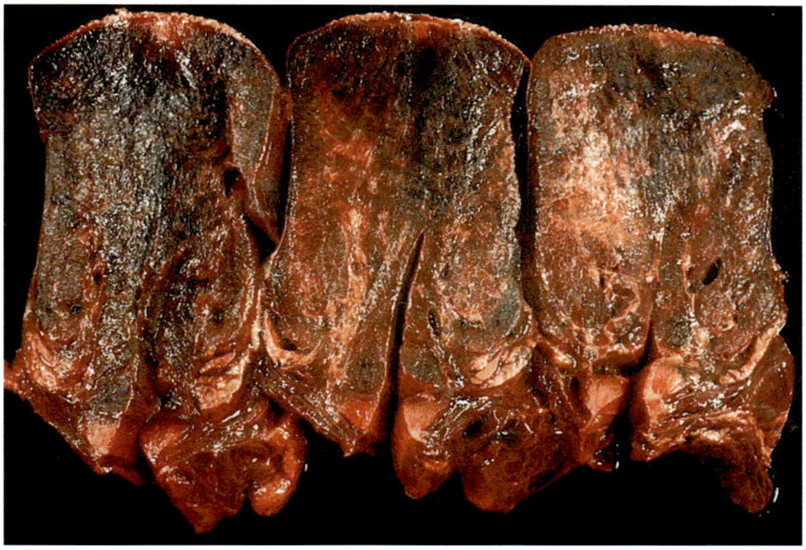

Fig. 5.19. Ox. Tongue. Blackleg. Hemorrhagic, necrotizing glossitis. The tongue is one of the visceral organs that can be infected with *Clostridium chauvoei*. Dark red foci suggest extensive tissue necrosis. Diagnosis can be established by direct immunofluorescence (DIF).

5.1.3 Dental diseases

Introduction. Dental disorders are relatively uncommon in cattle. Irregular molar wear or loss may lead to reduced foraging and weight loss, particularly in older cows. Excess of fluoride in water has an impact on enamel surface integrity, leading to pitting and erosions and periodontal inflammation. *In utero* infection with BVDV may result in enamel hypoplasia/dysplasia.

Clinical signs. Pathological fractures, excessive wear and brown discoloration of incisor teeth.

Differential diagnoses. Rickets, osteomalacia, other causes of enamel hypoplasia (e.g. intrauterine BVDV infection).

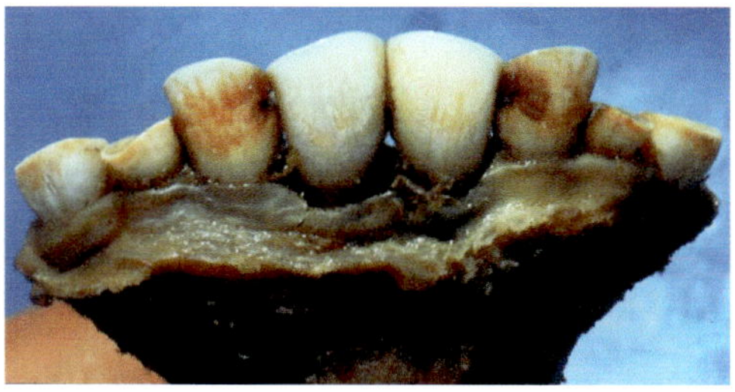

Fig. 5.20. Ox. Incisor teeth. Chronic fluorosis. Loss of enamel and discoloration. Affected teeth show accelerated wear, chalky white deposits in the enamel, and varying degrees of yellow to dark brown discoloration. (Courtesy of Dr F. Riet-Correa, National Institute for Agricultural Research, Uruguay.)

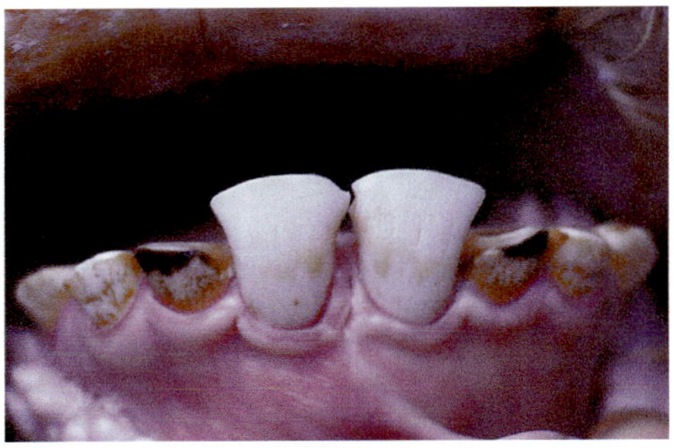

Fig. 5.21. Ox. Incisor teeth. Excessive wear and variable yellow/brown discoloration. The central incisors are only mildly affected, indicating that fluoride exposure was much lower when they were developing. Skeletal changes may resemble rickets and osteomalacia, presumably due to impaired mineralization in the presence of high fluoride concentration. Periosteal hyperostosis may also occur following prolonged exposure to toxic levels. (Courtesy of Dr K. Thompson, Massey University, North Palmerston, New Zealand.)

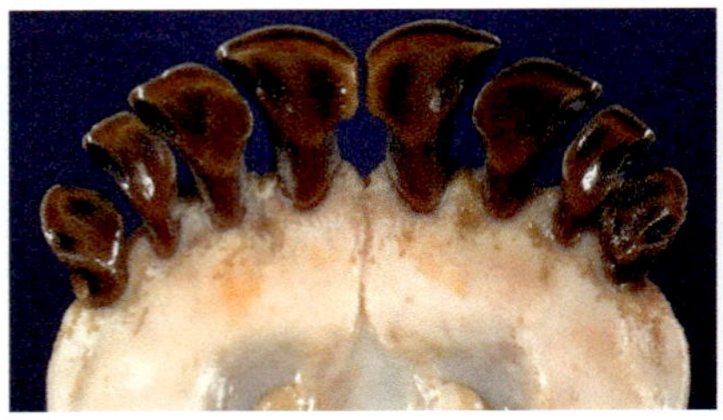

Fig. 5.22. Ox. Incisor teeth. Dental congenital erythropoietic porphyria (CEP). Usually seen under regular light as porphyrin deposition discoloring teeth pink to red, in this case deep brown.

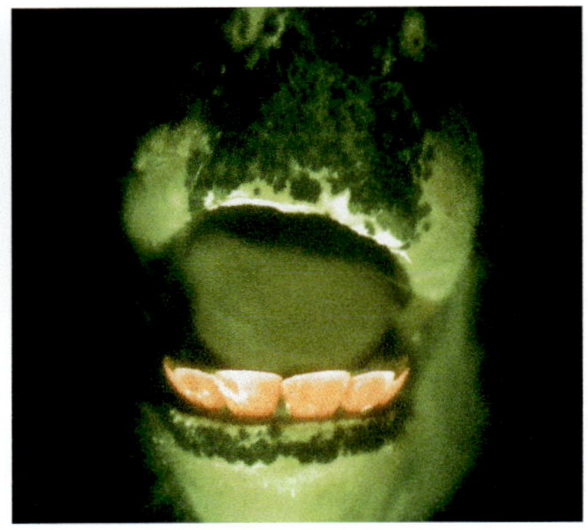

Fig. 5.23. Ox. Incisor teeth. Congenital erythropoietic porphyria (CEP). Teeth fluoresce under UV light in this genetic condition of porphyrin accumulation in teeth, bones, and other tissues. Porphyrin is a photodynamic substance. (For more of CEP, see Chapter 8: Diseases of the Musculoskeletal System and Chapter 11: Diseases of the Hematopoietic and Hemolymphatic System.)

5.1.4 Neoplasia

Tumors involving individual segments of the oral cavity are uncommon in cattle. Individual cases are reported as squamous cell carcinoma and ameloblastoma.

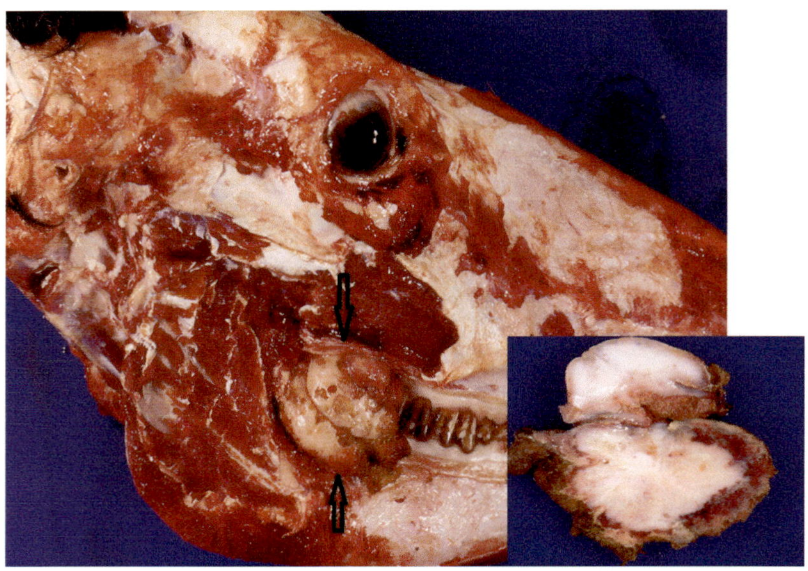

Fig. 5.24. Ox. Cheek. Oral fibroma. A discrete, round growth developed in the caudal oral cavity on the inside of the cheeks (arrows). The diagnosis is fibroma. Inset: on the cut section the growth has a glistening, uniform, white texture. Excess granulation tissue may be difficult to differentiate from fibroma.

5.2 DISEASES OF THE ESOPHAGUS

As a tubular organ, the esophagus provides passage for masticated food to reach the forestomachs and abomasum. Anatomically, it is divided into three segments: cervical, thoracic, and abdominal. There are three anatomic narrowings: at the larynx, the thoracic inlet, and the diaphragmatic hiatus. Esophageal disorders in cattle are relatively rare as compared to other compartments of the gastrointestinal tract.

5.2.1 Obstruction (choke)

Introduction. Food impaction and solid foreign bodies such as apples, beets, and turnips may become entrapped at the larynx or thoracic inlet. Compression of the mucosa beneath the objects results in pressure necrosis and, potentially, perforation.
Clinical signs. Head extension, salivation, dysphagia, bulge beneath the skin.
Differential diagnoses. Rabies, rumen tympany.

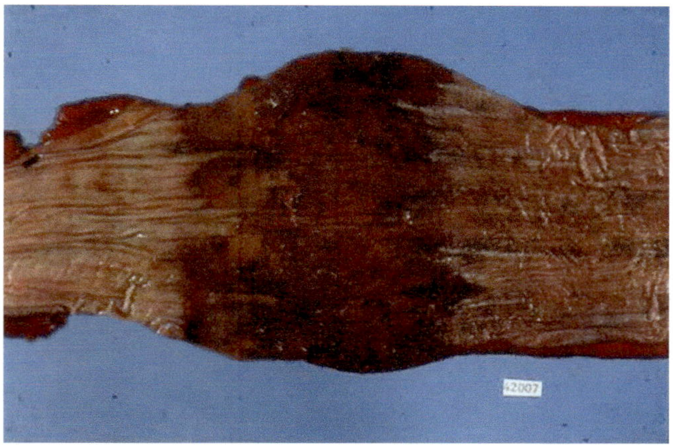

Fig. 5.25. Ox. Esophagus. Choke. Necrohemorrhagic esophagitis. Object entrapment in the esophageal lumen inflicted mucosal pressure necrosis and vascular congestion. (Courtesy of Ontario Veterinary College, Guelph, Canada.)

5.2.2 Trauma

Medical manipulations such as drenching and tubing may cause abrasions of the mucosa and, worse, perforations with severe complicating cellulitis of the adjacent soft tissue.

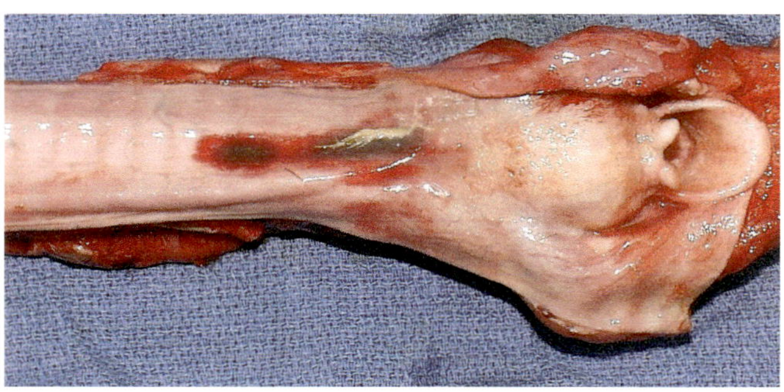

Fig. 5.26. Ox. Esophagus. Focal hemorrhagic-fibrinous esophagitis. A mucosal abrasion occurred during stomach tubing. (Courtesy of Dr P. Habecker, University of Pennsylvania, USA.)

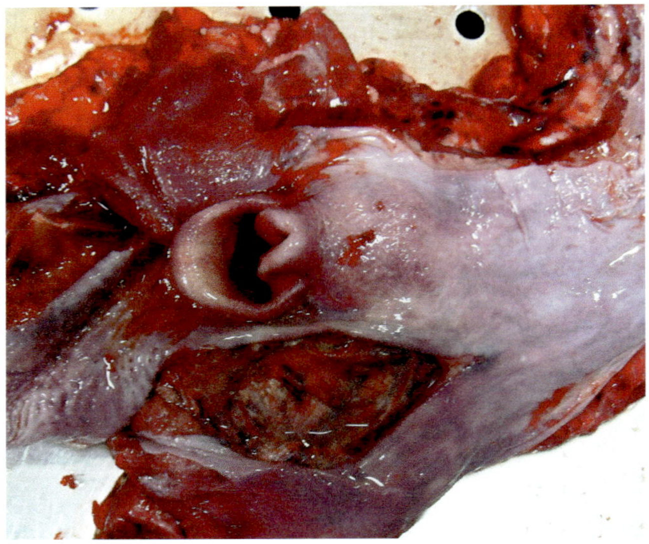

Fig. 5.27. Ox. Esophagus. Laceration. A mucosal perforation, possibly from a drenching gun, resulted in severe tissue necrosis, hemorrhage, and cellulitis. (Courtesy of Dr P. Habecker, University of Pennsylvania, USA.)

5.2.3 Inflammation

Introduction. The specific vesicular, erosive, and nodular viruses discussed under diseases of the oral cavity also inflict changes in the esophagus.

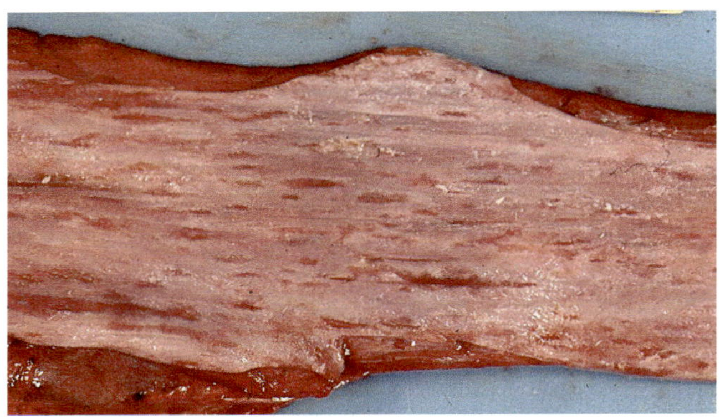

Fig. 5.28. Ox. Esophagus. Bovine viral diarrhea virus (BVDV). Erosive esophagitis. Linear erosions in the mucosa are highly suggestive of infection with BVDV.

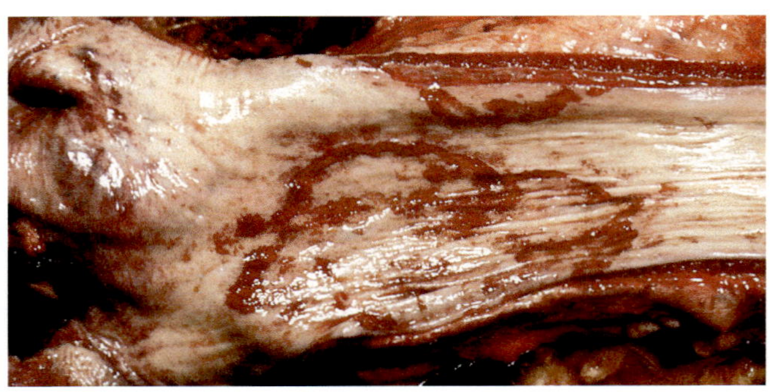

Fig. 5.29. Ox. Esophagus. Malignant catarrhal fever (MCF). Linear erosive-ulcerative hemorrhagic esophagitis. Changes are deeper in the mucosa, with evidence of hemorrhage surrounding the erosive foci and petechiae and ecchymoses in the mucosa.

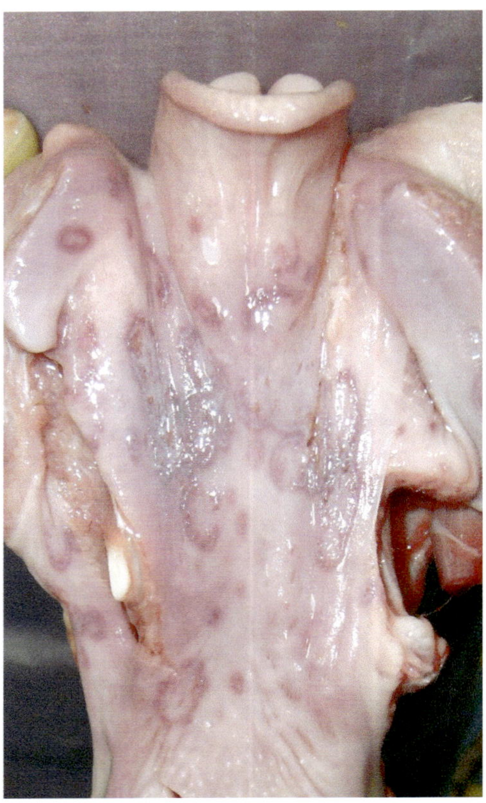

Fig. 5.30. Ox. Esophagus. Bovine papular stomatitis (BPS). Papular esophagitis. Gray nodules with red peripheral rings slightly raise the mucosa.

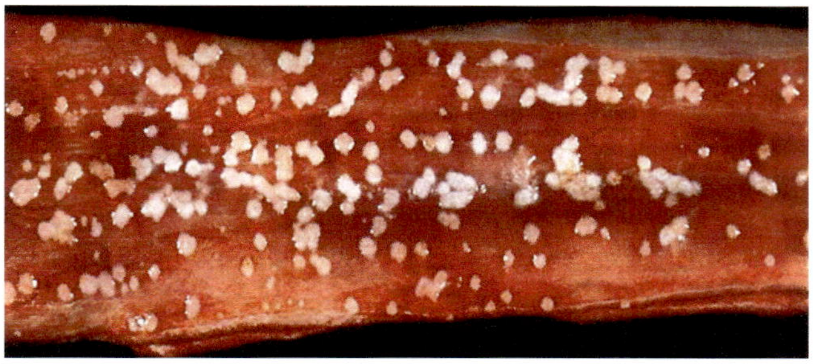

Fig. 5.31. Ox. Esophagus. Infectious bovine rhinotracheitis (IBR). Nodular esophagitis. Raised nodules represent proliferative changes induced by the virus.

5.2.4 Endoparasites

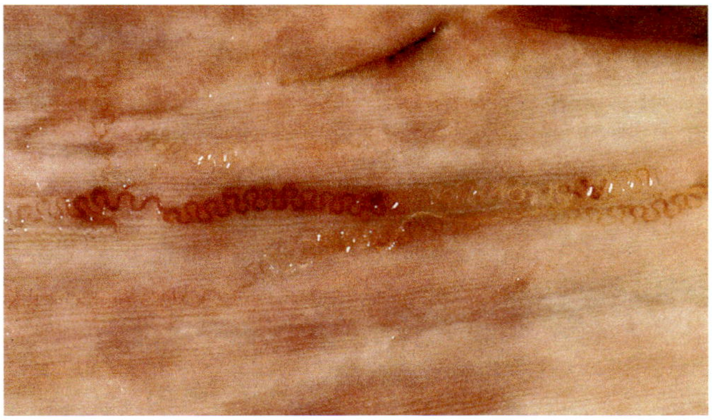

Fig. 5.32. Ox. Esophagus. *Gongylonema pulchrum*. Thin, serpentine, blood-sucking nematodes are located in the mucosa without inflammatory reaction. *Habronema* spp. may be present in the peri-esophageal tissue.

5.2.5 Neoplasia

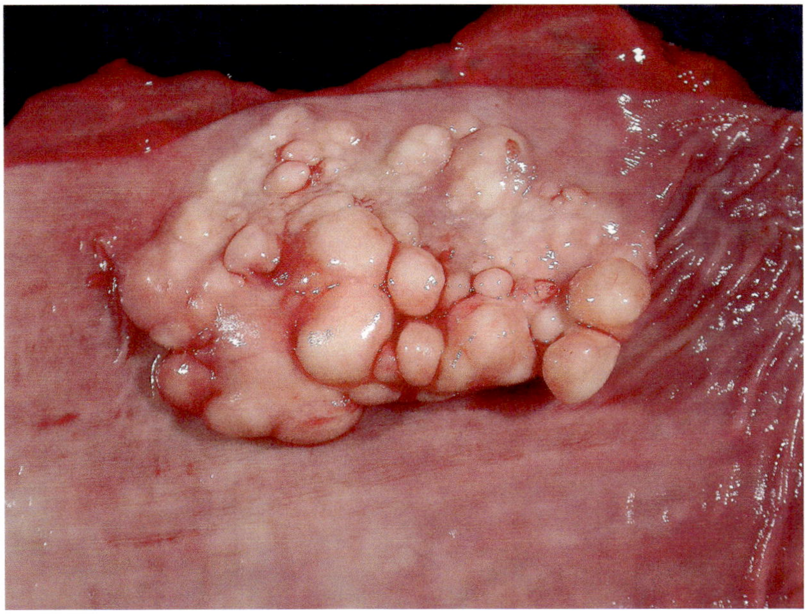

Fig. 5.33. Ox. Esophagus. Fibropapilloma. Multiple, confluent raised nodules occupy the surface of the mucosa. Induced by the bovine papilloma virus, the tissue reaction may be extensive, with near occlusion of the lumen.

5.3 DISEASES OF THE FORESTOMACHS

The forestomachs comprise rumen, reticulum, and omasum. They, particularly the rumen, are involved in bacterial digestion and fermentation to convert plant carbohydrates into fatty acids. During this process, gases are produced and eliminated from the rumen by eructation. The bacterial flora of the forestomachs is complex but well balanced under physiologic conditions. The rumen, representing the largest organ in the abdominal cavity, should be emptied or removed first during the necropsy procedure.

5.3.1 Metabolic disorders

Metabolic disorders are life threatening, interfering with homeostasis of the acid base and electrolytes, causing overproduction of lactic acids and pH changes of ruminal contents, and destabilization of the robust ruminal flora.

5.3.1.1 Rumen lactic acidosis

Introduction. Synonyms are 'overeating' disease or 'toxic' indigestion (grain overload). Feed rich in carbohydrates produce excessive amounts of lactic acid, which may drop the pH of the ruminal contents to as low as 4.0, at which time floral microbes are killed. Only a few survive and heavily replicate. These are *Fusobacterium necrophorum*, *Lactobacillus* spp., *Streptococcus bovis*, and fungi such as *Zygomycetes* spp. and *Aspergillus* spp. Other compartments of the forestomachs, such as the reticulum and omasum, may develop similar mucosal changes secondary to the condition of rumen lactic acidosis.

The diagnosis is difficult to make unless the carcass is very fresh and a low rumen pH is present, along with increased fluid contents in the rumen.

Clinical signs. Metabolic acidosis and circulatory shock, dehydration, diarrhea, laminitis.

Differential diagnoses. Hypocalcemia (periparturient milk fever), bloat, rumen atony.

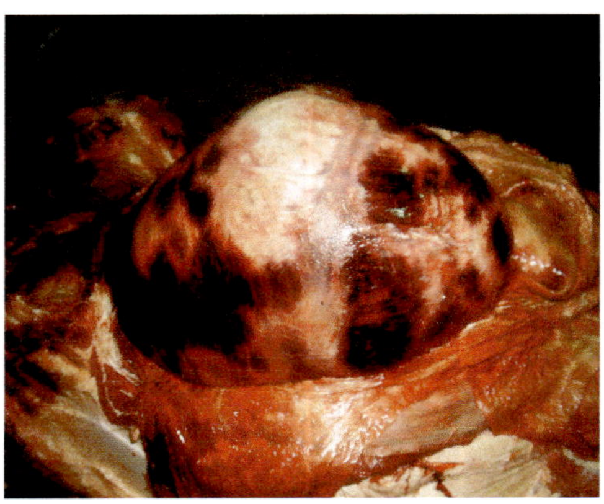

Fig. 5.35. Ox. Rumen. Grain overload. Mural hemorrhagic rumenitis. The rumen is markedly hemorrhagic due to secondary fungal invasion.

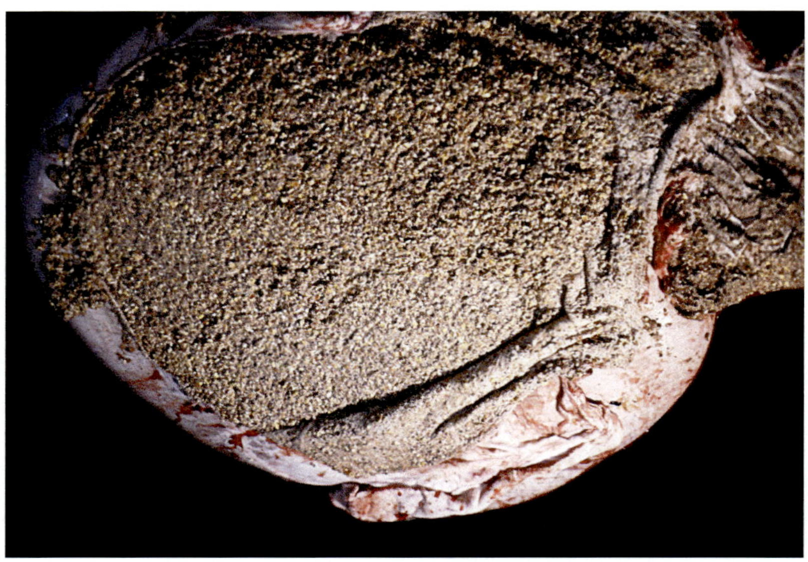

Fig. 5.34. Ox. Rumen. Grain overload. Heavy consumption of grain extends the rumen.

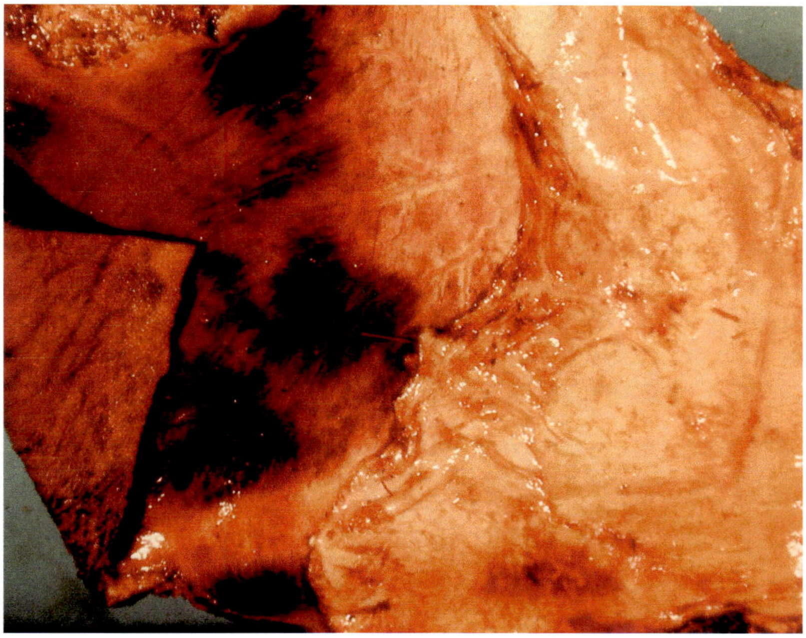

Fig. 5.36. Ox. Rumen. Grain overload. Mural hemorrhagic rumenitis. Hemorrhage extends through the wall, from the mucosa to the serosa.

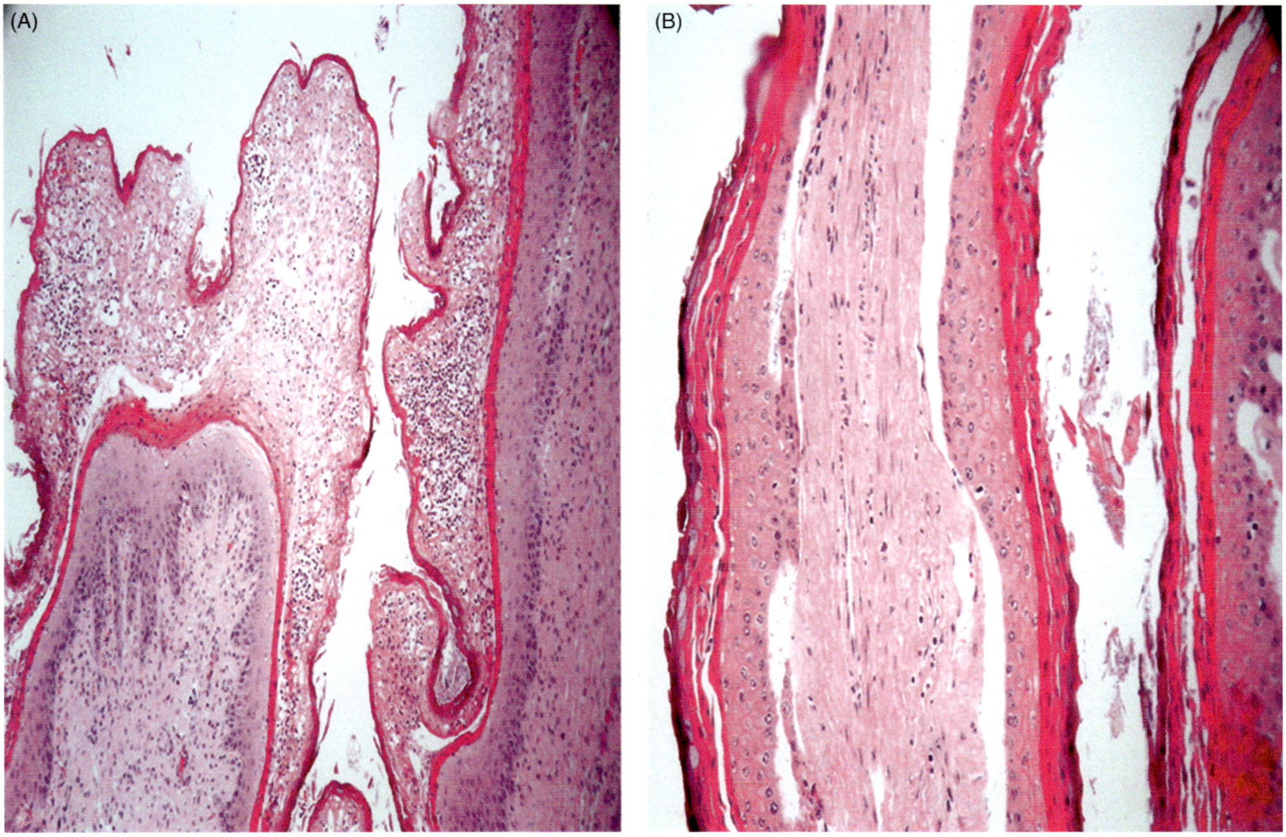

Fig. 5.37. Ox. Rumen. Mucosal lining. Lactic acidosis. (A) Vacuolar degeneration of the squamous epithelial lining with inflammation may aid the diagnosis of lactic acidosis microscopically in fresh cases. (B) Unaffected normal lining for comparison (H&E).

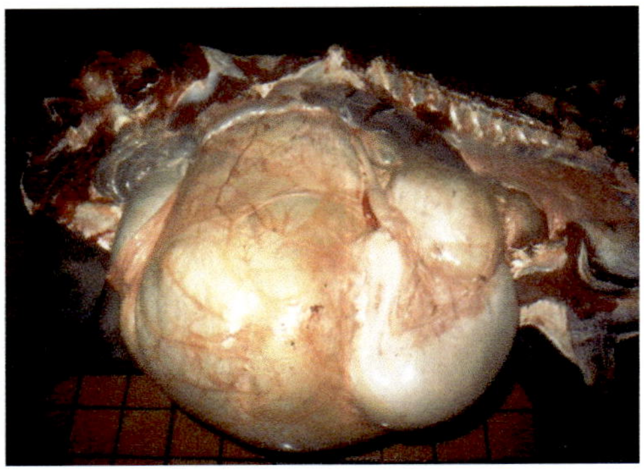

Fig. 5.38. Ox. Rumen. Tympany (bloat). The rumen is markedly distended by excessive gas.

5.3.1.2 Tympany (bloat)

Introduction. Rumen tympany, or bloat, is the result of excessive accumulation of gas in the lumen, leading to extensive ruminal distension. Primary bloat occurs in cattle pastured on legumes or succulent green forage. The excessive formation of gas leads to free gas or frothy ingesta in the rumen. Secondary tympany results from choke or functional neurogenic defects (vagal indigestion). The diagnosis of tympany is difficult to make due to the coexistence of other diseases and interference by varying degrees of post-mortem autolysis.

Clinical signs. Left-sided ruminal distension, dyspnea.

Differential diagnoses. Esophageal obstruction, rumen atony.

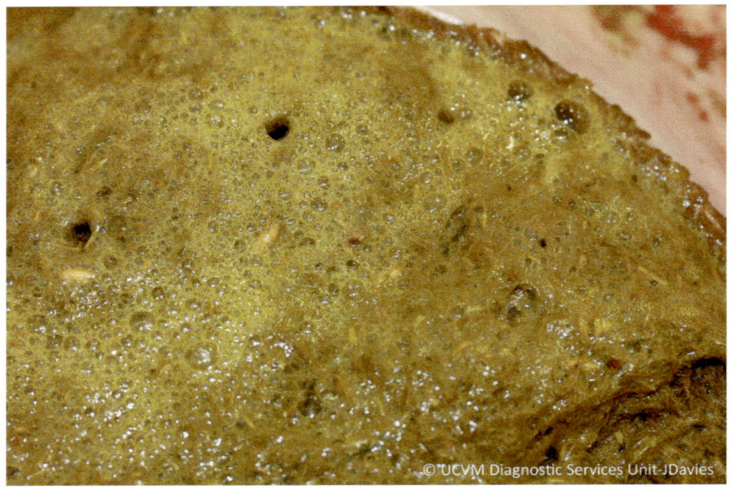

Fig. 5.39. Ox. Rumen. Frothy bloat. The ruminal contents are intermixed with gas, creating bubbles within the ingesta. (Courtesy of Dr J. Davies, UCVM Diagnostic Services, University of Calgary, Calgary, Canada.)

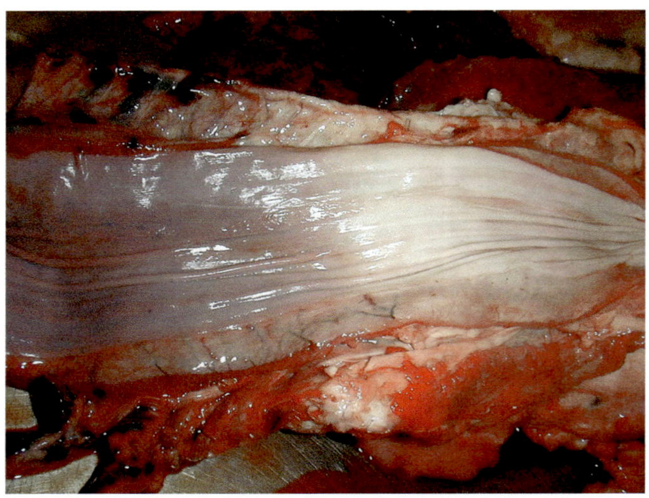

Fig. 5.40. Ox. Esophagus. Bloat line. There is a sharp color transition between a congested mucosa (cranial) and a pale mucosa at the site of the thoracic inlet. When present, it should not be used to make the final diagnosis as it is a common finding in many conditions, but it aids in conjunction with other findings for the diagnosis of intravitam tympany and differentiates from post-mortem gaseous extension of the rumen. The congestion is the result of an intrathoracic venous compression from increased pressure by an expanding tympanic rumen.

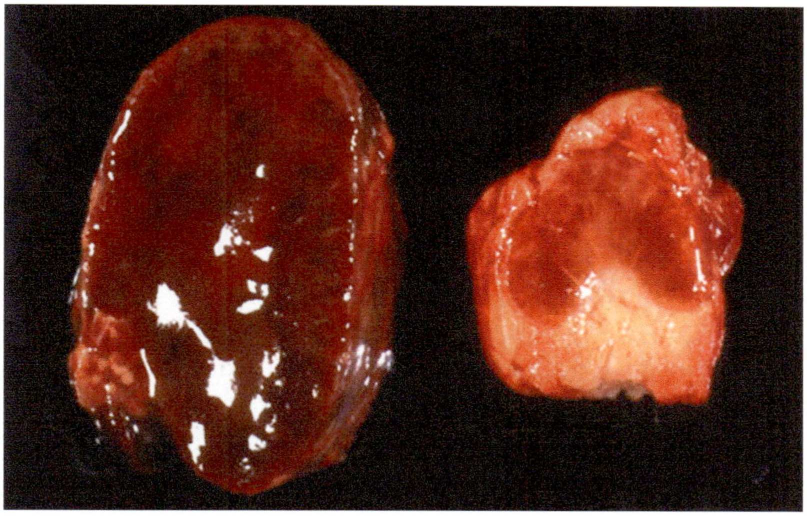

Fig. 5.41. Ox. Prescapular and prefemoral lymph nodes. Bloat. The prescapular lymph nodes are enlarged and congested, whereas the prefemoral lymph nodes are small and very pale. In a carcass with moderate to severe autolysis, this difference in peripheral lymph nodes cranial and caudal can be a highly useful supportive finding to bloat being responsible. In general, the carcass with bloat exhibits cranial congestion and caudal pallor.

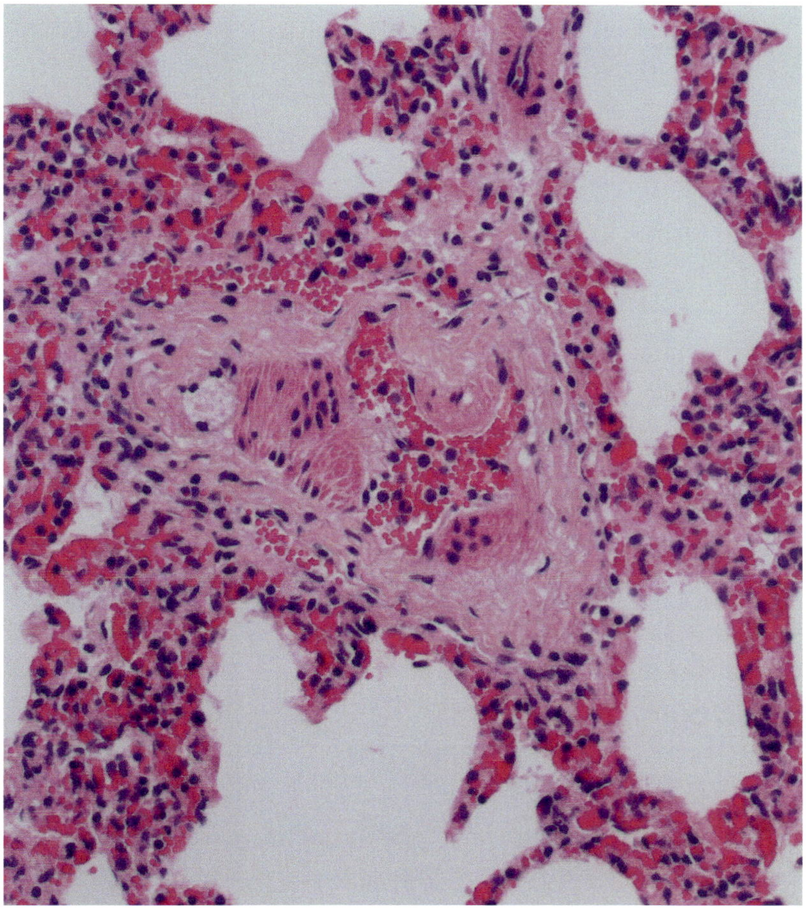

Fig. 5.42. Ox. Pulmonary vessel. Bloat. Smooth muscle hyperconstriction. One of the co-authors recommends taking a section of caudal lung for microscopic examination of the pulmonary vessels to see if there is segmental thickening of the smooth muscles in the media, to support the diagnosis of bloat. The bovine lung has normal spirals of smooth muscle in small vessels that, when hyperconstricted such as in bloat, make them distinctly visible (H&E).

Other gross findings lending support for the diagnosis of tympany include pallor of liver and kidneys, a congested and collapsed lung, and petechial or diffuse hemorrhage in the tracheal mucosa without blood clots. Intense congestion of nasal sinuses with or without varying degrees of hemorrhage is also quite a consistent finding with bloat.

5.3.1.3 Urea toxicity (ammonia toxicosis)

Introduction. A feed supplement when fed in too high concentrations (mixing error) in feed mixture (more than 3%) becomes toxic, causing sudden death on a larger scale. There is a relative lack of gross and microscopic findings in cases of urea poisoning, with the exception of ruminal bloat and a subjectively observed relatively advanced stage of post-mortem autolysis. Feed analysis and determination of urea concentration (non-protein nitrogen) in feed is recommended for the definitive diagnosis of urea poisoning. Also, determine blood and vitreous ammonia (>1.0 mg/dl).

Clinical signs. Paresis, recumbency, mucosanguinous nasal discharge, sudden death.

Differential diagnoses. Lightning, chemical or plant toxicoses.

5.3.1.4 Ruminal papillary hypertrophy/hyperplasia

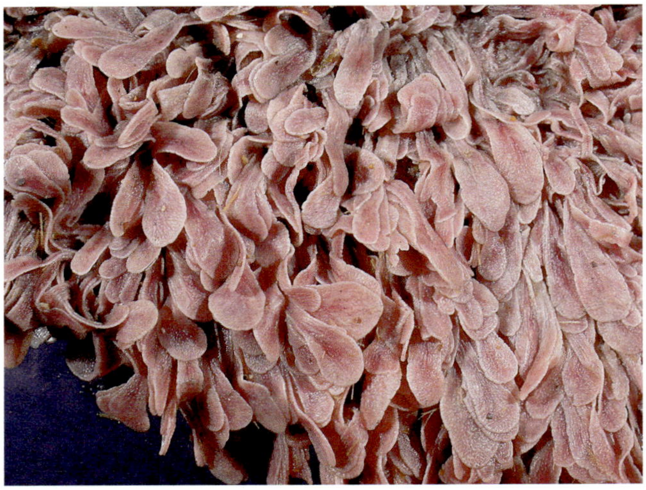

Fig. 5.43. Ox. Rumen. Hypertrophic papillae. Thickening and lengthening of ruminal papillae develop with a lack of fiber in the diet, whereas loss and lack of papillae occur when dietary roughage increases.

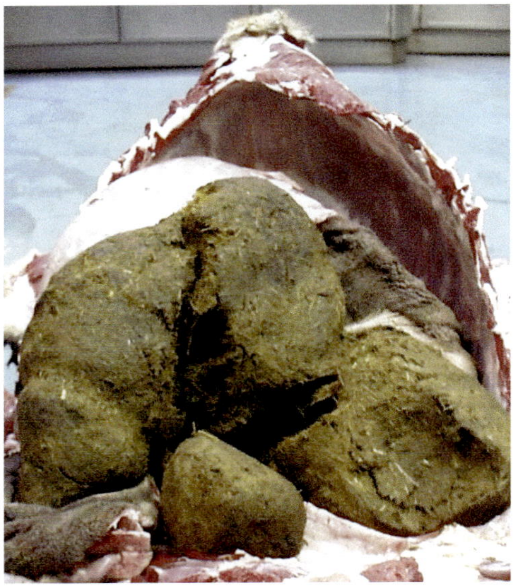

Fig. 5.44. Ox. Rumen. Impaction. The rumen is markedly distended with dry impacted ingesta.

5.3.2 Obstruction

5.3.2.1 Ruminal indigestion

Introduction. Events of overeating grain, poor-quality roughage such as straw, grass or silage lead to ruminal impaction, distension, and hypoactivity.

Clinical signs. Anorexia, gastrointestinal stasis, drop of milk production.

Differential diagnoses. Bloat, sudden feed changes.

5.3.3 Inflammation

Causes of inflammation range from toxic events (acute lead poisoning) to foreign bodies (hardware) and opportunistic pathogens (bacteria, fungi) secondary to lactic acidosis.

5.3.3.1 Traumatic reticulitis

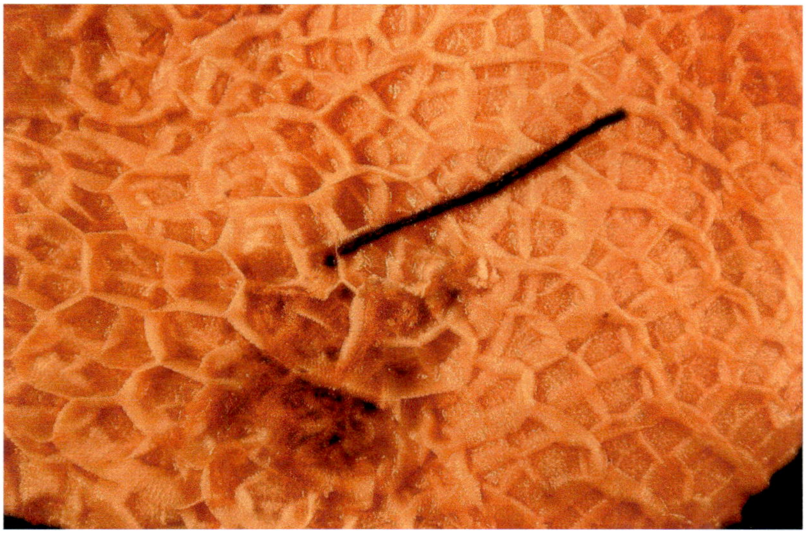

Fig. 5.45. Ox. Reticulum. Hardware. A nail is embedded in the mucosa without causing disease. If exceeding a certain length (>5 cm), a nail or piece of wire penetrates the wall of the reticulum to perforate it and to induce focal peritonitis. Further cranial hardware movement penetrates the diaphragm and pericardium. Multiple pyogenic bacteria travel along the path of the hardware to induce chronic traumatic reticulo-pericarditis (hardware disease) (also see Chapter 4: Diseases of the Cardiovascular System).

5.3.3.2 Opportunistic pathogens secondary to lactic acidosis

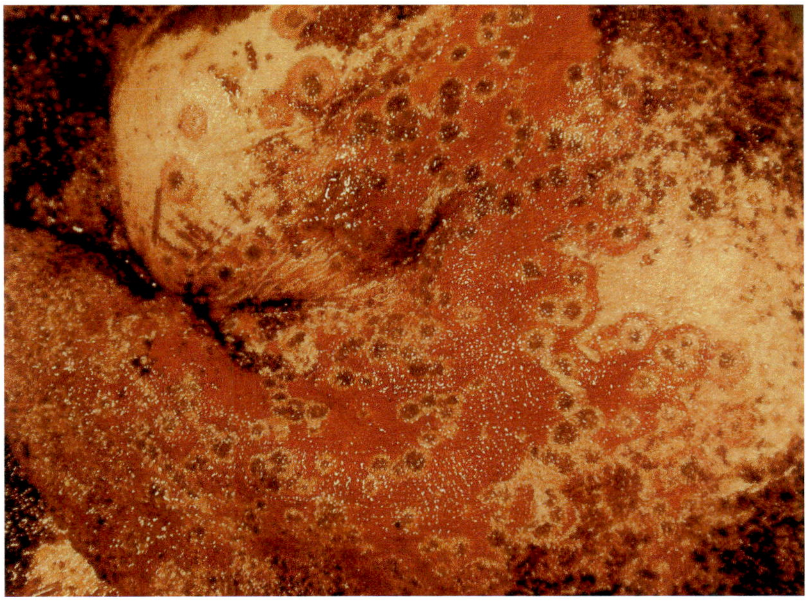

Fig. 5.47. Ox. Rumen. Necrohemorrhagic mycotic rumenitis. Secondary invasion of the mucosa by fungal organisms such as *Zygomycetes* spp. or *Aspergillus* spp. following lactic acidosis-created multifocal mucosal ulceration characterized by a central red zone and gray periphery. The remaining mucosa is deeply red.

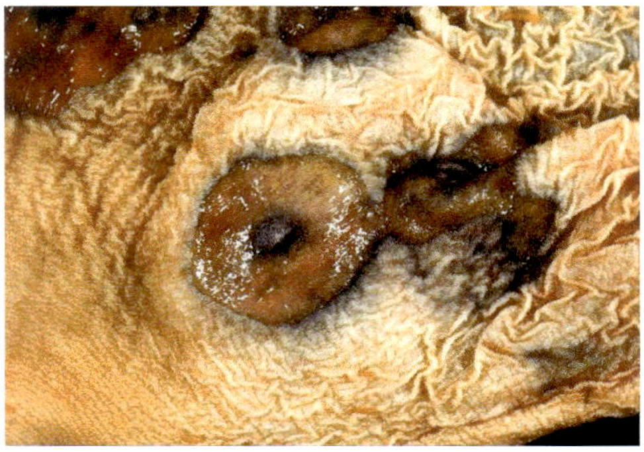

Fig. 5.46. Ox. Rumen. Necrobacillosis. Necrotizing, erosive-ulcerative rumenitis. Secondary changes in lactic acidosis due to proliferation of *Fusobacterium necrophorum*.

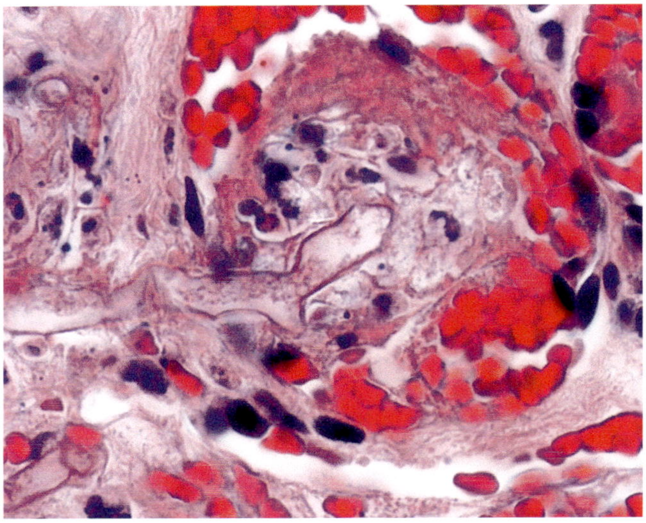

Fig. 5.48. Ox. Omasum. Vessel. Mycotic omasitis. Lactic acidosis. A thrombus containing a fungal hypha occludes a blood vessel (H&E).

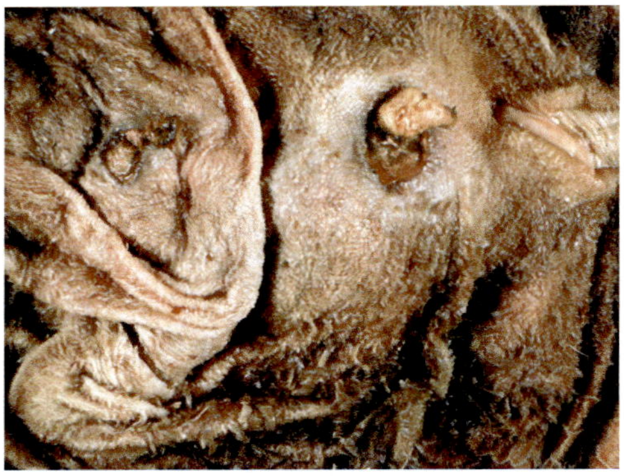

Fig. 5.50. Ox. Rumen. Chronic ulcers. These healed ulcers with scar tissue are indicative of transient lactic acidosis (acid indigestion).

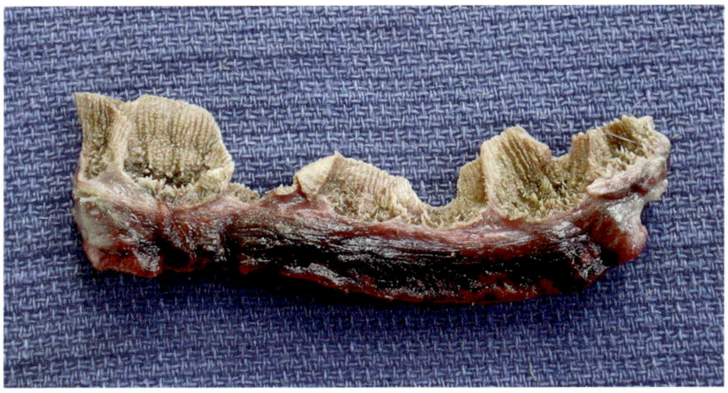

Fig. 5.49. Ox. Reticulum. Lactic acidosis. Transmural necrohemorrhagic reticulitis. Other compartments of the forestomachs may also be affected by secondary bacterial or mycotic invasion.

5.3.3.3 Rumen infected with BVDV

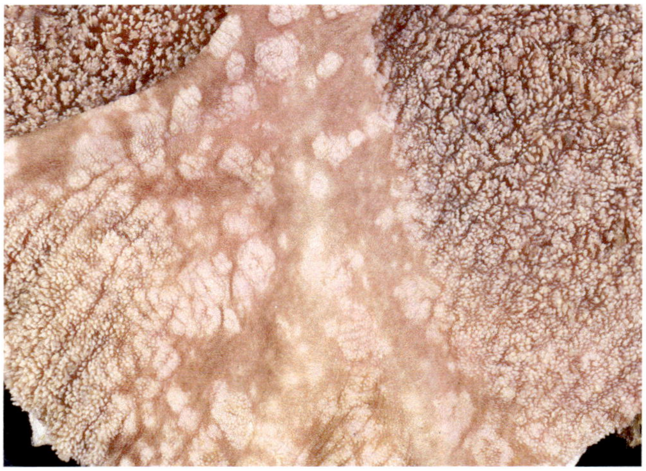

Fig. 5.51. Ox. Rumen. Bovine viral diarrhea virus (BVDV). Depigmented rumen pillars exhibit multiple white erosions and plaques.

5.3.4 Endoparasites

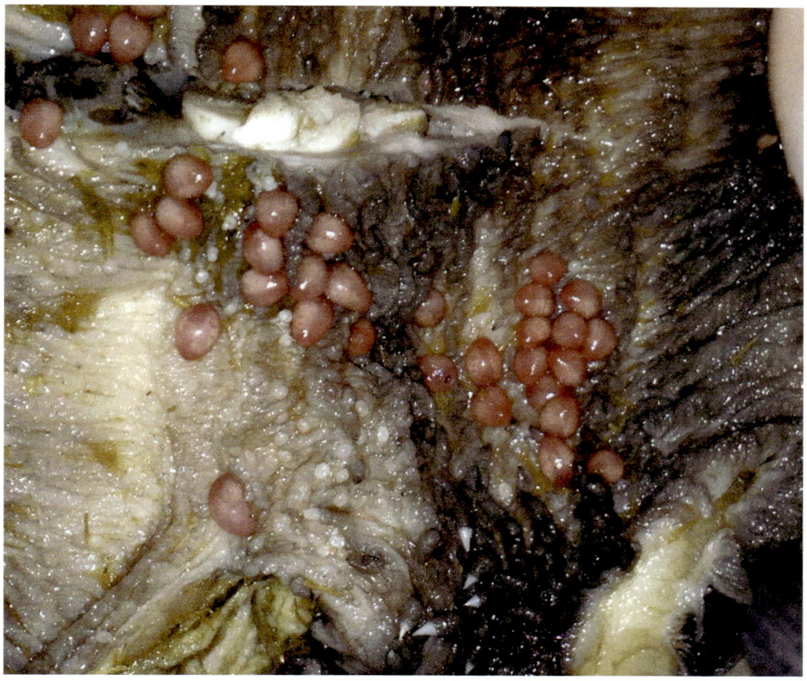

Fig. 5.52. Ox. Rumen. Ruminal flukes. *Paramphistomum cervi* are very small and easily overlooked. The conical, pale pink, droplet-shaped flukes blend in with the ruminal contents. They are incidental findings and usually non-pathogenic. Only heavy infestation causes clinical signs. (Courtesy of Dr F. Uzal, University of California, USA.)

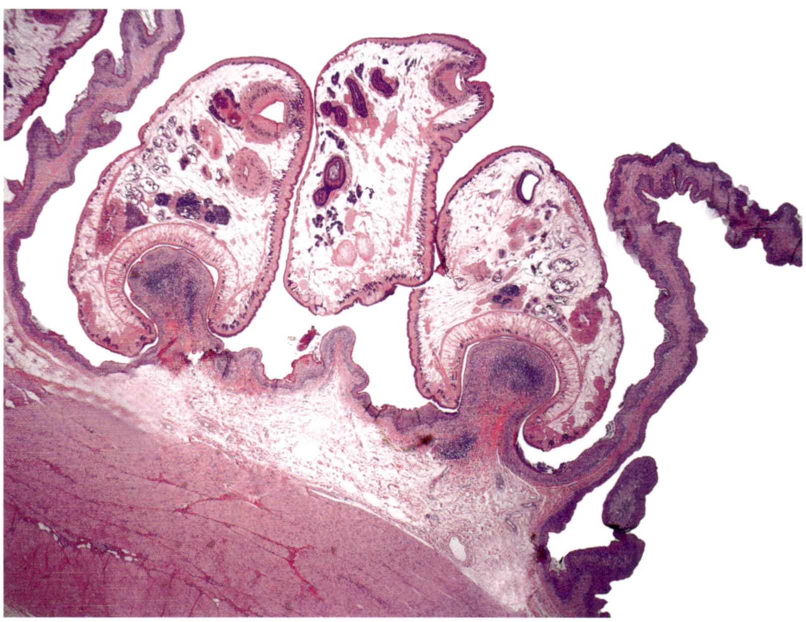

Fig. 5.53. Ox. Rumen. Ruminal flukes. Attachment site of *Paramphistomum cervi* to mucosa (H&E). (Courtesy of Dr F. Uzal, University of California, USA.)

5.3.5 Neoplasia

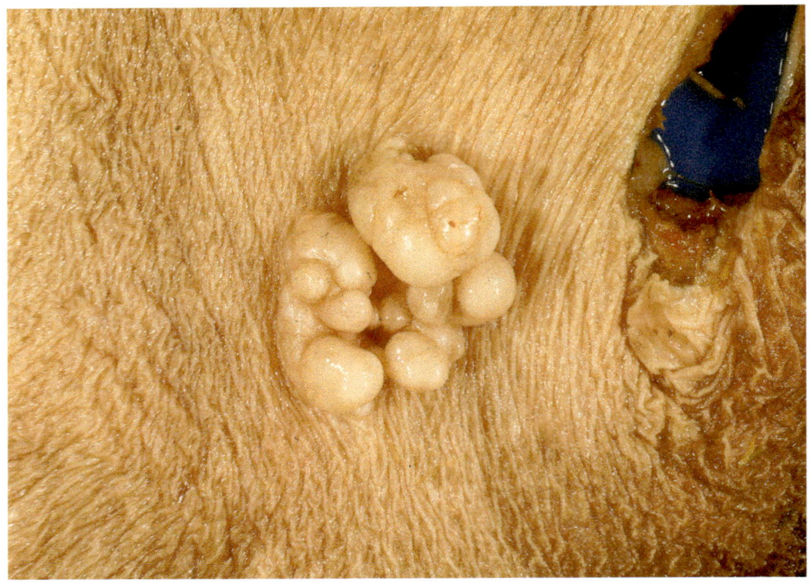

Fig. 5.54. Ox. Rumen. Viral fibropapillomas. Focal nodular growths are incidental findings that may be seen on occasions in the rumen and reticulum.

5.3.6 Miscellaneous disorders

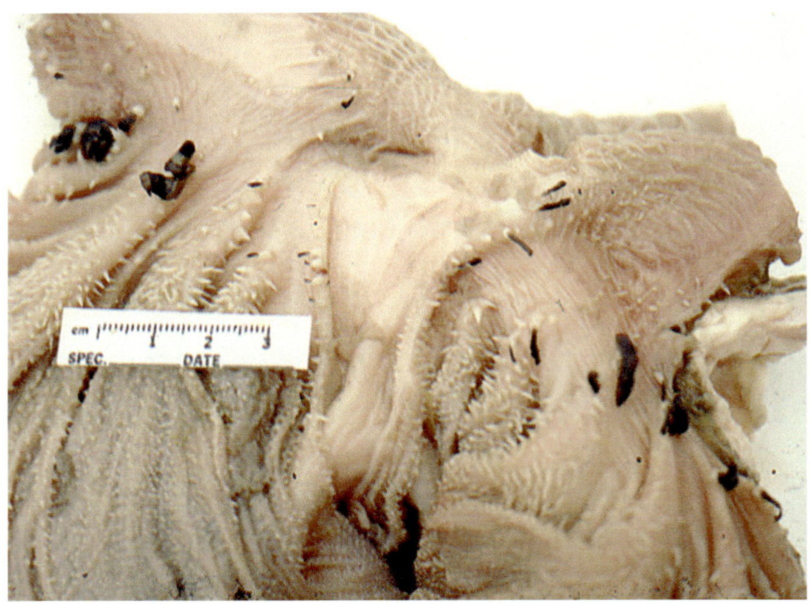

Fig. 5.55. Ox. Omasum. Unguiculliform papillae. These black, cornified structures near the reticular groove are normal incidental findings.

5.4 DISEASES OF THE ABOMASUM

Located to the right of the rumen and ventrally, the abomasum has the shape of a Pyrenese shepherd's wine bag. It is the true stomach in ruminants.

5.4.1 Changes in position

5.4.1.1 Abomasal displacement

Introduction. A condition in which the abomasum glides across the abdominal wall from right to left to a left-sided location (left-sided displacement, or LDA). Displacement may also occur to the right side (right displaced abomasum, or RDA). Most displacements are to the left side. Displacements may occur immediately following parturition or after high-concentrate feeding and increased volatile fatty acid production. Hypochloremia and metabolic alkalosis are serious clinic-pathologic complications.

Clinical signs. Distended rib cage, anorexia, reduced milk production, 'ping' sound on auscultation, ketosis.

Differential diagnoses. Abomasal torsion, primary ketosis.

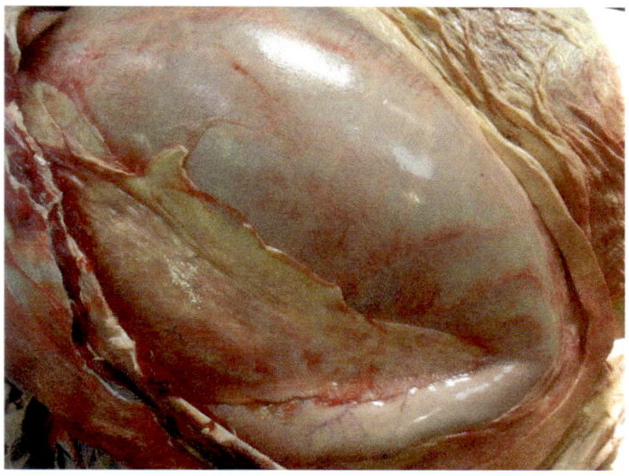

Fig. 5.56. Ox. Abomasum. Left displaced abomasum (LDA). The abomasum has rotated upwards. It is gas-filled and the wall is congested.

5.4.1.2 Abomasal torsion/volvulus

Introduction. Distention and rotation around duodenum. Fluid and feed movement into duodenum is interrupted.

Clinical signs. Dyspnea, pain, shock.

Differential diagnoses. Intestinal volvulus, intussusception, cecal torsion.

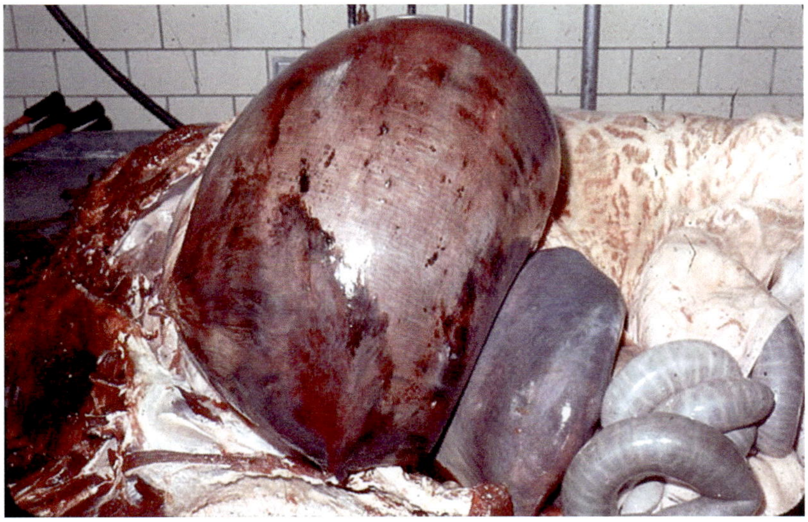

Fig. 5.57. Ox. Abomasum. Volvulus. The abomasum rotates around the duodenum. Its wall exhibits ischemic hemorrhagic necrosis. The compromised wall may rupture to cause acute peritonitis. (Courtesy of Dr J.M. King and the Anatomic Pathology Section,Cornell University, USA.)

5.4.2 Obstruction

5.4.2.1 Impaction

Introduction. Animals largely fed poor-quality fibrous feed, together with water deprivation, accumulate dry ingesta within the abomasum. Mechanical outflow obstructions are other pathologic conditions.
Clinical signs. Teeth grinding, pain.
Differential diagnoses. Vagal indigestion, perforating abomasal ulcer.

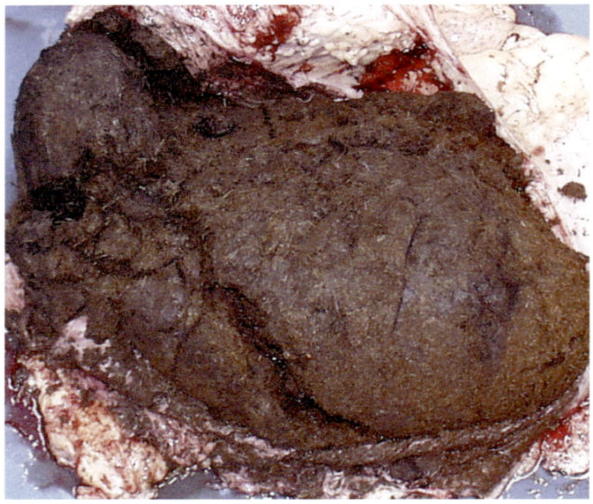

Fig. 5.58. Ox. Abomasum. Impaction. Ingesta are dry and hardened.

5.4.2.2 Vagal indigestion (Hoflund syndrome)

Introduction. Disease of the vagal nerve at its location within the abdominal cavity. A neurogenic, functional disturbance of motility of the forestomachs and abomasum is the consequence. Causes are chronic focal peritonitis, focal peritoneal abscess or neoplasia infringing on the nerve.
Clinical sign. Severe ruminal distension due to fluid or feed impaction.
Differential diagnoses. Tympany, ruminal or abomasal impaction through excessive feed uptake, perforating abomasal ulcer.

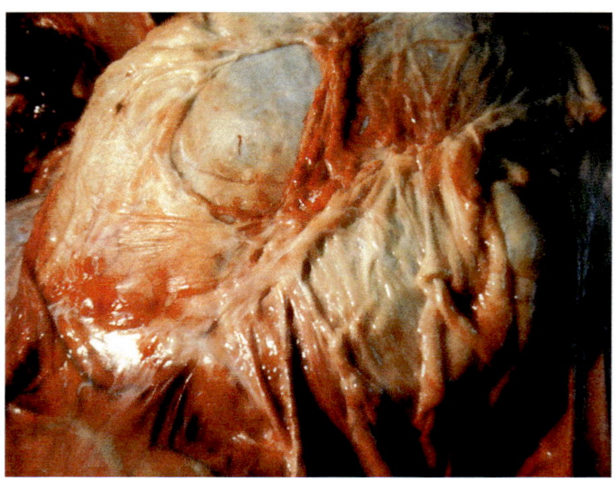

Fig. 5.59. Ox. Abomasum. Vagal indigestion. Focal chronic peritonitis. The omentum adheres to the abomasum and drapes around the vagal nerve.

5.4.3 Erosions and ulcers

Introduction. Erosions are defined as mucosal breaks above the basal lamina. Abomasal erosions have multiple causes such as corticosteroids, toxins (arsenic), infectious diseases (salmonellosis, thrombocytopenic strain of BVDV), or endoparasites (*Haemonchus placei*).

Ulcers are defined as mucosal breaks below the basal lamina. Abomasal ulcers are often incidental findings with no clinical signs and no reasonable explanation for the pathogenesis. Perforating ulcers in older animals are a common cause for generalized peritonitis. The topic is discussed in more detail in Chapter 1: Diseases of Neonates and Calves.

Clinical sign. Abdominal pain.

Differential diagnoses. Traumatic reticulitis, peritonitis.

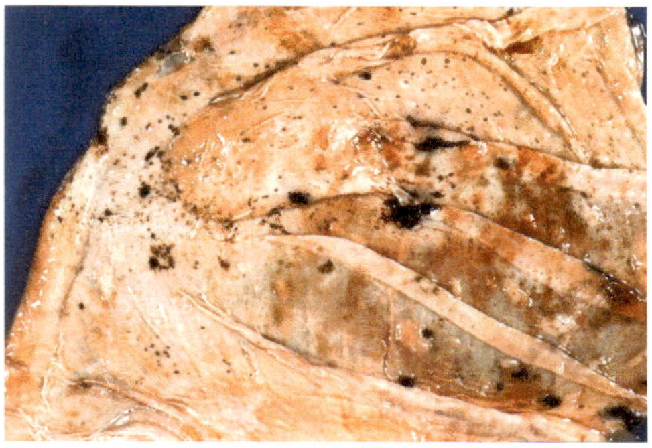

Fig. 5.60. Ox. Abomasum. Hemorrhagic erosions The mucosa is studded with ecchymoses, and shallow erosions covered by blood.

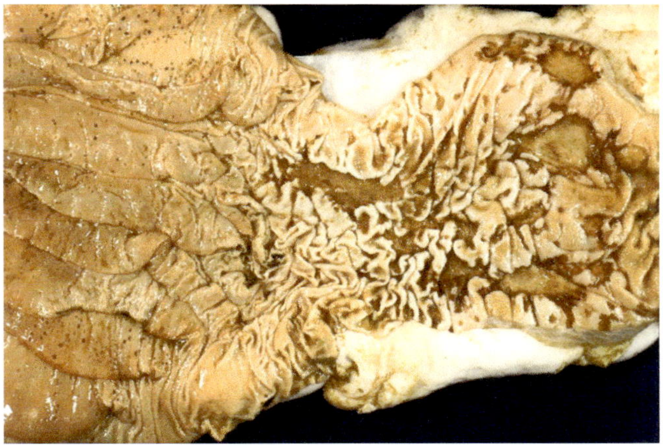

Fig. 5.61. Ox. Abomasum. Multiple ulcers. Various confluent ulcers seed the mucosa. They are suggestive of stress-related events. Abomasal rugal folds are edematous.

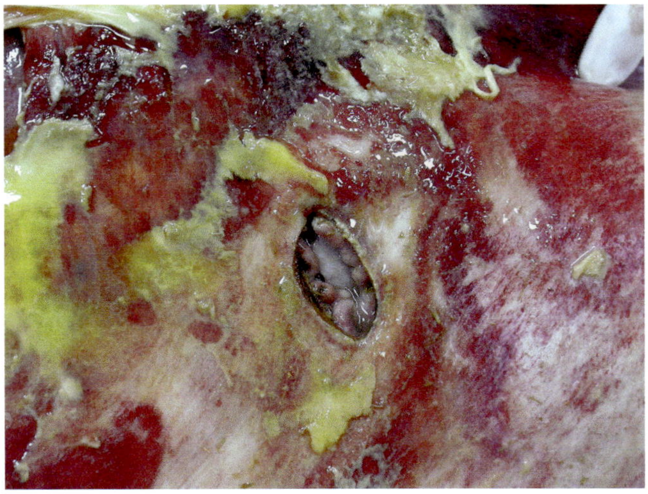

Fig. 5.62. Ox. Abomasum. Perforating ulcer and peritonitis. A septic, fibrinous peritonitis resulted from perforation of an abomasal ulcer. Abomasal content is usually mixed with peritoneal fibrin. This is a common problem in 1- to 3-month-old beef calves.

5.4.4 Inflammation

Introduction. Circumscribed or diffuse primary inflammations of the abomasum are relatively rare in cattle. Foreign bodies, chemical irritants, toxins, medications, endoparasites, or protozoa are causes to consider.
Clinical signs. Vary. Inappetence, dullness, weight loss, diarrhea.
Differential diagnoses. Abomasal ulcer, impaction, lymphoma.

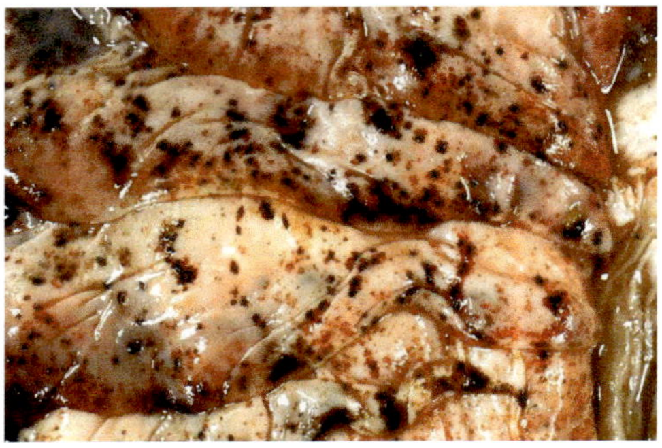

Fig. 5.63. Ox. Abomasum. Salmonellosis. Multifocal hemorrhagic abomasitis. Multiple foci of hemorrhage are disseminated throughout the mucosa. *Salmonella typhimurium* is usually isolated.

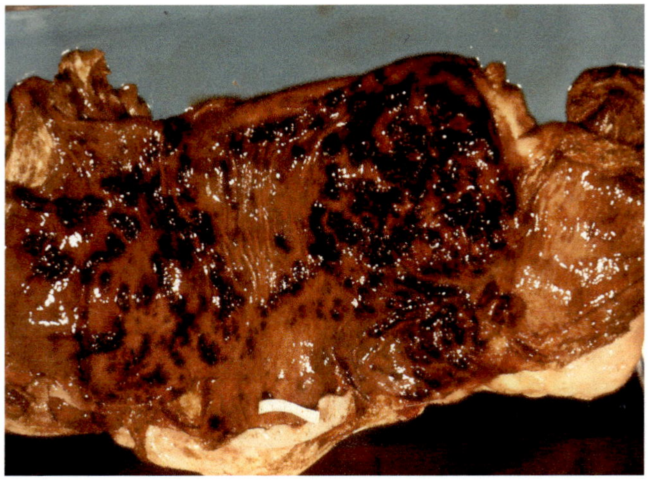

Fig. 5.64. Ox. Abomasum. Bracken fern toxicosis. Hemorrhagic abomasitis. Ingestion with *Pteridium aquilinum* invoked patches of hemorrhage in the mucosa. Arsenic toxicosis may induce similar changes. (For more, see Chapter 16: The Pathology of Select Poisonous Plant-induced Diseases in Cattle.)

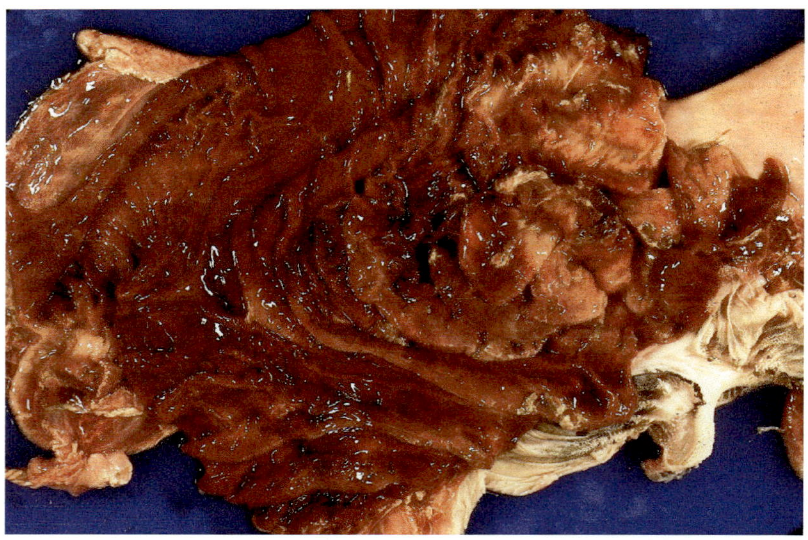

Fig. 5.65. Ox. Abomasum. Hemorrhagic abomasitis. Abomasal rugal folds are widened by edema, and the mucosa is covered markedly by blood. Infectious diseases or toxins are possible etiologic factors. Infestation with *Haemonchus placei* may provoke similar changes, as will infection with the thrombocytopenic strain of bovine viral diarrhea virus (BVDV). More on specific infectious causes of abomasitis can be found in Chapter 1: Diseases of Neonates and Calves.

5.4.5 Endoparasites

Introduction. Abomasal endoparasitism can inflict economic hardship under crowded environmental (intensive husbandry), moist weather, or poor hygienic and dietary conditions.

Clinical signs. Retarded growth, wasting, anemia, diarrhea.

Differential diagnoses. Bacterial and viral infectious gastroenteritis, toxins, other parasitoses.

5.4.5.1 Haemonchosis

Haemonchus placei, commonly referred to as 'barber pole' worm infestation, thrives in hot, humid climates. The bloodsucking parasite causes fatal anemia and hypoproteinemia. The life cycle is direct.

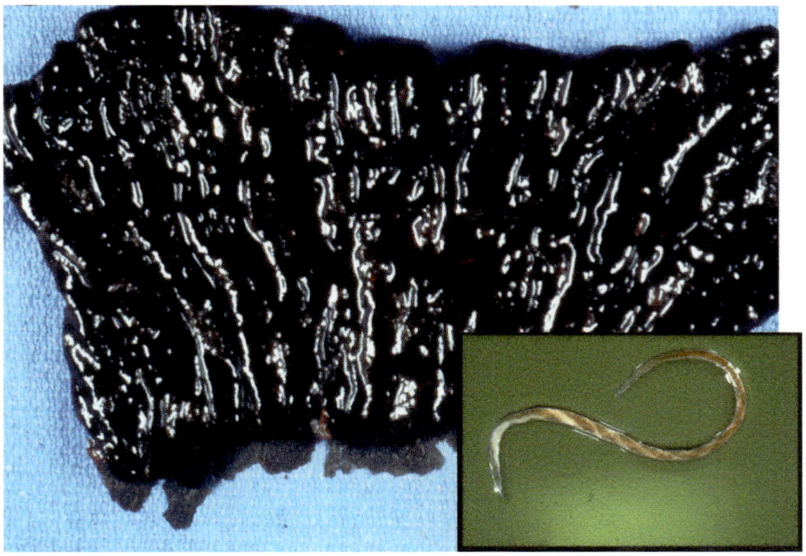

Fig. 5.66. Ox. Abomasum. Haemonchosis. Hemorrhagic abomasitis. Severe hemorrhagic effusion or punctate erosions in the mucosa can be inflicted by *Haemonchus placei*, depending on the load. Punctuate erosions in the mucosa reflect attachment sites. Spreading gastric contents over a white surface helps to identify individual parasites. Inset: individual 'barber pole' nematode.

5.4.5.2 Ostertagiosis

Ostertagia ostertagii is the most important parasite of grazing cattle in temperate climate zones. The life cycle is direct. Inflicted proliferating lesions in the abomasal mucosa cause hypoproteinemia and achlorhydria. Type I ostertagiosis results from ingestion of large numbers of larvae developing into adults. Type II disease is caused by hyperbiotic larvae in the abomasal glands from which they are shed in late winter or early spring.

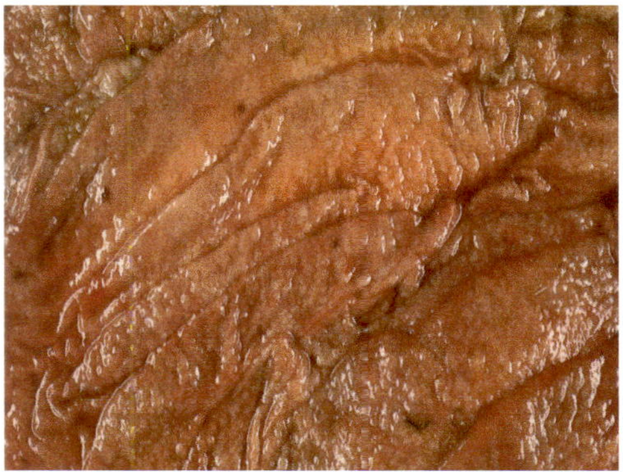

Fig. 5.67. Ox. Abomasum. Ostertagiosis. Proliferative abomasitis. Thickened rugal folds contain small cobblestone nodules of epithelial hyperplasia.

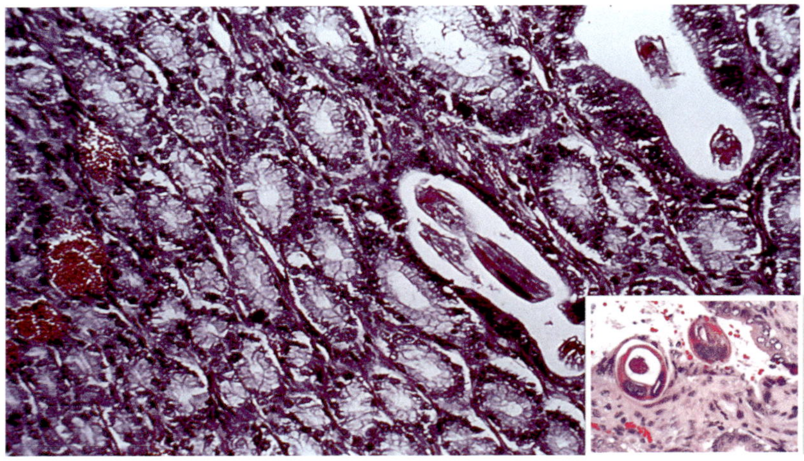

Fig. 5.68. Ox. Abomasum. Ostertagiosis. Proliferative abomasitis. Larvae of type II disease are burrowed within gastric pits of a hyperplastic mucosa. Inset: mucosa shows fibrosis with cross-sectioned nematodes present (H&E).

5.4.5.3 *Trichostrongylus axei*

The intraepithelial location of the small nematodes induces a diffuse thickening of the abomasal mucosa similar to *O. ostertagii*.

5.4.6 Neoplasia

Introduction. The abomasum is one of the three favorite non-lymphoid target sites for the bovine leukosis virus (BLV)-induced lymphoma to occur (heart and uterus are the other two non-lymphoid principal sites). Neoplastic involvement may be diffuse or nodular. Secondary tumor ulcers may develop.
Clinical signs. Weight loss, loss of appetite.
Differential diagnoses. Endoparasitism, impaction.

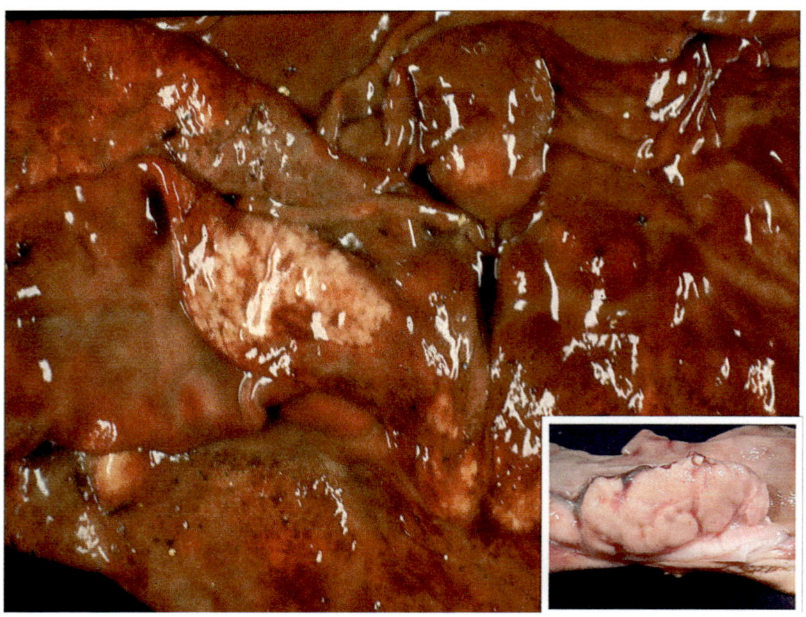

Fig. 5.69. Ox. Abomasum. Lymphoma (lymphosarcoma). Abomasal folds are distended and thickened by multiple pale, white, plaque-like elevations. Inset: the wall contains a glistening, lobulated focal growth compatible with lymphoma (lymphosarcoma).

5.5 DISEASES OF THE INTESTINAL TRACT

Digestion of food and protection from toxins and infectious agents are major functions of the intestinal tract. Nutrients, electrolytes, and water become part of the body only after they have crossed the intestinal lining of the gut and have entered the bloodstream. The intestinal mucosa is the most important stratum for digestion, absorption, and secretion. Most of this activity occurs in the small intestine. The principal function of the large intestine is absorption of sodium, chloride, and water, as well as secretion of mucus to facilitate fecal passing.

Morphologically, the small intestinal tract differs from the large intestinal tract by the presence of villi, which project into the intestinal lumen to increase the surface area.

The mucosal epithelium contains two main cell types: the enterocytes responsible for digestion and absorption, and the goblet cells secreting mucus for protection.

The intestinal tract has its own specialized immune system known as the gut-associated lymphoid tissue (GALT). Both cellular and humeral arms of the immune system represent important defense mechanisms. Peyer's patches in the mucosa of ruminants are compact and grossly visible structures of the cellular immune system. Peyer's patches are on the antimesenteric border of the ileum in a continuous line and multifocal in the jejunum.

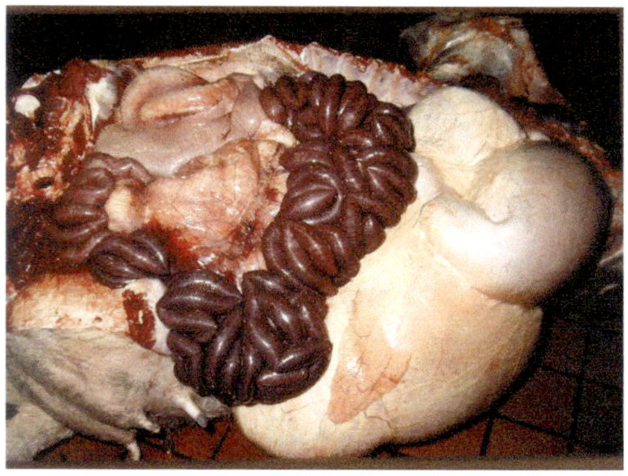

Fig. 5.70. Ox. Small Intestine. Volvulus. The loops of much of the jejunum are coiled and diffusely red-blue after rotation around the mesenteric attachment. Venous outflow obstruction devitalizes the intestinal wall, leading to ischemic necrosis and breakdown of the intestinal barrier system.

5.5.1 Anomalies

Examples are covered in Chapter 1: Diseases of Neonates and Calves.

5.5.2 Displacements and obstruction

Introduction. Twisting of small intestinal loops (volvulus), large intestinal rotation (torsion), or telescoping of intestinal segments (intussusception) interfere with the passage of digesta and invoke vascular compromise.

Clinical signs. Abdominal pain, abdominal distention, shock, lack of defecation.

Differential diagnoses. Ruminal displacement, abomasal torsion/volvulus, neoplasia, peritonitis.

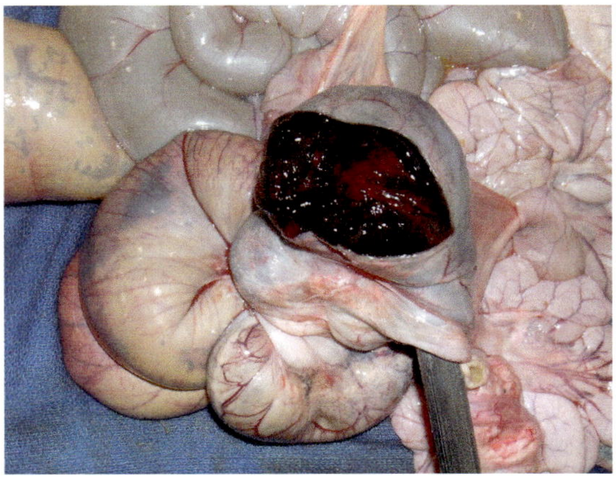

Fig. 5.72. Ox. Spiral colon. Intussusception. Segments of the colon are distended segmentally. The telescoped portion of the colon is markedly discolored and softened, indicating severe ischemic necrosis. This type of intussusception is rare; ceco-colonic intussusception occurs more frequently.

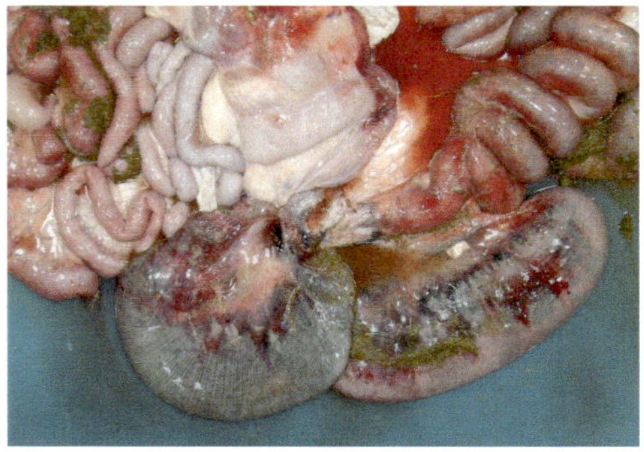

Fig. 5.71. Ox. Cecum. Torsion and ischemic infarction. The cecum on the right has rotated around its longitudinal axis, compromising its blood supply. As sequela, the wall is diffusely red due to venous stasis. During this process, the cecal wall ruptured, causing the release of ingesta. Portions of the colon on the left twisted as well.

5.5.3 Inflammation

Enteric inflammation conditions have overlapping morphologic features at the gross level. There are many classification schemes, one of which conveniently organizes enteric inflammation according to morphologic appearance, etiology, and time course (Table 5.1).

Table 5.1. Classification scheme for enteric inflammation.

Morphology	Etiology	Duration
Catarrhal (secretory)	Viral	Acute
Hemorrhagic	Bacterial	Subacute
Fibrinonecrotic	Mycotic (rare)	Chronic
Erosive-ulcerative-necrotic	Parasitic	
Granulomatous	Protozoal	
	Toxic	

Individual disease examples that are best applicable for each type of inflammation are presented.

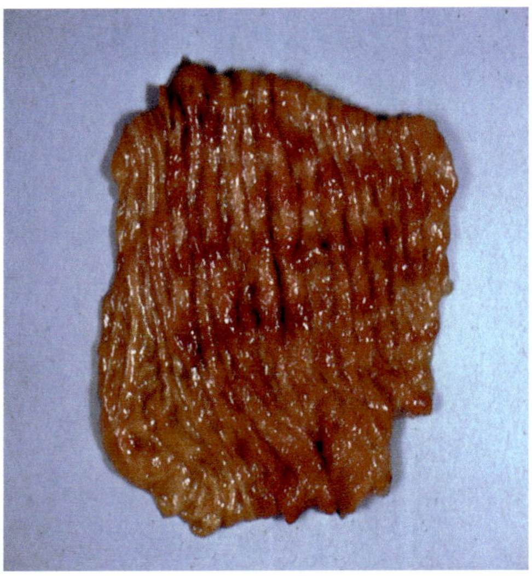

Fig. 5.73. Ox. Spiral colon. Winter dysentery. Mucosal congestion with multifocal hemorrhage. The mucosa is diffusely red and small hemorrhagic foci are embedded. Occasional blood clots are present in the lumen or are passed with feces. (Courtesy of Dr H. Van Kruiningen, University of Connecticut, USA.)

5.5.3.1 Catarrhal enteritis

Rotavirus, coronavirus, and adenovirus enteritis are viral diseases with gross manifestations of catarrhal inflammation. Colibacillosis exemplifies a bacterial enteric disease. Some endoparasites (*Trichuris* spp.) induce a similar intestinal inflammatory response. Some of these are introduced in Chapter 1: Diseases of Neonates and Calves.

5.5.3.2 Hemorrhagic enteritis

Winter dysentery

Introduction. A highly contagious disease that spreads rapidly within the establishment of adult cows in the winter months (has also been observed in summer months) has been associated with a coronavirus in the Northern American hemisphere. Mortality is low. The colon is mainly affected. Coronavirus can be demonstrated by culture in feces and by indirect immunohistochemistry in enteric tissue.

Clinical signs. Dysentery, hemorrhagic diarrhea, melena, temporary loss of milk production.

Differential diagnoses. Hemorrhagic bowel syndrome, coccidiosis, salmonellosis, poisons.

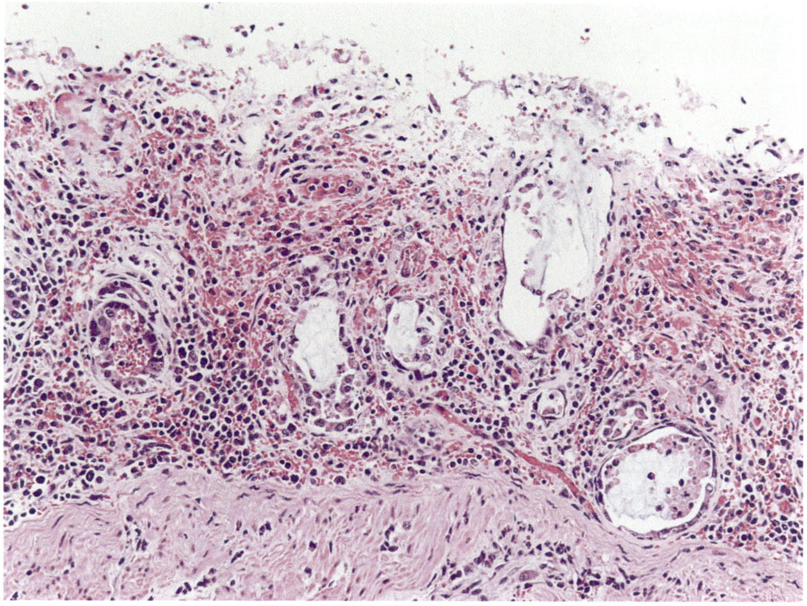

Fig. 5.74. Ox. Colon. Winter dysentery. Ulcerative, hemorrhagic colitis. Mucosal enterocytes are lost. Glands are distended by fibrin and have sequestered lining cells. Extravasation of red blood cells into the lamina propria is intense (H&E). (Courtesy of Dr S. Diab, University of California, USA.)

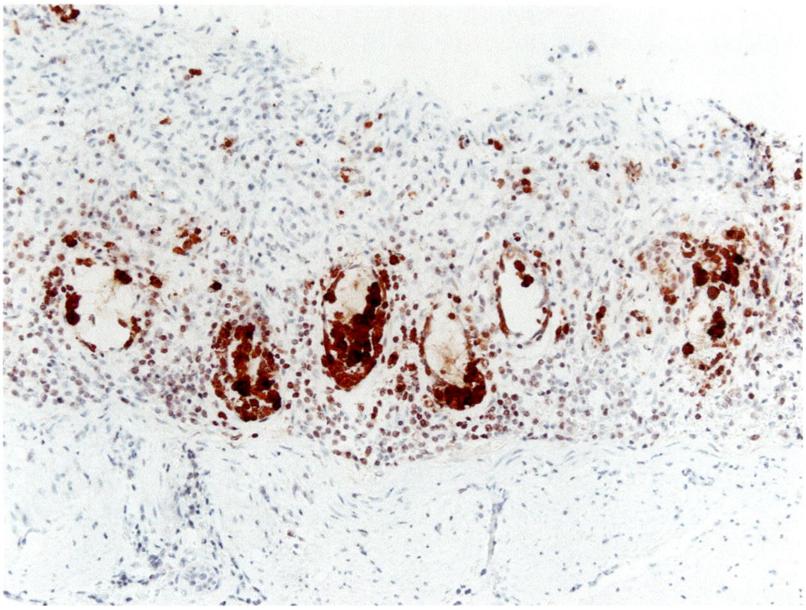

Fig. 5.75. Ox. Colon. Winter dysentery. Basal epithelial cells of glands exhibit dense labeling for coronavirus antigen by indirect immunohistochemistry (IHC). (Courtesy of Dr S. Diab, University of California, USA.)

Enterotoxemia

Introduction. Caused by *Clostridium perfringens* type D, it is a sporadic enteric disease in cattle, unlike in sheep. The causal relationship of *C. perfringens* type D in natural occurrence of diarrhea in cattle remains elusive. The clostridium produces alpha and epsilon toxins that can be analyzed in luminal contents.

Clinical signs. Dyspnea, ataxia, convulsions, recumbency.

Differential diagnoses. Neurologic diseases, nitrate toxicity.

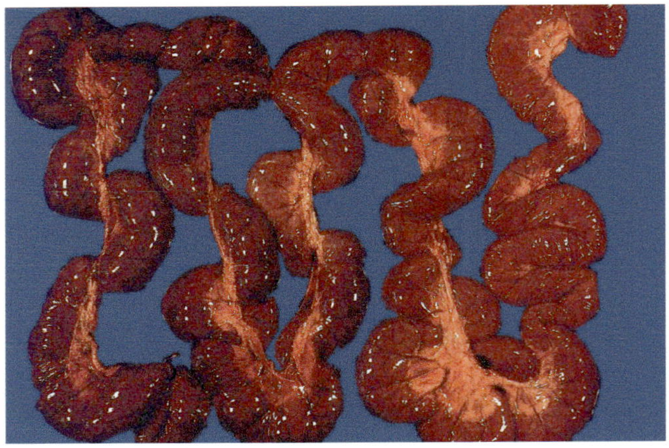

Fig. 5.76. Ox. Jejunum. Enterotoxemia. Hemorrhagic enteropathy. Loops of jejunum are manifesting severe, diffuse red discoloration.

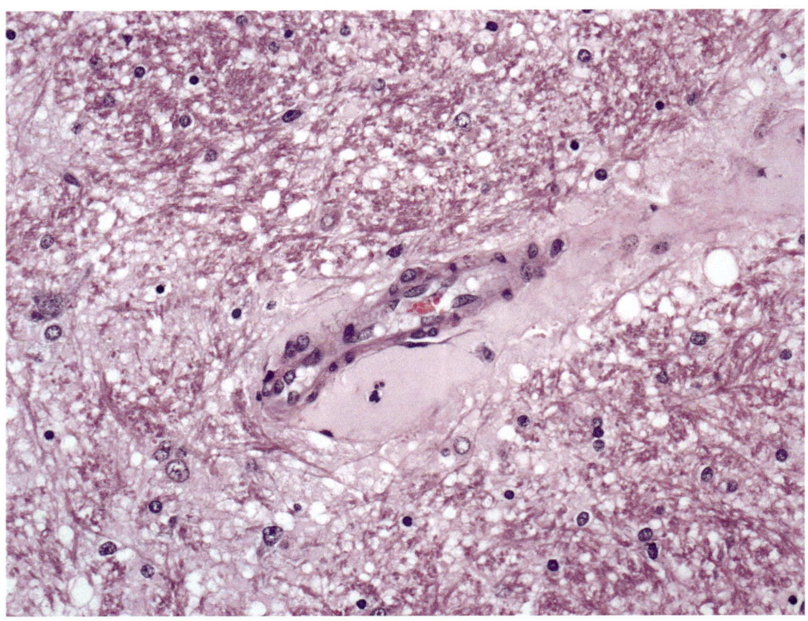

Fig. 5.77. Ox. Cerebral blood vessel. Enterotoxemia. Proteinaceous perivascular edema. In studies with calves experimentally inoculated with *Clostridium perfringens* type D, it has been shown that the neurologic signs exhibited in these animals have resulted from microangiopathy of cerebral blood vessels leading to fibrinoid vascular wall necrosis and vascular permeability disturbances. Histologic examination of brain tissue is recommended to support the diagnosis of enterotoxemia (H&E). (Courtesy of Dr F. Uzal, University of California, USA.)

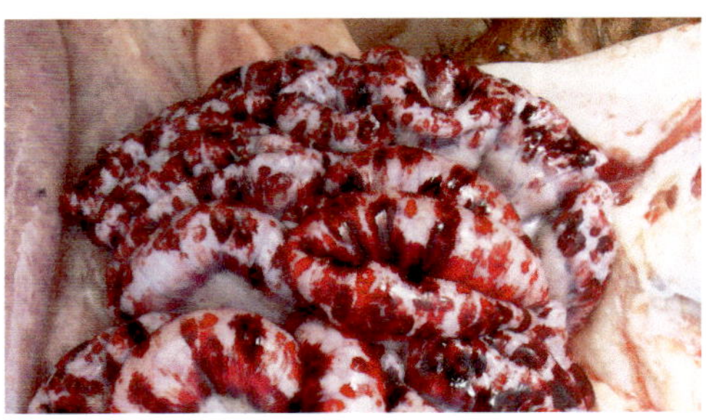

Fig. 5.78. Ox. Intestine. Tiger striping. Ecchymoses and patches of hemorrhage in the serosa of intestinal tissue can be encountered in agony, winter dysentery, bovine viral diarrhea virus (BVDV) infection, and rinderpest (presumably eradicated morbillivirus).

5.5.3.3 *Fibrinonecrotic enteritis*

Also defined as pseudomembranous enteritis, the hallmark changes are the formation of fibrin casts from necrotic enteric mucosa. An example of this type of inflammation occurs in salmonellosis.

Salmonellosis

Introduction. Outbreaks of salmonellosis occur from changes in management (free-stall housing), concurrent infection with the BVDV or other pathogens, contaminated feed and feed supplements, carrier animals other than ruminants shedding the organism into the environment, environmental stressors, and other risk factors. Young animals have a greater susceptibility to infection with *Salmonella* spp. than adult animals. Young animals more likely suffer from sepsis. Adults are frequently colonizing the bacterium without developing disease, thus serving as carriers. There are 2500 serotypes of *Salmonella* organisms, with varying strain virulence. Varying virulence factors are responsible for enteric and systemic lesions. Uptake of organisms occurs by absorptive enterocytes and M-cells. A frequent isolate is *Salmonella enterica* serovar *typhimurium*. Fecal–oral transmission is the usual route of infection. The organism is a facultative intracellular agent residing in macrophages. Most infections are confined to the intestinal tract and draining mesenteric lymph nodes, particularly in feedlot cattle. Sepsis ensues when the organisms are shed into other organs, including the udder. *Salmonell*a spp. are zoonotic. The bacilli produce endotoxins, enterotoxins, and cytotoxins. There are acute and chronic forms of salmonellosis. The acute disease is associated more with a catarrhal or hemorrhagic enteritis. As the disease progresses, the mucosa becomes necrotic, and sloughs to form casts or pseudo (diphtheritic) membranes in the enteric lumen. The chronic form features a scabby, crusty mucosa. Draining lymph nodes are enlarged. Transient BVDV infection may exist concurrently in infected animals. Salmonellosis of calves is presented in Chapter 1: Diseases of Neonates and Calves.

Clinical signs. Fever, diarrhea, odiferous feces.

Differential diagnoses. Coccidiosis, winter dysentery, endoparasitism.

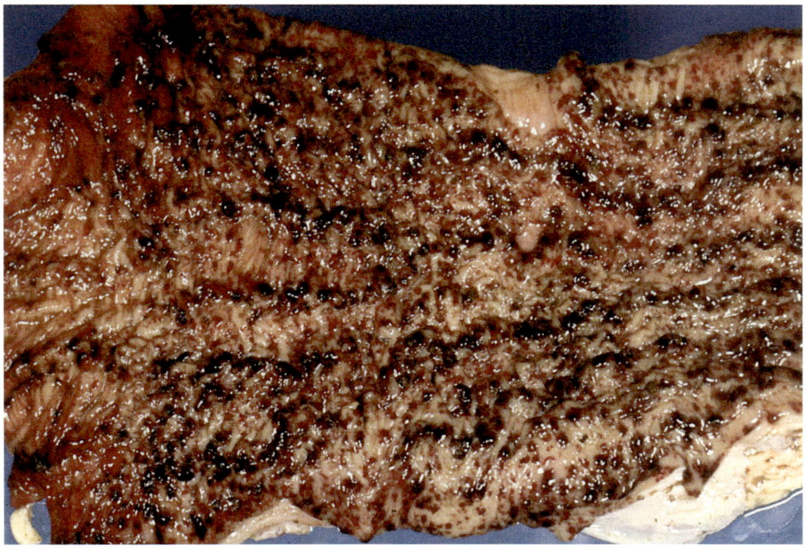

Fig. 5.79. Ox. Intestine. Salmonellosis. Hemorrhagic enteritis. The pale red mucosa is covered by multiple discrete, deep red patches of hemorrhage, suggestive of acute infection.

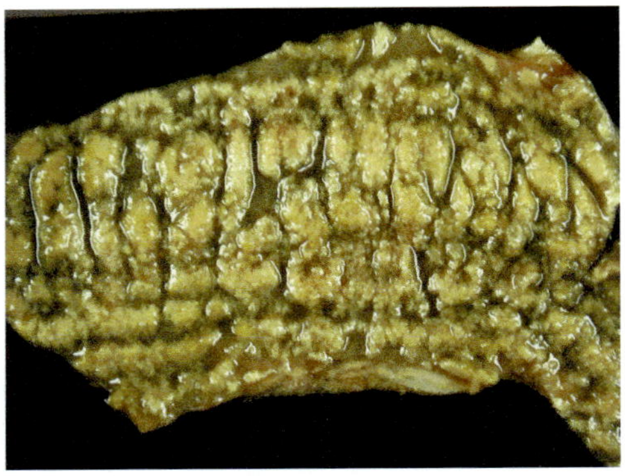

Fig. 5.81. Ox. Colon. Salmonellosis. Pseudomembranous (diphtheritic) enterocolitis. The mucosa is diffusely covered by inspissated fibrin representing the chronic type of salmonellosis.

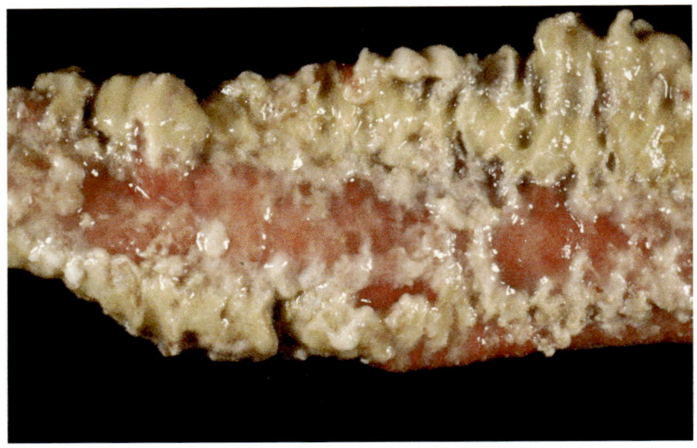

Fig. 5.80. Ox. Colon. Salmonellosis. Diphtheritic colitis. Collections of fibrin bands cover a slightly red mucosa. The animal was co-infected with transient bovine viral diarrhea virus (BVDV). This represents the subacute form of infection.

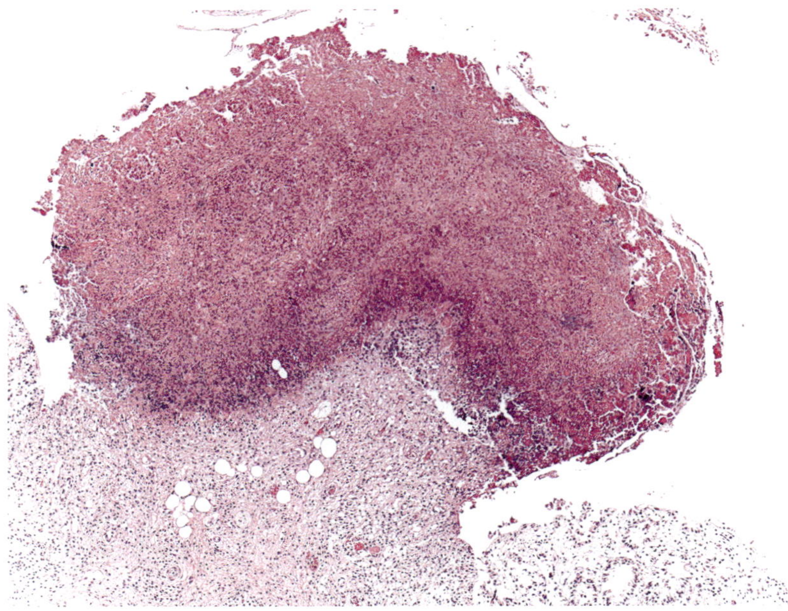

Fig. 5.82. Ox. Colon. Salmonellosis. Necro-ulcerative colitis with diphtheritic membrane. The colon mucosa is ulcerated, partially absent, and replaced by a fungiform, thick layer of fibrin and necrotic cells containing basophilic bacterial colonies. The underlying submucosa is effaced by edema and mononuclear cells. Fibrin thrombi are found within the capillary lumina.

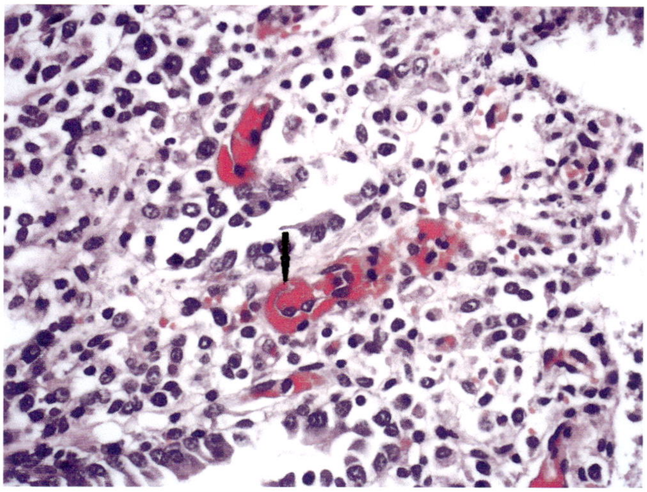

Fig. 5.83. Ox. Intestine. Salmonellosis. Vascular fibrin thrombi. Small arteries and capillaries in the lamina propria often contain fibrin thrombi (arrow). The thrombi may also develop in the lymphatics. Toxins secreted by *Salmonella* spp. are responsible for fibrin thrombi in small enteric blood vessels by causing endothelial damage and initiating the fibrin cascade. An alternative mechanism is disseminated intravascular coagulopathy (DIC). The lamina propria contains moderate numbers of lymphocytes and plasma cells (H&E).

5.5.3.4 Erosive-ulcerative-necrotizing enteritis

Bovine viral diarrhea

Introduction. BVDV infection when presenting as mucosal disease (MD) in a persistently infected animal induces ulceration of Peyer's patches and mucosal erosions in the small intestine. These changes are not pathognomonic for BVDV as they can also be seen with *Salmonella* spp. On occasion in the colon, one may encounter a diffuse, fibrinous, necrotizing typhlitis with intraluminal fibrinous casts and crypt abscesses. Special attention should be paid to vascular changes (submucosal vasculitis) at histologic examination of small intestinal tissue, and to immunohistochemical demonstration of BVDV antigen in the inflamed vessel wall, to confirm the presence of virus antigen. To best observe Peyer's patches, the ileum should be opened close to the mesenteric attachment.

Clinical signs. Diarrhea, sialorrhea, lameness, stunting, wasting, compromised immunity (immunosuppression).

Differential diagnoses. Salmonellosis, endoparasitism, gastrointestinal lymphosarcoma.

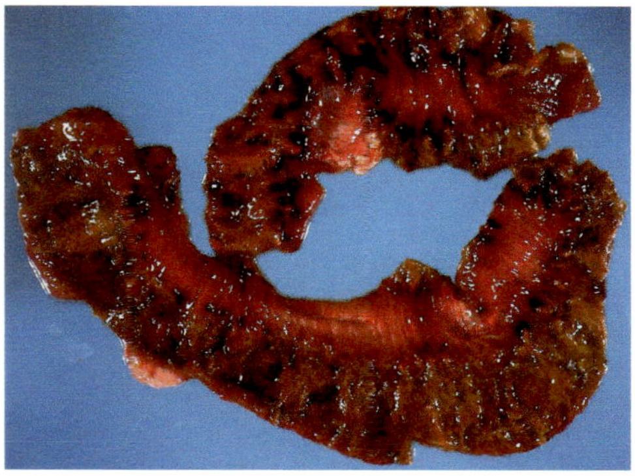

Fig. 5.84. Ox. Intestine. Bovine viral diarrhea virus (BVDV). Fibrino-necrotizing enteritis. Rarely, severe BVDV infection may cause a fibrino-necrotizing enteritis indistinguishable from salmonellosis. (Courtesy of the Government of Alberta, Canada.)

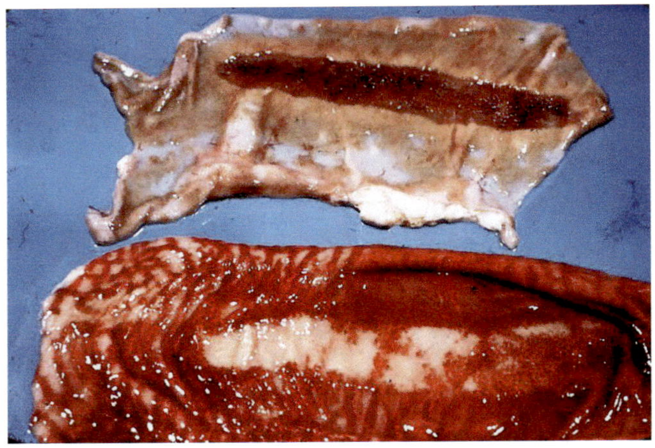

Fig. 5.85. Ox. Small intestine. Bovine viral diarrhea virus (BVDV). Peyer's patches. Necrosis and normal. The upper Peyer's patch has lost its smooth surface and is covered by fibrin and blood. The normal Peyer's patch below has maintained its smooth, intact, white surface.

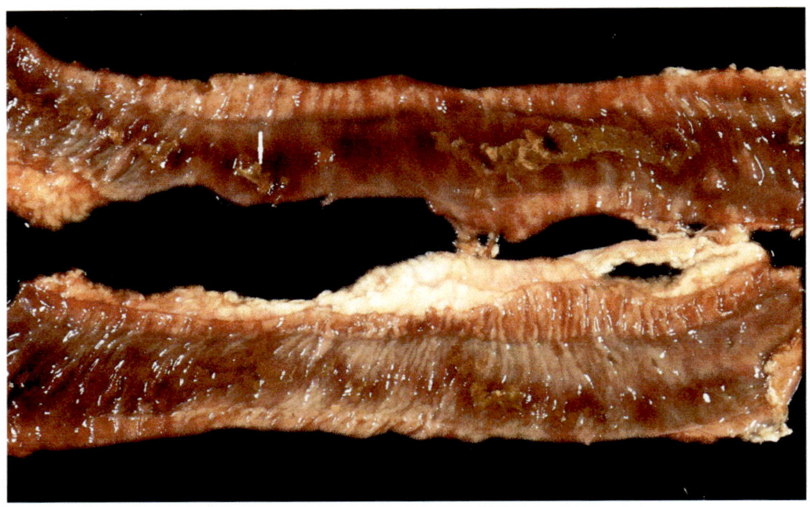

Fig. 5.86. Ox. Small intestine. Bovine viral diarrhea virus (BVDV). Peyer's patches necrosis. These are covered by fibrin; so are other parts of the mucosa (arrow). Co-infection with *Salmonella* spp. has to be considered in the differential diagnosis.

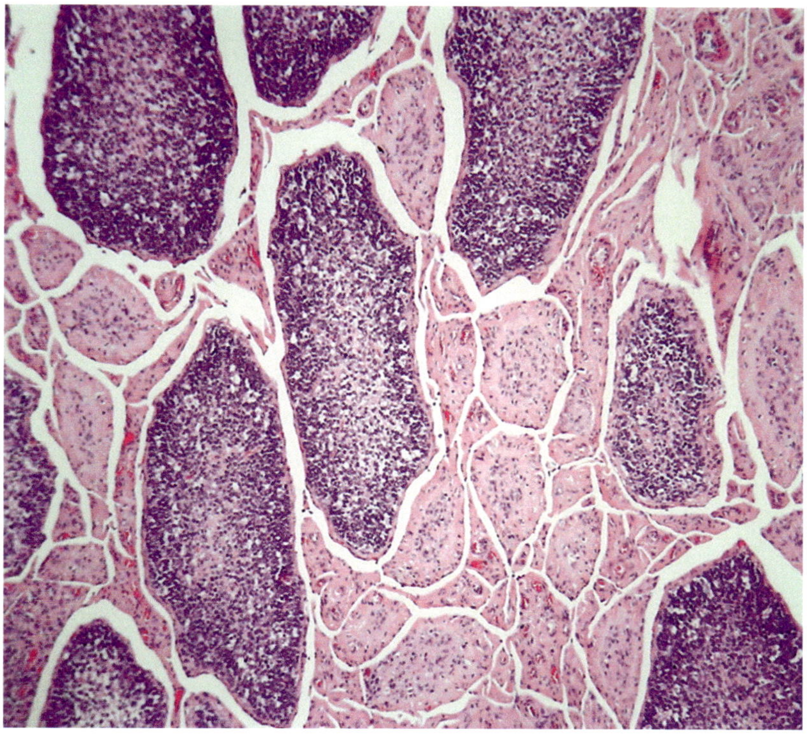

Fig. 5.87. Ox. Small intestine. Bovine viral diarrhea virus (BVDV). Peyer's patch. Follicles are atrophic and depleted from lymphocytolysis. In transient infections, it is common to see some of the follicles beginning to regenerate, as seen in this image (H&E).

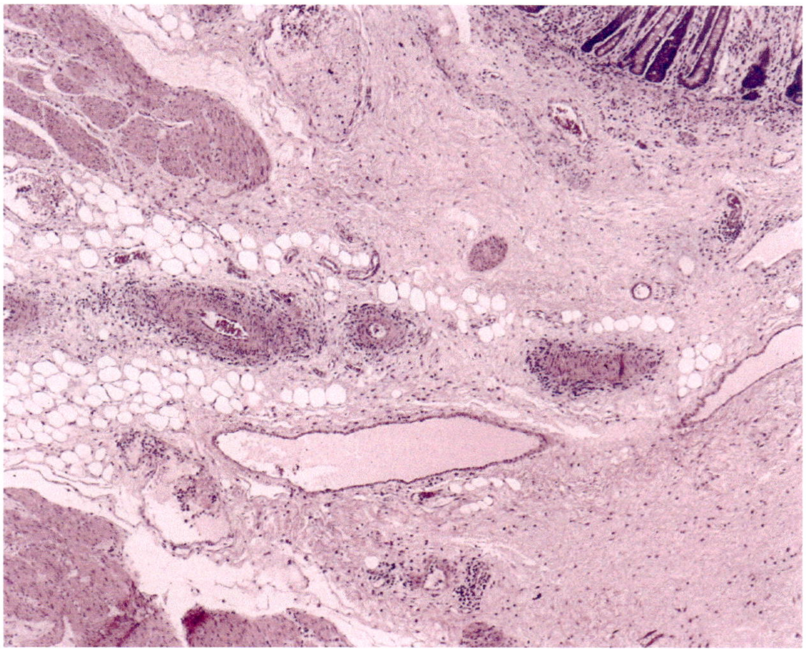

Fig. 5.88. Ox. Colon. Bovine viral diarrhea virus (BVDV). Vasculitis. Several arteries in the submucosa are infiltrated and surrounded by lymphocytes. This is occasionally seen in mucosal disease cases, but is much more common in transient infections (H&E).

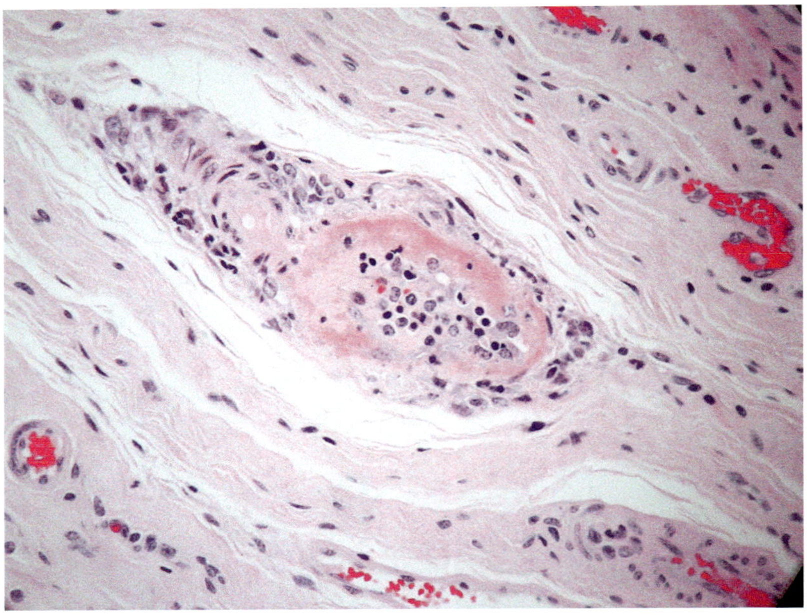

Fig. 5.89. Ox. Ileum. Bovine viral diarrhea virus (BVDV). Necrotizing vasculitis. Small arteries in the submucosa of the small intestine frequently show fibrinoid necrosis in the media with intramural and perivascular lymphocyte collections. Lymphocytic vasculitis and perivasculitis occur in multiple organ systems in BVDV infection, particularly in transient infection. The vascular changes are thought to be type III immune hypersensitivity reactions. The vascular changes should not be confused with ones induced by malignant catarrhal fever (MCF) (H&E).

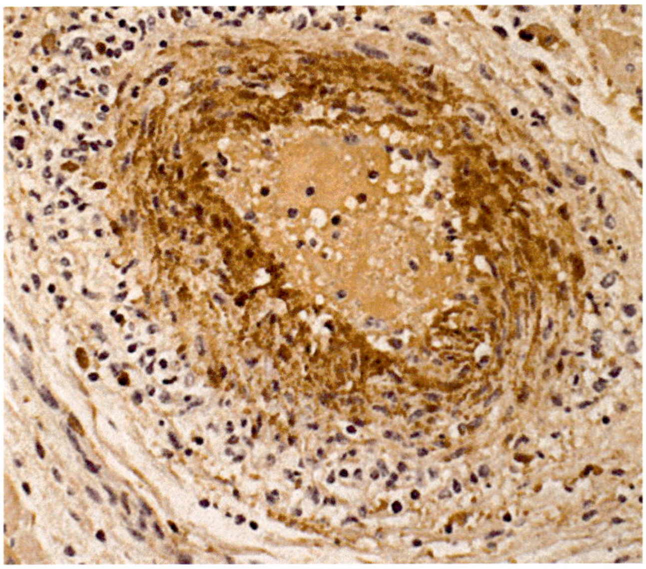

Fig. 5.90. Ox. Blood vessel. Bovine viral diarrhea virus (BVDV). Cytoplasmic viral antigen is detected in the media of a small artery and in histiocytes in the perivascular location (IHC).

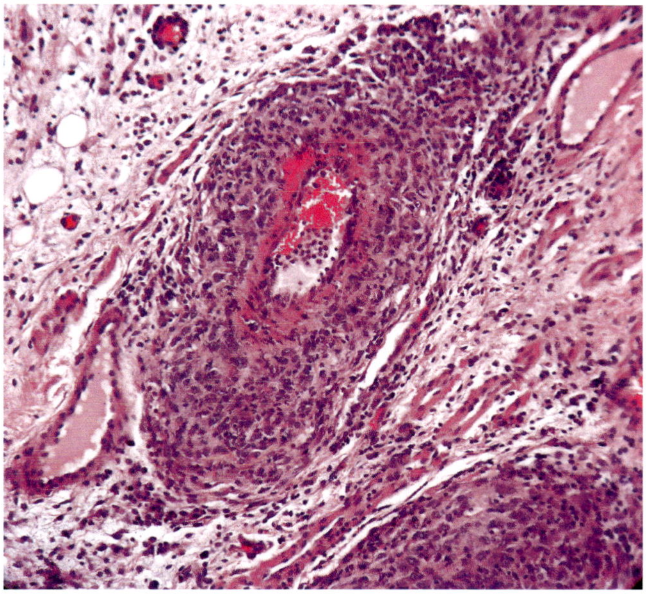

Fig. 5.91. Ox. Blood vessel. Bovine viral diarrhea virus (BVDV). Necrotizing lymphocytic panvasculitis. The vasculitis can be quite intensive, involving all layers of the vessel wall. Heart, lung, and kidneys are recommended organs to look for these dense vascular lymphocytic populations, especially when transient BVDV infection is involved.

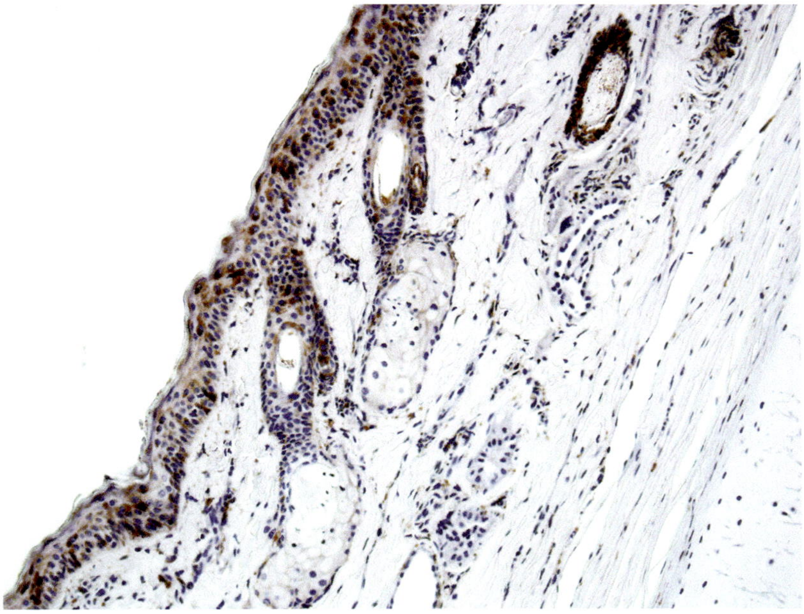

Fig. 5.92. Ox. Bovine viral diarrhea virus (BVDV). Skin test. Most conveniently, skin from the ear notch or from other sites in the body can be subjected to indirect immunohistochemistry for BVD viral antigen demonstration in the cytoplasm of epithelial cells (keratinocytes) of epidermis and adnexa (follicular epithelium), blood vessel endothelium, myocytes and pericytes, nerves, and Langerhans antigen-presenting cells. If antigen is demonstrated in all these sites, then the animal is most likely a persistently infected (PI) individual. Focal staining is typical of a transient infection, but if the infection is too chronic, the skin may be totally negative (IHC).

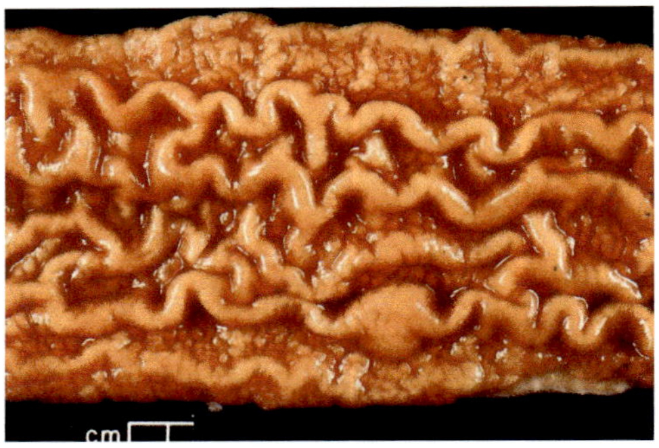

Fig. 5.93. Ox. Ileum. Paratuberculosis. Granulomatous ileitis. The intact mucosal surface has a corrugated, thickened appearance. In cases of intestinal tuberculosis, one should expect a multifocal ulcerative enteritis.

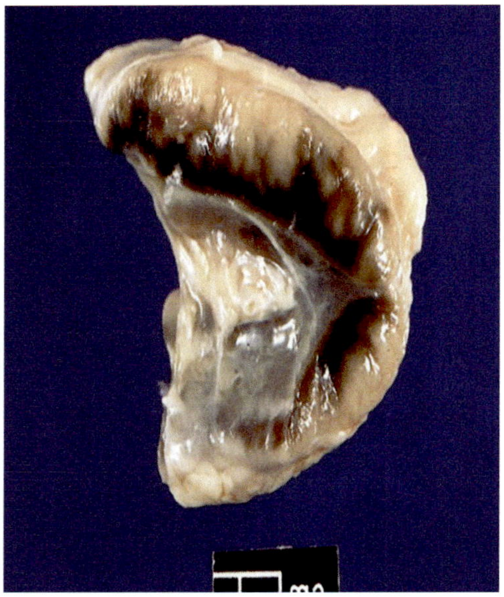

Fig. 5.94. Ox. Mesenteric lymph node. Paratuberculosis. Lymphadenopathy. After phagocytosis of *Mycobacterium avium* subsp. *paratuberculosis* (MAP) bacilli, macrophages and inflammatory giant cells are permanently drained into adjacent mesenteric lymph nodes (reactive lymph nodes). For paratuberculosis screening purposes, it is recommended to collect the ileocecal lymph node in addition to intestinal (ileum) samples.

5.5.3.5 Granulomatous enteritis

Bovine paratuberculosis and tuberculosis are infectious disease examples fitting the clinical and morphologic criteria of chronic granulomatous enteric inflammation.

Granulomatous inflammation affecting the intestinal tract is associated with protein-losing enteropathy and malabsorption. Its duration is chronic. The intestinal mucosa grossly is markedly thickened due to intense diffuse inflammatory cell infiltration, primarily macrophages and inflammatory giant cells. Associated lymph nodes are enlarged by draining inflammatory cells from intestinal tissue.

Bovine paratuberculosis (Johne's disease)

Introduction. Domestic and wild ruminants are susceptible to natural infection with *Mycobacterium avium* subsp. *paratuberculosis* (MAP), a facultative intracellular acid-fast bacillus. Paratuberculosis has a worldwide distribution. The oral–fecal route is mainly responsible for the transmission of the organisms. Other routes of transmission are via colostrum and *in utero*. The organism is shed into semen. In a herd situation, most animals are subclinically infected and shedders of MAP; only few show signs of clinical disease ('tip of the iceberg' concept). Currently, the disease is controlled by 'test-and-cull' programs, as the bacilli resist treatment and preventative vaccination is not an option in cattle.

Clinical signs. Persistent diarrhea, progressive weight loss.

Differential diagnoses. BVDV, salmonellosis, endoparasitism, intestinal tuberculosis, gastrointestinal lymphosarcoma, and subtotal intestinal obstruction.

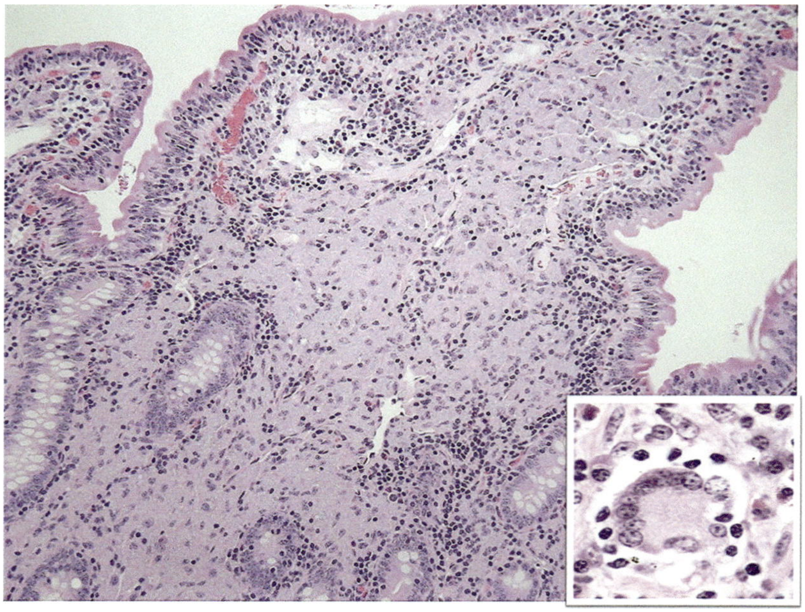

Fig. 5.95. Ox. Ileum. Paratuberculosis. Granulomatous ileitis. The villus is markedly widened by epithelioid macrophages occupying the lamina propria partially replacing mucosal glands. Inset: inflammatory giant cells participate in the granuloma formation. Early in the infection, individual inflammatory giant cells (Langhans type), when detected in the superficial lamina propria, are supportive of the diagnosis of paratuberculosis (H&E).

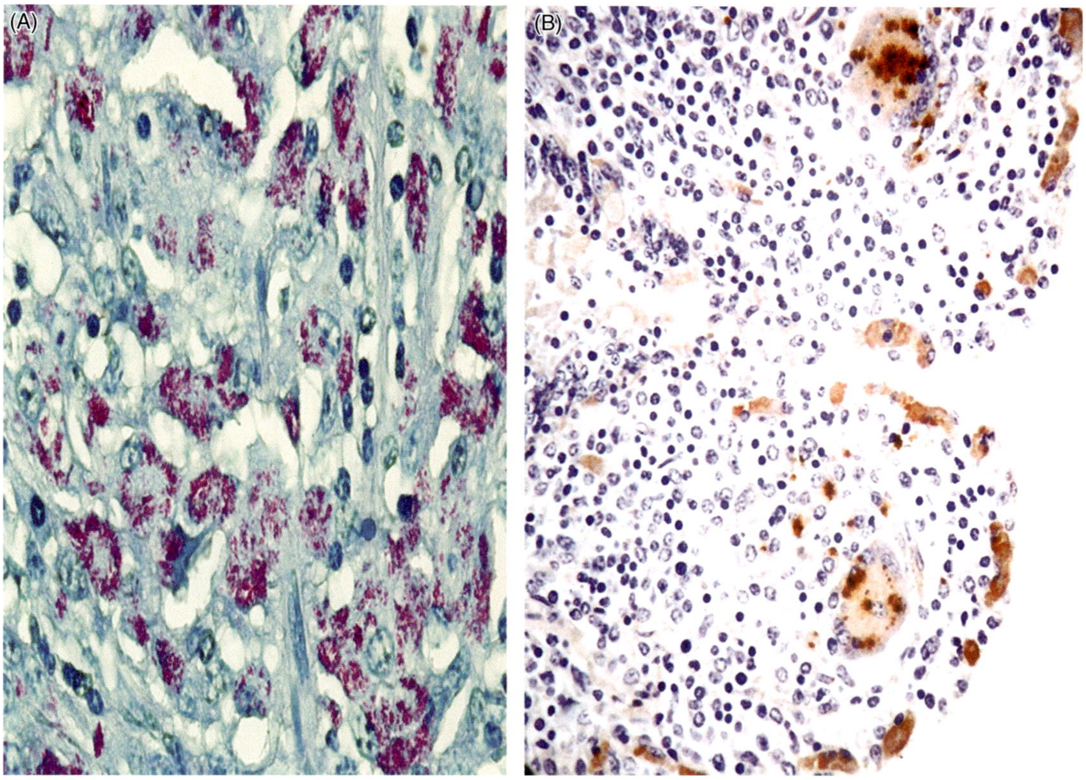

Fig. 5.96. Ox. Ileum. Paratuberculosis. (A) A plethora of acid-fast bacilli can be demonstrated in macrophages and inflammatory giant cells by special stain, as an example of the multibacillary form of the disease. A paucibacillary form of paratuberculosis exists, but to a lesser incidence (Ziehl–Neelsen). (B) Immunohistochemical labeling of populations of bacilli in the cytoplasm of macrophages and inflammatory giant cells (IHC).

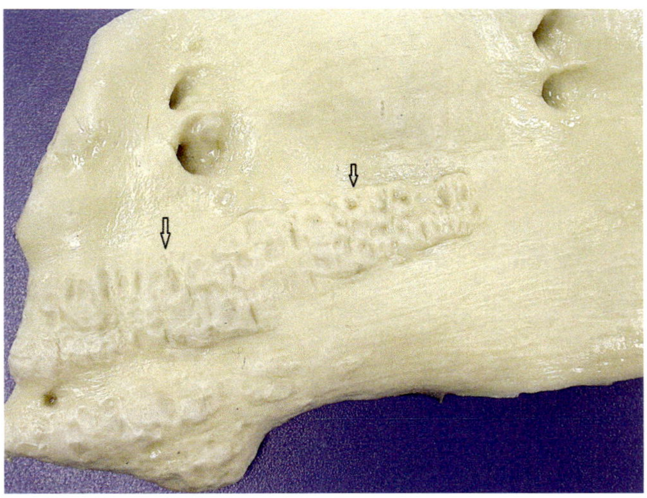

Fig. 5.97. Ox. Aorta. Paratuberculosis. Mineralization. The intima contains firm, elevated plaques (arrows). A few clinical cows have aorta intima and/or left atrium endocardial mineral deposits, hypothesized to represent vitamin D3 metabolites produced by activated macrophages.

5.5.4 Intestinal endoparasites

Introduction. The contribution of gastrointestinal endoparasites to unthriftiness in growing and newly pastured livestock should not be overlooked, and should be listed high on the list as a cause of intestinal disease. Nematode spp., Cestode spp. can be encountered in intestinal segments. Their contribution to disease depends on the number of worms present and the injury that each of them inflicts on the host tissue. Generally, clinical signs developing from intestinal parasites are less severe when compared with gastric parasites.

5.5.4.1 *Nematodes*

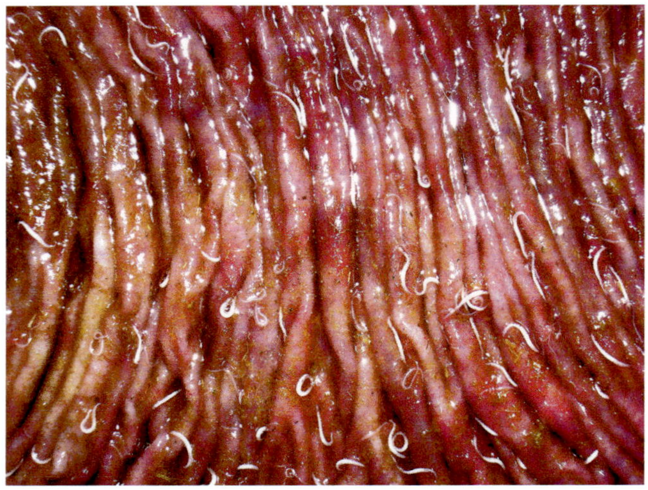

Fig. 5.98. Ox. Cecum. *Trichuris discolor*. Catarrhal typhlitis. The anterior end of the parasites burrows into the mucosa. The irritated mucosa is moist and congested. The life cycle is direct.

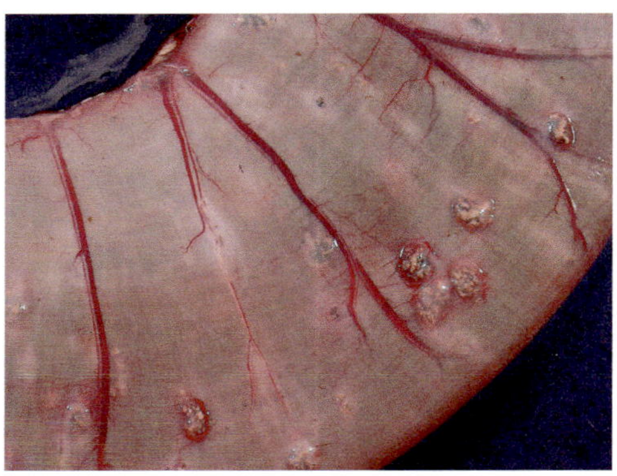

Fig. 5.100. *Ox. Large intestine. Oesophagostomum radiatum*. Serosal calcified granulomas. Adults of *O. radiatum* (nodular worm) live in the large intestine. Larvae develop in the small and large intestinal wall, where they inflict mineralized, caseating nodules on the serosal surface.

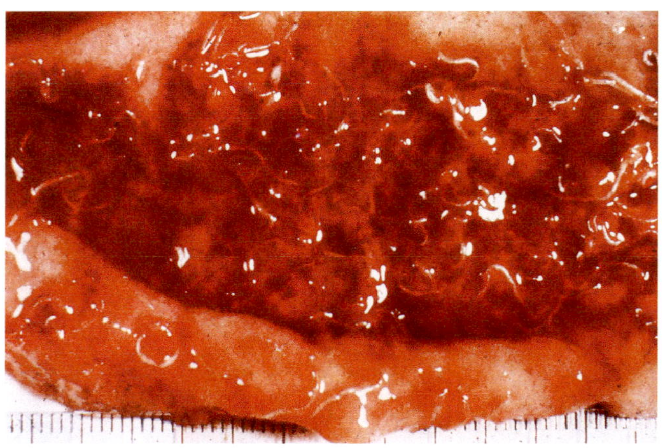

Fig. 5.99. Ox. Small intestine. *Bunostomum phlebotomum*. Hemorrhagic enteritis. Bloodsucking strongyloid nematode ('hookworm'). (Courtesy of the Government of Alberta, Canada.)

5.5.4.2 *Ascarids*

Adults of *Toxocara vitulorum* reside in the small intestine and are shown in Chapter 1: Diseases of Neonates and Calves. Usually, calves are infected at 4–6 months of age. The parasite prefers tropical climates.

5.5.4.3 Cestodes

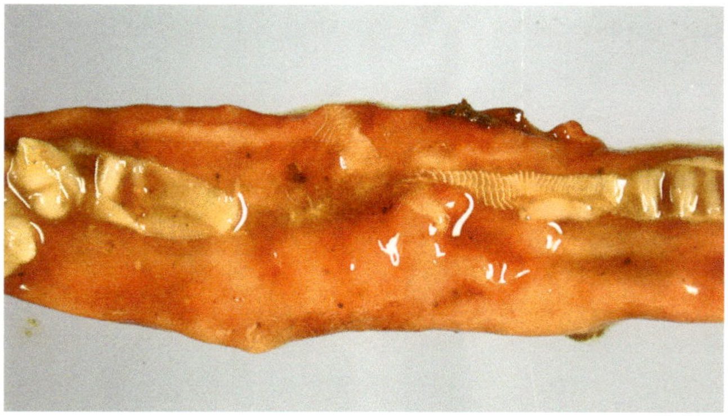

Fig. 5.101. Ox. Intestine. Cestodiasis. *Monezia expansa*. Verminous catarrhal enteritis. An oribatic mite is the intermediate host. Cattle accidentally ingest mites when grazing. Adult parasites with proglottids reside in the small intestine.

5.5.4.4 Protozoa

Introduction. The topic of coccidiosis is also discussed in Chapter 1: Diseases of Neonates and Calves as being one of the causes of calf scours. *Eimeria bovis* and *Eimeria zurnii* are the most pathogenic species of the genus *Eimeria* in adult cattle. Gametogony develops in the terminal ileum, and especially in the colon and cecum. Nervous coccidiosis in beef calves being affected by a heavy load of parasites has been reported from Canada and the USA. The pathogenesis is poorly understood, but is thought to be caused by a toxin produced by the parasites. No brain lesions are present histologically.

Clinical signs. Diarrhea, dysentery, tenesmus, anemia, rectal prolapse.

Differential diagnoses. Viral and bacterial enteric diseases, hemorrhagic bowel syndrome, gastrointestinal lymphosarcoma, toxicities.

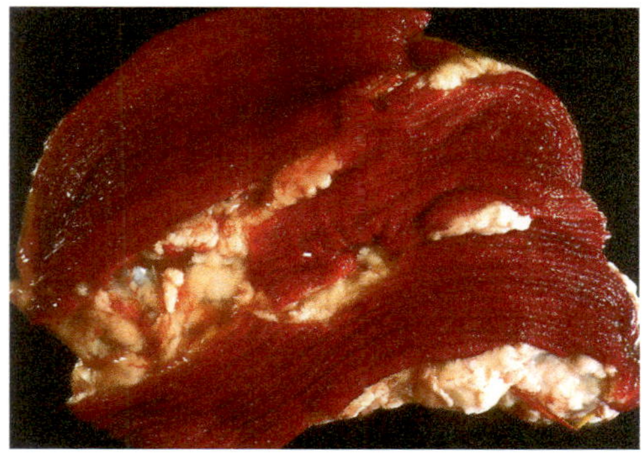

Fig. 5.102. Ox. Spiral colon. Coccidiosis. Hemorrhagic colitis. The mucosa is reddened diffusely. The intestinal lumen can be filled with bloody fluid. Infestation with *Eimeria zurnii* causes the most severe clinical signs. (Courtesy of the Government of Alberta, Canada.)

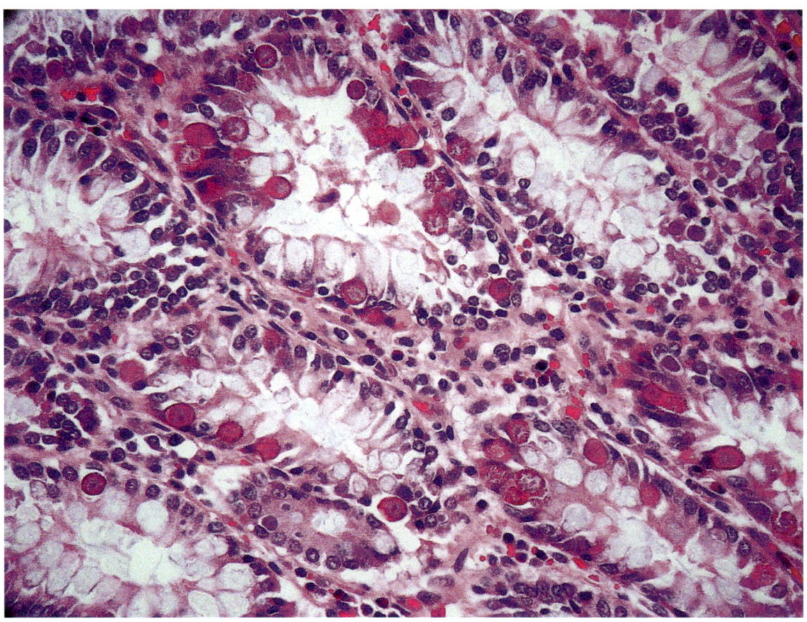

Fig. 5.103. Ox. Coccidiosis. Gametogony. Sexual and asexual stages of *Eimeria* spp. occupy the mucosal enterocytes (H&E).

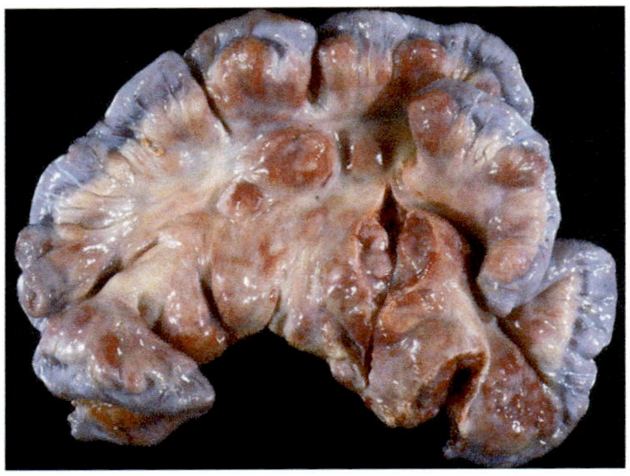

Fig. 5.104. Ox. Small intestine and mesenteric lymph nodes. Lymphosarcoma. Multiple tan brown nodes arise from the serosal surfaces of the intestine, and a similar pattern of growth is noticed in the mesenteric lymph nodes. In a young animal, this type of lymphosarcoma might represent the juvenile form.

5.5.5 Neoplasia

Epithelial or mesenchymal tumors are rare and sporadic in the digestive tract of cattle.

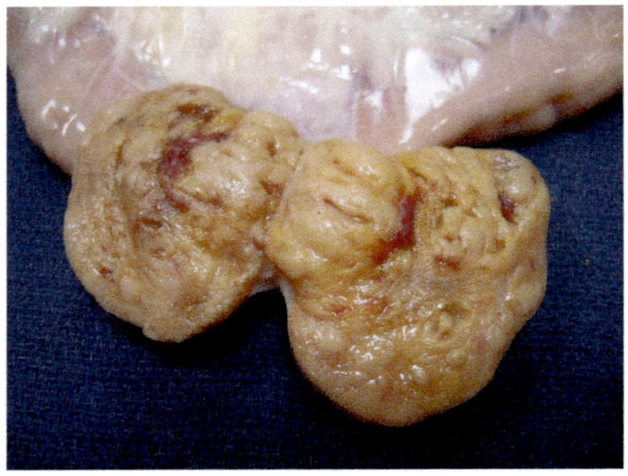

Fig. 5.105. Ox. Small intestine. Leiomyosarcoma. A small, sessile, multilobulated, bulging neoplasm is attached to the serosal surface.

5.5.6 Miscellaneous

5.5.6.1 Hemorrhagic bowel syndrome (HBS)

Introduction. A disorder of adult dairy cattle, also referred to as jejunal hemorrhagic syndrome, has emerged as one of the most frequent causes of small intestinal ileus. Its etiology remains obscure, but some association with toxigenic strains of *Clostridium perfringens* type A has been proposed as a cause. Experimental reproduction of the disease with toxigenic *C. perfringens*, or with its toxins (alpha toxin and beta2 toxin), has failed thus far, despite the clostridial pathogen or its toxins being isolated in most of the clinical studies. Microbiologists have considered *C. perfringens* type A as part of the normal bovine intestinal flora. The disease is seasonal (winter/spring).

Clinical signs. Inappetence, abrupt loss of milk production, colic, abdominal distension, passing of blood or blood clots with feces.

Differential diagnoses. Abomasal and intestinal displacement, intussusception, winter dysentery, bleeding abomasal ulcer.

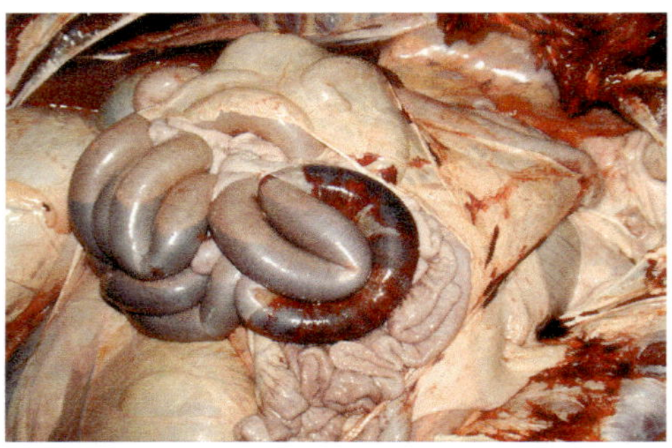

Fig. 5.106. Ox. Jejunum. Hemorrhagic bowel syndrome (HBS). Segmental hemorrhagic jejunitis. Jejunal loops are distended by gas and red-tinged, watery fluid.

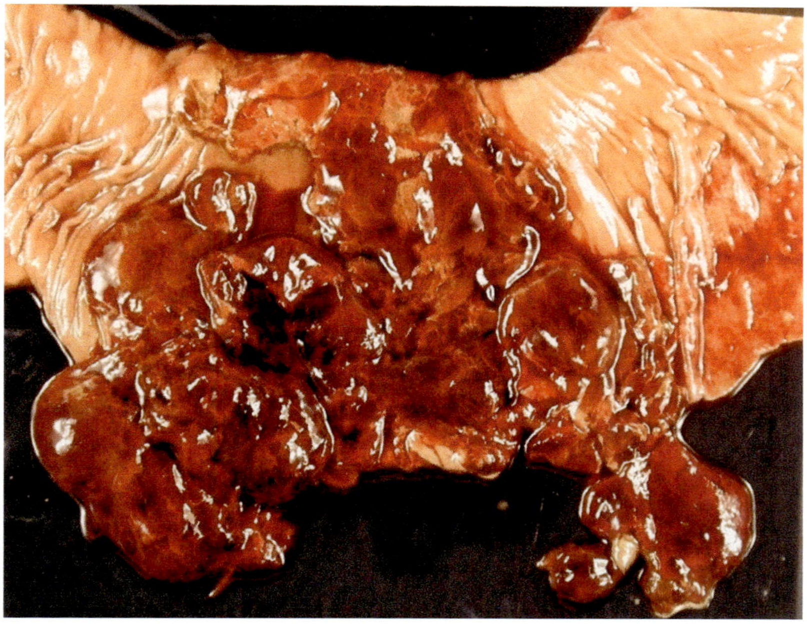

Fig. 5.107. Ox. Jejunum. Hemorrhagic bowel syndrome (HBS). Focal hemorrhagic ulcer. When opened, a circumscribed segment of the mucosa is covered by coagulated blood, overlying a linear ulcer usually hidden underneath.

5.5.6.2 Rectal perforation

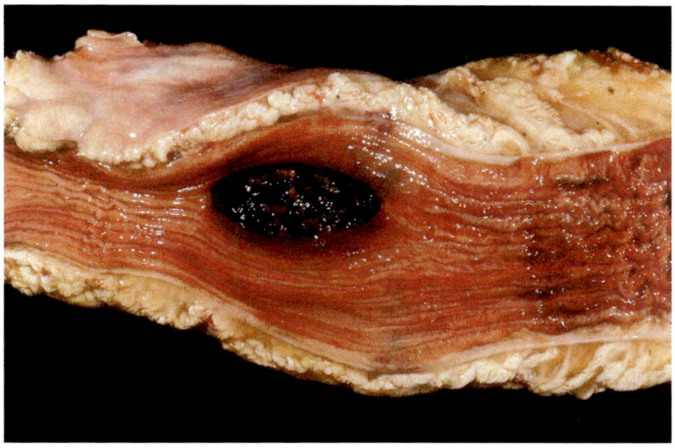

Fig. 5.108. Ox. Rectum. Laceration. Traumatic in origin, the site of laceration is usually the dorsal rectum. Rectal palpation, obstetric intervention or sadism may cause tearing of the rectum, with a varying degree of tissue destruction. Full wall perforation will lead to perirectal cellulitis or peritonitis in the pelvic canal. The perirectal fat is necrotic. (Courtesy of Dr P. Habecker, University of Pennsylvania, USA.)

5.5.6.3 Diaphragmatic hernia

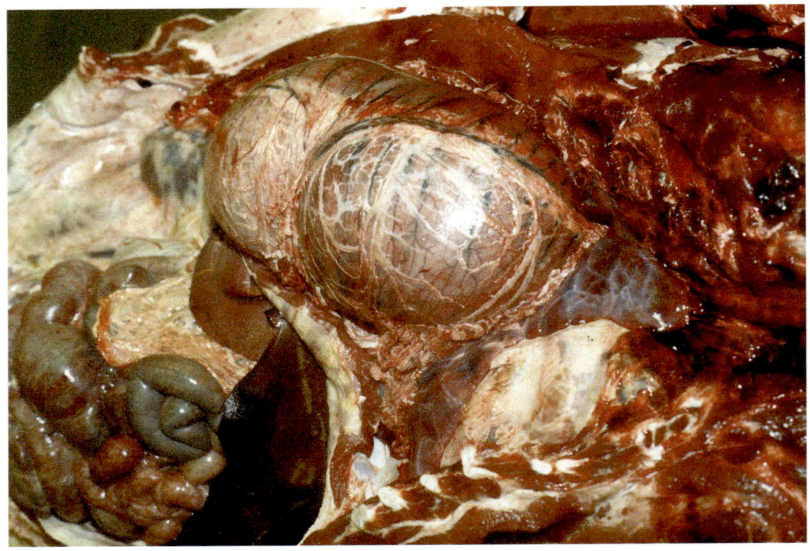

Fig. 5.109. Ox. Body cavities. Diaphragmatic hernia. Gaps following trauma allowed portions of the abomasum to slip into the dorsal thorax.

5.5.6.4 Intestinal droplets

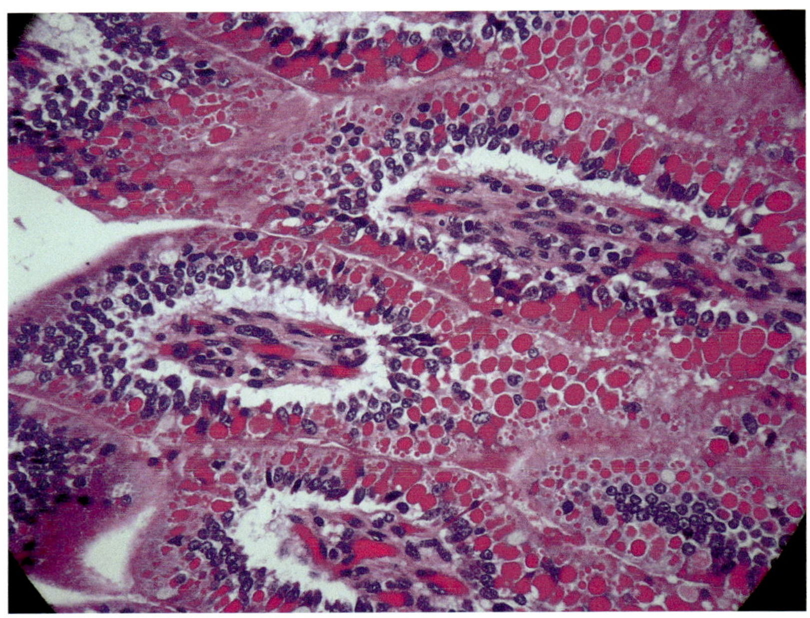

Fig. 5.110. Ox. Jejunum. Mucosa. Eosinophilic droplets. Magnitude of colostral immunoglobulins in neonates (Periodic acid-Schiff (PAS) stain).

5.6 DISEASES OF THE PERITONEUM

The normal peritoneum is a smooth, thin, glistening membrane that is kept moist by small amounts of straw-colored fluid. If abundant, distinction should be made between ante-mortem and post-mortem effusion. Excessive ante-mortem effusion, depending on its origin and color, may lead to the diagnosis of hydroperitoneum, hemoperitoneum or uroperitoneum.

5.6.1 Fat necrosis

Introduction. Excessive fat accumulation in the abdominal cavity interferes with adequate blood supply to the adipose tissue, resulting in ischemic necrosis and saponification of abdominal fat. The condition may be breed dependent (Channel Island breed) or may develop following consumption of fescue grass. The diffuse, hard masses of fat when developing close to the rectum and descending colon lead to extraluminal compression and obstruction of these tubular organs. The masses may encase both kidneys.

Clinical signs. Low production of feces, abdominal distension.

Differential diagnoses. Intrapelvic abscesses, pelvic hematomas, intrapelvic adhesions.

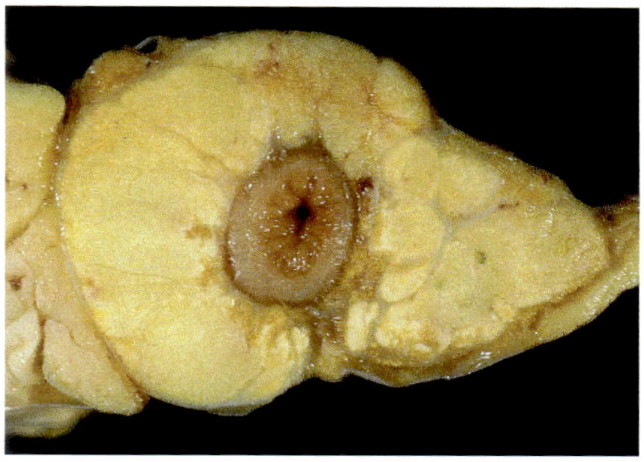

Fig. 5.111. Ox. Rectum. Perirectal fat necrosis. Lobulated, hardened, saponified appearance of excessive fat may be compared to a space-occupying mass with a potential for intestinal obstruction and feels firm on rectal palpation.

5.6.2 Inflammation

Introduction. Peritonitis in cattle is nearly always septic, particularly when generalized. It creates a serious clinical condition. It is usually the result of a perforation, laceration or rupture of a viscus within the abdominal cavity, from which it spreads diffusely. There may be a direct extension through an inflamed wall of a portion of the intestinal tract, resulting in a more focal peritonitis with fibrous adhesions.

Clinical signs. Fever, weight loss, anorexia, abdominal tension, extension of head and neck, intestinal dysmotility.

Differential diagnoses. Rumenitis, abomasitis, abomasal dislocation, pneumonia, obstetric complications.

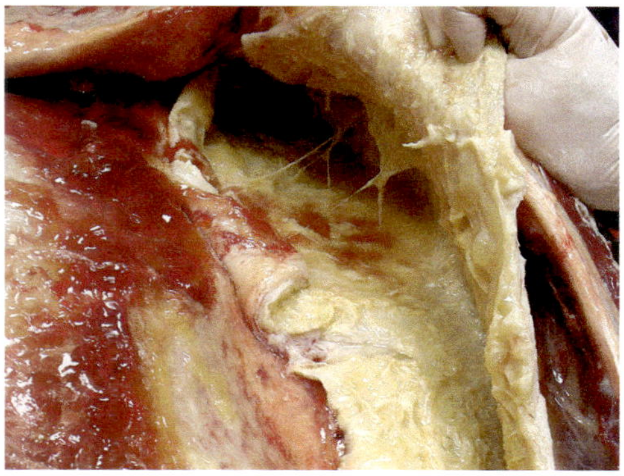

Fig. 5.112. Ox. Abdomen. Generalized fibrinous septic peritonitis. A thick, tenacious, fibrinous exudate covers the parietal and visceral peritoneal surfaces.

SUGGESTED READING

Bianchi, M.V., Konradt, G., de Souza, S.O., Bassuino, D.M., Silveira, S., *et al.* (2017) Natural outbreak of BVDV-Id-induced mucosal disease lacking intestinal lesions. *Veterinary Pathology* 54, 242–248.

Brodersen, B.W. (2014) Bovine viral diarrhea virus infections: manifestations of infection and recent advances in understanding pathogenesis and control. *Veterinary Pathology* 51, 453–464.

Cornish, T.E., van Olphen, A.L. and Cavender, J.L. (2005) Comparison of ear notch immunohistochemistry, ear notch antigen capture ELISA and buffy coat virus isolation for the detection of calves persistently infected with bovine viral diarrhea virus. *Journal of Veterinary Diagnostic Investigation* 17, 110–117.

Elhanafy, M.M., French, D.D. and Braun, U. (2013) Understanding jejunal hemorrhagic syndrome. *Journal of the American Veterinary Association* 243, 352–358.

Filho, E.J.F., Carvalho, A.U., Assis, R.A., Laboto, F.F., Rachid, M.A., *et al.* (2009) Clinicopathologic features of experimental *Clostridium perfringens* type D enterotoxemia in cattle. *Veterinary Pathology* 46, 1213–1220.

Garrett, E.F., Po, E., Bichi, E.R., Hexum, S.K., Melcher, R. and Hubner, A.M. (2015) Clinical disease associated with epizootic hemorrhagic disease virus in cattle in Illinois. *Journal of the American Veterinary Association* 247, 190–195.

Kane, S.E., Holler, L.D., Braun, L.L., Neil, J.D., Young, D.B., *et al.* (2015) Bovine viral diarrhea outbreak in a beef cow herd in South Dakota. *Journal of the American Veterinary Association* 246, 1358–1362.

Njaa, B.L., Panciera, R.J., Clark, E.G. and Lamm, C.G. (2012) Gross lesions of alimentary disease in adult cattle. *Veterinary Clinics of North America: Food Animal Practice* 28, 483–513.

O'Toole, D. and Li, H. (2014) The pathology of malignant catarrhal fever, with emphasis on ovine herpesvirus 2. *Veterinary Pathology* 51, 437–452.

Uzal, F.A., Kelly, W.R., Morris, W.E. and Assis, R.A. (2002) Effects of intravenous injection of *Clostridium perfringens* type D epsilon toxin in calves. *Journal of Comparative Pathology* 126, 71–75.

Weiss, D.J. and Souza, C.D. (2008) Review paper: modulation of mononuclear phagocyte function of *Mycobacterium avium* subsp. *paratuberculosis*. *Veterinary Pathology* 45, 829–841.

CHAPTER 6

Diseases of the Hepatobiliary System and Pancreas

6.1 **Liver**
- 6.1.1 Metabolic and toxic disorders
  - 6.1.1.1 Hepatic lipidosis
  - 6.1.1.2 Hepatotoxicity
- 6.1.2 Inflammation
  - 6.1.2.1 Bacterial hepatitis
  - 6.1.2.2 Mycotic hepatitis
  - 6.1.2.3 Parasitic hepatitis
- 6.1.3 Neoplasia
- 6.1.4 Miscellaneous
  - 6.1.4.1 Telangiectasia
  - 6.1.4.2 Vascular tension lipidosis
  - 6.1.4.3 Intrahepatic cholestasis
  - 6.1.4.4 Citrus pulp toxicosis

6.2 **Gall Bladder**
- 6.2.1 Inflammation

6.3 **Exocrine Pancreas**
- 6.3.1 Pancreolithiasis

INTRODUCTION

The liver is involved in a variety of metabolic and detoxification processes. The organ possesses a large functional reserve and regeneration capacity. If the liver fails, a variety of organ systems will fail as well. Clinical liver disease may be present long before liver failure develops. Increased serum liver enzyme activity is often the first clinicopathologic change noticed in liver disease. The liver responds to insults with a limited number of pathologic changes. Multiple foci of necrosis suggest recent damage, with inflammation responding to dead cells. Replacement occurs with new hepatocytes or fibrosis, depending on the severity of the damage. Zonal dropout of hepatocytes with or without necrosis occurs in conjunction with toxicosis. Megalocytosis occurs in mycotoxicosis and pyrrolizidine alkaloid toxicosis. Abscess formations are the result of preceding disease in forestomachs and abomasum.

6.1 LIVER

6.1.1 Metabolic and toxic disorders

6.1.1.1 Hepatic lipidosis

Introduction. Metabolic accumulation of lipids within the liver is the result of both increased mobilization of lipids from adipose tissue and decreased export of lipoprotein from the liver into the circulation. Various

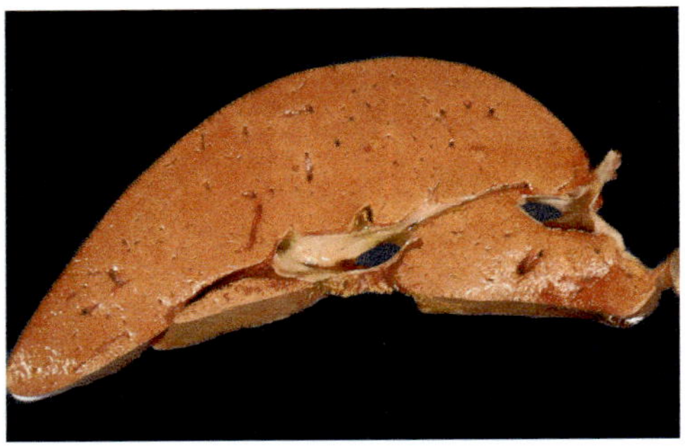

Fig. 6.1. Ox. Liver. Lipidosis. Cut section shows diffuse yellow discoloration. Such liver is enlarged, soft, and friable to touch.

disturbances of the normal lipid metabolism lead to increased deposition of lipids in the liver. Fatty liver syndrome occurs in obese dairy cows at the time of parturition, or due to excessive carbohydrate intake during the dry period. Dietary restriction (starvation) is another cause for hepatic lipidosis. Ketosis resulting in lipidosis develops in late-term pregnant cows or cows in early lactation, from negative energy balance or high energy demand. Toxemia and hypoxia are other pathogenic principles for hepatic lipidosis to occur.

Clinical signs. Anorexia, ataxia (neurologic ketosis), overweight, recumbency.

Differential diagnoses. Primary neurologic diseases, other metabolic and toxic diseases.

6.1.1.2 Hepatotoxicity

Introduction. Main hepatotoxins in cattle are metabolites produced by fungi (mycotoxins) or cyanobacteria (*Microcystis aeruginosa*), plant-derived pyrrolizidine alkaloids, excess of chemicals (coal tar), and excess of mineral elements. It should be kept in mind that many hepatotoxins have simultaneous damaging effects on other organs, particularly kidney and gastrointestinal tract.

Clinical signs. Anorexia, diarrhea, weight loss, icterus, photosensitization, edema, head pressing, blindness, heart failure.

Differential diagnoses. Bacterial hepatitis, hepatic endoparasites (flukes), endotoxemia.

Aflatoxicosis

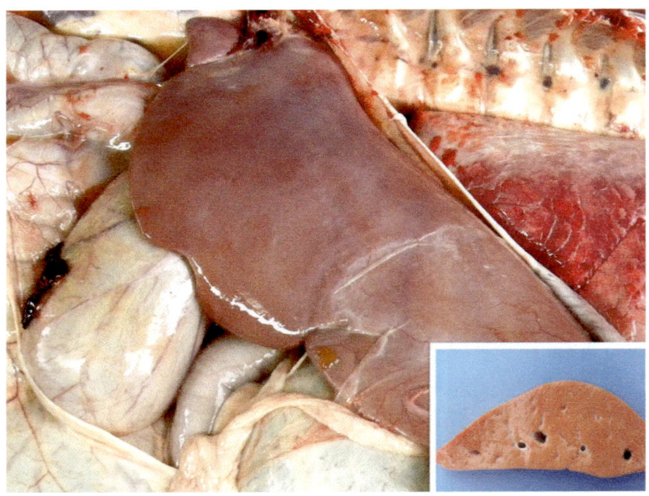

Fig. 6.2. Ox. Liver. Aflatoxicosis. Hepatic pallor. Inset: the cut section is dry and of mahogany color. Originating from products of feed-contaminating fungi such as *Aspergillus flavus*, aflatoxin-affected livers may be grossly swollen with rounded edges, pale; nodular and firm in chronic conditions.

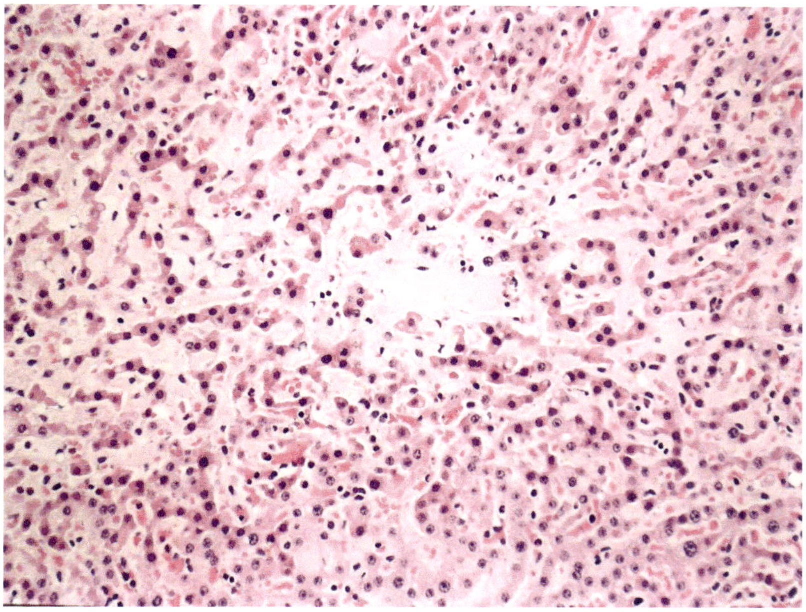

Fig. 6.3. Ox. Liver. Aflatoxicosis. Centrilobular hepatocellular dissociation and necrosis. Hepatocytes are sequestered from plates, and individual hepatocytes have undergone early necrosis (H&E).

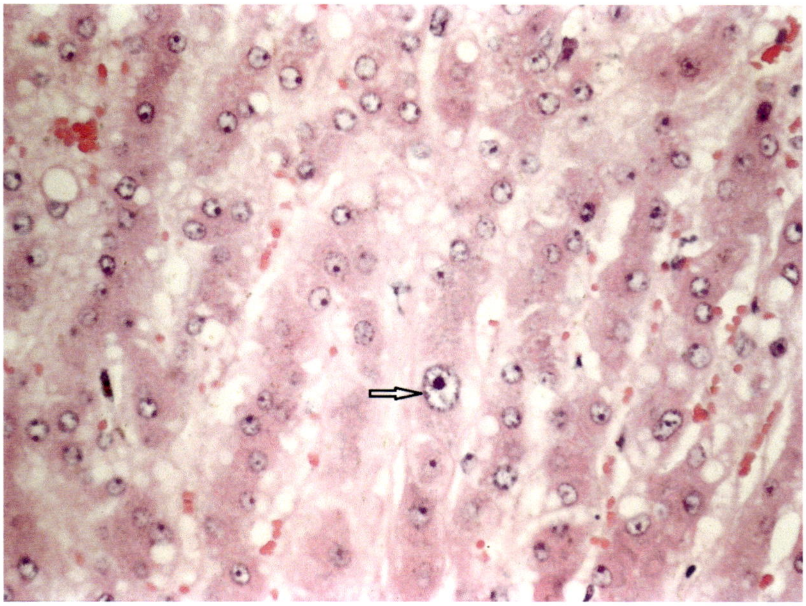

Fig. 6.4. Ox. Liver. Megalocyte. The microscopic finding of enlarged hepatic nuclei (arrow) is suggestive, but not pathognomonic, of aflatoxicosis. Megalocytes developing from mitosis inhibition also form in pyrrolizidine alkaloid and nitrosamine toxicoses. Other microscopic findings include lobular necrosis, lipidosis, fibrosis, bile ductular epithelial proliferation, nodular regeneration, and cholestasis (H&E) (also see Chapter 16: The Pathology of Select Poisonous Plant-induced Diseases in Cattle).

Blue-green algae toxicosis

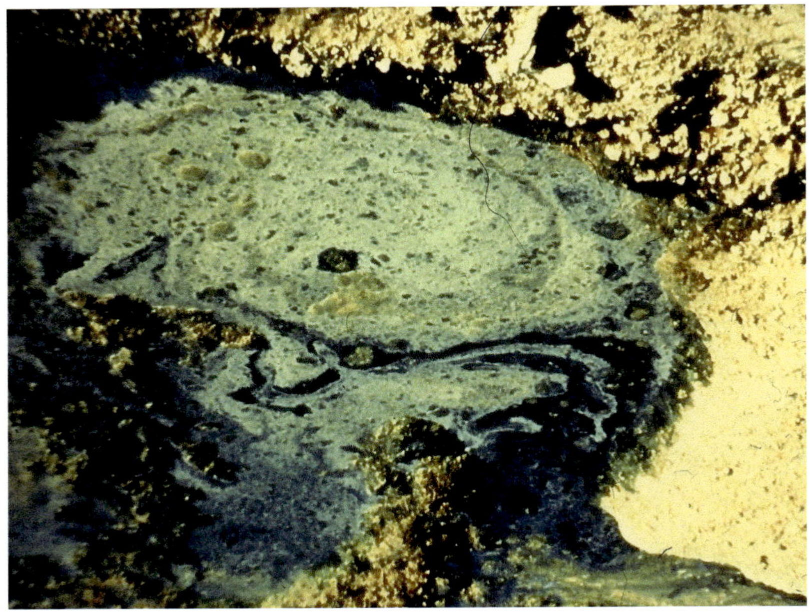

Fig. 6.5. Ox. Blue-green algae (cyanobacterium) toxicosis. Stock pond. Blue-green sludge is heavily contaminated with the cyanobacterium of the genus *Microcystis aeruginosa*. Blue-green algae cover the surface of stagnant lakes, ponds, rivers, and brackish waters. The cyanobacterium in blooming formation produces the cyanotoxin microcystin, a cyclic peptide, which causes severe liver necrosis. Cyanobacteria can produce neurotoxins, cytotoxins, endotoxins, and hepatotoxins, and as a group they are called cyanotoxins. Affected livers are enlarged, friable, and dark red.

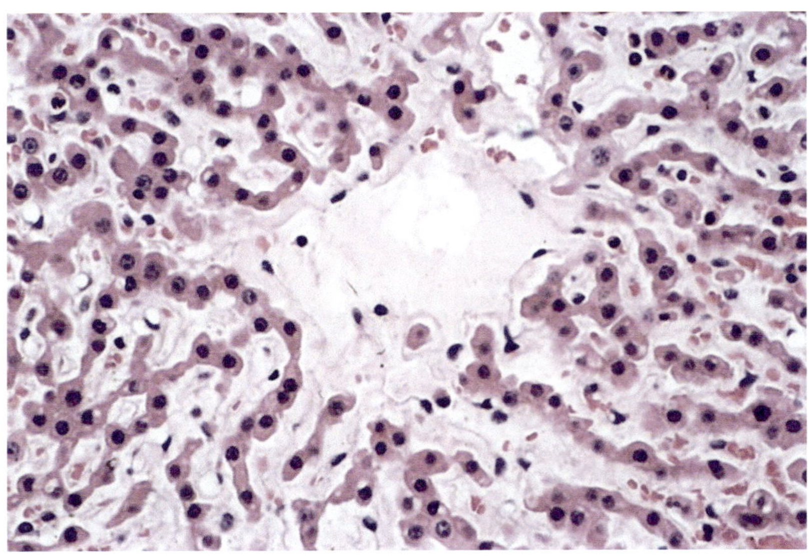

Fig. 6.6. Ox. Liver. Blue-green algae toxicosis. Dissociation of centrilobular hepatocytes. Other microscopic changes include hepatocyte degeneration and necrosis (H&E).

Lantana poisoning

Introduction. Lantana (*Lantana camara*) is a widespread toxic plant that grows in tropical and subtropical regions of the world. It is hepatotoxic to grazing ruminants. The hepatotoxins called lantadenes are triterpene acids. The kidneys may be involved in developing nephrosis in lantana toxicosis. In addition to the plant structure and leaves, both ripe and unripe Lantana berries are potentially lethal, despite claims that ripe berries are not poisonous (see Chapter 16: The Pathology of Select Poisonous Plant-induced Diseases in Cattle).

Clinical signs. Jaundice, secondary photosensitization, anorexia.

Differential diagnoses. Other hepatotoxins, metabolic disorders.

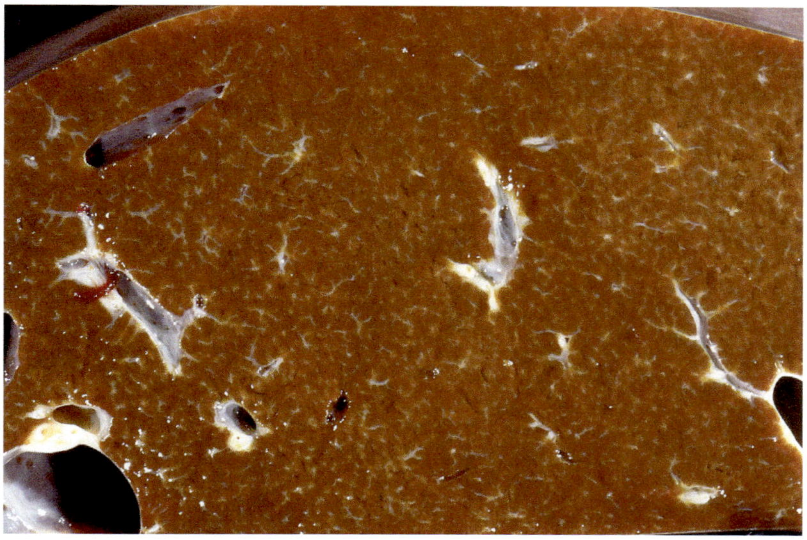

Fig. 6.7. Ox. Liver. Lantana hepatosis. The liver has a reticulate pattern. Bronze discoloration suggests intrahepatic cholestasis. (Courtesy of Dr J. Edwards, Texas A&M University, USA.)

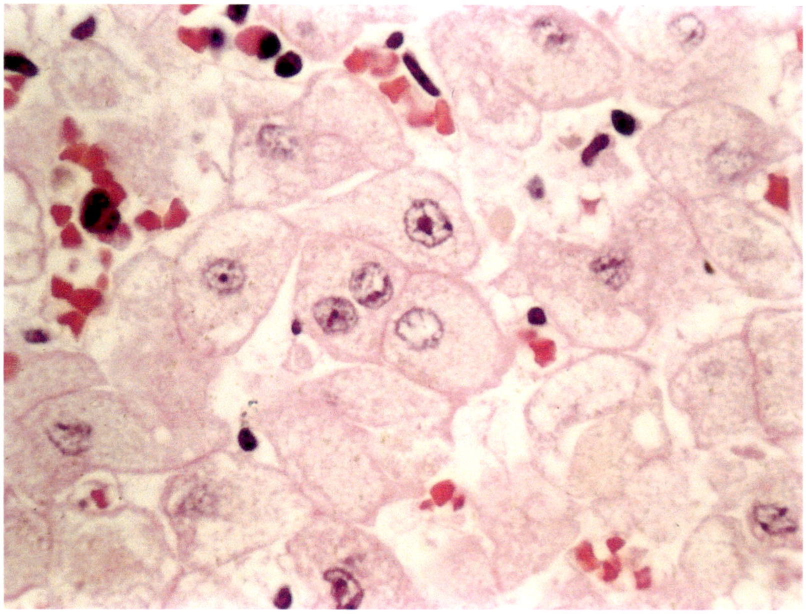

Fig. 6.8. Ox. Liver. Lantana poisoning. Hepatocellular ballooning degeneration. Hepatocytes are markedly swollen, with feathery cytoplasmic degeneration and double nuclei (H&E).

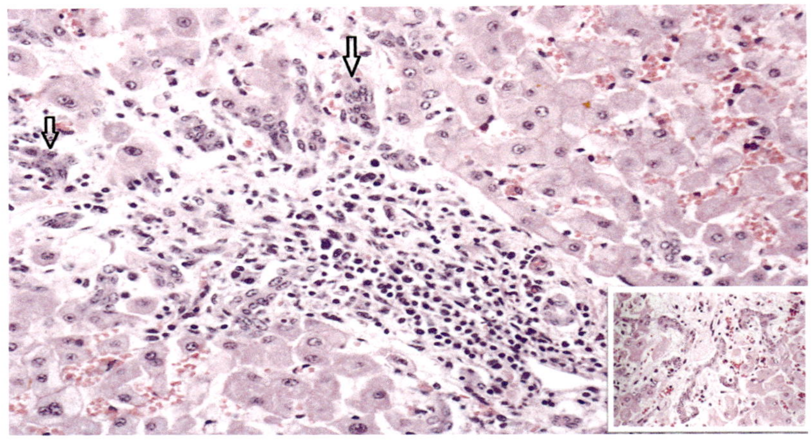

Fig. 6.9. Ox. Liver. Lantana poisoning. Portal triaditis. Peripheral hepatocytes are dissociated from limiting plates. Some are individualized. A moderate infiltration of lymphocytes and plasma cells is present in portal tracts. Portal ductules show epithelial proliferation (arrows). Inset: portal ductules have proliferating epithelial lining cells, and there is evidence of collagen deposition within portal triads (H&E).

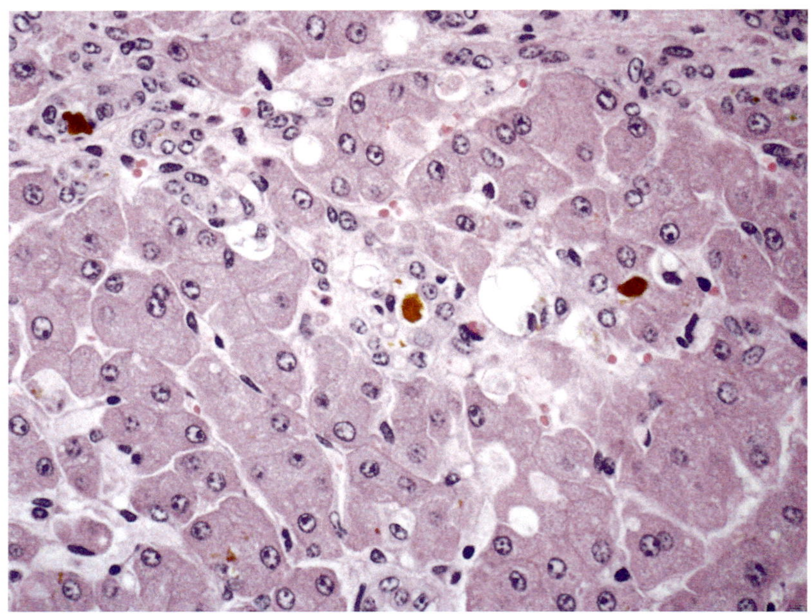

Fig. 6.10. Ox. Liver. Lantana poisoning. Biliary cholestasis. Accumulation of yellow bile pigment in sinusoids, hepatocytes, and ductules. The mechanism by which lantana induces cholestasis remains obscure, but swelling of hepatocytes might lead to plugging of biliary canaliculi (H&E).

Fact Sheet: Lantana Poisoning

Cause:	weed *Lantana camara*
Species affected:	ruminants, horses, humans
Toxicity:	triterpene acids lantadene A and lantadene B
Toxic dose:	20 kg fresh leaves for 500 kg cow
Clinical signs:	hepatogenous photosensitization (exudative dermatitis) jaundice swelling of ears and eyes anorexia depression
Gross findings:	hepatomegaly with bronze discoloration (cholestasis) hepatic lipidosis with multifocal necrosis enlarged gall bladder generalized icterus swollen, pale kidneys ulcerations of cheeks, muzzle, nostrils, and tongue
Microscopic findings (liver):	ballooning hepatocellular degeneration bile canalicular and ductular cholestasis bile ductular epithelial proliferation portal triaditis and fibrosis

Photosensitization

Introduction. Photosensitization occurs when ultraviolet light of a specific wavelength acts upon fluorescent pigment that has accumulated in tissues, mainly the skin, to induce photochemical action to release energy causing tissue damage.

There are three types of photosensitization: (i) primary, in which photodynamic chemicals, or plant toxins, reach the skin through the circulation; (ii) bovine congenital porphyria, in which there is a metabolic defect in porphyrin metabolism; (iii) hepatogenous (secondary) photosensitization, in which there is a disturbance of normal secretion of phylloerythrin, a metabolite of chlorophyll. The liver normally conjugates phylloerythrin and excretes it into bile. Hepatotoxic plants (*Lantana camara*, *Nolina texana*, *Agave lechugilla*, and *Phyllanthus abnormis*), or hepatotoxic mycotoxins (sporidesmin) produced by *Pithomyces chartarum*, are the primary cause of hepatogenous photosensitization.

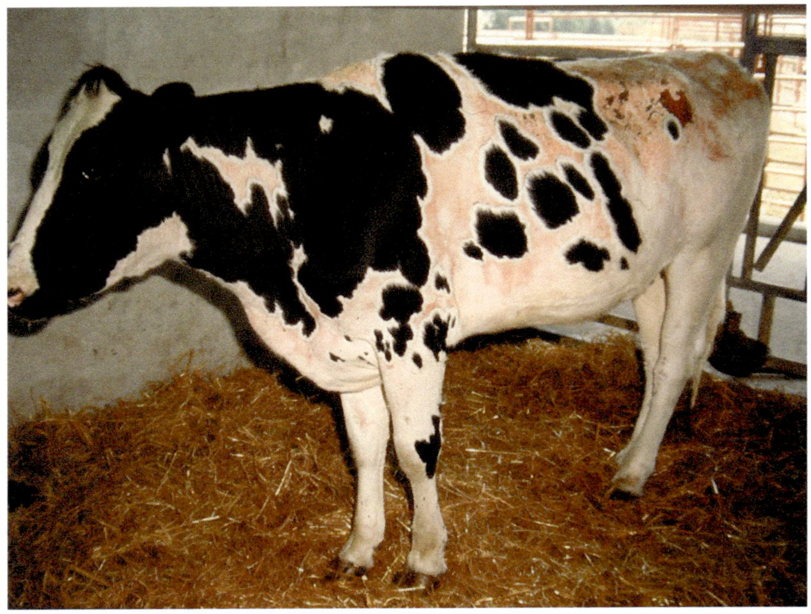

Fig. 6.11. Ox. Photosensitization. Exudative dermatitis. Erythematous lesions are limited to the non-pigmented parts of the skin. Removal of affected animals from exposure to sunlight will alleviate skin condition (see Chapter 12: Diseases of the Integument).

6.1.2 Inflammation

Introduction. Primary hepatitis is usually of infectious origin following bacterial, fungal, or endoparasite exposure. Secondary hepatitis is the reaction to primary toxic liver damage. Bovine hepatitis has acute or chronic forms, depending on the nature of the initiating agent and survival of the affected animal.

Clinical signs. Anorexia, decreased milk production, weight loss, diarrhea, intermittent fever, hemoglobinuria, icterus, encephalopathy.

Differential diagnosis. Hepatotoxins.

6.1.2.1 Bacterial hepatitis

Bacillary hemoglobinuria (redwater, black disease, infectious necrotic hepatitis). The disease is caused by *Clostridium haemolyticum*, also known as *Clostridium novyi*. The anaerobic bacterium is a normal resident of the liver, with spores germinating within damaged liver segments secondary to injury such as trauma, presence of flukes, or other parasitic migration. The organism elaborates toxins that cause hepatic necrosis and hemolysis. Differential diagnoses include post-parturient hemoglobinuria, leptospirosis, bracken fern toxicosis (enzootic hematuria), and babesiosis.

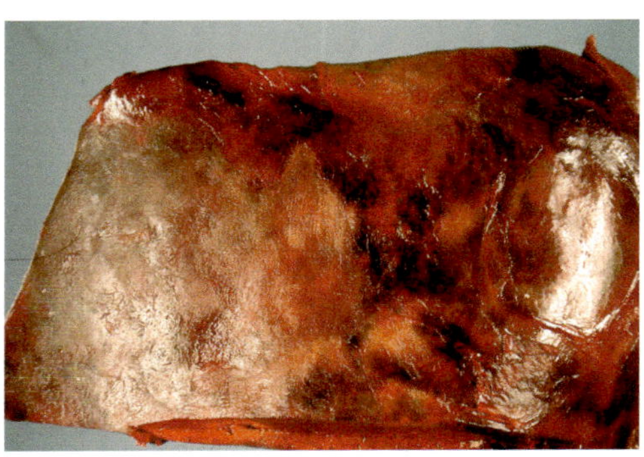

Fig. 6.12. Ox. Liver. Bacillary hemoglobinuria. Necrotizing, hemorrhagic hepatitis. Large zones of the hepatic parenchyma when viewed through the Glisson's capsule are mottled yellow, dark red.

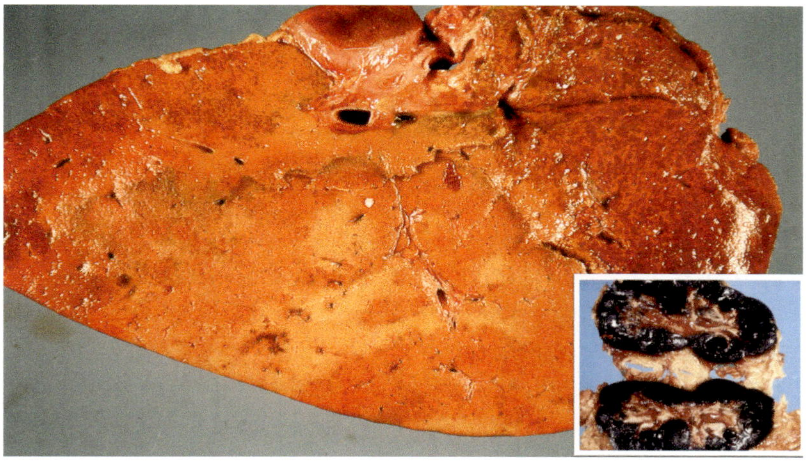

Fig. 6.13. Ox. Liver. Bacillary hemoglobinuria. Necrotizing hepatitis. On cross section, a large zone of liver has undergone yellow-tan mottling, and has effaced the normal lobular pattern. There is a sharp transition into uninvolved liver tissue leading to the descriptive term of pseudoinfarction for this tissue damage. Inset: pigmentary nephrosis. Black discoloration of the kidney after severe hemolysis caused by *Clostridium haemolyticum* (*novyi*).

Leptospirosis. In adult cattle, leptospirosis caused by *Leptospira interrogans* serovar *pomona* or *hardjo* usually leads to abortions and stillbirths. Hematogenous spread of the organism leads to the development of kidney or liver changes (see Chapter 7: Diseases of the Urinary System).
Clinical signs. Complications are sepsis, hemolysis, hemoglobinuria, anemia, and icterus.
Differential diagnoses. Post-parturient hemoglobinuria, bacillary hemoglobinuria, babesiosis, enzootic hematuria, malignant catarrhal fever (MCF) cystitis.

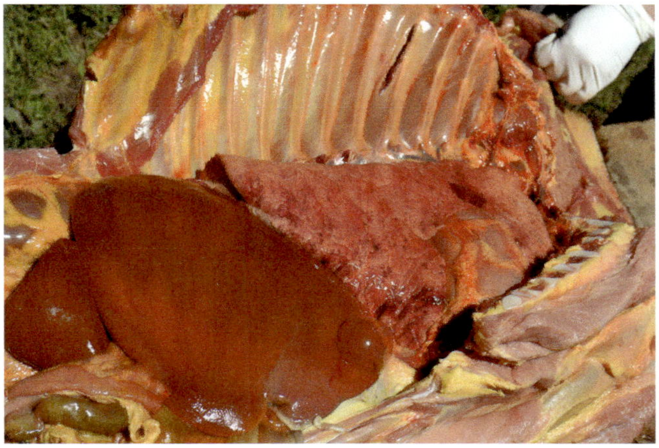

Fig. 6.14. Ox. Liver. Leptospirosis. Cholestasis. The liver has a bronze tinge and is enlarged. The carcass is characterized by yellow discoloration (jaundice). Feces will have a green discoloration. (Courtesy of Dr D. Driemeier, Universidade Federal do Rio Grande do Sul, Brazil.)

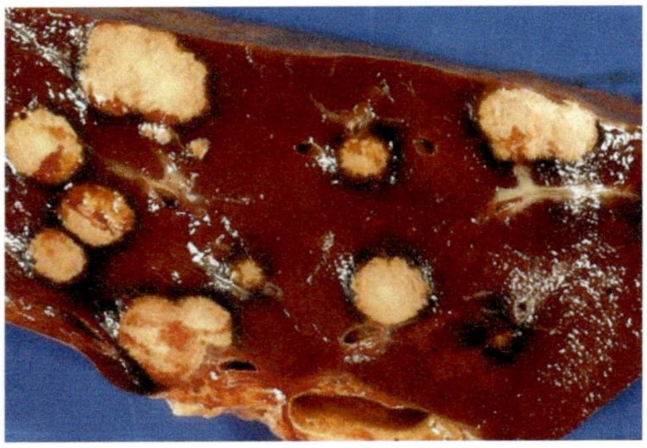

Fig. 6.15. Ox. Liver. Hepatic necrobacillosis. Necrotizing hepatitis. Hepatic colonization by *Fusobacterium necrophorum*, a member of the ruminal anaerobic bacterial flora, resulted in multiple foci of coagulative necrosis surrounded by peripheral red rings of hemorrhage. Hematogenous dissemination of the bacterium to the liver is a complication of rumenitis or abomasitis following overeating disease.

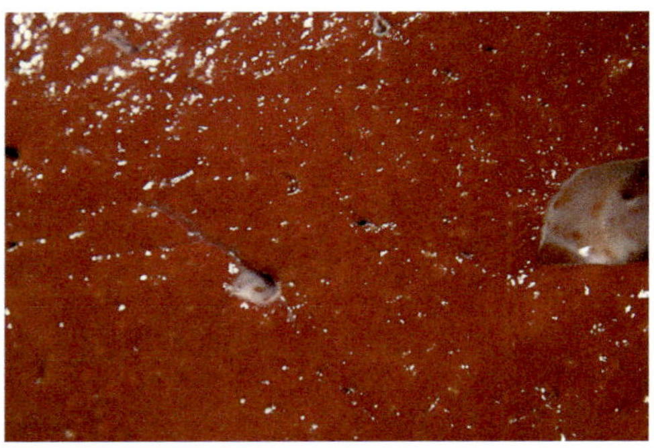

Fig. 6.16. Ox. Liver. Microabscesses. Multiple, miliary, pinpoint white foci are scattered throughout the liver parenchyma. These foci generally suggest non-specific bacteremia, but also can occur specifically in salmonellosis or in conjunction with listeriosis. Differential morphologic diagnosis: multifocal necrotizing hepatitis.

Hepatic necrobacillosis

Abscesses

Introduction. Hepatic abscesses may be single or multiple, small or large, and are usual findings at slaughter. Route of transmission is hematogenous from a preceding rumenitis or abomasitis through the portal system. An alternate portal of entry of infectious agents is ascending from the intestinal tract up the biliary tree. Enteric pathogens such as *Salmonella* spp. or *Escherichia coli* use the ascending biliary route of transmission during episodes of gastroenteritis. In neonates, a third portal of entry is umbilical, through the ductus venosus.

Abscesses are frequently located in the mid-dorsal diaphragmatic or dorsocranial area of the liver. Location of abscesses adjacent to the overriding caudal vena cava results in the caudal vena cava syndrome (thromboembolic disease) and is discussed in Chapter 3: Diseases of the Respiratory System.

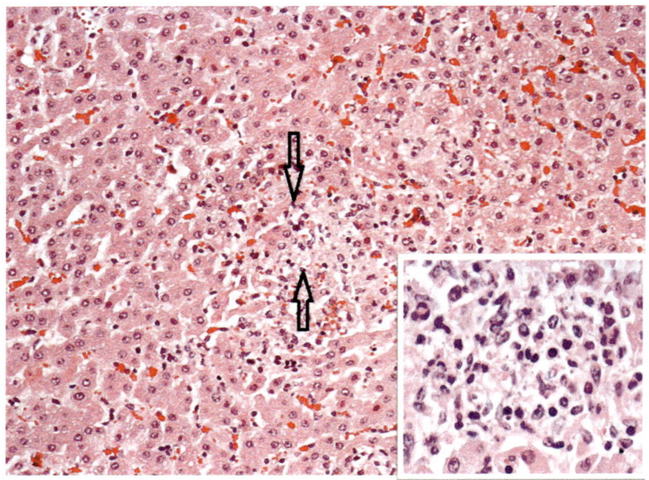

Fig. 6.17. Ox. Liver. Typhoid nodule. In the case of *Salmonella* spp. infection, discrete foci of necrotizing hepatitis named typhoid nodules (arrows) morphologically support the etiologic diagnosis. Typhoid nodules are a pathologic change in human typhoid fever after infection with *Salmonella typhi*. Inset: the typhoid nodule is composed of lymphocytes, histiocytes, and occasional plasma cells replacing dropped-out hepatocytes (H&E).

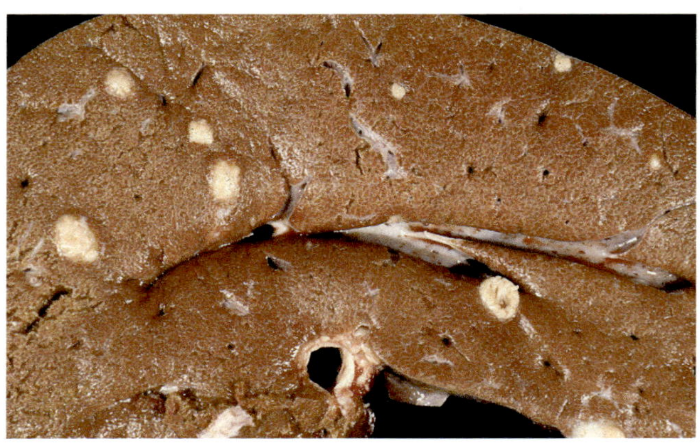

Fig. 6.18. Ox. Liver. Abscesses. Multiple mid-sized, almost uniform, abscesses are present. These are the result of *Trueperella pyogenes* showering the liver from a primary rumenitis. (Courtesy of Dr P. Habecker, University of Pennsylvania, USA.)

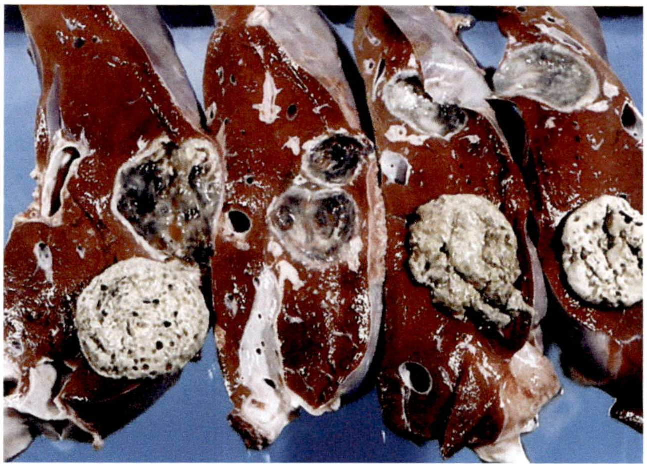

Fig. 6.19. Ox. Liver. Abscesses. Multiple nodular configurations with a creamy, purulent exudate surrounded by a thin capsule occupy much of the parenchyma. *Fusobacterium necrophorum* is a likely cause. The liver, with its portal circulation, is seeded hematogenously by bacterial pathogens originating within the gastrointestinal tract.

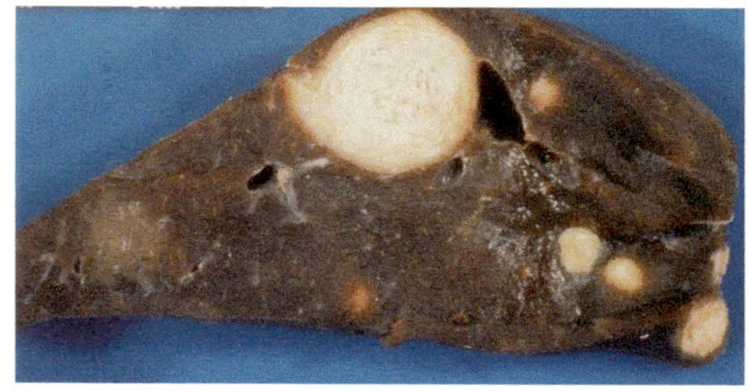

Fig. 6.20. Ox. Liver. Mycobacteriosis. Caseous granulomatous hepatitis. *Mycobacterium bovis* is the infectious strain affecting cattle. Depending on the portal of entry, inhalation or ingestion, different organ systems become infected with *M. bovis.* Primary lesions occur as caseous, calcified granulomas in infected organs and draining lymph nodes (see Chapter 11: Diseases of the Hematopoietic and Hemolymphatic System, and Chapter 3: Diseases of the Respiratory System).

6.1.2.2 Mycotic hepatitis

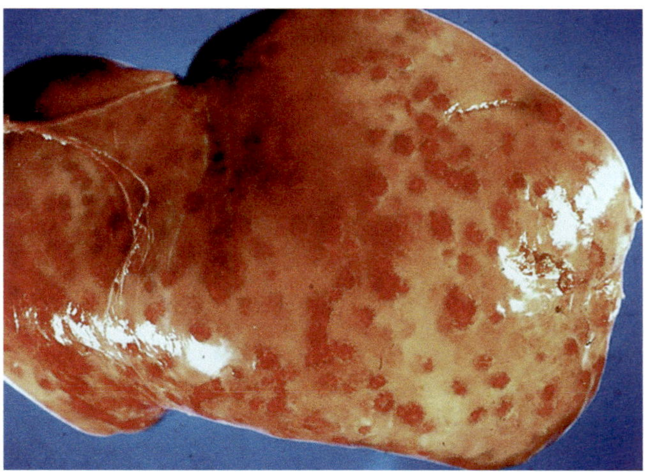

Fig. 6.21. Ox. Liver. Mycotic hepatitis. Multiple, uniformly sized, red foci are disseminated throughout the hepatic parenchyma. These foci, with a two-color pattern of a pale center and a red periphery, suggest fungal etiology. Preceding mycotic rumenitis or abomasitis should be considered as the primary site of infection. *Aspergillus* spp. or *Zygomycetes* spp. are frequently involved.

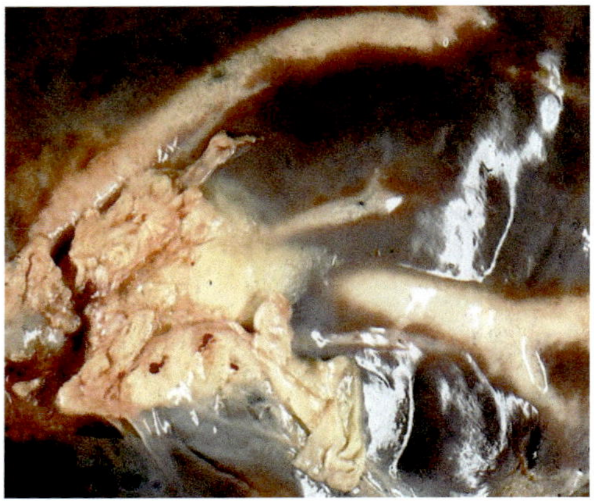

Fig. 6.22. Ox. Liver. Fascioliasis. Fibrosing cholangitis. Major bile ducts are markedly thickened, due to residing mature flukes. This condition is also defined as 'pipestem' liver.

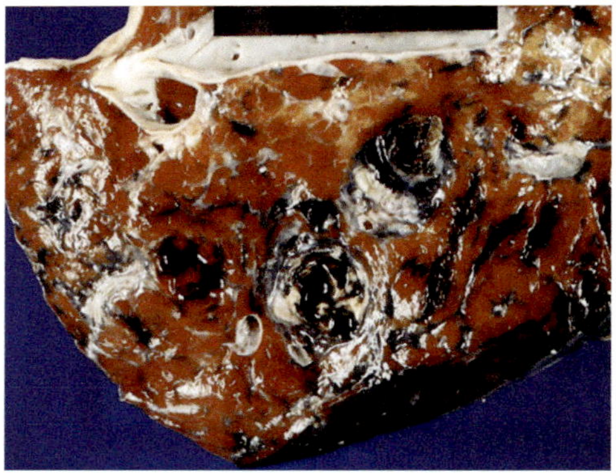

Fig. 6.23. Ox. Liver. Fascioliasis. Parasitic migration tracts. Necrotizing, hemorrhagic hepatitis. The cavitations are seen in conjunction with migration of *Fascioloides magna* fluke larvae and may be extensive. The black pigment is an excretory product deposited into the migration tracts.

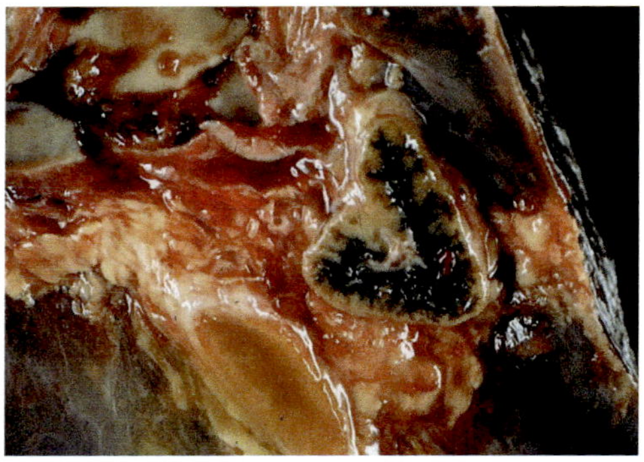

Fig. 6.24. Ox. Hepatic lymph node. Fascioliasis. Excretory pigment deposition. The black pigment drained into lymph nodes nearby points to fluke infestation.

6.1.2.3 Parasitic hepatitis

Fascioliasis (distomatosis)

Introduction. Liver fluke infestation occurring in cattle are due to *Fasciola hepatica* and *Fascioloides magna* (deer fluke). Adult parasites live in bile ducts, where they invoke cholangitis, bile duct obstruction, and cholestasis. Immature flukes migrate within the liver to produce hemorrhagic tracts that are resolved by fibrosis. Fluke transmission is seasonal during the cooler months. Ruminants are usually the final host, with lymnaeid snails the intermediate host. Massive infestation may lead to severe anemia, hypoproteinemia, and high mortality.

Clinical signs. Weight loss, reduced milk production, loss of condition.

Differential diagnoses. Inflammatory, metabolic and toxic liver disorders.

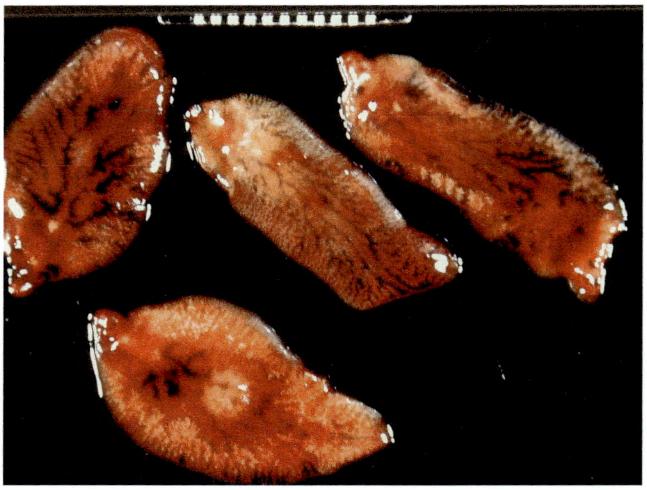

Fig. 6.25. *Fascioloides magna* (deer fluke). The giant liver fluke may reach a size of 10 cm in length and 3.5 cm in width. The fluke has two suckers (one oral, one ventral), and no external signs of segmentation.

Cestodes

Hydatid liver disease is the result of *Echinococcus granulosus* infestation. It is manifested by the presence of thin-walled cysts in or nearby the liver. Another species of intermediate cestode forming encapsulating, granulomatous structures in the liver and abdominal wall is *Cysticercus tenuicollis*, caused by the larval stage of the adult *Taenia hydatigena* residing in dogs as the definitive host.

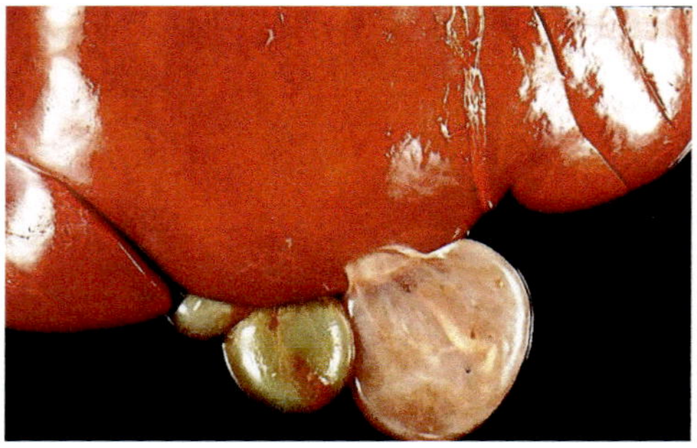

Fig. 6.26. Ox. Liver. Hydatid disease. A thin-walled, spherical cyst containing a watery fluid and a parasitic second-stage larva (metacestode) is attached to the margin of the liver next to the gall bladder. Notice gall bladder duplication.

6.1.3 Neoplasia

Primary tumors of the liver are rare in cattle and are designated as either hepatocellular or cholangiocellular neoplasms. As a secondary tumor, lymphoma (lymphosarcoma) occurs with some frequency.

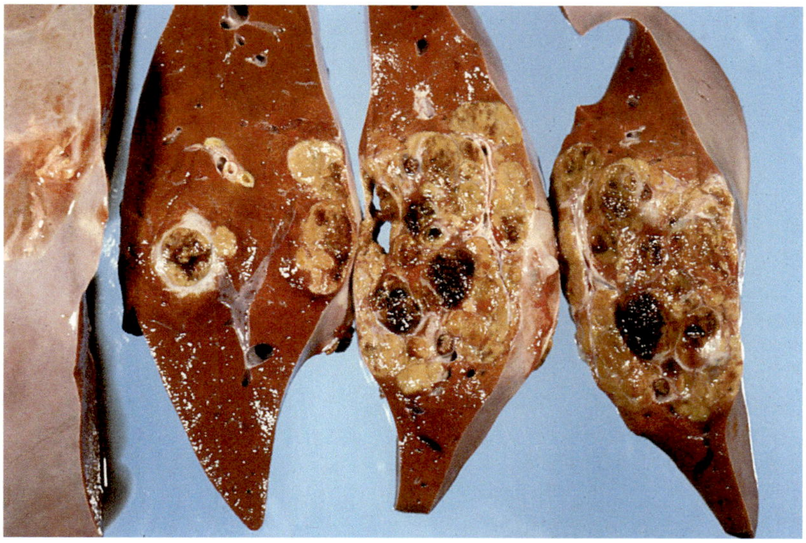

Fig. 6.27. Ox. Liver. Hepatocellular carcinoma. Multiple, partially coalescing, hemorrhagic, necrotic, encapsulated foci are present on cut section. Differential diagnoses: abscesses, liver flukes.

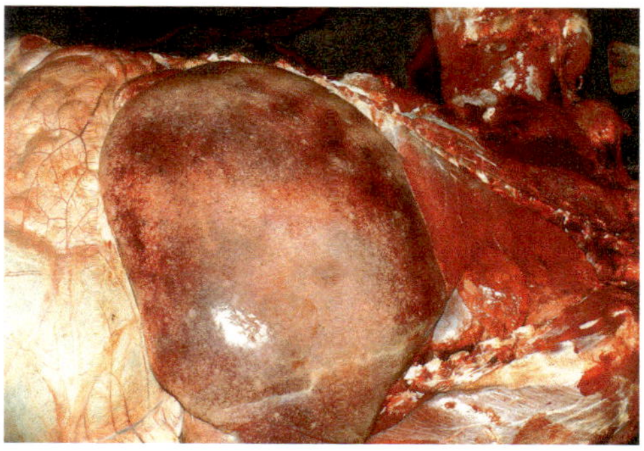

Fig. 6.28. Ox. Liver. Lymphoma (lymphosarcoma). Diffuse form. The liver is markedly enlarged, with multiple uniform gray-tan foci disseminated throughout organ. (Courtesy of the Government of Alberta, Canada.)

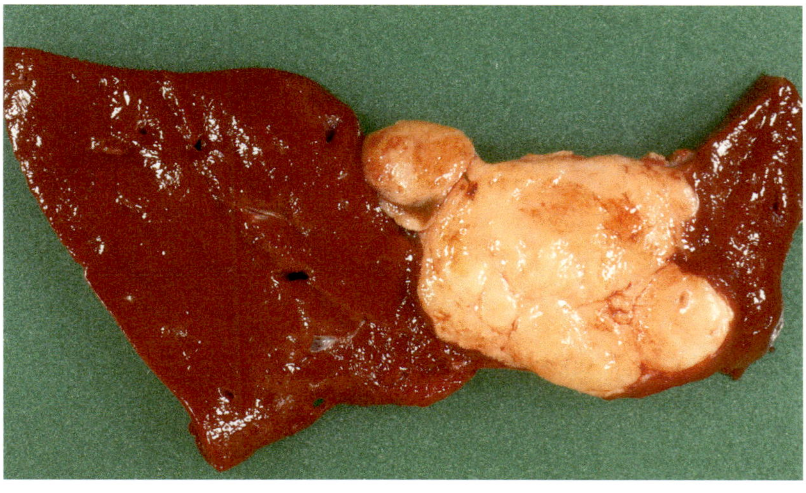

Fig. 6.29. Ox. Liver. Lymphoma (lymphosarcoma). The cut section contains a lobulated, bulging, gray, glistening nodule. This is an example of the nodular (multinodular) type of lymphoma.

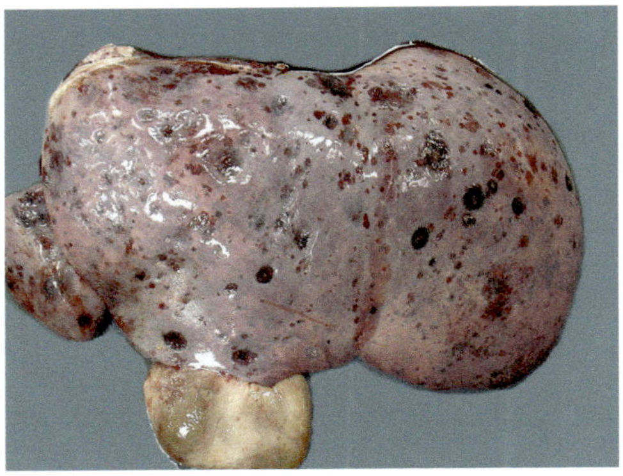

Fig. 6.31. Ox. Liver. Metastatic hemangiosarcoma. Multiple, uniform, red foci are disseminated throughout liver parenchyma. Differential diagnosis: telangiectasia.

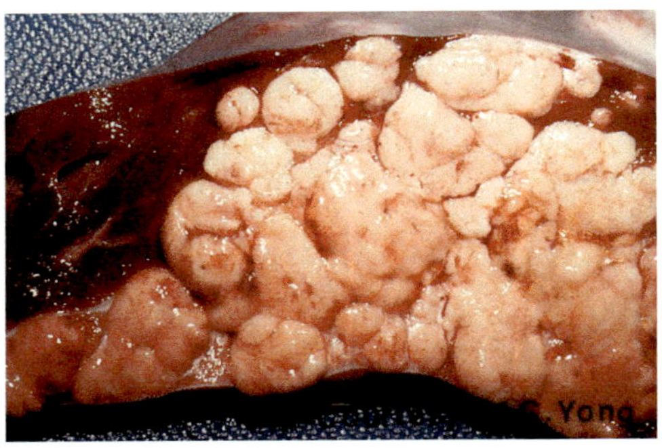

Fig. 6.32. Ox. Liver. Metastatic pheochromocytoma. A multilobular, white, bulging neoplasm should be differentiated from multinodular hepatic lymphoma (lymphosarcoma).

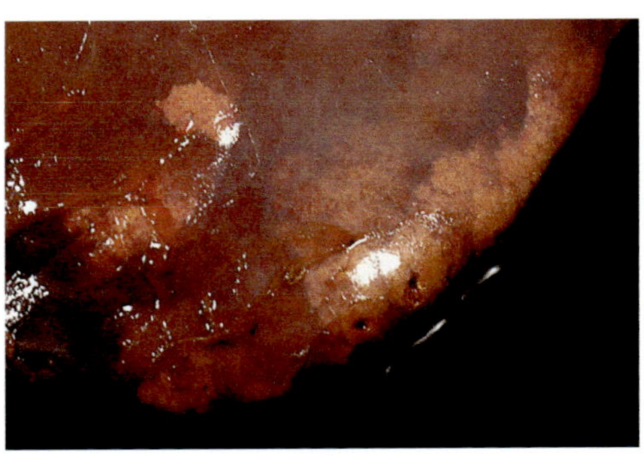

Fig. 6.34. Ox. Liver. Multifocal subcapsular hepatocellular lipidosis (vascular tension lipidosis). Circumscribed yellow foci of lipidosis are located at the edge of the liver below the Glisson's capsule. Notice fibrous adhesion on capsule. Differential diagnosis: pallor due to autolysis from clostridial overgrowth.

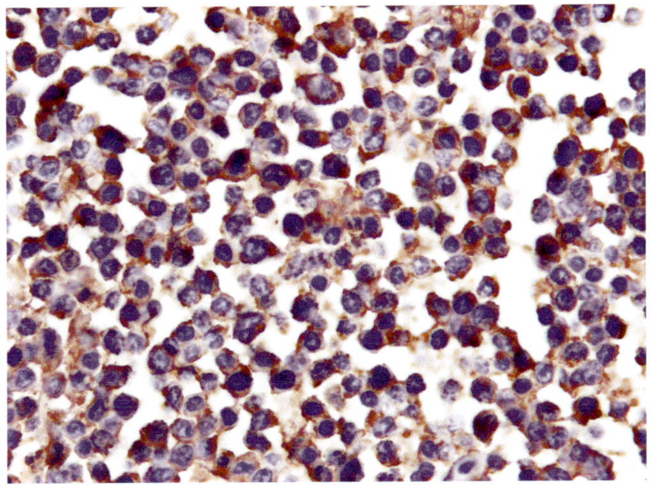

Fig. 6.30. Ox. Liver. Lymphoma (lymphosarcoma). Phenotypically, bovine lymphoma is of the B-cell type. Retroviral antigen is scattered diffusely within the cytoplasm. BLA36 marker (IHC).

6.1.4 Miscellaneous

6.1.4.1 Telangiectasia

Incidental finding that leads to condemnation of the liver at slaughter. Hepatic sinusoids become focally dilated and filled with blood. There is a loss of hepatocytes, and sinusoids become ectatic. The condition may be estrogen related. It is also known as peliosis hepatis.

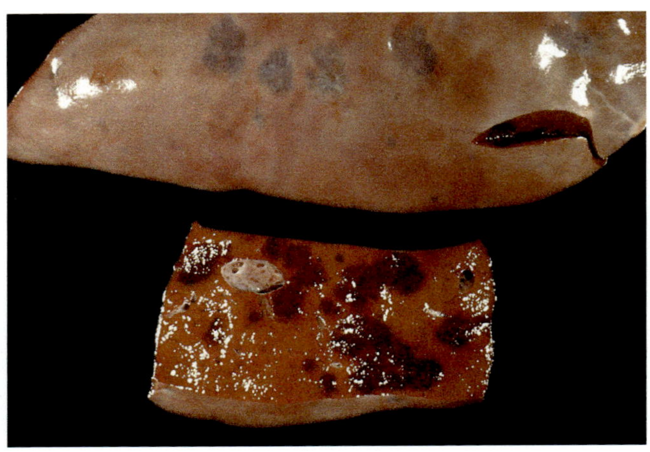

Fig. 6.33. Ox. Liver. Telangiectasia. Focal sinusoidal dilatation. Discrete, dark red foci are disseminated throughout cross section and liver surface. (Courtesy of Dr P. Habecker, University of Pennsylvania, USA.)

6.1.4.2 Vascular tension lipidosis

Focal ischemic lipidosis due to adhesion of the Glisson's capsule to neighboring organs resulting from hypoperfusion of adhered liver segment upon traction. Incidental finding at necropsy.

6.1.4.3 *Intrahepatic cholestasis*

Acute severe hemolysis such as in babesiosis or anaplasmosis leads to excessive bilirubin production and retention in bile canaliculi. Alternatively, severe liver injury disables hepatocytes to metabolize and excrete bile.

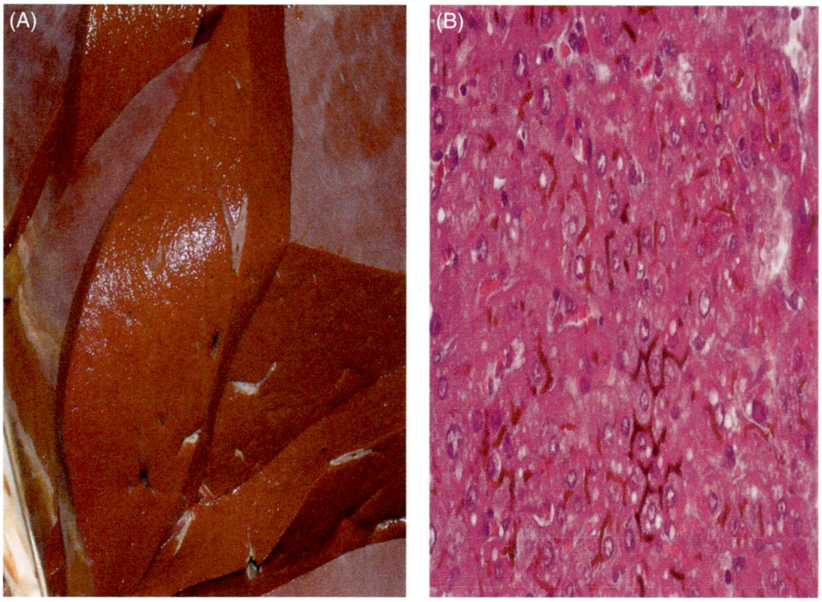

Fig. 6.35. Ox. Liver. Intrahepatic cholestasis. Anaplasmosis. Hepatic bile retention. (A) Grossly, the liver has a typical bronze tinge, indicating intrahepatic bile retention. (Courtesy of Dr D. Driemeier, Universidade Federal do Rio Grande do Sul, Brazil.) (B) Numerous bile plugs are retained within canaliculi (H&E). (Courtesy of Dr D. Driemeier, Universidade Federal do Rio Grande do Sol, Brazil.)

6.1.4.4 *Citrus pulp toxicosis*

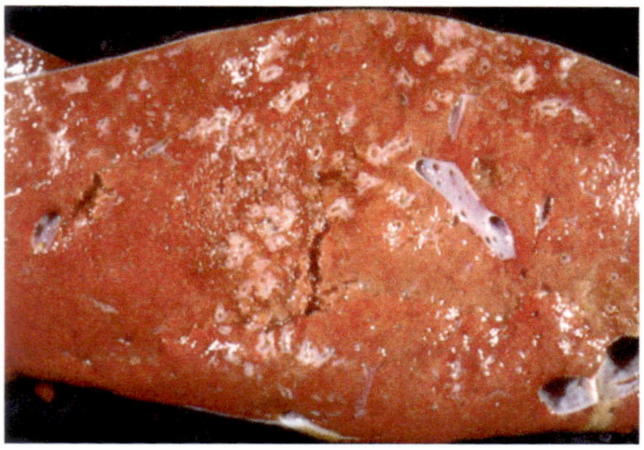

Fig. 6.36. Ox. Liver. Citrus pulp toxicosis. Hypertrophy of portal veins and granulomatous hepatitis. Citrus pulp, when fed as an energy-rich by-product to the diet of dairy cows, exhibits toxic effects on multiple organs such as the liver (for more, see Chapter 9: Diseases of the Endocrine System). (Reprinted with permission of the *Journal of Veterinary Diagnostic Investigation*, vol 12, p. 269, Fig. 2, 2000.)

6.2 GALL BLADDER

6.2.1 Inflammation

Introduction. Cholecystitis is usually the result of bacterial infection, rarely viral (bovine adenovirus) or toxic (arsenic). Cholecystitis may develop secondary to calculi (choleliths).

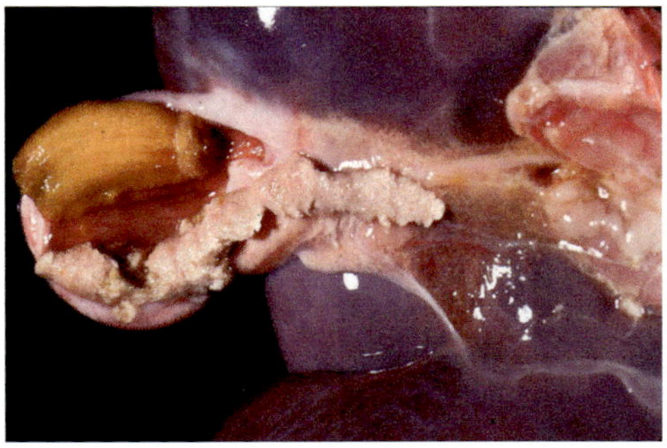

Fig. 6.38. Ox. Gall bladder. Fibrinous cholecystitis. A yellow fibrin cast and a large strand of fibrin occupy an enlarged, opened gall bladder and bile duct. The finding is highly indicative of enteric salmonellosis. (Courtesy of Dr J.M. King and the Anatomic Pathology Section, Cornell University, USA.)

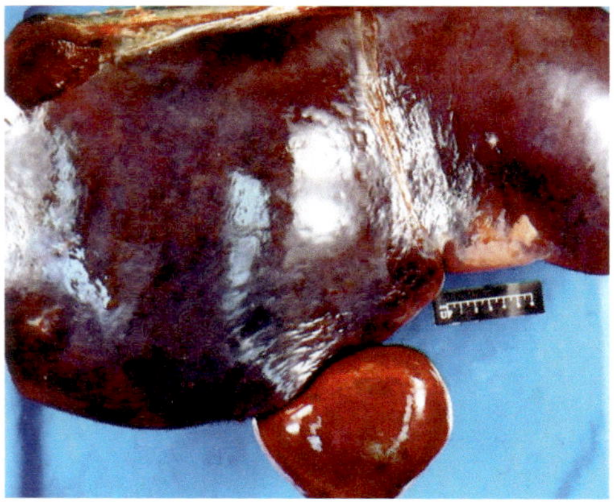

Fig. 6.37. Ox. Gall bladder. Hemorrhagic cholecystitis. The wall of the gall bladder is diffusely red. *Escherichia coli* was isolated from the bile. Arsenic toxicosis should be considered in the differential diagnosis, in conjunction with concurring hemorrhagic gastroenteritis.

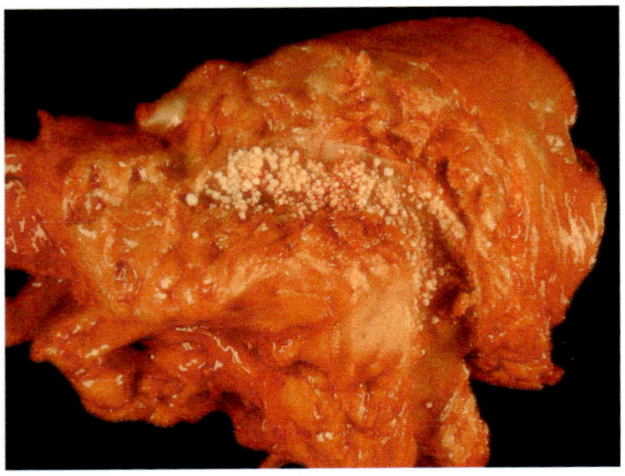

Fig. 6.39. Ox. Pancreas. Pancreolithiasis. Numerous small, white rice grain-sized calculi are located in the pancreatic bile duct. Inflammatory processes are responsible for their development.

6.3 EXOCRINE PANCREAS

The bovine pancreas is rarely involved in disease.

6.3.1 Pancreolithiasis

Pancreatic calculi are incidental findings in cattle. They are of calcium-carbonate or calcium-phosphate composition and contain an organic matrix.

SUGGESTED READING

Allen, J.K. (1981) An evaluation of lupinosis in cattle in Western Australia. *Australian Veterinary Journal* 57, 212–215.

Bertin, F.R., Baseler, L.J., Wilson, C.R., Kritchevsky, J.E. and Talor, S.D. (2013) Arsenic toxicosis in cattle: meta-analysis of 156 cases. *Journal of Veterinary Internal Medicine* 27, 977–981.

De Barros, C.S., Driemeier, D., Pilati, C., Barros, S.S. and Castilhos, L.M. (1992) Senecio spp. poisoning in cattle in southern Brazil. *Veterinary and Human Toxicology* 34, 241–246.

Galey, F.D., Beasley, V.R., Carmichael, W.W., Kleppe, G., Hooser, S.B. and Haschek, W.W. (1987) Blue-green algae (*Microcystis aeruginosa*) hepatotoxicosis in dairy cows. *American Journal of Veterinary Research* 48, 1415–1420.

Johnson, J.H. and Jensen, J.M. (1998) Hepatotoxicity and secondary photosensitization in a red kangaroo (*Megaleia rufus*) due to ingestion of *Lantana camara*. *Journal of Zoo and Wildlife Medicine* 29, 203–207.

Nagaraja, T.G. and Chengappa, M.M. (1998) Liver abscesses in feedlot cattle: a review. *Journal of Animal Science* 76, 287–298.

Neiger, R., Nelson, N., Miskimins, D. and Caster, L. (2004) Bovine arsenic toxicosis. *Journal of Veterinary Diagnostic Investigation* 16, 436–438.

O'Sullivan, E.N. (1999) Two-year study of bovine hepatic abscessation in 10 abattoirs in County Cork, Ireland. *Veterinary Record* 145, 389–393.

Puschner, B., Galey, F.D., Johnson, B., Dickie, C.W., Vondy, M., *et al.* (1998) Blue-green algae toxicosis in cattle. *Journal of the American Veterinary Medical Association* 213, 1605–1607.

Scruggs, D.W. and Blue, G.K. (1994) Toxic hepatopathy and photosensitization in cattle fed moldy alfalfa hay. *Journal of the American Veterinary Association* 204, 264–266.

Sharma, O.P., Sharma, S., Pattabhi, V., Mahato, S.B. and Pharma, P.D. (2007) A review of the hepatotoxic plant *Lantana camara*. *Critical Review of Toxicology* 37, 313–352.

Van Apeldoorn, M.E., van Egmond, H.P., Speijers, G.J. and Bakker, G.J. (2007) Toxins of cyanobacteria. *Molecular Nutritional Food Research* 51, 7–60.

West, H.J. (1997) Clinical and pathological studies in cattle with hepatic disease. *Veterinary Research Communication* 21, 169–185.

CHAPTER 7

Diseases of the Urinary System

7.1 Kidney
- 7.1.1 Anomalies
  - 7.1.1.1 Dysplasia
- 7.1.2 Circulatory disturbances
  - 7.1.2.1 Hemorrhage
  - 7.1.2.2 Infarcts
- 7.1.3 Necrosis and degeneration
  - 7.1.3.1 Nephrotoxicosis
  - 7.1.3.2 Amyloidosis
- 7.1.4 Inflammation
  - 7.1.4.1 Nephritis
  - 7.1.4.2 Chronic nephritis
  - 7.1.4.3 Pyelonephritis
- 7.1.5 Neoplasia
- 7.1.6 Miscellaneous
  - 7.1.6.1 Calculi
  - 7.1.6.2 Cysts

7.2 Lower Urinary Tract
- 7.2.1 Inflammation
- 7.2.2 Urolithiasis
- 7.2.3 Neoplasia
- 7.2.4 Miscellaneous
  - 7.2.4.1 Enzootic hematuria

INTRODUCTION

The main function of the urinary system is the elimination of nitrogen metabolites (waste products) and maintaining homeostasis of water, electrolytes, and acid-base balance. As an endocrine organ, the kidney produces erythropoietin and renin/angiotensin. The nephron is the anatomic and physiologic unit of the kidney. It consists of glomerulo-tubular structures. The kidney has a high functional capacity; a loss of up to 75% of nephrons maintains normal renal function.

About 40% of aortic blood passes through the human kidneys, the rich blood supply to the kidney making it highly susceptible to injury, infections, toxins, ischemia, and metabolic disorders.

7.1 KIDNEY

7.1.1 Anomalies

Introduction. The embryologic structures that develop into the nephron are the mesonephros and metanephros. Branches of the metanephric duct system come into contact by budding with the mesenchyme of the mesonephros to form the glomerulo-tubular apparatus. The potential for malformations is high in a development system that requires the uniting of two complex separate systems during nephrogenesis.

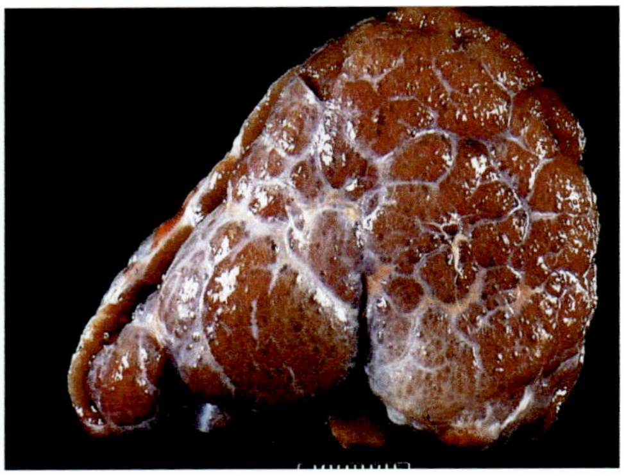

Fig. 7.1. Ox. Kidney. Dysplasia. The kidney is misshapen and lobules are of uneven size. The interlobular tissue shows fibrosis.

Agenesis, hypoplasia, dysplasia, and congenital polycystic kidneys are examples of inherited developmental disturbances. They occur unilaterally or bilaterally.

7.1.1.1 Dysplasia

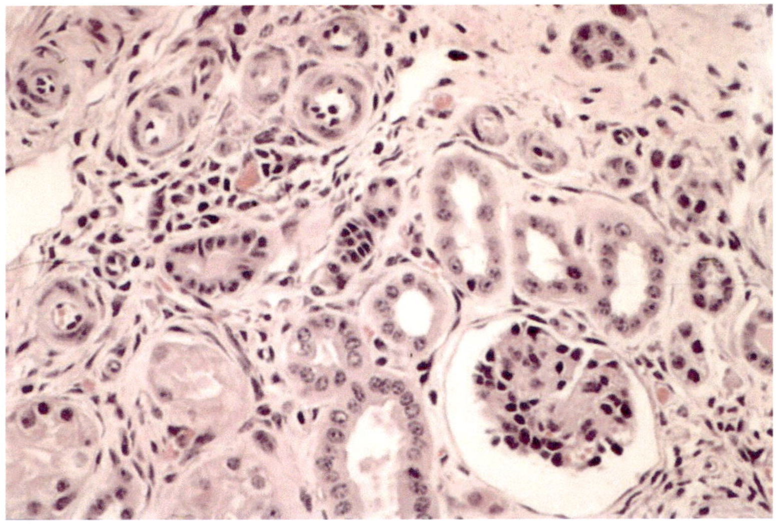

Fig. 7.2. Ox. Kidney. Dysplasia. Microscopically, the glomerulus has a fetal appearance. The intertubular connective tissue is fibrotic. Tubules are underdeveloped and of various diameter. Small collections of lymphocytes surround a small interstitial blood vessel. Blood vessels are generally unapparent (H&E).

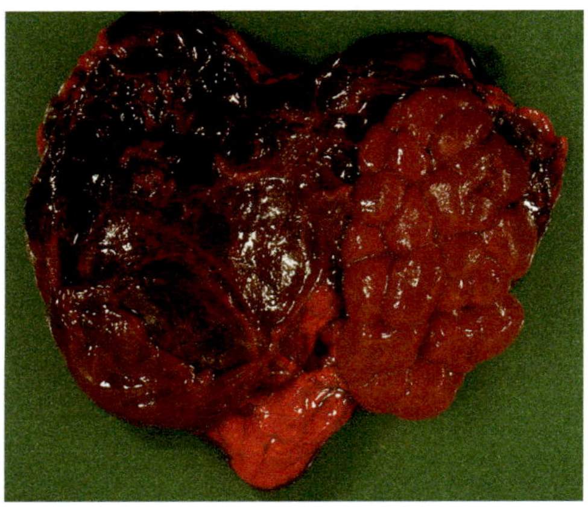

Fig. 7.3. Ox. Kidney. Perirenal hemorrhage. One pole is markedly covered by clotted blood. Sweet clover (*Melilotus officinalis*) consumption.

7.1.2 Circulatory disturbances

7.1.2.1 Hemorrhage

Hemorrhage results from trauma, bleeding disorders, or vascular insults. Petechiae and ecchymoses may suggest bacterial and viral infections.

7.1.2.2 Infarcts

Thromboemboli showering from a nidus somewhere else in the body are entrapped in the rich vascular network of the kidney at the terminal circulation. Infarcts are red when acute and pale when chronic. They typically exhibit a wedge shape on cross section. The size of the infarct depends on the caliber of the occluded vessel.

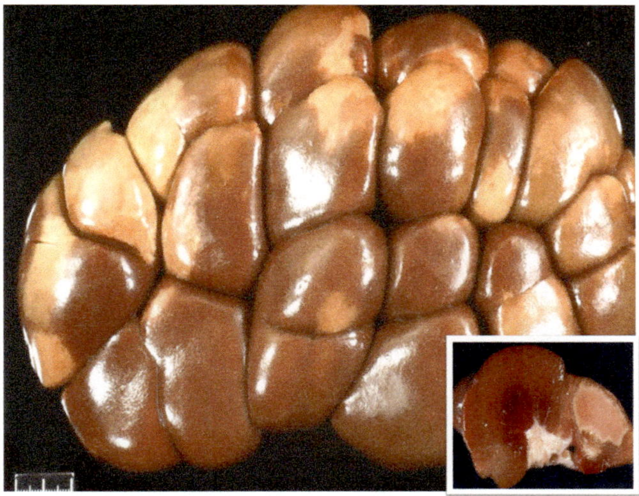

Fig. 7.4. Ox. Kidney. Infarcts. Multiple, well circumscribed, tan areas in the cortex of the lobules reflect chronic infarcts. A common source for infarcts is bacterial valvular or endocardial vegetative inflammation in the heart. In many instances, renal infarctions are not recognized clinically since they do not damage much of the renal parenchyma. Inset: pale infarct. On cut section, the surface of the kidney has an uneven, shrunken appearance. The parenchyma contains a circumscribed, rectangular tan area. (Courtesy of Department of Veterinary Pathology, WCVM, University of Saskatchewan, Saskatoon, Canada.)

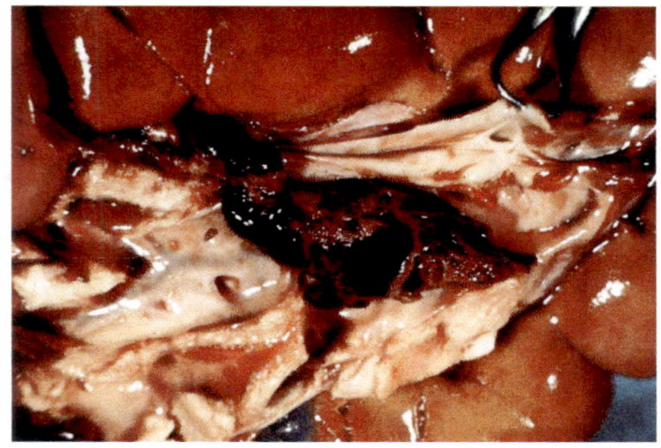

Fig. 7.5. Ox. Kidney. Renal vein thrombosis. Cows treated intravenously with high-glucose solutions occasionally develop thrombosis of deep renal veins.

7.1.3 Necrosis and degeneration

7.1.3.1 Nephrotoxicosis

Introduction. Tubular (cortical) nephrosis is a synonym used for necrotic and degenerative renal changes. The proximal convoluted tubules are the most susceptible to ischemia and toxic damage. Renal failure is a frequent fatal outcome. Hypoperfusion associated with shock, hemorrhage, and systemic sepsis deprives tubular epithelial cells of oxygen and metabolite exchange. Heavy metals such as lead, mercury, and cadmium; toxic plants such as pigweed (*Amaranthus retroflexus*), oak (*Quercus* spp.), plant oxalates; mycotoxins (*Aspergillus* spp.); and drugs such as aminoglycosides, tetracycline, and sulfonamides have a direct damaging effect on tubular epithelium. Endogenous pigments such as hemoglobin, myoglobin, and bilirubin are internal toxic causes.

Clinical signs. Anorexia, oliguria, azotemia, isosthenuria, dehydration.

Differential diagnosis. Renal amyloidosis.

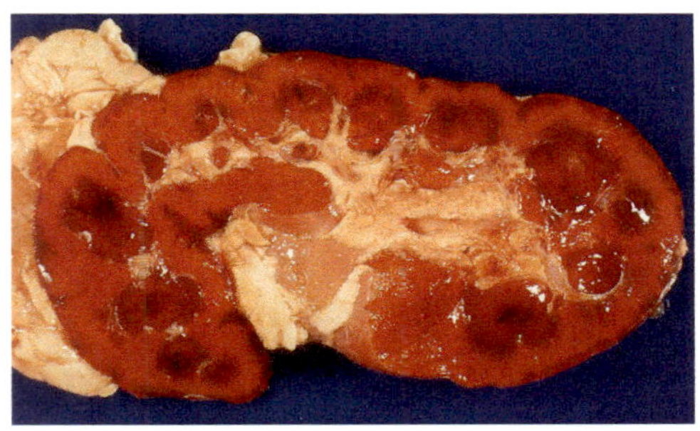

Fig. 7.6. Ox. Kidney. Diffuse to subtotal cortical necrosis. The distinct cortical pallor resulted from hypoperfusion due to shock.

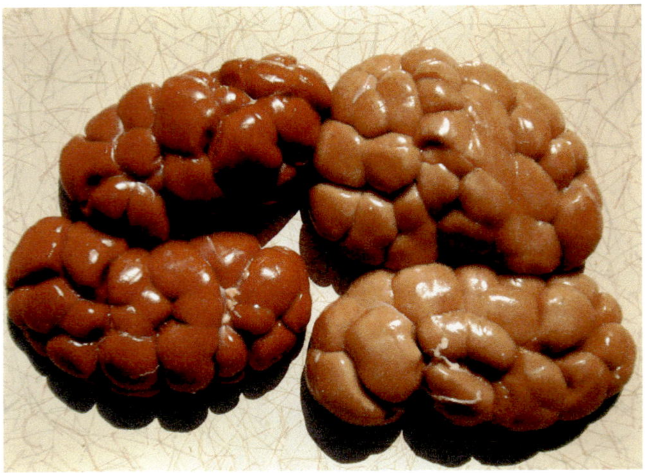

Fig. 7.7. Ox. Kidneys. Nephrosis and glomerulitis. The set of kidneys on the left has a normal dark brown color and small white foci of inflammation on the cortical surface. The set of kidneys on the right diagnosed as nephrosis is pale and enlarged. Perirenal edema is a common finding in nephrosis. Differential diagnoses for renal pallor are anemia, lipidosis, and amyloidosis.

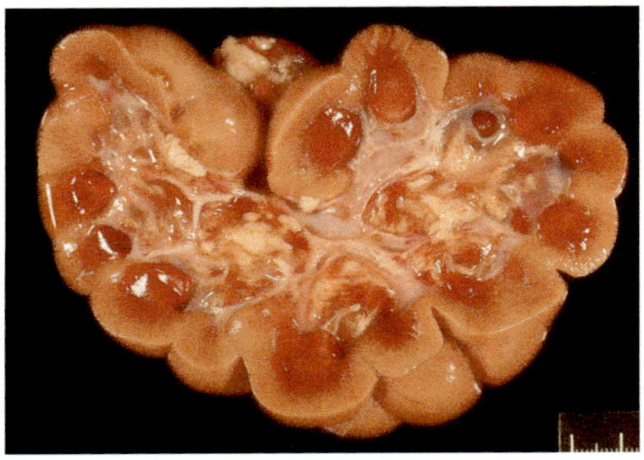

Fig. 7.9. Ox. Kidney. Oxalate nephrosis. Develops after ingestion of oxalate-containing plants such as *Halogeton glomeratus*, *Amaranthus retroflexus*, *Brassica* spp. and others. On cut section, the cortex is pale, moist, and bulges slightly. Differential diagnoses: amyloidosis, anemia. (Courtesy of Department of Veterinary Pathology, WCVM, University of Saskatchewan, Saskatoon, Canada.)

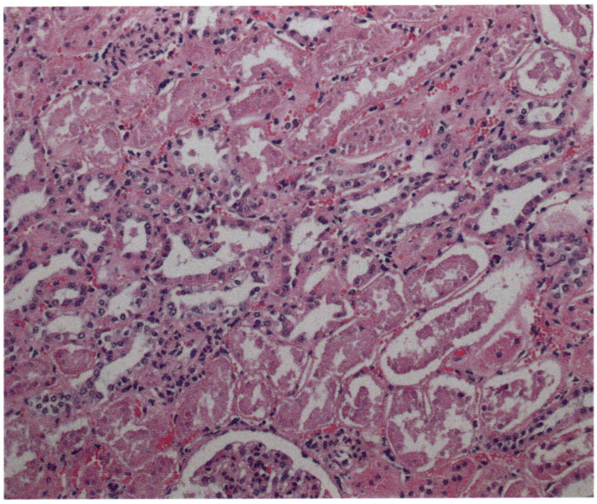

Fig. 7.8. Ox. Kidney. Lead nephrosis. Acute tubular necrosis. Cortical tubular epithelial cells next to the normal ones are sequestered from the basement membrane, causing luminal obstruction. Regeneration of affected tubular epithelium is only possible on an intact basement membrane. Tubulorrhexis results in fibrosis and scarring (H&E). (Courtesy of Department of Veterinary Pathology, WCVM, University of Saskatchewan, Saskatoon, Canada.)

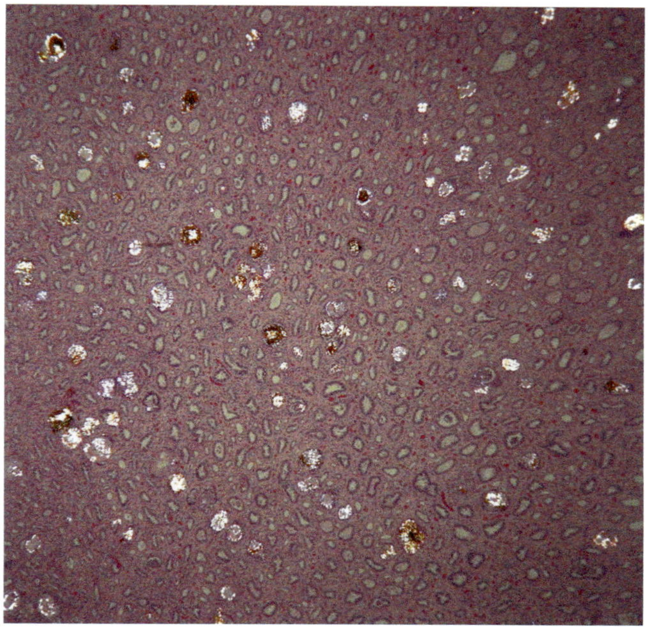

Fig. 7.10. Ox. Kidney. Oxalate nephrosis. Birefringent oxalate crystals are lodged within tubules. Polarized light (H&E).

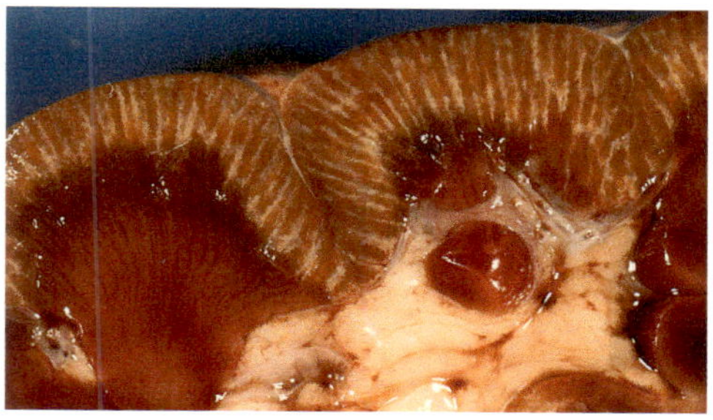

Fig. 7.11. Ox. Kidney. Cortical calcification. Unknown etiology. Ingestion of calciferous plants such as *Cestrum diurnum*, *Trisetum flavescens*, or *Solanum malacoxylon* causes calcification and nephrosis. Also occurs due to excess vitamin D, by either ingestion or injection. Notice the streaky, white appearance of calcified tubules.

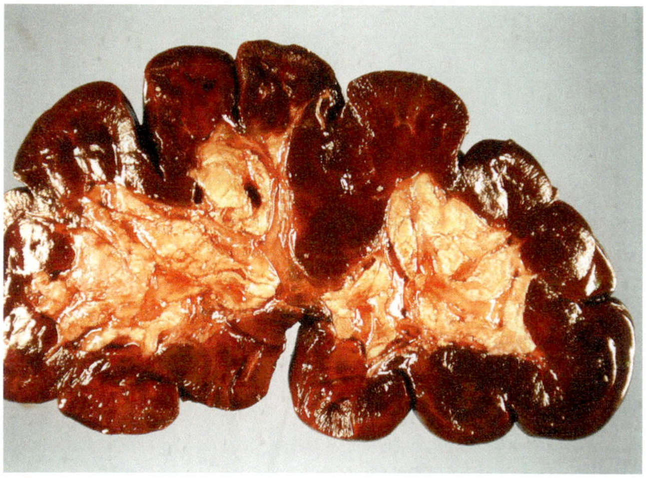

Fig. 7.12. Ox. Kidney. Pigmentary nephrosis. On cut section, the renal cortex markedly and diffusely manifests a red-brown discoloration suggestive of a hemolytic crisis. Hemoglobinuria or myoglobinuria are responsible for the color change. Diseases to consider are babesiosis, anaplasmosis, bacillary hemoglobinuria, post-parturient hemoglobinuria, and leptospirosis. *Staphylococcus aureus* toxins can cause this condition as well. Acute skeletal myopathies due to various causes will result in myoglobinuria.

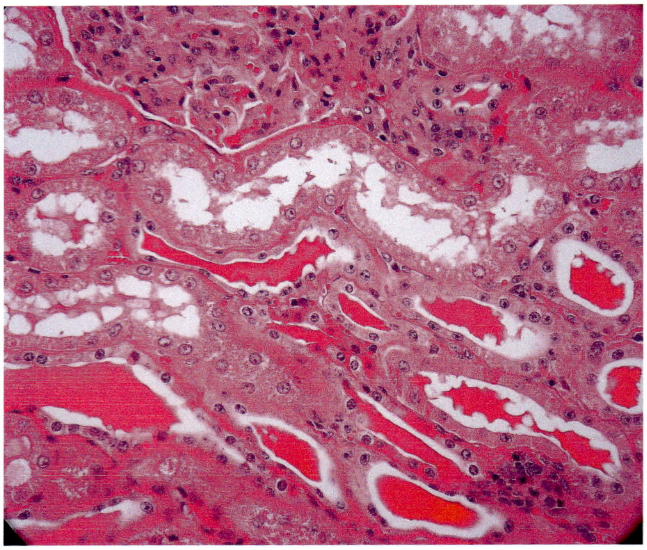

Fig. 7.13. Ox. Kidney. Hemoglobinuric (pigmentary) nephrosis. Hemoglobin casts are lodged within dilated tubules (bacillary hemoglobinuria) (H&E).

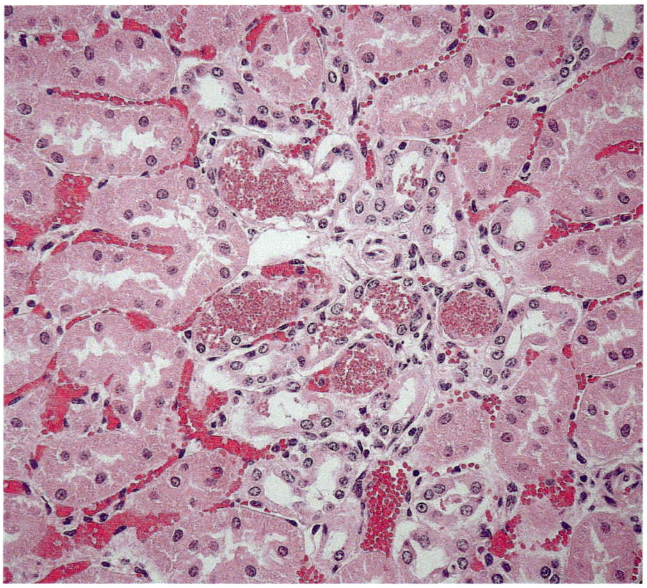

Fig. 7.14. Ox. Kidney. Myoglobinuric (pigmentary) nephrosis. Red myoglobin granules are distributed within the cytoplasm of proximal tubular epithelial cells. A few myoglobin casts are within the lumen. Individual epithelial lining cells are necrotic (H&E).

7.1.3.2 *Amyloidosis*

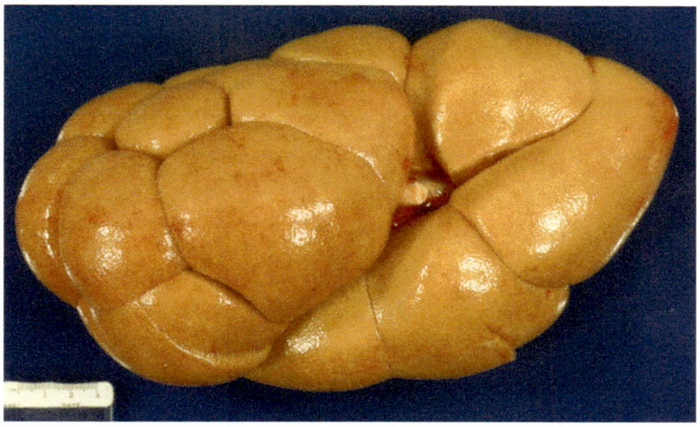

Fig. 7.15. Ox. Kidney. Amyloidosis. The image exhibits a uniform, yellow, glistening appearance mimicking changes encountered in nephrosis or lipidosis. Amyloid, an abnormal and insoluble protein, is deposited in glomeruli, causing proteinuria and hypoproteinemia. Kidneys are frequently grossly enlarged. The make-up of amyloid is either reactive serum amyloid (SAA) or atypical amyloid protein (AA). Proteinuria is a clinical hallmark of the disease. (Courtesy of Department of Veterinary Pathology, WCMV, University of Saskatchewan, Saskatoon, Canada.)

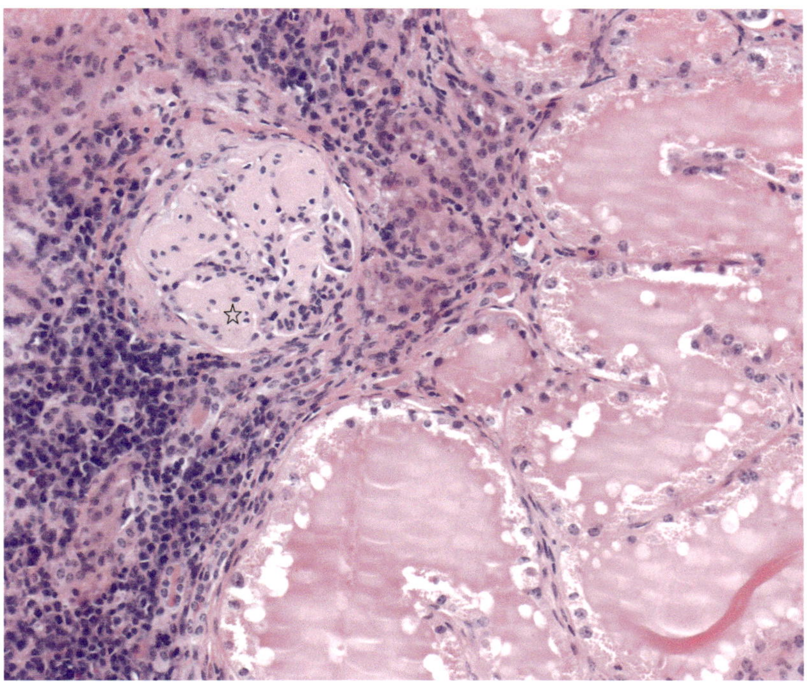

Fig. 7.16. Ox. Kidney. Amyloidosis. An enlarged glomerulus (asterisk) is obliterated by pink deposits lodged in the mesangium. Adjacent tubules are distended by proteinaceous fluid (proteinuria). The interstitium is infiltrated by marked numbers of lymphocytes and plasma cells (H&E).

7.1.4 Inflammation

Introduction. Primary inflammation of the kidney is commonly the result of infectious agents. These may spread to the kidney via hematogenous or ascending (urogenous) pathways. Ascending infection extending from the lower urinary tract induces a pyelitis first, which continues to develop into a pyelonephritis. Main causes for ascending infection in cattle are *Trueperella pyogenes* and *Corynebacterium renale*. Gram-negative bacteria such as *Proteus* spp., *Pseudomonas aeruginosa* and *Escherichia coli* may also participate. Infectious agents hematogenously spread to the kidneys become entrapped in glomeruli to induce a glomerulitis. Adjacent tubules quickly become inflamed, and further extension of inflammation to the tubular apparatus and interstitium results in tubulo-interstitial nephritis. An alternative mechanism for the development of tubulo-interstitial nephritis is infectious agent invasion of interstitial blood vessels, with secondary migration into interstitium and tubules. The latter route of infection is chosen by *Leptospira* spp.

7.1.4.1 Nephritis

Leptospirosis

Introduction. The genus Leptospira consist of many species that can only be distinguished by genotyping. The genospecies *Leptospira interrogans* serovar *pomona*, *hardjo*, and *grippotyphosa* are the main pathogens in North American cattle. Septicemia and reproductive disease develop following infection after skin penetration or ingestion. From there, the spirochetes localize in the liver, where primary replication takes place. Hematogenous spread establishes renal disease.

Clinical signs. Fever, icterus, anemia (extravascular hemolysis), hemoglobinuria, reduced milk production, abortion.

Differential diagnoses. Bacillary hemoglobinuria, post-parturient hemoglobinuria, babesiosis, anaplasmosis.

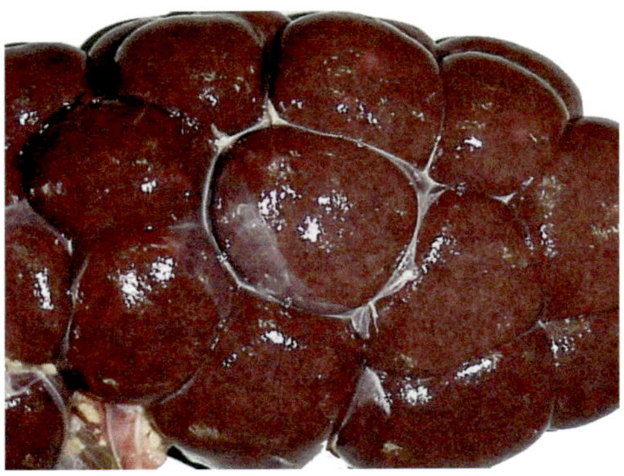

Fig. 7.17. Ox. Kidney. Leptospirosis. Interstitial nephritis. Multiple small white foci of inflammation are present on cortical surface. (Courtesy of Dr D. Driemeier, Universidade Federal do Rio Grande do Sul, Brazil.)

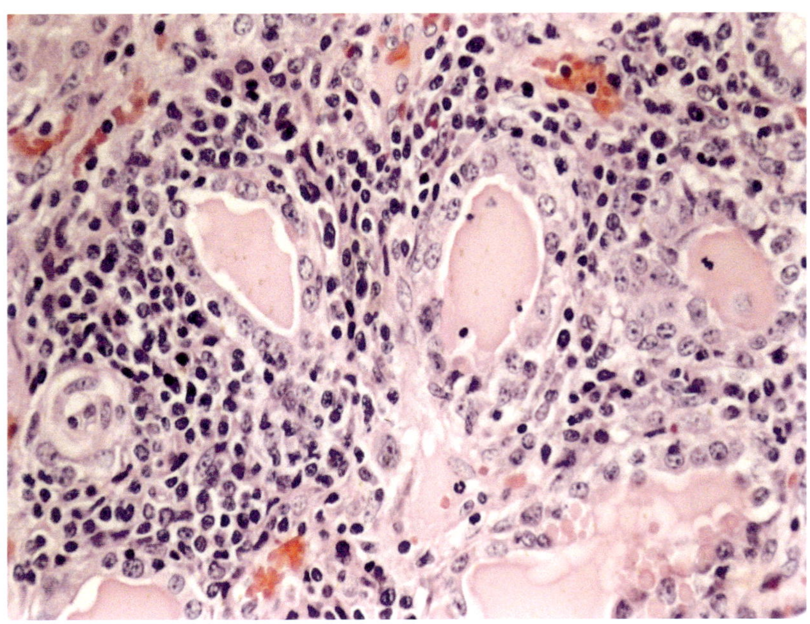

Fig. 7.18. Ox. Kidney. Leptospirosis. Lymphoplasmacytic, tubulo-interstitial nephritis. Moderate collections of lymphocytes and plasma cells infiltrate the interstitium. Tubules contain protein casts. Tubular epithelial cells have sequestered and are infiltrated mildly by lymphocytes (H&E).

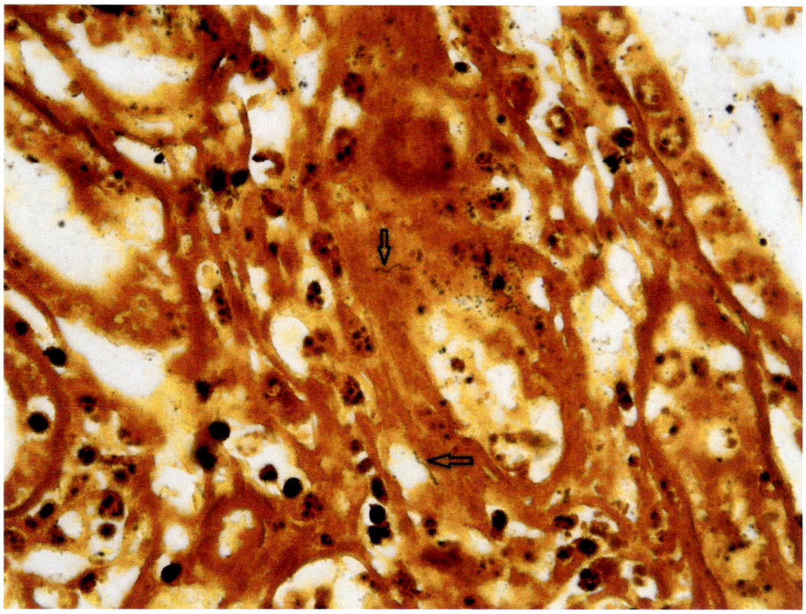

Fig. 7.19. Ox. Kidney. Leptospirosis. Intralesional spirochetes. A special stain outlines spirochetes in the tubular wall (arrows) (Warthin-Starry silver stain). Indirect immunohistochemistry (IHC) also can be applied as diagnostic tool. (Courtesy of Dr.R.Moeller, UC Davis, Tulare, USA)

Fact Sheet: Bovine Renal Leptospirosis

■ Agent:	*Leptospira interrogans* serovars: *pomona*, *hardjo*, *grippotyphosa*
■ Transmission:	cutaneous, oral, venereal, aerosol
■ Main reservoir:	rodents, bats, wild carnivores, deer
■ Clinical forms:	acute – septicemic, hemolytic subacute – jaundice chronic-abortions
Renal gross pathology:	mottled gray-brown cortical surface gray confluent cortical foci on cross section focal corticomedullary fibrosis
■ Renal histology:	aggregates of lymphocytes and plasma cells in interstitium necrotic and inflamed tubular epithelium interstitial fibrosis
■ Health aspect:	zoonosis

Histophilus somni

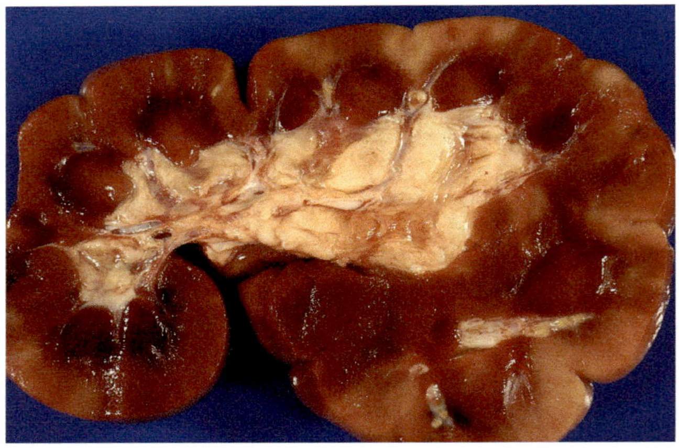

Fig. 7.20. Ox. Kidney. Chronic multifocal nephritis. The cortex contains multiple pale confluent patches. This is an example of multicentric bacterial hematogenous dissemination of *Histophilus somni*.

Malignant catarrhal fever

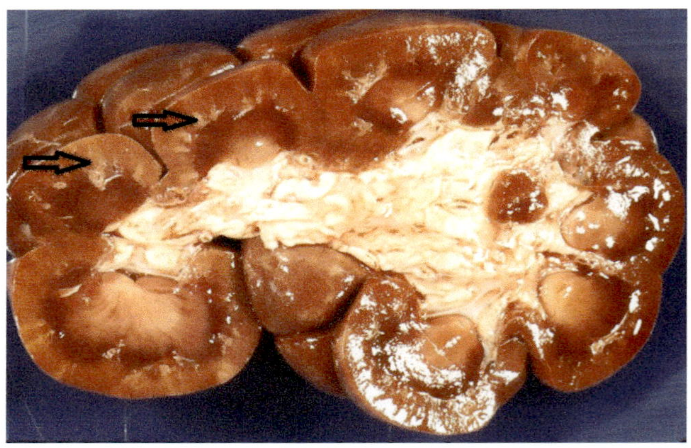

Fig. 7.21. Ox. Kidney. Malignant catarrhal fever (MCF). Cortical vasculitis and nephritis. Multiple blood vessels (arrows) are accentuated as white spots and small white streaks, indicating interstitial nephritis.

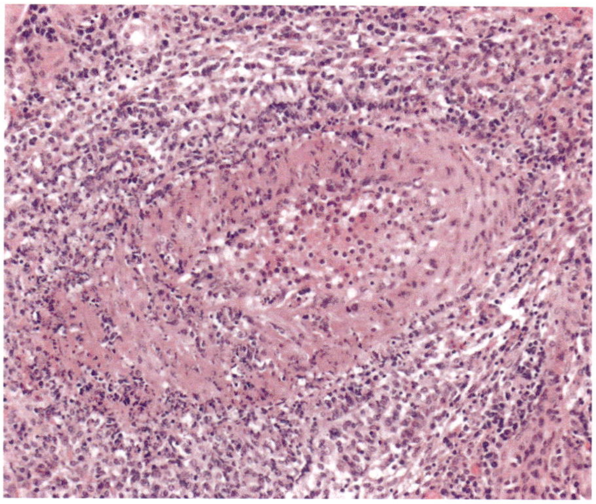

Fig. 7.22. Ox. Kidney. Malignant catarrhal fever (MCF). Fibrinoid necrotizing panvasculitis. Intraluminal mononuclear cells, mural degenerating neutrophils, and fibrinoid necrosis, as well as perivascular mononuclear cells, are present (H&E).

Hairy vetch (Vicia villosa Roth)

Hairy vetch constituents (lectins) invoke a multisystemic type-IV hypersensitivity reaction characterized by a granulomatous inflammatory response involving dermis, renal cortex, adrenal gland cortex, lymph nodes, and liver.

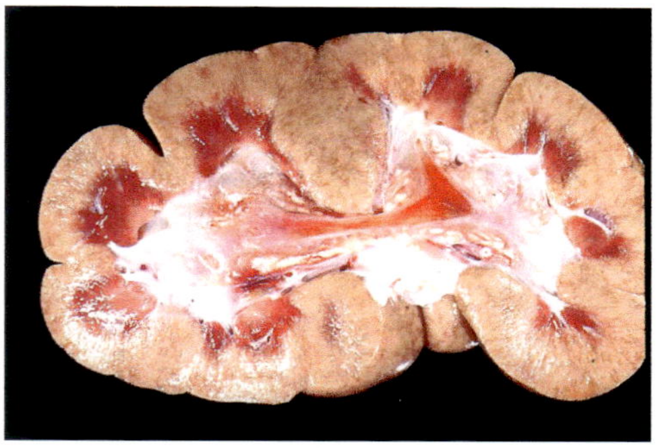

Fig. 7.23. Ox. Kidney. Granulomatous nephritis Cut section of the kidney contains multiple confluent bulging nodules. Differential diagnoses: citrus pulp toxicosis, tuberculosis, lymphosarcoma. (Courtesy of J. Edwards, Texas A&M University, USA.)

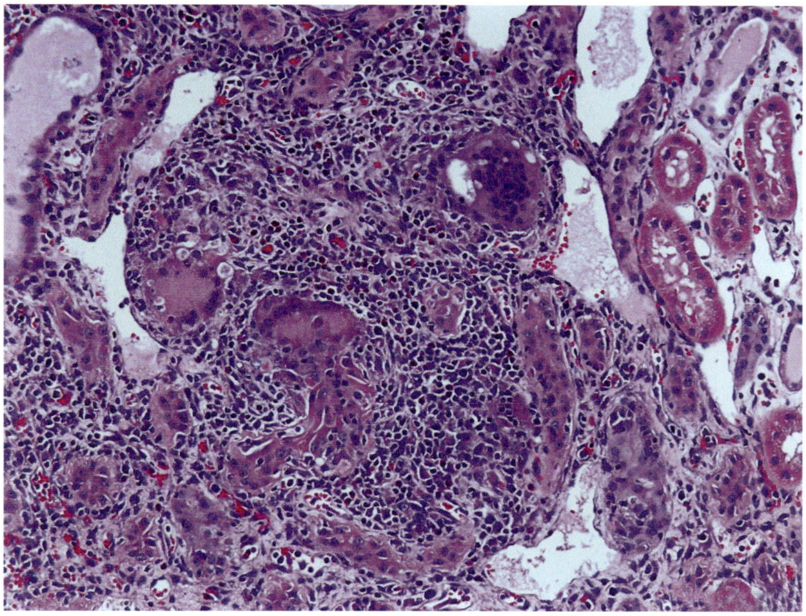

Fig. 7.24. Ox. Kidney. Granulomatous nephritis. The intertubular interstitium has been replaced by an inflammatory infiltrate composed of lymphocytes, plasma cells, and multinucleate giant cells (H&E). (Courtesy of Dr L. Woods, University of California, USA.)

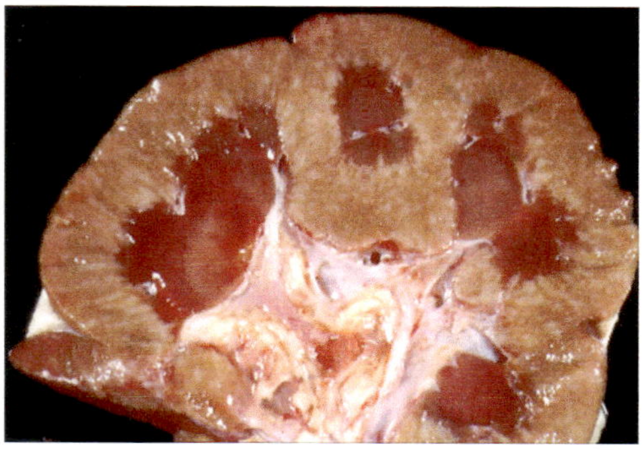

Fig. 7.25. Ox. Kidney. Citrus pulp toxicosis. Granulomatous nephritis. The cortex contains multiple discrete white foci. (Reprinted with permission of *Journal of Veterinary Diagnostic Investigation* 12, 269, figure 1, 2009.)

Citrus pulp toxicosis

Citrus pulp is fed as energy-rich supplement to dairy cows. Its toxic effects on multiple organs results in lesions similar to vetch poisoning. (For more, see Chapter 9: Diseases of the Endocrine System.)

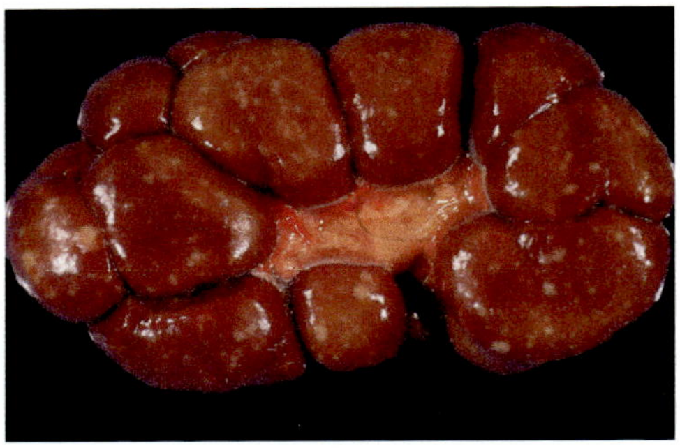

Fig. 7.26. Ox. Kidney. Embolic nephritis. Often an incidental finding at necropsy. Multiple white spots are scattered throughout the cortical surface. Hematogenous spread of mainly gram-negative bacteria has been implicated in the literature, but has also been ruled out by some authors. Specifically, the role of leptospires in the induction of 'white-spotted kidneys' has not been clearly established. The spotty arrangement of the changes fits the concept of 'white-spotted kidney' disease, which is introduced in Chapter 1: Diseases of Neonates and Calves.

7.1.4.2 Chronic nephritis

Introduction. In chronic renal disease, the kidneys are affected bilaterally and are of varying size and shapes. They are pale and firm. The capsule is difficult to strip because of adhesions. Often, the original cause is obscure, but bacteria as the initiating cause should be considered.

Clinical signs. Weight loss, edema, diarrhea, anorexia.

Differential diagnoses. Pyelonephritis, renal amyloidosis, leptospirosis.

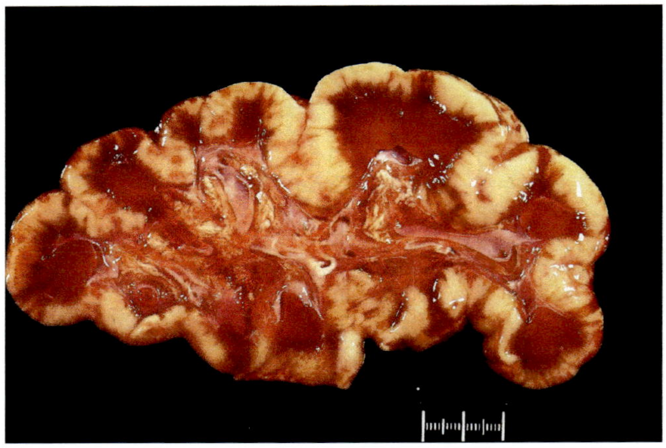

Fig. 7.27. Ox. Kidney. Cortical nephritis. On cut section, the cortex contains tan confluent, glistening, slightly bulging nodules.

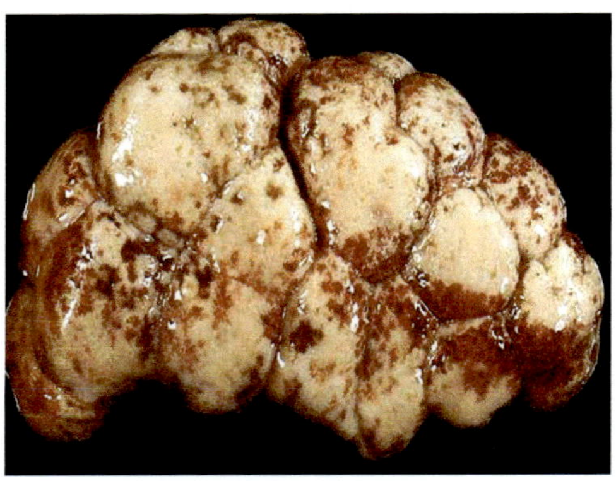

Fig. 7.29. Ox. Kidney. Interstitial nephritis. Lobules are of irregular size. There is pitting of the cortical surface. The majority of the renal lobular parenchyma is replaced by white texture suggestive of fibrous connective tissue.

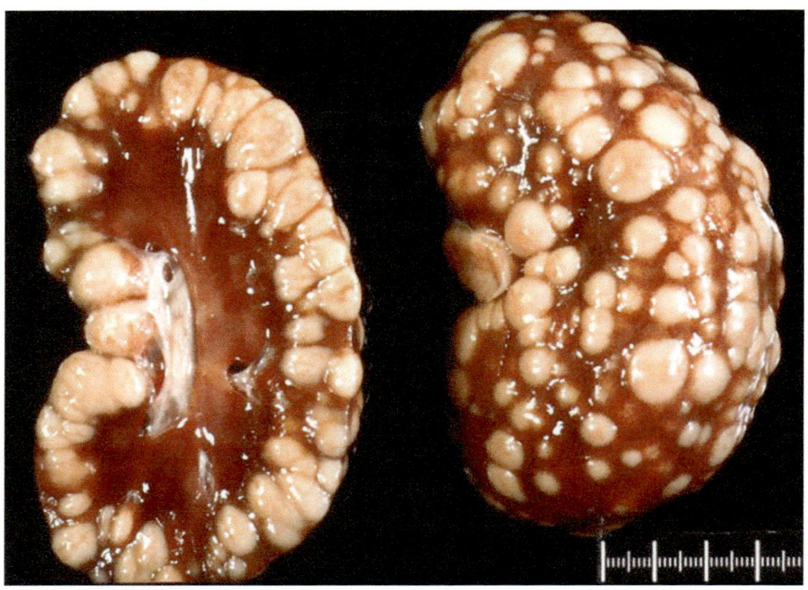

Fig. 7.28. Ox. Kidney. Interstitial nephritis. Tumor-like arrangement of multiple nodules in the cortex mimics neoplasia such as lymphosarcoma.

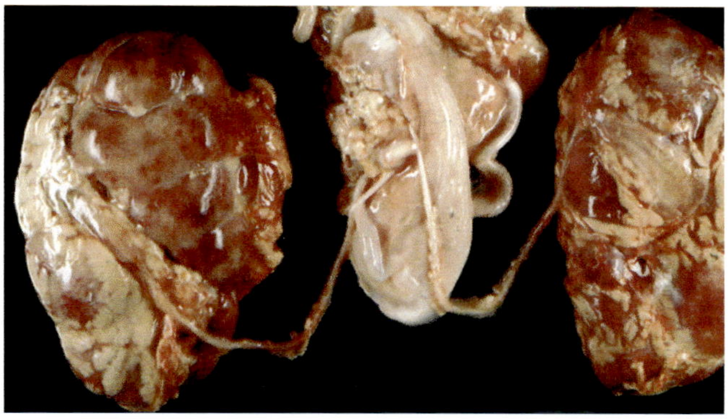

Fig. 7.30. Ox. Kidneys. Chronic renal disease. The kidneys are reduced in size and have irregular, discolored lobules. The capsules are adherent.

7.1.4.3 Pyelonephritis

Introduction. The result of ascending bacterial infection from the lower urinary tract or genitalia, pyelonephritis is a common disease of dairy cows. Ureters also become inflamed in this process, and concurrent cystitis may be present. *C. renale*, possessing special pili for attachment to the urothelium, and *E. coli* are the principal infectious agents responsible for the condition. Less frequent causes are *T. pyogenes*, *Corynebacterium pilosum*, *Streptococcus* spp. and *Enterococcus faecalis*. Acute pyelonephritis begins with necrosis and inflammation of the renal crest. Chronic pyelonephritis extends into the medulla and cortex. Vesicoureteral reflux is the mechanism for transporting bacteria from the lower urinary passages to the kidney.

Clinical signs. Fever, colic, stranguria, hematuria, pyuria.

Differential diagnoses. Renal and urethral calculi, cystitis.

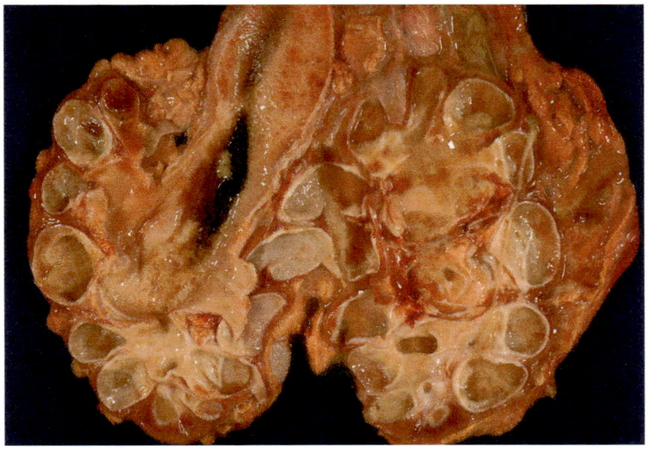

Fig. 7.32. Ox. Kidney. Chronic pyelonephritis and ureteritis. Ascending infection is evident by markedly thickened ureter, with hemorrhagic urothelium and distended renal calyces containing a watery exudate and some fibrin.

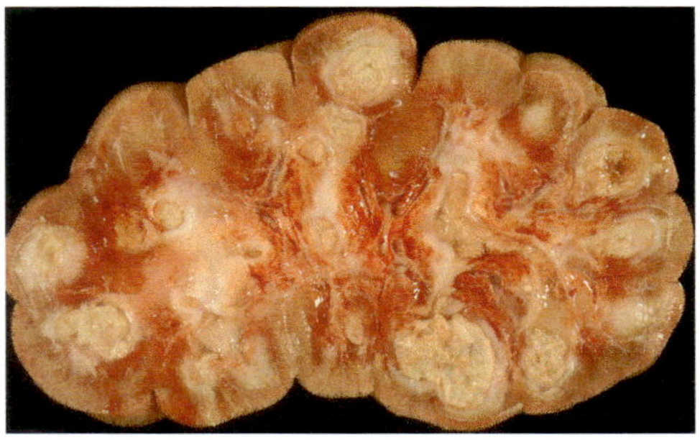

Fig. 7.31. Ox. Kidneys. Suppurative pyelonephritis. Calyces are distended and filled with inspissated pus. (Courtesy of Department of Veterinary Pathology, WCVM, University of Saskatchewan, Saskatoon, Canada.)

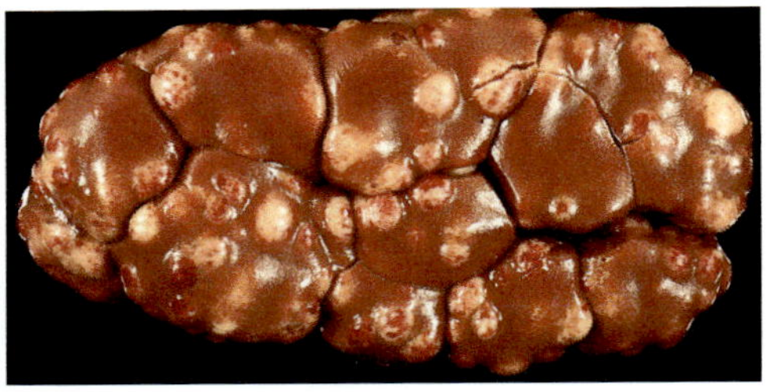

Fig. 7.33. Ox. Kidney. Lymphosarcoma. Uniform-sized, white-gray nodules are often spread throughout the cortex. Differential diagnoses: metastasizing carcinoma, granulomas.

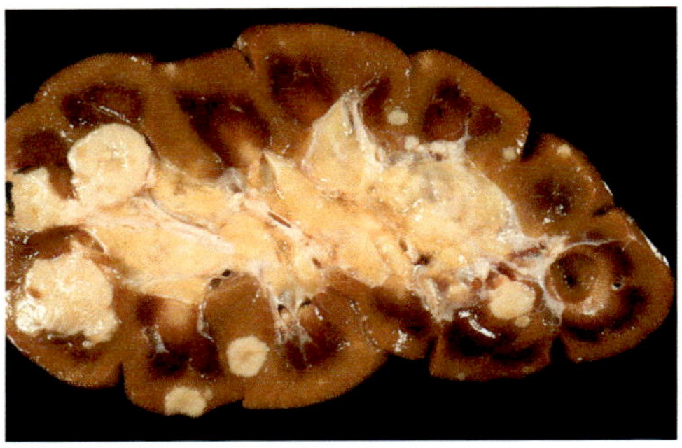

Fig. 7.34. Ox. Kidney. Metastasizing uterine carcinoma. Multiple small, regular-sized, slightly raised nodules are disseminated throughout the cortical surface. The pelvis is covered by extensive adipose tissue. Malignant pheochromocytomas have a tendency to metastasize to the kidneys as well.

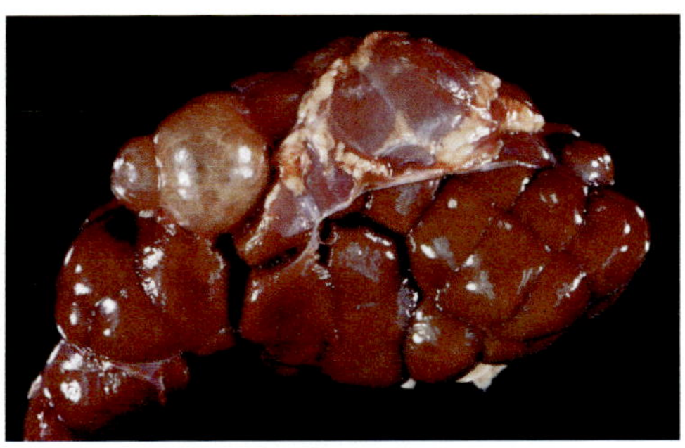

Fig. 7.36. Ox. Kidney. Renal cysts. Several thin-walled, spherical, fluid-filled structures bulge from the cortical surface.

7.1.5 Neoplasia

Primary neoplasms are extremely rare in cattle. Multicentric lymphosarcoma is the most commonly observed neoplasm. Metastatic neoplasia is occasionally encountered.

7.1.6 Miscellaneous

7.1.6.1 Calculi

Urethral obstruction can be serious, leading to oliguria or bladder rupture with urine in the abdomen, resulting in uroperitoneum.

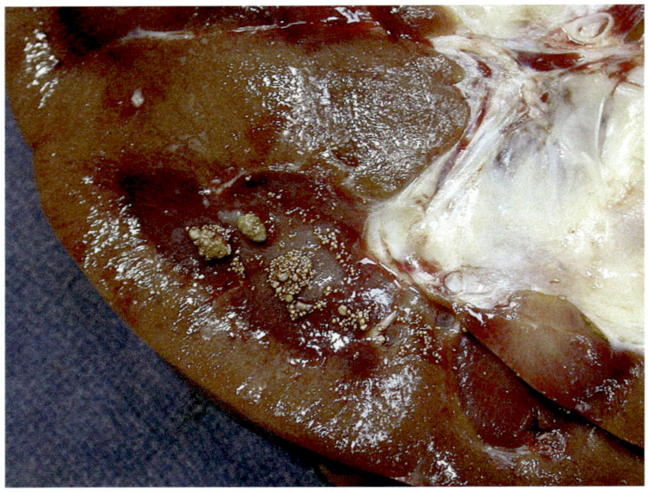

Fig. 7.35. Ox. Kidney. Microcalculi. Small, green, gritty, sand-like and a few medium-sized green particulate formations are located in the pelvis. Incidental findings with no evidence of obstructive changes (see Section 7.2 Lower Urinary Tract).

7.1.6.2 Cysts

Kidneys develop single or multiple cysts that arise from obstruction anywhere in the nephron. They may be congenital as well, particularly in young animals. Increased luminal pressure creates a thin-walled structure filled with a watery fluid. Frequent incidental finding.

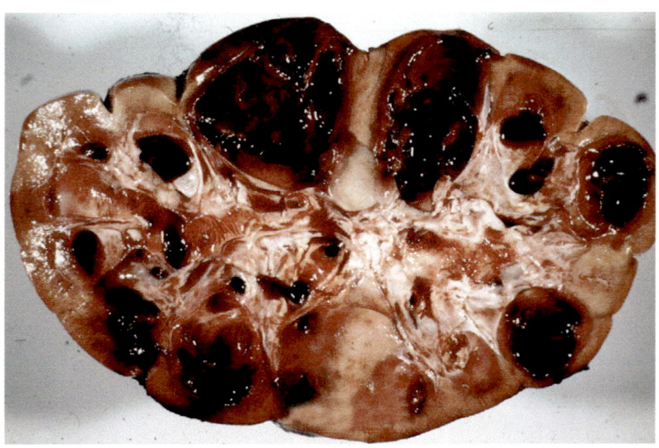

Fig. 7.37. Ox. Kidney. Hemorrhagic cysts. Multiple large, blood-filled cysts occupy and obliterate renal lobules. Hematuria should be an expected clinical sign in this case.

7.2 LOWER URINARY TRACT

The lower urinary tract comprises ureters, urinary bladder, and urethra. Together, they share the urothelium as a mucosal lining.

7.2.1 Inflammation

Introduction. Cystitis develops from ascending infection of the urethra, or from irritation by pre-existing calculi.
Clinical signs. Stranguria, urine dribbling, hematuria.
Differential diagnosis. Pyelonephritis.

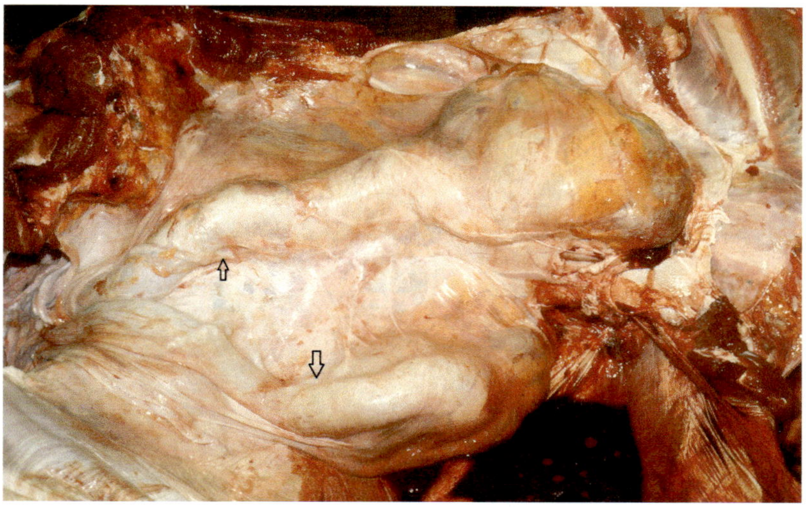

Fig. 7.40. Ox. Ureters. Pyoureters and pyelonephritis. Both inflamed ureters are markedly thickened (arrows). Distension reaches the renal pelvis.

7.2.2 Urolithiasis

Introduction. Urinary calculi are mineral concretions forming anywhere in the urinary passages from supersaturation of urine solutes. Calculi are composed of a central proteinaceous nidus that becomes enveloped by concentric crystals. As calculi grow, they may become entrapped in narrow segments of the lower urinary tract, such as the ischial arch of bulls, or ureters when dislodged from the original site (renal pelvis, urinary bladder). The composition of urinary calculi varies depending on husbandry; the calculi are silica when animals are pastured; they are struvite (magnesium ammonium phosphate hexahydrate) in feedlot cattle on high grain ration; they are oxalate calculi in animals consuming plants high in soluble oxalate. Entrapped calculi cause luminal obstruction, pressure necrosis, and rupture of the urinary passages. Expected secondary and occasional fatal complications are hydronephrosis, hydroureters, and uroperitoneum from a ruptured urinary bladder.

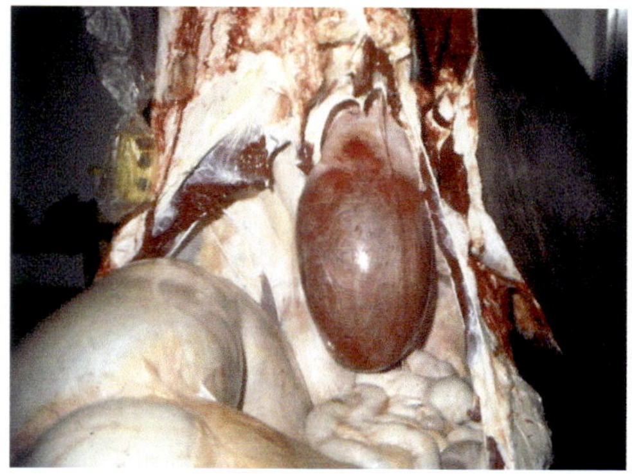

Fig. 7.38. Ox. Urinary bladder. Hemorrhagic cystitis. The urinary bladder is distended by blood-tinged urine. The animal (bull) had a calculus obstructing the urethra at the site of the sigmoid flexure.

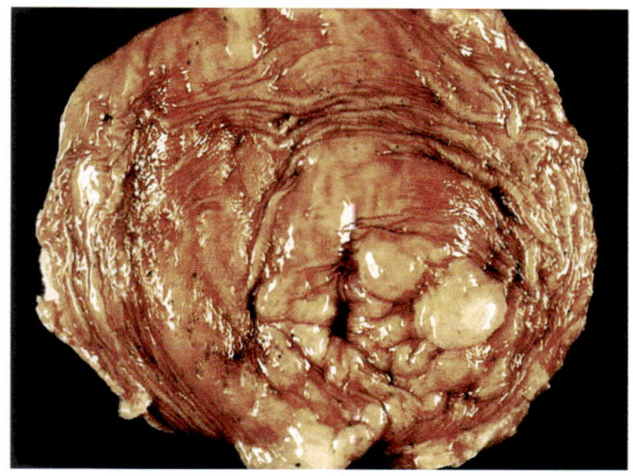

Fig. 7.39. Ox. Urinary bladder. Emphysematous cystitis. Multiple gas spheres occupy the mucosa. Excessive glucose treatment and/or gas-producing bacteria are responsible for the gas production.

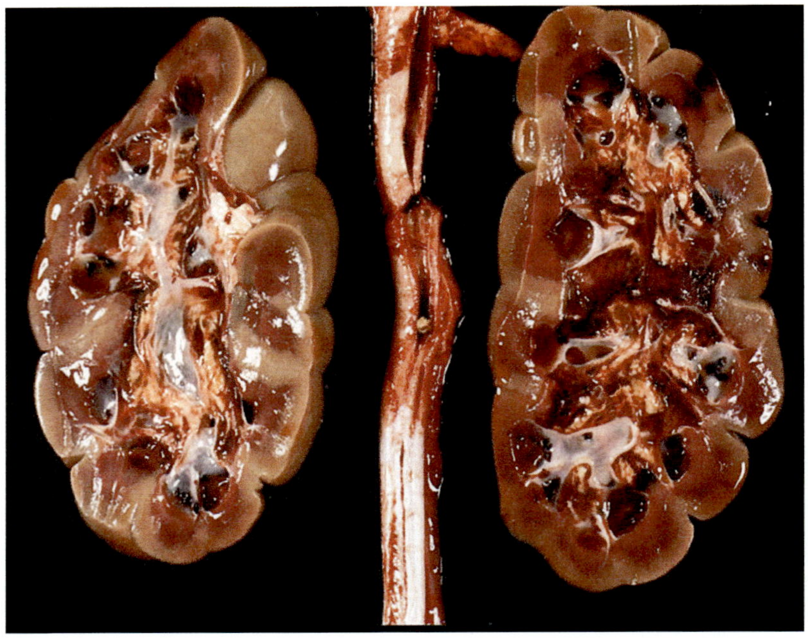

Fig. 7.41. Ox. Kidneys and urethra. Renoliths and urolith. Multiple calculi are lodged within renal calyces. One small calculus flushed into the urethra.

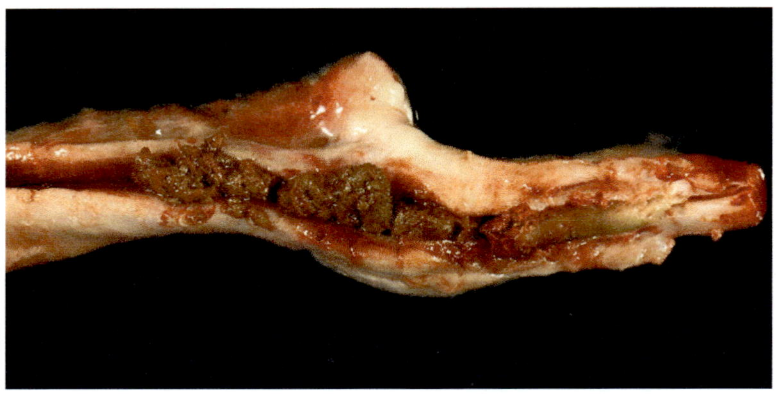

Fig. 7.42. Ox. Urethra. Urolithiasis. Marked obstruction of the urinary passage by calculi.

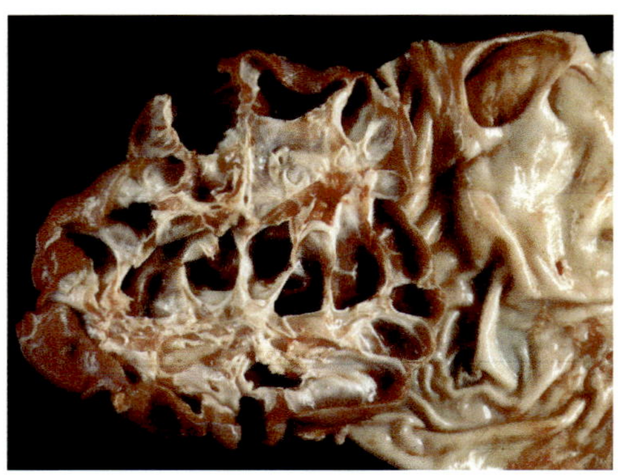

Fig. 7.43. Ox. Kidney. Hydronephrosis. Calyces are markedly distended with compression loss of the medulla and atrophy of the cortical parenchyma. The condition is a common complication following obstruction of lower urinary tract sites.

7.2.3 Neoplasia

Tumors of the urinary bladder are associated with the enzootic hematuria syndrome. If sporadic, they are part of multicentric lymphosarcoma.

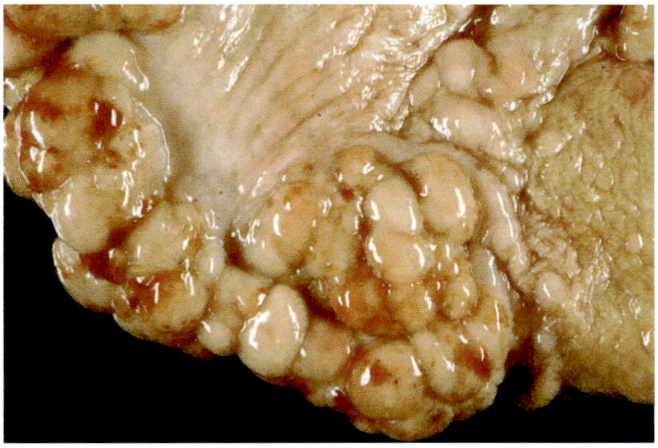

Fig. 7.44. Ox. Urinary bladder. Lymphosarcoma. Multiple confluent, white, glistening nodules protrude from the mucosa.

7.2.4 Miscellaneous

7.2.4.1 *Enzootic hematuria*

Introduction. Bovine enzootic hematuria is a syndrome that develops in cattle foraging on pastures contaminated with bracken fern (*Pteridium aquilinum*). Bracken fern contains compounds toxic to the bone marrow, gastrointestinal tract, and urinary bladder, and the glucoside ptaquiloside, which is carcinogenic to the urinary bladder and mucosa of gastrointestinal tract. Animals with access to bracken fern develop cystitis first, followed by urinary bladder neoplasia after prolonged consumption. Bovine papilloma virus-2 (BPV-2) has been implicated as a co-factor in the pathogenesis of bracken-fern-induced cystitis and urinary bladder tumors, which include benign and malignant epithelial and vascular neoplasms (for more, see Chapter 16: The Pathology of Select Poisonous Plant-induced Diseases in Cattle).

Clinical signs. Fever, diarrhea, diathesis, hematuria, anemia, septicemia.

Differential diagnoses. Pyelonephritis, anthrax, furazolidine toxicity, pruritus–pyrexia–hemorrhagic syndrome (presumptive citronin toxicity).

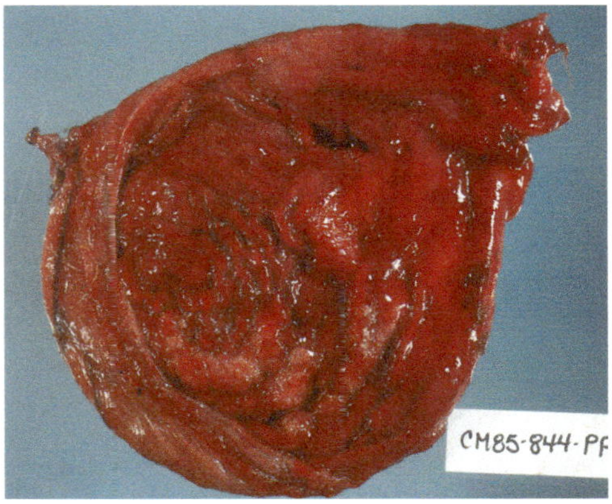

Fig. 7.45. Ox. Urinary bladder. Hemorrhagic cystitis. The thickened mucosa is extensively and diffusively hemorrhagic. (Courtesy of the Government of Alberta, Canada.)

SUGGESTED READING

Azizi, S., Tajbakhsh, E., Hajimirzael, M.R., Gholami Varmamkhast, M., Sadeghian, H. and Oryan, A. (2012) Evaluation of 'white-spotted kidneys' associated with leptospirosis by polymerase chain reaction based LipL32 gene in slaughtered cows. *Journal of the South African Veterinary Association* 83(1), doi: 10.4102/sava.v83i1.69.

Azizi, S., Kheirandish, R. and Rahimi, E. (2014) Comparison of polymerase chain reaction with Warthin–Starry techniques to detect *Leptospira* spp. in kidneys of slaughtered cattle. *Onderstepoort Journal of Veterinary Research* 81(1), doi: 10.4102/ojvr.v81i1.821.

Carvalho, T., Pinto, C. and Peleteiro, M.C. (2006) Urinary bladder lesions in bovine enzootic haematuria. *Journal of Comparative Pathology* 134, 336–346.

Elitok, O.M., Elitok, B. and Unver, O. (2008) Renal amyloidosis in cattle with inflammatory diseases. *Journal of Veterinary Internal Medicine* 22, 450–455.

Marakami, T., Inoshima, Y., Kobayashi, Y., Matsui, T., Inokuma, H. and Ishiguro, N. (2012) Atypical AA amyloid deposits in bovine AA amyloidosis. *Amyloid* 19, 15–20.

Miller, D.A., Wilson, M.A. and Beran, G.W. (1991) Survey to estimate prevalence of leptospiral interrogans infection in mature cattle in the United States. *American Journal of Veterinary Research* 52, 1761–1765.

Panciera, R.J., Mosier, D.A. and Ritchey, J.W. (1992) Hairy vetch (*Vicia villosa* Roth) poisoning in cattle: update and experimental induction of disease. *Journal of Veterinary Diagnostic Investigation* 4, 318–325.

Resendes, A.R., Roperto, S., Trapani, F., Urraro, C., Rodrigues, A., *et al.* (2011) Association of bovine papillomavirus type 2 (BPV-2) and urinary bladder tumours in cattle from the Azores archipelago. *Research in Veterinary Science* 90, 526–529.

Somvanshi, R., Pathania, S., Nagarajan, N., Pangty, K. and Kumar, P. (2012) Pathological study of non-neoplastic urinary bladder lesions in cattle and buffaloes: a preliminary report. *Tropical Animal Health Production* 44, 855–861.

Uzal, F.A., Dobrenov, B., Smythe, L., Norris, M., Dohnt, M., *et al.* (2002) A study of 'white spotted kidneys' in cattle. *Veterinary Microbiology* 86, 369–375.

CHAPTER 8

Diseases of the Musculoskeletal System

Keith G. Thompson (contributed Section 8.2 Skeletal System)
Institute of Veterinary, Animal and Biomedical Sciences, Massey University, Palmerston North, New Zealand

8.1 Muscular System
- 8.1.1 Myodegeneration/myonecrosis
  - 8.1.1.1 Nutritional
  - 8.1.1.2 Toxic
  - 8.1.1.3 Downer cow myopathy
- 8.1.2 Inflammation
  - 8.1.2.1 Clostridial myositis
  - 8.1.2.2 Parasitic myositis
  - 8.1.2.3 Protozoal myositis
  - 8.1.2.4 Miscellaneous
- 8.1.3 Hyperplasia

8.2 Skeletal System
- 8.2.1 Genetic abnormalities
  - 8.2.1.1 Chondrodysplasias
  - 8.2.1.2 Osteogenesis imperfecta
  - 8.2.1.3 Osteopetrosis
  - 8.2.1.4 Localized abnormalities
- 8.2.2 Nutritional and metabolic bone diseases
  - 8.2.2.1 Osteoporosis
  - 8.2.2.2 Rickets and osteomalacia
  - 8.2.2.3 Manganese deficiency
- 8.2.3 Inflammatory and infectious diseases of bone
  - 8.2.3.1 Osteomyelitis
  - 8.2.3.2 Toe-tip necrosis
  - 8.2.3.3 Intrauterine bovine viral diarrhea virus infection
- 8.2.4 Miscellaneous bone diseases
  - 8.2.4.1 Juvenile lymphoma
  - 8.2.4.2 Tetracycline deposition
- 8.2.5 Arthritis
- 8.2.6 Degenerative joint disease
- 8.2.7 Osteochondrosis

8.1 MUSCULAR SYSTEM

Introduction. Diseases involving any muscle group affect intended function and impede locomotion. Metabolic, nutritional, toxic, infectious, genetic, and neurogenic etiologies have to be taken into consideration.

There are two types of skeletal muscle fibers. Type 1, the aerobic fiber, is rich in myoglobin and oxidative enzymes, and resists fatigue. Type 2, the anaerobic fiber, is rich in glycogen and fatigues rapidly. Its energy supply is derived from the glycolytic pathway. Most muscles contain both type 1 and type 2 fibers.

8.1.1 Myodegeneration/myonecrosis

8.1.1.1 Nutritional

Introduction. Also known as 'white muscle disease' (WMD) and 'enzootic myopathy', the metabolic disorder affects young, fast-growing animals.

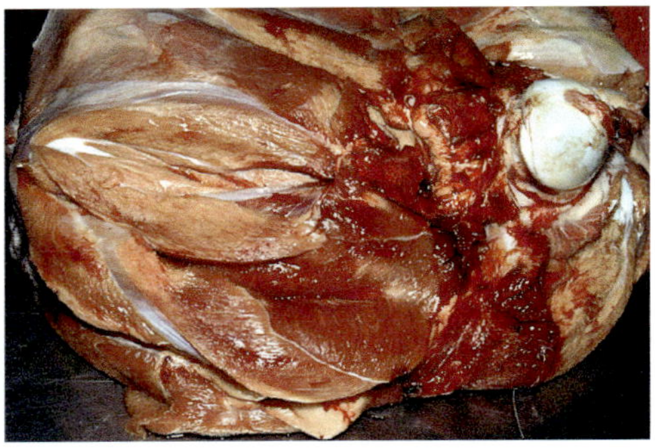

Fig. 8.1. Ox. Skeletal muscle. White muscle disease (WMD). Locally extensive and multifocal pallor of hind-leg muscles. Toxic myodegeneration or chronic myodegeneration from trauma should be considered in differential diagnosis. (Courtesy of Department of Veterinary Pathology, WCVM, University of Saskatchewan, Saskatoon, Canada.)

Historically, it is associated with vitamin E/selenium deficiency, either from selenium-deficient soil, diet or binding by minerals (sulfur). Selenium and vitamin E function synergistically, and have similar actions. Selenium-containing enzymes of the glutathione oxidase system are cell membrane protective. In their absence, membranes are damaged by uncontrolled free radicals. Vitamin E protects against superoxide damage.

Clinical signs. Non-specific. Weakness in locomotion, stiff gait, recumbency.

Laboratory findings. Elevated muscle enzymes, myoglobinuria.

Differential diagnoses. Laminitis, toxic myopathies, growth promotors (monensin).

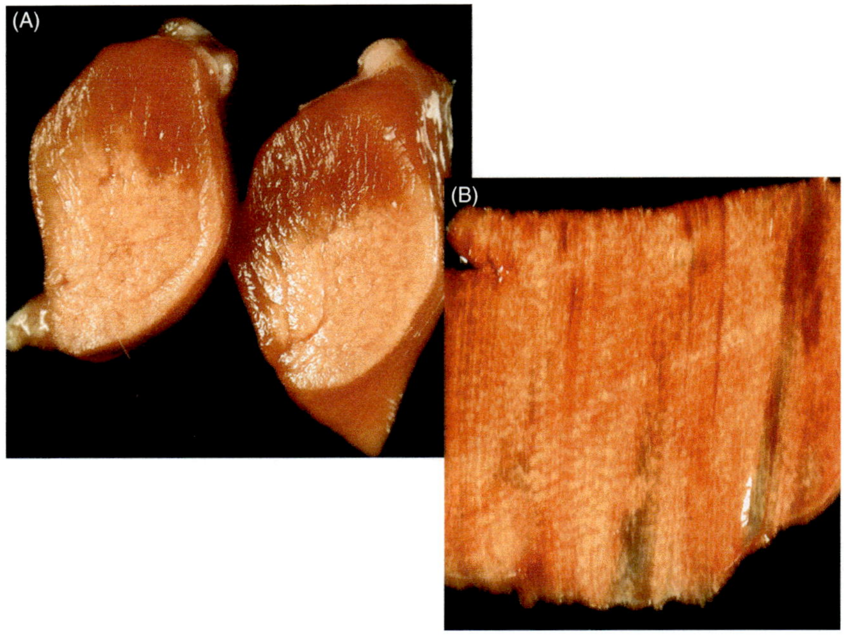

Fig. 8.2. Ox. Skeletal muscle. White muscle disease (WMD). (A) Iliopsoas muscle. Cut section. Diffuse pallor. (B) Diaphragm. Typical paintbrush, streak-like appearance of one of the most active muscle groups, and therefore commonly affected.

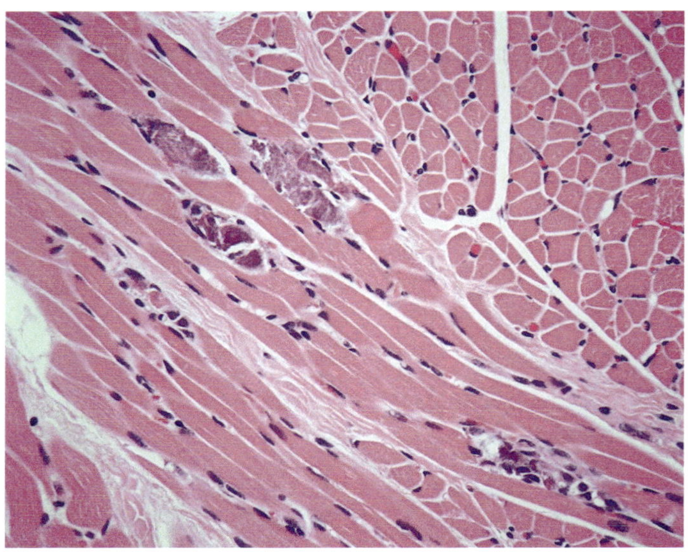

Fig. 8.3. Ox. Skeletal muscle. White muscle disease (WMD). Histologic features of fragmentation and dystrophic mineralization of myofibers. Additional microscopic changes may include sarcoplasmal hypereosinophilia and loss of striation. Type 1 fibers are principally affected (H&E).

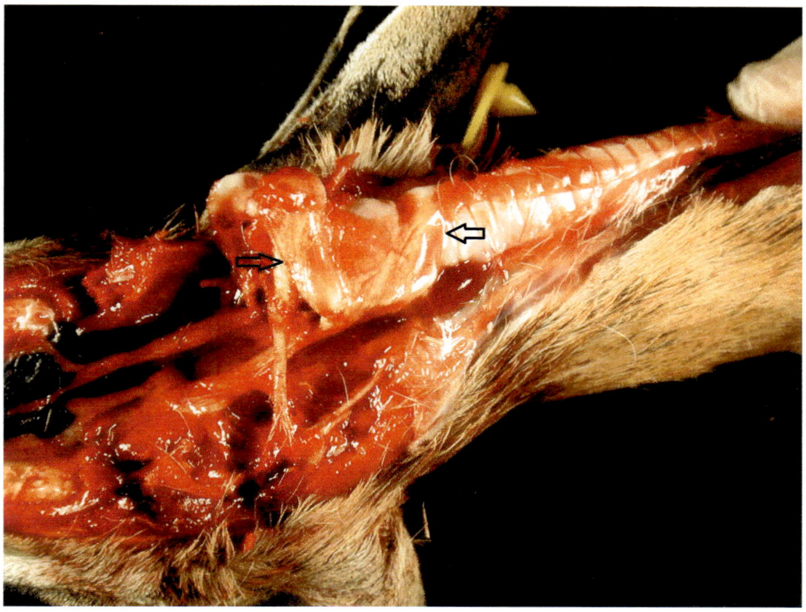

Fig. 8.4. Ox. Muscles of deglutition. White muscle disease (WMD). In veal calves, this muscle group (arrows) is actively involved in suckling or drinking milk from buckets. When developing myodegeneration, aspiration pneumonia is a fatal complication. Beef calves born weak with vitamin E or selenium deficiency will often have tongue lesions as well, but usually only recognized histologically.

8.1.1.2 Toxic

Similar changes occur as with those of nutritional myopathy, thus making distinction difficult. Etiologic examples are monensin and *Senna* (*Cassia*) *occidentalis* (coffee senna), Coyotillo plant spp. (*Karwinskia humboldtiana*). (Also see Chapter 16: The Pathology of Select Poisonous Plant-induced Diseases in Cattle.)

Senna (Cassia) occidentalis *myopathy*

Introduction. *Senna (Cassia) occidentalis* is a shrub from the Leguminosae family. Consumption of fresh or dried bean pods is toxic to large animals, rodents, chicken, and humans. Toxicity is thought to be associated with anthraquinones and their derivatives. Affected organs are skeletal muscles, liver, kidney, and heart in a minimal fashion. Muscle and liver changes result in biochemical abnormalities. Death results from metabolic complications such as hyperkalemia. *Senna obtusifolia* (sicklepod) is a similar shrub, but less toxic to cattle.

Clinical signs. Diarrhea, recumbency with alertness, gait abnormalities, tremor, and incoordination of hind legs.

Differential diagnoses. Nutritional myopathy, trauma, fractures, spinal cord lymphosarcoma, rupture of pubic tendon, peripheral neuropathy, babesiosis, bacillary hemoglobinuria.

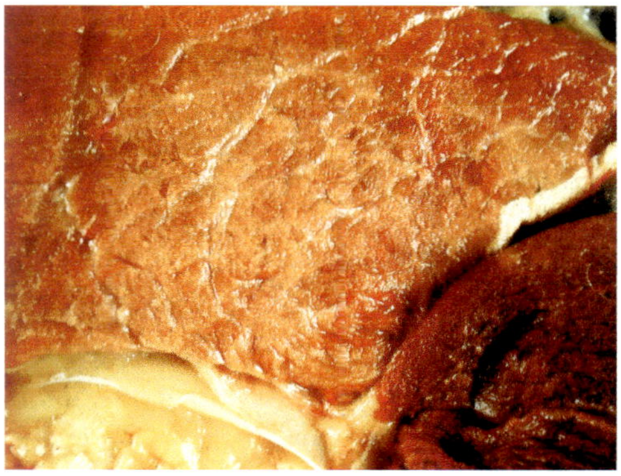

Fig. 8.5. Ox. Skeletal muscle. *Senna occidentalis*. Diffuse pallor. Myopathy of thigh-region muscles is reflected by demarcated discoloration

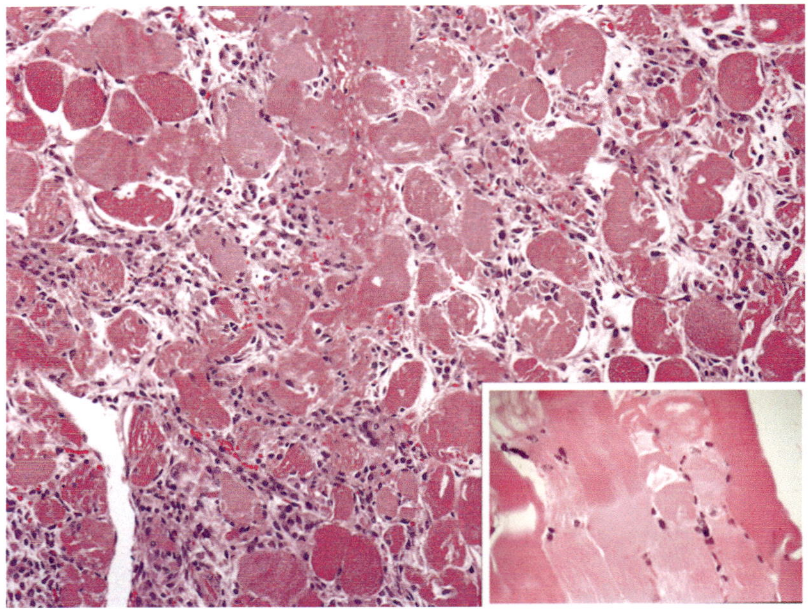

Fig. 8.6. Ox. Skeletal muscle. *Senna occidentalis*. Necrotizing myositis. Muscle fibers are hypereosinophilic, swollen, fragmented, and vacuolar. Sarcolemmal inflammation is mononuclear and moderate. Inset: myonecrosis and vacuolar myodegeneration. There is loss of striation, but no mineralization. Swelling of mitochondria with loss of cristae results from the toxic effect of *S. occidentalis* (H&E).

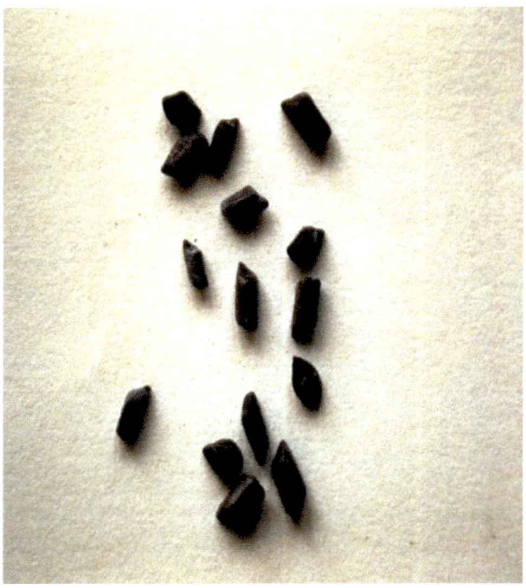

Fig. 8.8. Ox. Seeds of *Senna occidentalis*. Resemblance to coffee beans.

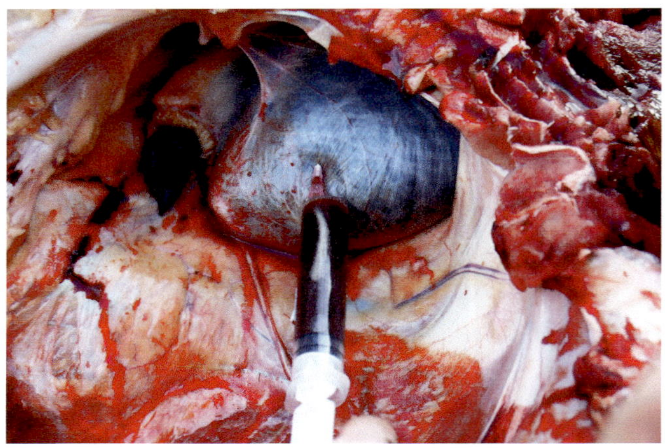

Fig. 8.7. Ox. Urinary bladder. *Senna occidentalis*. Myoglobinuria. The urinary bladder is markedly distended by burgundy-red urine (see contents of syringe).

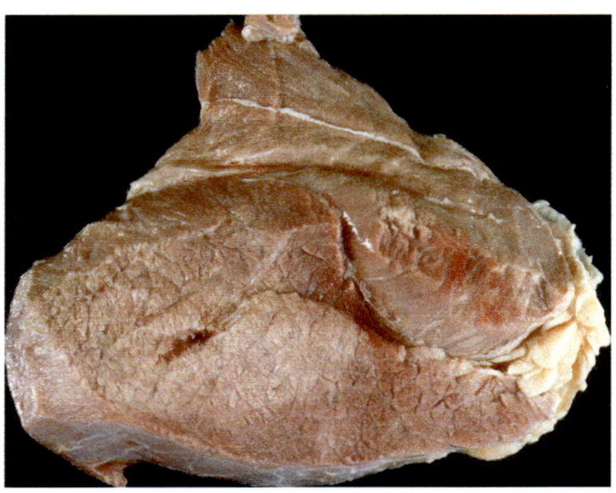

Fig. 8.9. Ox. Hind-leg muscle. Downer cow. Myonecrosis. Diffuse pallor. (Courtesy of the Government of Alberta, Canada.)

8.1.1.3 Downer cow myopathy

Various metabolic, neurologic, and musculoskeletal diseases and disorders contributing to prolonged recumbency will result in ischemic muscle necrosis. Muscle enzymes are significantly elevated. Such animals are unable to rise. If the primary cause of recumbency is not established and treatment instituted, recumbency may become permanent due to severe hind-leg muscle pathology (compartment syndrome).

8.1.2 Inflammation

Bacteria, parasites, and protozoa have to be taken into consideration as pathogens for myositis.

8.1.2.1 Clostridial myositis

Introduction. Caused by various *Clostridium* spp., including *Clostridium septicum*, *Clostridium sordelli*, *Clostridium chauvoei*, or *Clostridium perfringens*, animals die quickly from blood invasion of the organisms or exposure to the potent toxins produced by them. Wound infections or other exogenous routes (intramuscular (IM) injection, tail docking) are preceding events. Affected tissues exhibit edema, necrosis, serosanguinous exudate, gas formation, or a rancid to foul odor (blackleg).
Clinical signs. Lameness, muscle swelling, crepitus, fever, lethargy.
Differential diagnoses. Autolysis, cellulitis, snake bite, trauma.

Malignant edema. *C. septicum* is the major pathogen. Edematous and blood-tinged muscles are common gross findings.

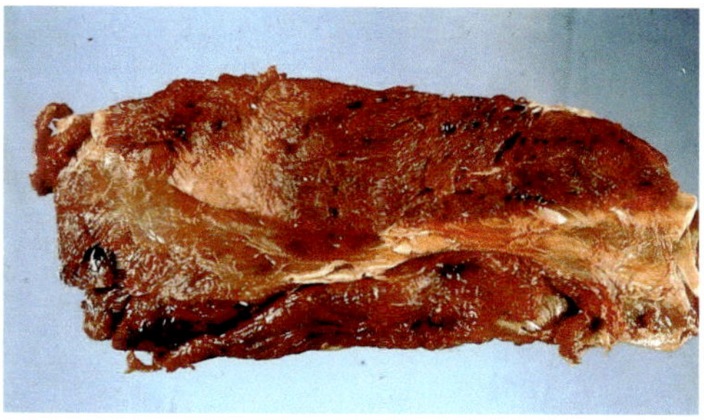

Fig. 8.10. Ox. Malignant edema. Skeletal muscle. Necrotizing myositis. Affected muscles are soft, wet, and discolored. *Clostridium septicum* was isolated.

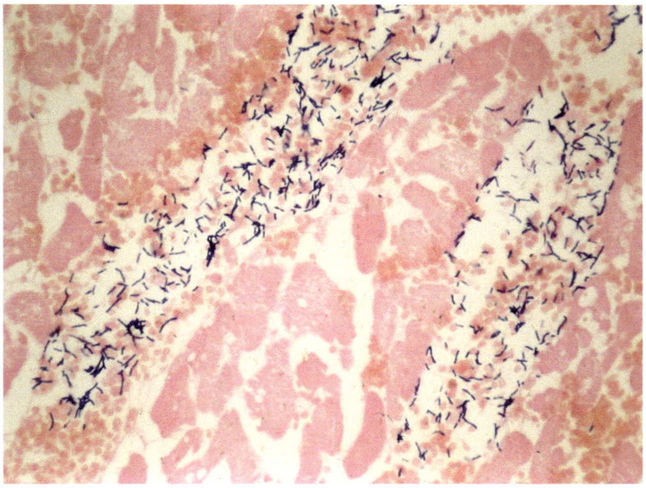

Fig. 8.11. Ox. Skeletal muscle. Clostridial necrotizing myositis. Multiple long rods are demonstrated in the interstitium. Muscle fibers are necrotic and hemorrhagic (myonecrosis) (H&E).

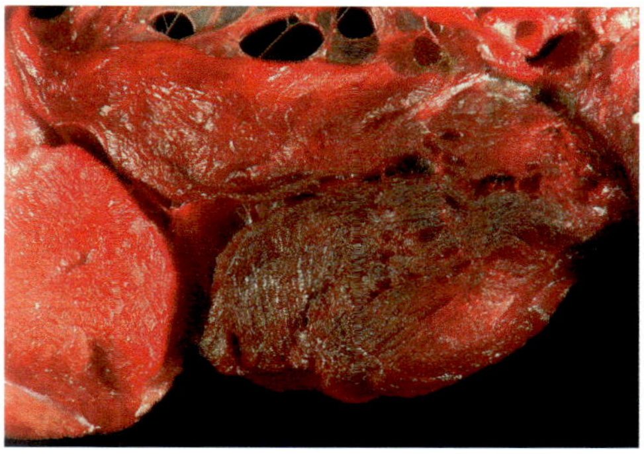

Fig. 8.12. Ox. Blackleg. Skeletal muscle. Gangrenous myositis. Dry, red-brown discoloration of muscle tissue with gas bubble formation. (Courtesy of Department of Veterinary Pathology, WCVM, University of Saskatchewan, Saskatoon, Canada.)

Blackleg. Caused by *C. chauvoei*, affected muscle groups, particularly those of the pectoral and pelvic girdle, are deep red, soft, and dry, with gas bubbles visible. Other organs involved are tongue and heart (visceral blackleg). Rancid smell is elicited from necrotic muscles. The disease strikes the best fattened, pastured animals without major preceding clinical signs. Post-parturient occurrence of blackleg has been described with pelvic muscles.

Histophilosis. *Histophilus somni* is a disseminating bacterial disease with targets in several organ systems (central nervous system (CNS), respiratory, pleura, reproductive system, eye, and heart). As an infectious

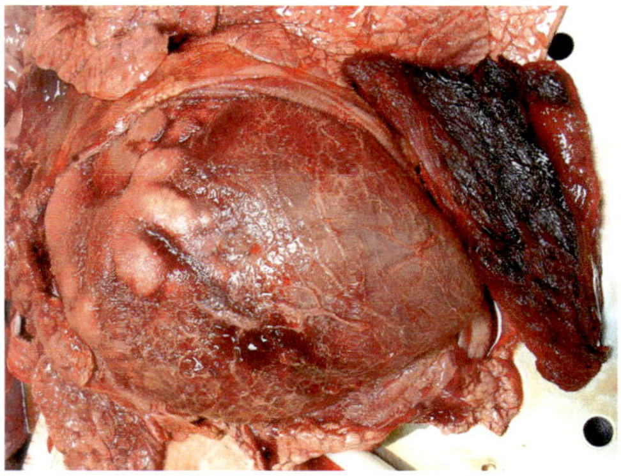

Fig. 8.13. Ox. Blackleg. Skeletal muscle and pericardium. Gangrenous myositis and fibrinous pericarditis. This case is an example of concurrent muscular and visceral blackleg associated with *Clostridium chauvoei* infection. Deep, red, dry discoloration of muscle on the right. Fibrin deposition of pericardium developed in association with clostridial myocarditis.

disease of cattle, it is underdiagnosed. Its spread to the skeletal muscular system may be rare, and may not be pursued on a regular basis at necropsy, but should not be overlooked. Microscopic findings of thrombotic vasculitis help to make a presumptive etiologic diagnosis, but IHC can be used to confirm the diagnosis as well. *H. somni* has also been isolated from arthritis–synovitis in cattle.

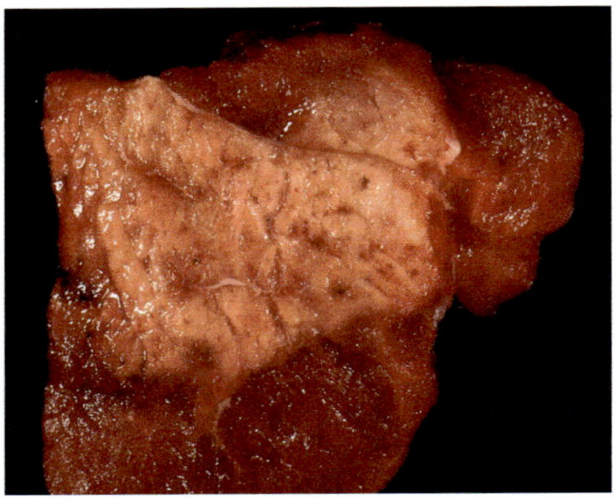

Fig. 8.14. Ox. Skeletal muscle. *Histophilus somni*. Necrotizing myositis. Pale muscle bundles reflect necrosis and inflammation.

8.1.2.2 Parasitic myositis

Cysticercosis. The larval forms of *Cysticercus bovis* reside as the intermediate stage of *Taenia saginata* (syn. *Taeniarhynchus saginata*) in selective skeletal muscles, as they do in the heart. It is commonly called the beef tapeworm.

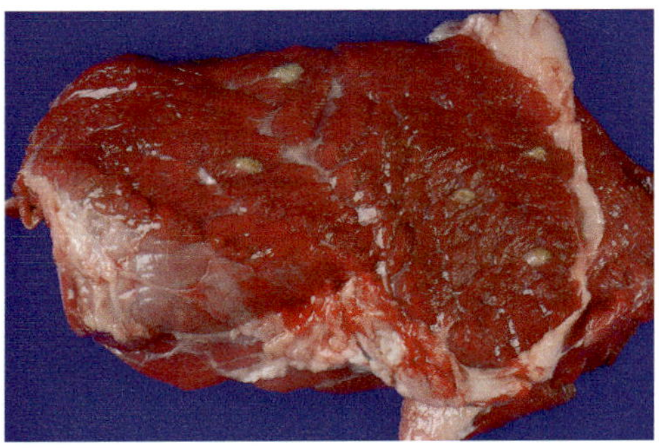

Fig. 8.15. Ox. Skeletal muscle. Cysticercosis. Parasitic myositis. Small, white cysts are present in the muscle parenchyma. (Courtesy of Prof F. Guarda, University of Turin, Italy.)

8.1.2.3 Protozoal myositis

Sarcocystosis. Intracytoplasmic cysts of *Sarcocystis* spp. are common, incidental findings in the myofibers of skeletal muscles and the myocardium. Gross lesions are usually absent, except in the condition of eosinophilic myositis, in which the musculature is discolored at the gross level. The lesions are thought to be the result of a hypersensitivity reaction to disintegrating, dead Sarcocystis protozoa. Cattle are intermediate hosts for the three species of Sarcocystis: *Sarcocystis cruzi* or *bovicanis*, *Sarcocystis hominis* or *bovihominis*, *Sarcocystis hirsuta* or *bovifelis*. *S. bovicanis* has a thin wall, *S. bovihominis* and *S. bovifelis* have a thicker and septate wall. The CNS and reproductive tract (abortions) are other organ systems affected in clinical sarcocystosis.

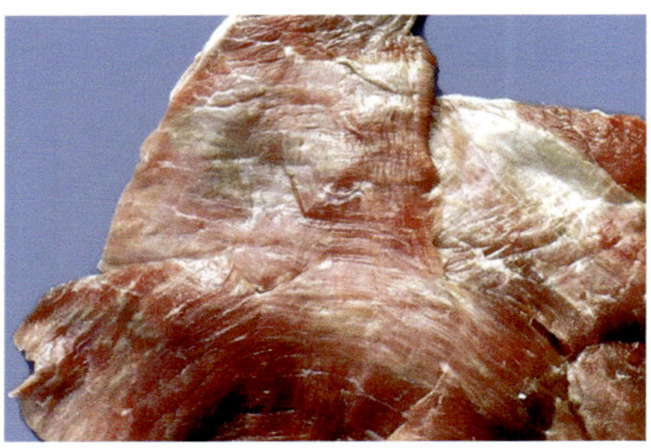

Fig. 8.16. Ox. Skeletal muscle. Sarcocystosis. Eosinophilic myositis. White, green discoloration of various muscle groups. (Courtesy of Dr J.M. King and Section of Anatomic Pathology, Cornell University, USA.)

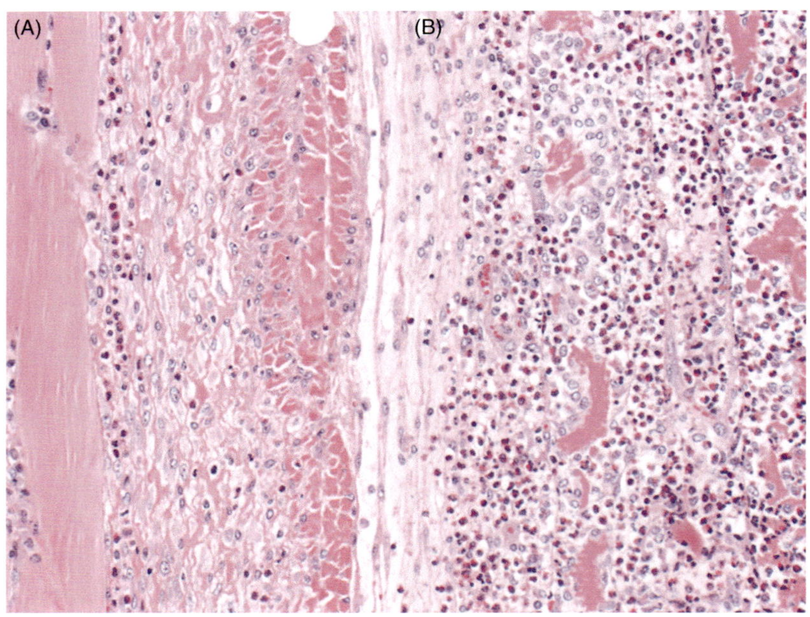

Fig. 8.17. Ox. Skeletal muscle. Sarcocystosis. Eosinophilic myositis. An inflammatory infiltrate of predominantly eosinophils admixed with lymphocytes and plasma cells has replaced myofibers on the right (B). Residual dissociated myofibers are fragmented and have lost striation. Intact myofibers on the left (A) are surrounded by eosinophils, as is the perimyseal tissue (H&E). (Courtesy of Dr J. Edwards, Texas A&M University, USA.)

8.1.2.4 *Miscellaneous*

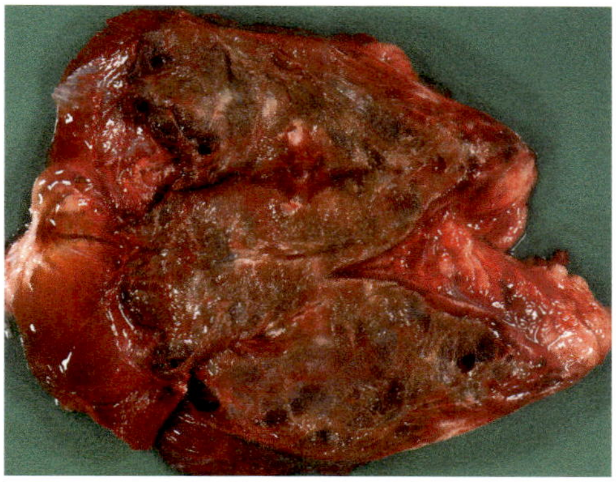

Fig. 8.18. Ox. Skeletal muscle. Antibiotic injection site. Necrotizing and hemorrhagic myositis found at slaughterhouse. Injected material needs to be differentiated from infectious agents.

8.1.3 Hyperplasia

Doubling of muscles is an autosomal recessive genetic disorder seen in Belgian Blue, Charolais, Angus, Santa Gertrudis and other beef-cattle breeds. The gene abnormality is located on chromosome 2 in Belgian Blue cattle. The increased muscle volume (about 20%) leads to dystocia and hind-leg lameness of affected animals.

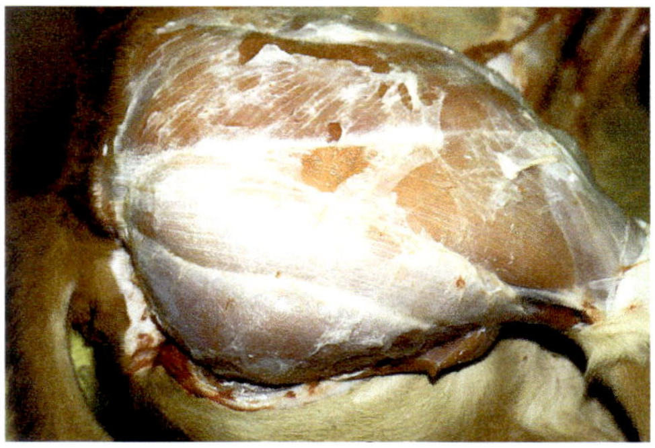

Fig. 8.19. Ox. Skeletal muscles. Doubling. Phenotype of doubling of the gluteal muscles.

8.2 SKELETAL SYSTEM

Introduction. Many skeletal diseases can be diagnosed with confidence on the basis of gross lesions, but can easily be missed if the skeleton is not examined thoroughly during autopsy. Examination of the entire skeleton is impractical, but should include areas of most rapid growth or remodelling in young animals and bones that develop by both intramembranous and endochondral ossification. Longitudinal sectioning of key bones with a bandsaw to reveal growth plates, cortical thickness, and density of trabecular bone is crucial.

Radiography of whole bones or sawn slabs can be a valuable adjunct to gross examination, particularly in identifying areas of bone lysis, healing fractures, or the severity of demineralization.

8.2.1 Genetic abnormalities

8.2.1.1 Chondrodysplasias

Introduction. Several forms of inherited chondrodysplasia, characterized by disproportionate dwarfism, are reported in different breeds of cattle. All bones that develop by endochondral ossification are affected as a result of defective cartilage formation. The most severe form of bovine chondrodysplasia is the lethal 'bulldog' type, which is best known in Dexter cattle. Affected calves are usually aborted before 7 months of gestation, but are occasionally carried to full term. Dexter chondrodysplasia is caused by one of two different mutations in the aggrecan (*ACAN*), which encodes the protein aggrecan (cartilage-specific proteoglycan core protein (CSPCP) or chondroitin sulfate proteoglycan), and testing for carriers is commercially available. Bulldog-type chondrodysplasia is also reported in several other miniature breeds and in Holstein-Friesians (see Chapter 1: Diseases of Neonates and Calves).

Less severe forms of chondrodysplasia include 'snorter' dwarfism in Hereford and Angus cattle, and Ellis van Creveld syndrome 2 in Japanese Brown and Tyrolean grey cattle.

Clinical sign. Disproportionate dwarfism of varying severity, depending on form of chondrodysplasia.

Differential diagnoses. Non-genetic causes of defective cartilage formation such as intrauterine manganese deficiency.

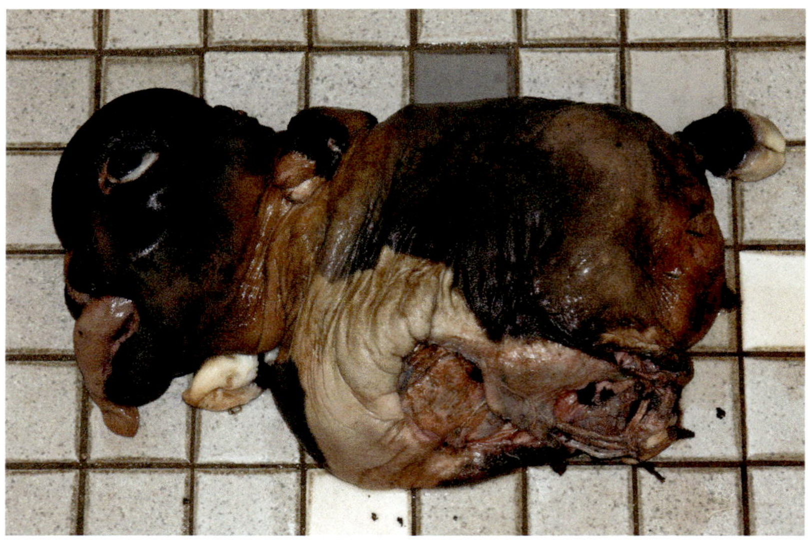

Fig. 8.20. Ox. Aborted Dexter calf. Bulldog-type chondrodysplasia. The limbs are partly rotated and markedly reduced in length. The shortened, dome-shaped skull and protruding tongue are consistent features of this form of chondrodysplasia and are typically accompanied by a cleft palate. Also note the large umbilical hernia, which is presumably secondary to reduced length of the vertebral column.

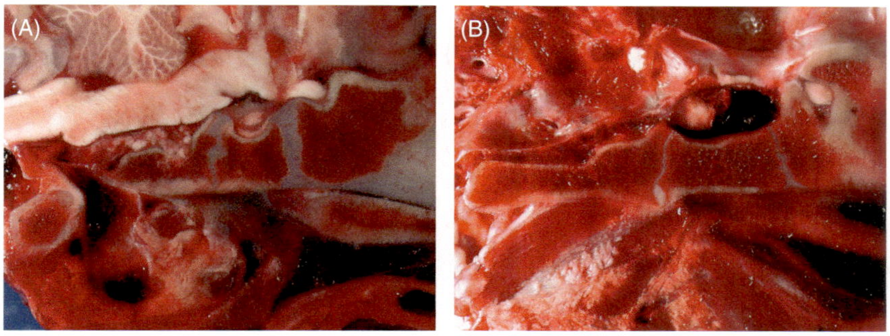

Fig. 8.21. Ox. (A) Newborn Holstein-Friesian calf. Bulldog-type chondrodysplasia. Sagittal section through the skull. Shortened, abnormally-shaped basocranial bones, which develop by endochondral ossification, result in a reduction in size of the cranial cavity and the typical dome-shaped skull. (B) Normal newborn calf. Sagittal section through the skull (with brain removed). The basocranial bones are longer, more regular in shape, and have narrower growth plates than the chondrodysplastic calf illustrated in (A).

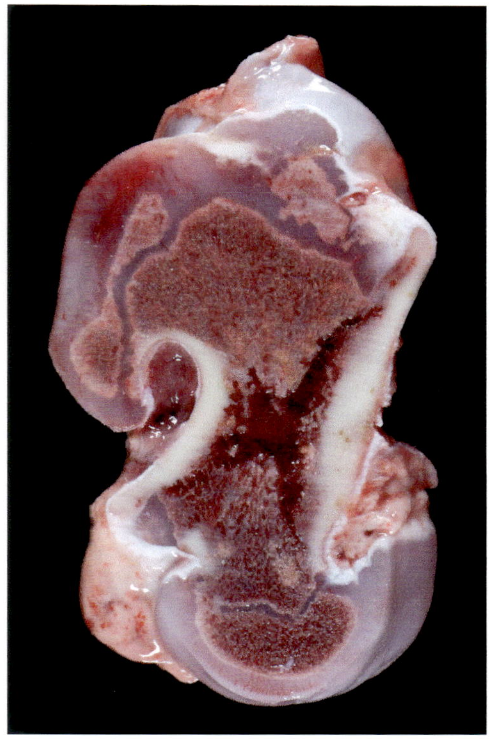

Fig. 8.22. Ox. Newborn Holstein-Friesian calf. Bulldog-type chondrodysplasia. Sagittal section through a humerus. Defective endochondral ossification has resulted in marked reduction in bone length and an abnormally flattened proximal epiphysis. Cortical thickness is relatively normal since intramembranous ossification beneath the periosteum is unaffected in this disease.

8.2.1.2 *Osteogenesis imperfecta*

Introduction. Osteogenesis imperfecta (OI), characterized by marked bone fragility in newborn calves, is caused by a mutation in either *COL1A1* or *COL1A2*, the genes encoding the two chains of type I collagen. The disease is usually inherited as an autosomal dominant trait secondary to a new mutation in germ cell lines, and may occur in 'outbreak' form in the progeny of a clinically normal bull. As a result, the disease is not breed specific and is just as likely to occur in cross-bred as in pure-bred calves. Other abnormalities include joint laxity, poorly erupted pink teeth (dentinogenesis imperfecta), and dark blue sclera, reflecting the predominance of type I collagen in tendons, ligaments, teeth, and the ocular sclera. Forms of OI with only mild bone fragility are recognized in humans and probably occur also in cattle, but are difficult to diagnose. Skin fragility is a feature of OI in lambs, but not calves.

Clinical signs. Newborn calves of normal size but with multiple recent and intrauterine fractures. Usually unable to stand due to marked joint laxity. Dark blue sclera and pink teeth.

Differential diagnoses. Osteopetrosis and intrauterine copper deficiency may be associated with bone fragility in newborn calves, but the bones are less fragile than in OI and would not be accompanied by joint laxity or the dentinal and ocular lesions.

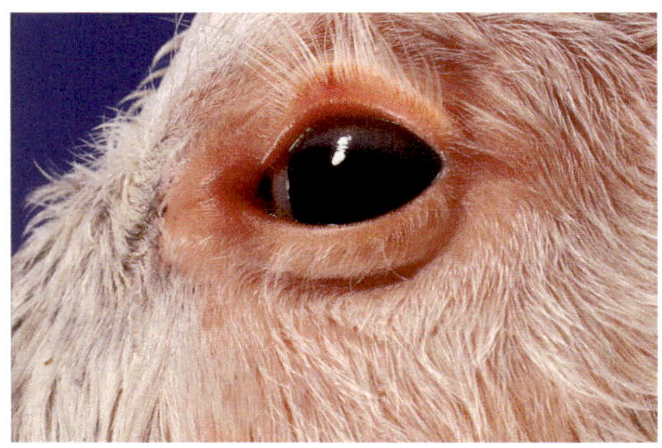

Fig. 8.23. Ox. Sclera. Newborn calf. Osteogenesis imperfecta. The sclera is dark blue because of its markedly reduced thickness – approximately 20% of that in normal calves.

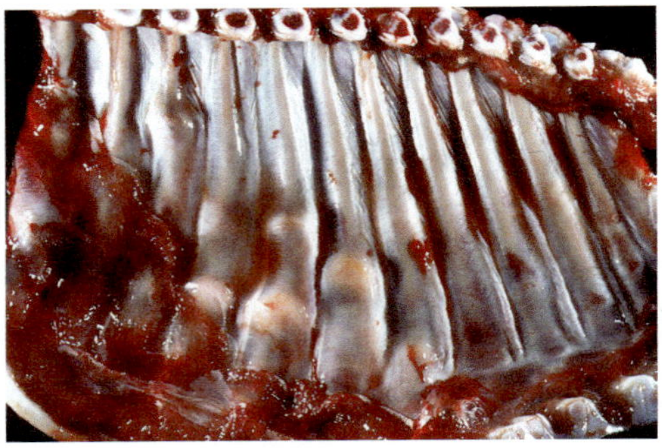

Fig. 8.24. Ox. Ribs. Newborn calf. Osteogenesis imperfecta. Multiple calluses on the ribs indicate intrauterine fractures due to extreme bone fragility.

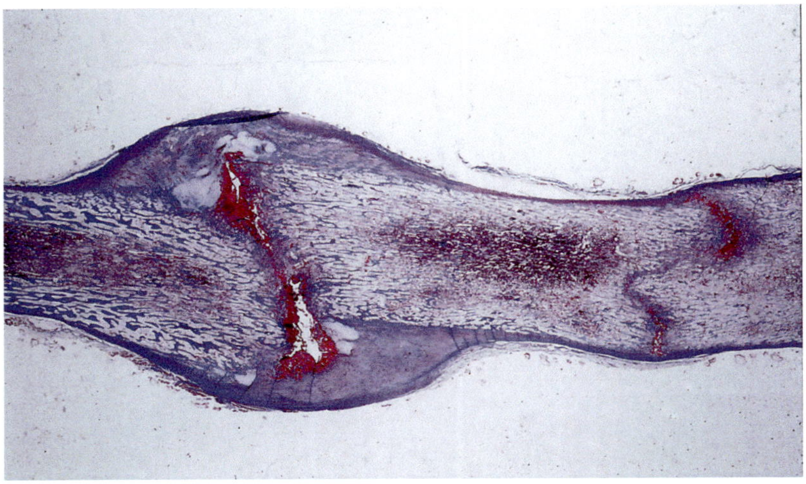

Fig. 8.25. Ox. Rib. Newborn calf. Osteogenesis imperfecta. Subgross histology illustrating two intrauterine rib fractures, one with callus formation and the other with an intact periosteum ('greenstick' fracture). Cortical bone is extremely porous and almost non-existent in some areas (Masson's trichrome stain).

8.2.1.3 Osteopetrosis

Introduction. In this disease, an inherited defect in osteoclastic bone resorption results in accumulation of primary spongiosa in the medullary cavities of bones throughout the body. Inheritance is usually autosomal recessive. Breeds affected include Black Angus, Red Angus, Simmental, Hereford, and Belgian Blue. Osteoclasts are sparse or absent in some forms of the disease, but may be abundant in others, depending on the genetic defect. A deletion in the anion exchange gene *SLC4A2* has been identified in Red Angus calves with osteopetrosis, but not in other breeds.

Clinical signs. Affected calves are usually stillborn, have brachygnathia inferior, impacted molars, reduced length of long bones, and moderately increased bone fragility.

Differential diagnoses. OI, intrauterine bovine viral diarrhea virus (BVDV) infection.

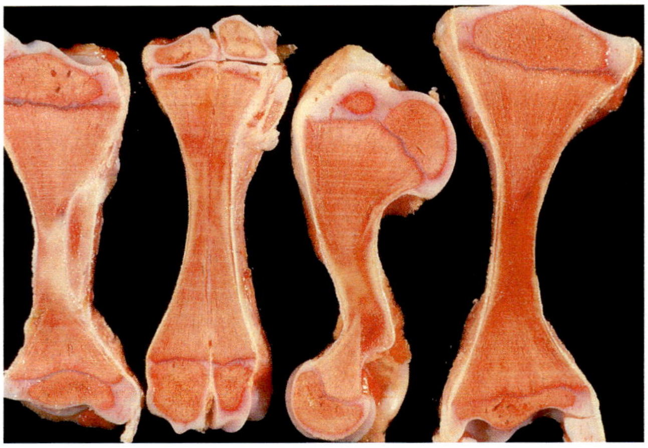

Fig. 8.26. Ox. Newborn calf. Osteopetrosis. Cone-shaped cores of unresorbed primary spongiosa extend into the metaphyses from distal and proximal growth plates in these long bones from an affected calf. Medullary cavities are non-existent. (Courtesy of Dr R. Fairley and Department of Pathology, WCVM, University of Saskatchewan, Saskatoon, Canada.)

8.2.1.4 *Localized abnormalities*

Introduction. A wide variety of localized skeletal defects have been described in cattle. In individual cases, proving an inherited basis is often difficult or impossible since similar defects can be associated with intrauterine exposure to teratogenic agents. Furthermore, some defects appear to have a polygenic mode of inheritance. (Also see Chapter 13: Diseases of the Claw and Foot Skin.)

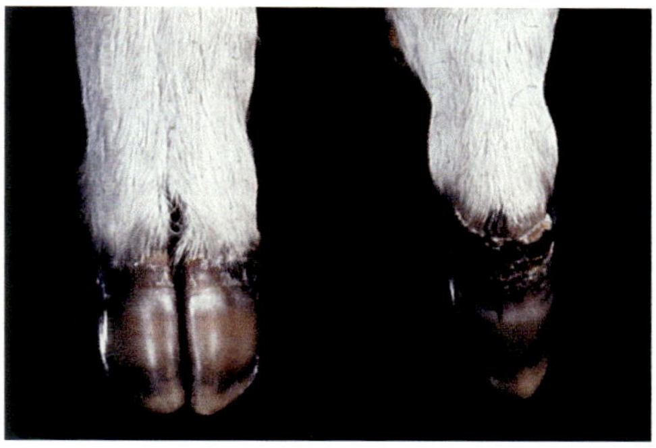

Fig. 8.27. Ox. Digit. Newborn Holstein-Friesian calf. Syndactyly. Fusion of digits in one foot. Inherited as an autosomal recessive trait with variable expression, the defect became common in the Holstein-Friesian breed following the use of a heterozygous bull for artificial breeding, but is now rare in all breeds of cattle.

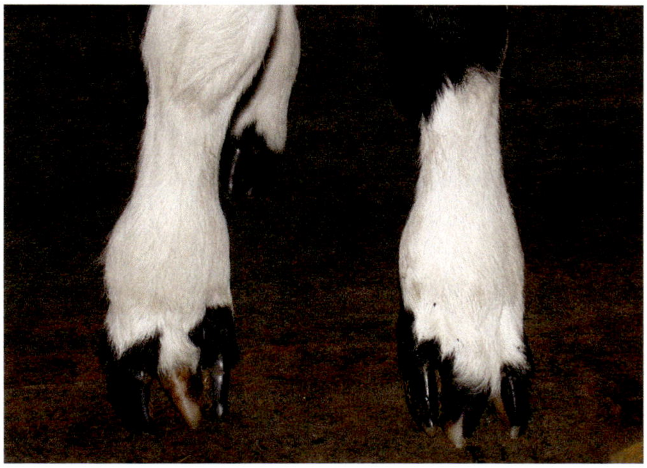

Fig. 8.28. Ox. Digit. Newborn Holstein-Friesian calf. Polydactyly. Increased number of digits in both forelimbs. Believed to be inherited as a polygenic trait in some breeds of cattle.

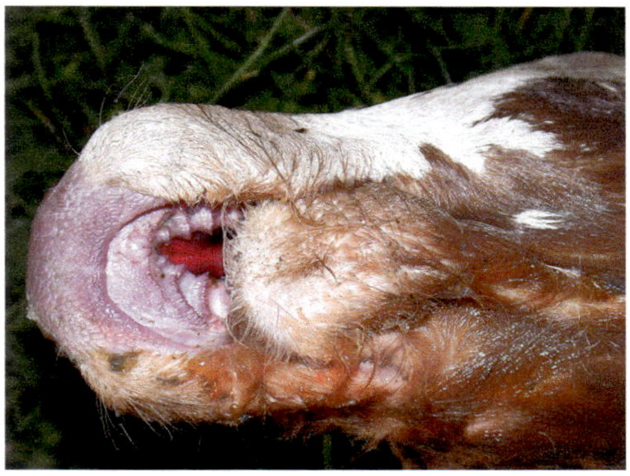

Fig. 8.29. Ox. Oral cavity. Newborn Gelbvieh calf. Severe brachygnathia inferior and palatoschisis. This combination of lesions often occurs together in ruminants and may be either genetic or teratogenic in origin. The syndrome is believed to have an inherited etiology in Red Boer goats, but this has not been established in cattle.

8.2.2 Nutritional and metabolic bone diseases

8.2.2.1 *Osteoporosis*

Introduction. Osteoporosis is common in cattle and other grazing animals, but most mild cases are undiagnosed. It is the result of an imbalance between bone formation and resorption in favour of the latter. Bone shape is normal but strength is reduced due to depletion of bone tissue. Because of its greater surface area, the reduction in trabecular bone is greater than cortical bone. Common causes of osteoporosis in cattle include starvation, gastrointestinal parasitism, and other chronic wasting diseases, such as Johne's disease. Lactation may accelerate bone loss in heifers, resulting in significant osteoporosis in animals with low initial bone mass. Osteoporosis also occurs in animals with severe copper deficiency and is associated with increased bone fragility due to lysyl oxidase deficiency and reduced cross-linkage of collagen in bone tissue.
Clinical signs. Pathological fracture, severe lameness.
Differential diagnoses. Osteomalacia, arthritis, osteomyelitis.

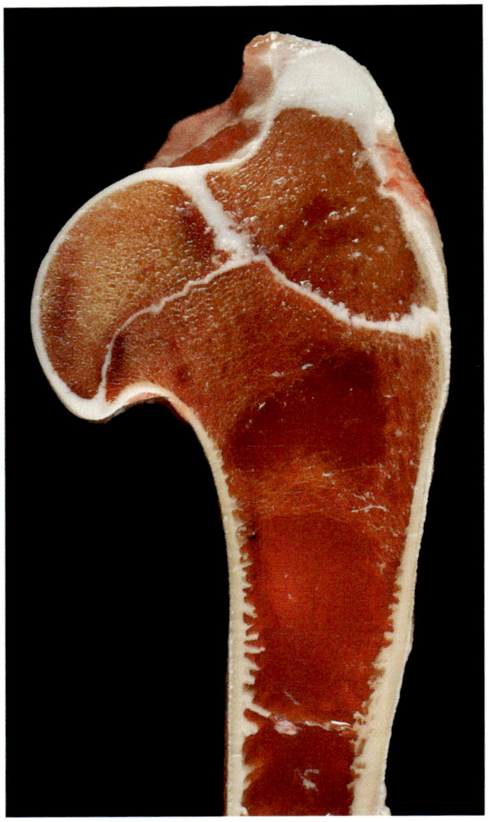

Fig. 8.31. Ox. Humerus. One-year-old. Osteoporosis. In addition to thin cortices and depletion of trabecular bone, there is serous atrophy of medullary fat. This indicates mobilization of body fat reserves, likely due to either starvation or chronic gastrointestinal parasitism. In the metaphysis beneath the humeral head, there are multiple transverse trabeculae parallel to the physis. These are 'growth arrest lines' and represent periods where physeal growth ceased then recommenced.

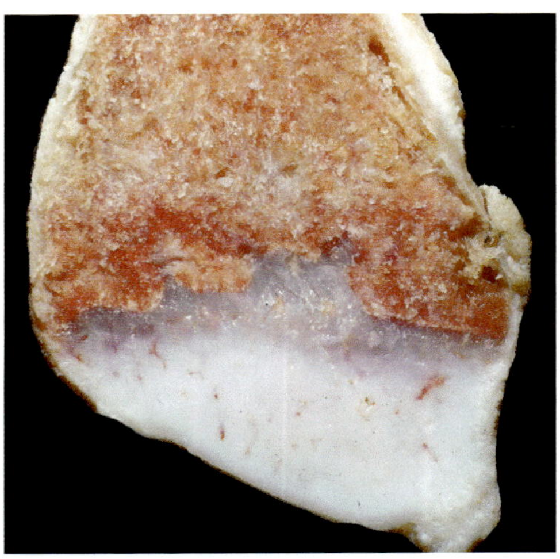

Fig. 8.32. Ox. Rib. One-year-old steer. Costochondral junction. Rickets. Broad tongues of unresorbed physeal cartilage extend into the metaphysis. The steer had been fed on a swede crop during winter and would have been deficient in both phosphorus and vitamin D.

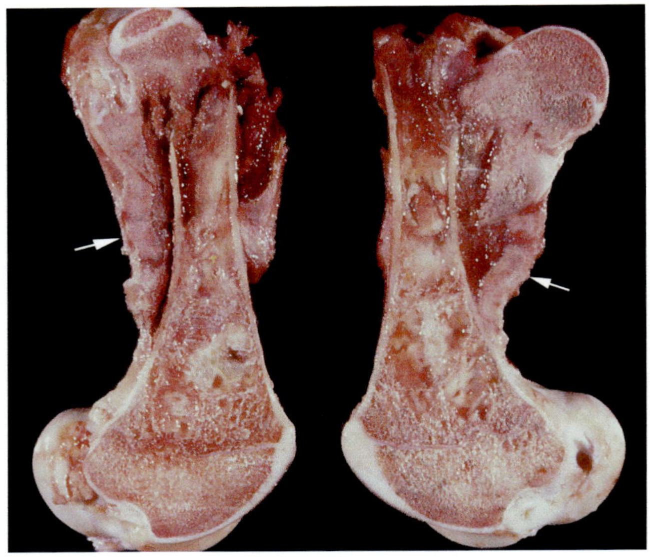

Fig. 8.30. Ox. Femur. Four-month-old calf. Osteoporosis. Bilateral pathological femoral fractures. The cortices are thin, and trabecular bone in the metaphyses and epiphyses is more porous than normal. Attempted callus formation between the displaced femoral heads and the femoral shafts (arrows) indicates that the fractures occurred 2–3 weeks before euthanasia.

8.2.2.2 Rickets and osteomalacia

Introduction. The pathogenesis of both rickets and osteomalacia involves defective mineralization caused by deficiency of either vitamin D or phosphorus. Rickets is a disease of the developing skeleton and is characterized by defective endochondral ossification at growth plates, in addition to impaired mineralization of newly formed osteoid. Osteomalacia occurs in adults following physeal closure, and lesions are therefore confined to areas of new bone formation during remodelling (osteomalacia results from a defect in the bone-building process, while osteoporosis develops due to a weakening in previously constructed bone). As a result, the skeletal effects of osteomalacia are generally more subtle than in rickets and may not be apparent until there has been pathological fracture of a weakened bone.

Phosphorus deficiency typically occurs in cattle grazing phosphorus-deficient pastures or crops. Vitamin D deficiency is usually associated with inadequate exposure to UV irradiation during winter. Young cattle housed during the winter and not supplemented with vitamin D are at risk of developing rickets.

Clinical signs. Lameness, reluctance to stand, pathological fractures. In rickets, swelling and pain at the ends of long bones, swollen costochondral junctions.

Differential diagnoses. Osteoporosis, fluorosis, osteomyelitis, arthritis.

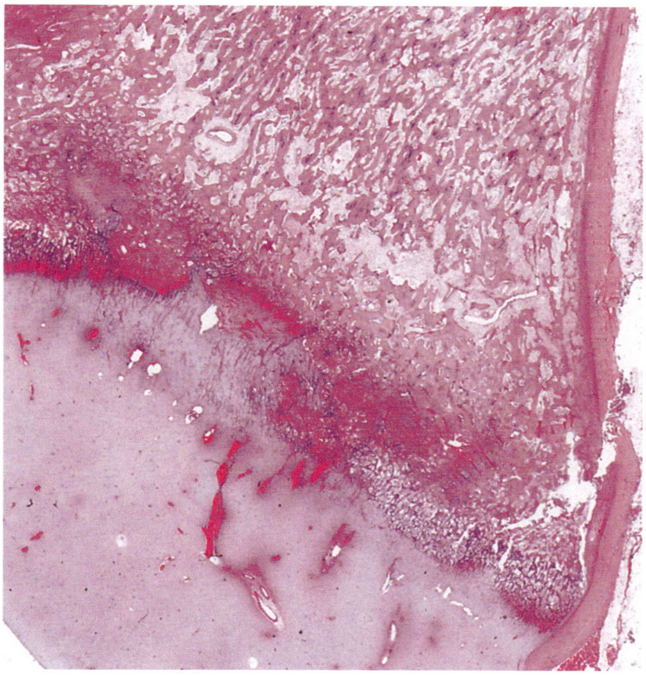

Fig. 8.33. Ox. Rib. One-year-old steer. Costochondral junction. Rickets. Subgross histologic preparation from the same animal illustrated in Fig. 8.32. In addition to the irregularly thickened physeal cartilage, there is disruption of weakened trabeculae in the primary spongiosa, with associated hemorrhage (H&E).

8.2.2.3 Manganese deficiency

Introduction. Manganese is required for the activation of glycosyltransferase enzymes, which are crucial for the synthesis of sulfated glycosaminoglycans, and therefore cartilage. As a result, deficiency during development may affect any bones formed by endochondral ossification. Adult cattle are not affected, but calves born to cows fed a manganese-deficient diet during pregnancy may show a range of skeletal deformities, including disproportionate dwarfism, short, twisted limb bones, enlarged ends of long bones, and spinal stenosis. The deficiency typically occurs when pregnant cows are fed an unusual ration, as may occur during a drought.
Clinical signs. Newborn calves unable to stand in severe cases, or with variable shortening and twisting of limbs.
Differential diagnosis. Inherited chondrodysplasias.

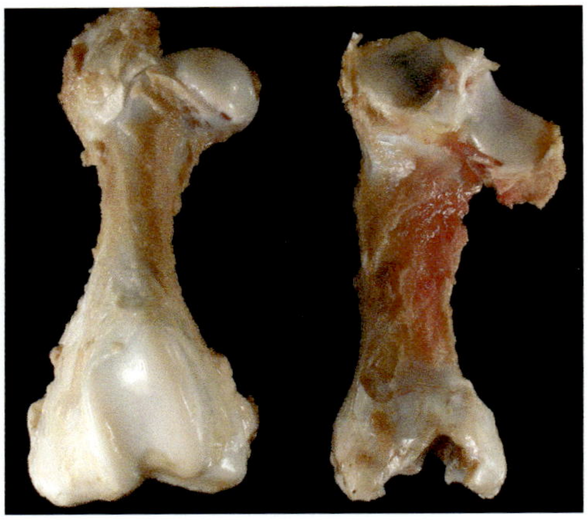

Fig. 8.35. Ox. Newborn calf. Manganese deficiency. The femur and tibia are shorter than normal and there is abnormal alignment of the articular surfaces of the distal femur and proximal tibia, resulting in varus deformity of the limb.

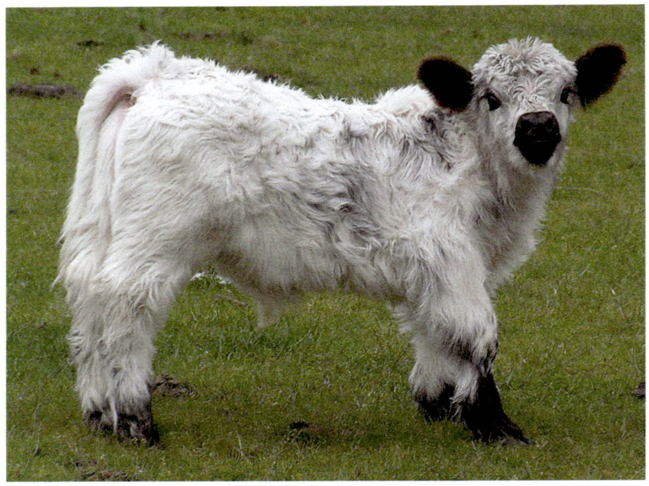

Fig. 8.34. Ox. Manganese deficiency. Shortened limbs with enlarged epiphyses in a calf whose dam was fed a manganese-deficient ration during pregnancy because of a drought. Several other calves in the herd were affected to varying degrees. (Courtesy of S.A. Atkinson, Blenheim, New Zealand.)

8.2.3 Inflammatory and infectious diseases of bone

8.2.3.1 Osteomyelitis

Introduction. Hematogenous osteomyelitis is relatively common in young cattle following neonatal bacteremia and often occurs in association with bacterial polyarthritis. Infection most frequently localizes in the metaphyses and epiphyses of several long bones. Vertebral bodies and/or intervertebral disks may also be involved. Adult cattle are also susceptible to hematogenous osteomyelitis. *Salmonella* spp. are frequently the cause of hematogenous osteomyelitis in calves less than 3 months of age, but a variety of other bacteria can be involved. *Trueperella pyogenes* is most commonly involved in older cattle.

Mandibular osteomyelitis ('lumpy jaw') caused by *Actinomyces bovis* is a classical lesion of adult cattle following the spread of infection from an oral injury or periodontitis to the underlying bone, most likely via lymphatics.

Clinical signs. Severe lameness, reluctance to stand, bone swelling. Sudden-onset hindlimb paralysis following collapse of weakened bone in vertebral osteomyelitis.

Differential diagnoses. Arthritis, rickets/osteomalacia.

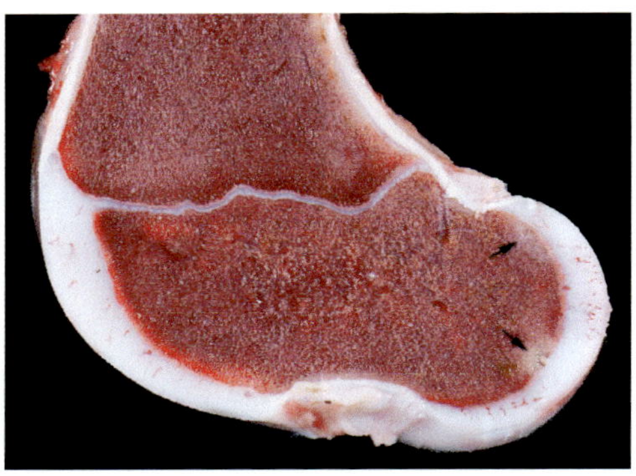

Fig. 8.36. Ox. Suppurative osteomyelitis. Two foci of early epiphyseal infection (arrows) are apparent in the distal femoral condyle of this 8-day-old calf. Cartilage canal blood vessels in the adjacent articular–epiphyseal cartilage complex have been destroyed.

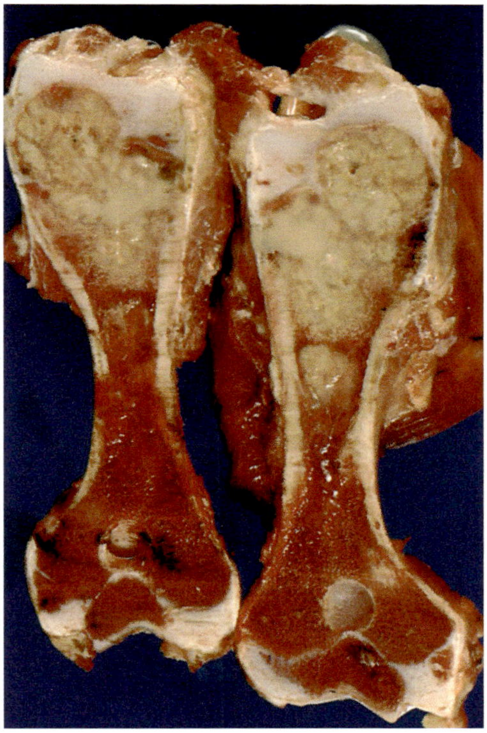

Fig. 8.37. Ox. Humerus. Suppurative osteomyelitis. Extensive loss of metaphyseal trabecular bone and replacement with suppurative exudate in the proximal humerus of an older animal with chronic osteomyelitis. *Trueperella pyogenes* was isolated from the lesion.

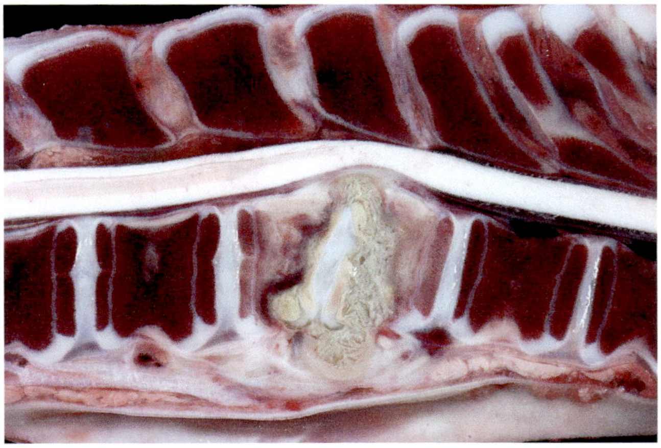

Fig. 8.38. Ox. Vertebral column. Suppurative diskospondylitis. Two adjacent vertebral bodies and the associated intervertebral disk have been largely destroyed by a chronic bacterial infection, resulting in vertebral collapse and sudden-onset paralysis due to compression of the spinal cord. The artefactual clefts in the suppurative exudate surrounding the remains of the disk are due to freezing of the specimen prior to sagittal sectioning.

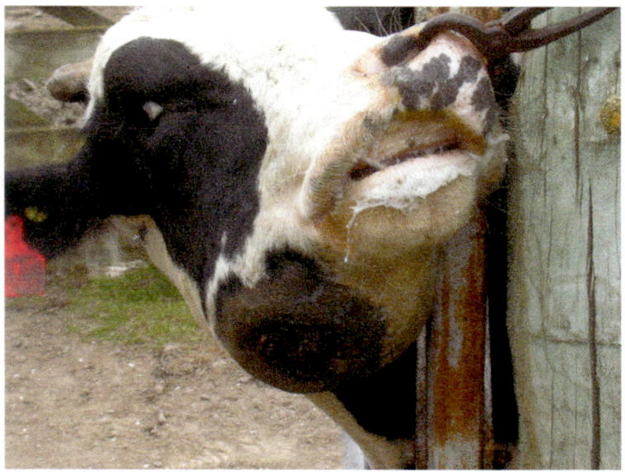

Fig. 8.39. Ox. Mandibular osteomyelitis ('lumpy jaw'). Massive swelling of the mandible due to chronic infection by *Actinomyces bovis*. In this case, there is fistulation to the skin surface, with a large ulcer and swelling of surrounding soft tissues (see Chapter 5: Diseases of the Gastrointestinal Tract, and Chapter 12: Diseases of the Integument).

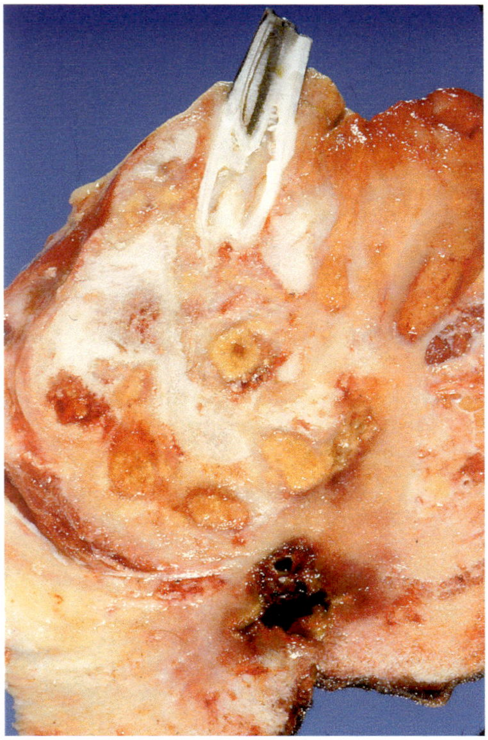

Fig. 8.40. Ox. Mandibular osteomyelitis ('lumpy jaw'). Section through enlarged mandible containing several yellow foci of suppurative inflammation surrounded by sclerotic bone. The 1–2 mm diameter yellow-white flecks in the pockets of inflammation are so-called 'sulfur granules', which consist of colonies of *Actinomyces bovis* surrounded by Splendore–Hoeppli material

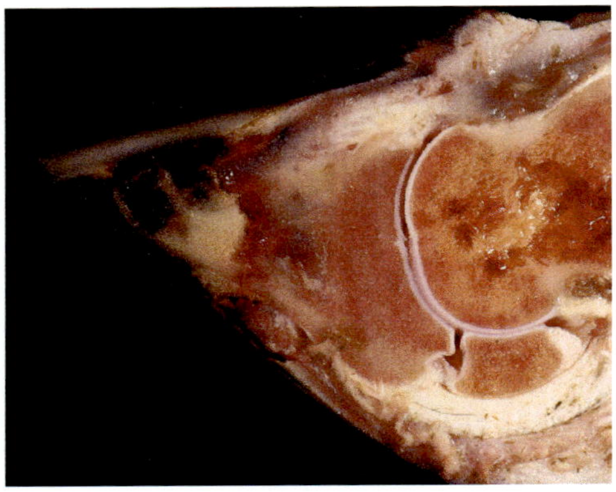

Fig. 8.41. Ox. Digit. Toe-tip necrosis. The sharply demarcated, necrotic distal portion of P3 is separated from the remainder of the bone by a hyperemic rim and early cleft formation. A lytic focus containing dark grey-black exudate is present near the tip of the bone. Similar exudate is present in clefts between the necrotic segment of bone and the wall and sole of the claw. (Courtesy of Department of Veterinary Pathology, WCVM, University of Saskatchewan, Saskatoon, Canada.)

8.2.3.2 *Toe-tip necrosis*

Introduction. This syndrome, which occurs most often in the lateral claw of the hind feet in feedlot beef cattle around 10–12 months of age, is characterized by necrosis of the apex of the distal phalanx (P3). Arthritis of the distal interphalangeal joint, flexor tendonitis and osteomyelitis of P2 and P1 may also be present, and embolic spread of infection to the lungs, liver, and kidneys is described in some cases. The pathogenesis is believed to involve ascending bacterial infection to the distal phalanx following traumatic damage to the white line at the tip of the claw. Another possibility is that ischemic damage to the tip of P3 is the primary lesion, and separation of the wall with secondary bacterial infection is a secondary change.

Clinical sign. Lameness.

Differential diagnoses. Laminitis, foot rot, interdigital dermatitis, arthritis.

8.2.3.3 *Intrauterine bovine viral diarrhea virus infection*

Introduction. Intrauterine BVDV infection has been associated with one or more narrow bands of metaphyseal sclerosis parallel to the physes in aborted or newborn bovine fetuses. These are referred to as growth retardation lattices and are considered to reflect viral destruction of osteoclasts. The pathogenesis resembles that of osteopetrosis, but in this case the impaired osteoclastic resorption of primary spongiosa is transient. Similar lesions have also been described in older calves up to 4 months of age.

Differential diagnoses. Osteopetrosis, growth arrest.

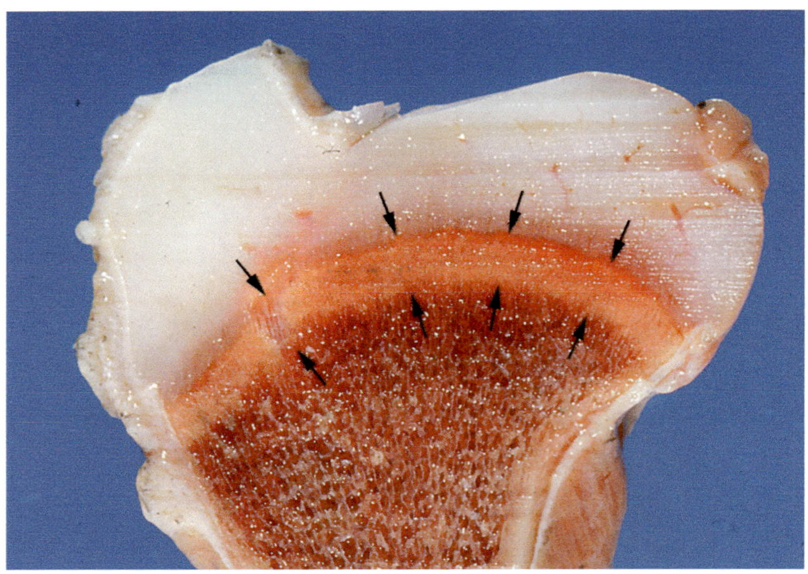

Fig. 8.42. Ox. Bone. Aborted bovine fetus. Persistence of the primary spongiosa (between arrows) in a bovine viral diarrhea virus (BVDV)-positive aborted calf. A temporary reduction in osteoclastic activity, presumably due to viral destruction of osteoclasts, has resulted in a zone of metaphyseal sclerosis, parallel to the physis, referred to as a growth retardation lattice. All growing bones will be similarly affected, and in some cases the sclerotic bands are multiple. Growth retardation lattices differ from growth arrest lines in pathogenesis and histological appearance.

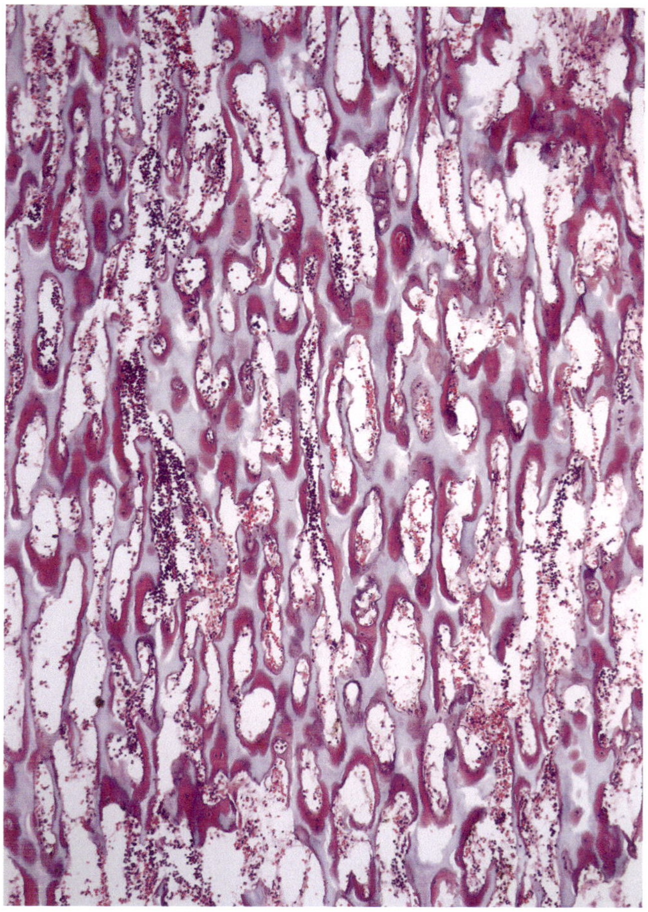

Fig. 8.43. Ox. Bone. Aborted bovine fetus. Histology of growth retardation lattice in a calf with intrauterine bovine viral diarrhea virus (BVDV) infection. Note the persistence of calcified cartilage of physeal origin and the lack of osteoclastic activity (H&E). (Also see Chapter 1: Diseases of Neonates and Calves, and Chapter 10: Diseases of the Reproductive System.)

8.2.4 Miscellaneous bone diseases

8.2.4.1 Juvenile lymphoma

Introduction. Multifocal bone marrow infarction is associated with infiltration with neoplastic lymphocytes in calves with the juvenile form of sporadic malignant lymphoma. The infarcts are readily visible grossly in sectioned bones and typically involve multiple sites. Calves most affected also have generalized lymph node enlargement and variable involvement of other tissues, such as liver, kidney, and spleen. In this form of lymphoma, the lesions may be present at birth or develop during the first 6 months of life.

Clinical signs. Newborn or young calf with multiple enlarged lymph nodes, sometimes causing dystocia. Diffuse thymic enlargement in some cases.

Differential diagnosis. Bacterial osteomyelitis with sequestration of bone.

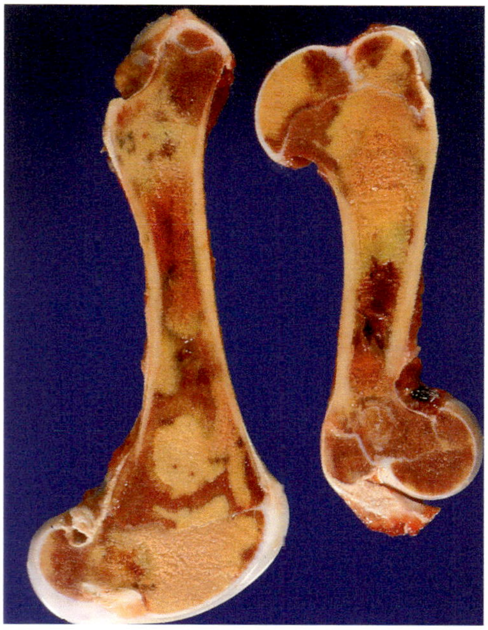

Fig. 8.44. Ox. Calf. Six weeks old. Juvenile form of sporadic malignant lymphoma. Multiple discrete, locally extensive foci of medullary infarction in the metaphyses and epiphyses of the humerus and femur (see Chapter 11: Diseases of the Hematopoietic and Hemolymphatic System).

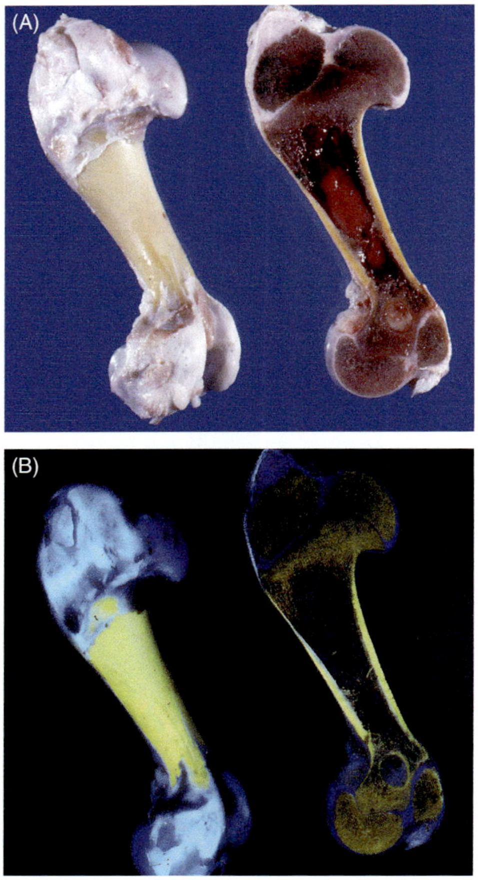

Fig. 8.45. Ox. Humerus. Calf, 8 weeks old. (A) Tetracycline deposition in bone. Yellow discoloration of the shaft of the humerus and extending through most of the cortex. All other bones examined from the calf showed similar discoloration. (B) Tetracycline deposition in bone. Bright yellow fluorescence of the yellow areas is apparent when viewed under UV light. This confirms long-term administration of tetracycline, as the antibiotic is only deposited at sites of active mineralization.

8.2.4.2 Tetracycline deposition

Introduction. Tetracycline is deposited in bone and dentine at sites of active mineralization and has been used as a bone marker of bone growth in research projects. The antibiotic has a characteristic yellow color and fluoresces bright yellow when viewed under UV light in a dark room. A single dose is unlikely to be visible grossly as deposition in bone will be confined to sites of active growth. However, if it is administered as a feed additive to young growing animals for several weeks or months, it can cause yellow discoloration of bones. This practice is now discouraged or banned in many countries because of the risks of antibiotic resistance. If there is a suspicion of inappropriate tetracycline use in a young animal, examination of bones under UV light, ideally a cut surface including sites of active growth, should allow confirmation or exclusion.

8.2.5 Arthritis

Introduction. Infectious arthritis is a common sequel to neonatal bacteremia in calves, often secondary to inadequate colostral transfer of immunity. The synovial membrane is richly vascular, and is a favoured site for localization of hematogenous infection. Multiple joints are usually affected, at least initially. Concurrent localization in the bones occurs in most calves with infectious arthritis, resulting in osteomyelitis. Opportunistic bacteria commonly isolated from neonatal calves with septic arthritis include: *Escherichia coli*, *Salmonella* spp., *Streptococcus* spp, and *T. pyogenes.* Other agents, such as *H. somni*, *Chlamydophila pecorum*, and *M. bovis* have a special predilection for synovial joints and cause polyarthritis (and other lesions) in older cattle. Osteomyelitis is not a feature in these cases.

Clinical signs. Lameness, hot, swollen, painful joints, pyrexia.

Differential diagnoses. Rickets, foot injuries, or infections.

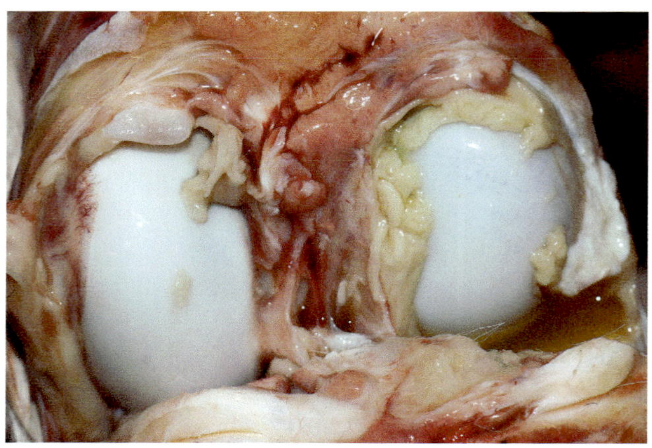

Fig. 8.46. Ox. Joint. Acute fibrinous arthritis. Stifle joint from a 7-day-old calf with polyarthritis and osteomyelitis. Note the slightly turbid synovial fluid and the sheets of pale yellow fibrin partly surrounding one of the femoral condyles. Also note the injected blood vessels starting to encroach on the other condyle from the edematous synovium near the left margin of the image. (Also see Chapter 1: Diseases of Neonates and Calves.)

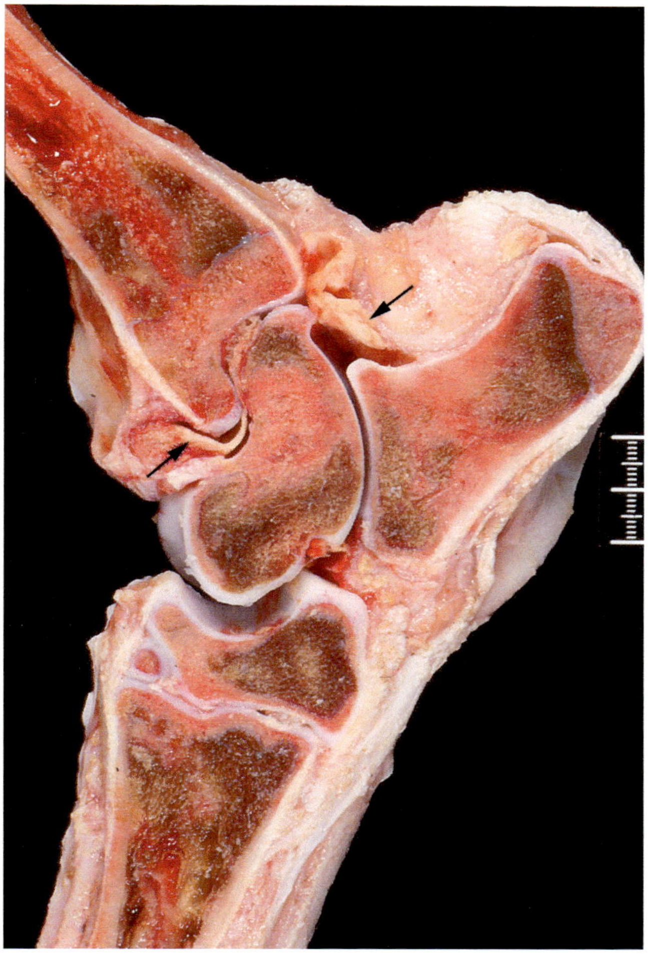

Fig. 8.47. Ox. Joint. Fibrinous arthritis and multifocal osteomyelitis with bone necrosis. Sheets of fibrin (arrows) are attached to the synovial membrane in the tibiotarsal joint and extend between the articular surfaces in one area. Multiple large, yellow-brown foci of necrotic bone are present in the distal tibial metaphysis, tarsal bones and metatarsal, reflecting concurrent localization of hematogenous bacterial infection in the synovium and bones. (Courtesy of Dr R. Fairley, Gribbles Veterinary Pathology, Christchurch, New Zealand.)

8.2.6 Degenerative joint disease

Introduction. In cattle, degenerative joint disease is most common in adult dairy cows and stud dairy or beef bulls, particularly those in artificial breeding centers. Predisposing factors include poor conformation, previous septic arthritis, osteochondrosis, and ligament damage secondary to trauma, especially in bulls. Stifle and hip joints are most commonly affected, and the lesions are often bilateral. Since the lesions are usually advanced by the time they are available for examination at autopsy, the predisposing cause is seldom obvious.

Clinical signs. Chronic lameness, abnormal gait, reluctance to stand, muscle atrophy.

Differential diagnoses. Arthritis, osteochondrosis.

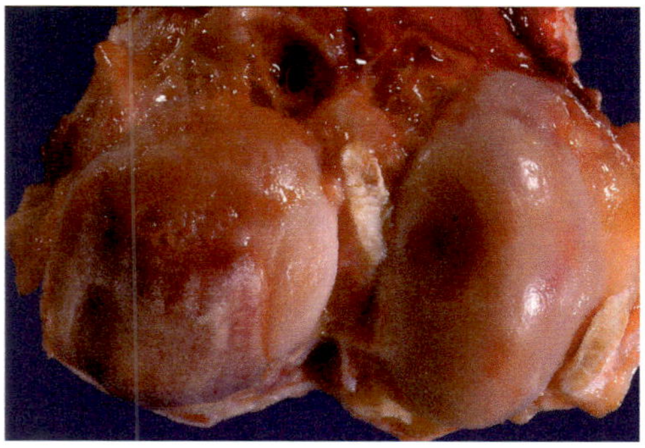

Fig. 8.48. Ox. Femur. Adult Jersey cow. Chronic degenerative joint disease. Complete loss of articular cartilage on the medial condyle, with eburnation of exposed bone and grooves in the direction of joint movement. The medial meniscus was shredded and there was similar cartilage loss and eburnation on the corresponding articular surface of the tibia. A smaller area of cartilage degeneration and erosion is present on the lateral femoral condyle.

8.2.7 Osteochondrosis

Introduction. Although only reported occasionally in cattle, osteochondrosis is probably more common than is recognized. The pathogenesis involves localized defects in endochondral ossification in the physes and/or articular–epiphyseal cartilage complex of growing animals, secondary to focal vascular impairment. As such, the disease is most likely to occur in well-grown young bulls during their first year of life. The lesions often involve several joints and are sometimes bilaterally symmetrical. Early lesions are seldom detected in cattle but are characterized by a flap of articular cartilage which often detaches, leaving a discrete defect in the articular surface. Detached cartilage fragments may enlarge within the joint space and may become firmly attached to the synovium. Predilection sites include the lateral trochlear ridge of the stifle joint, humeral head, distal radius, elbow joint, tibial tarsal and occipital condyles. In severe cases, osteochondrosis predisposes to degenerative joint disease.

Clinical signs. Mild lameness, becoming more severe if the lesion progresses to degenerative joint disease.

Differential diagnoses. Arthritis, degenerative joint disease, ligament damage.

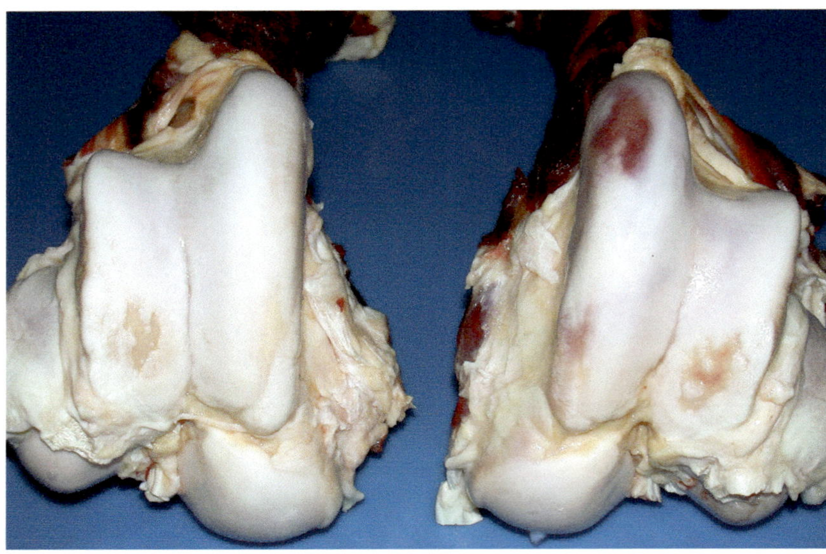

Fig. 8.49. Ox. Stifle joint. Osteochondrosis. Bilaterally symmetrical lesions involving the trochlear groove and ridges of both stifle joints in a 2-year-old Holstein-Friesian bull. Similar lesions were also present in the shoulder, elbow, carpal and tarsal joints of the bull.

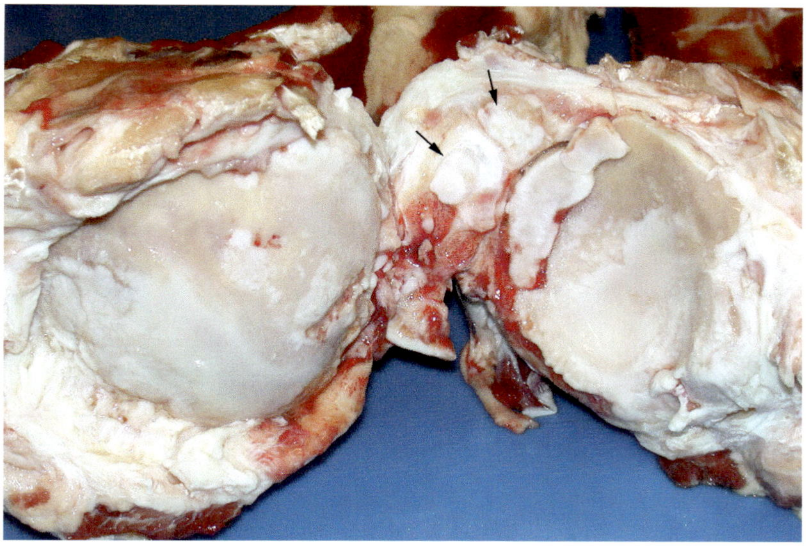

Fig. 8.50. Ox. Shoulder joint. Osteochondrosis with secondary degenerative joint disease in the shoulder joint of a 3-year-old Holstein-Friesian bull. Extensive loss of articular cartilage on the humeral head and glenoid fossa. Several irregular-shaped chondro-osseous nodules are embedded in the thickened synovial membrane (arrows) and also encroaching on the articular surface of the glenoid fossa. The nodules most likely originated from flaps of articular cartilage that detached during the early stages of the disease and became ossified following attachment to the synovium. Similar but milder lesions were also present in the other shoulder joint and a radiocarpal joint.

SUGGESTED READING FOR MUSCLE

Bagge, E., Lewerin, S.S. and Johansson, K.E. (2009) Detection and identification by PCR of *Clostridium chauvoei* in clinical isolates, bovine faeces and substrates from biogas plant. *Acta Veterinaria Scandinavia* 51, 8–17.

Barth, A.T., Kommers, G.D., Alles, M.S., Wouters, F. and de Barros, C.S. (1994) Coffee Senna (*Senna occidentalis*) poisoning in cattle in Brazil. *Veterinary and Human Toxicology* 35, 541–545.

Calore, E.E., Weg, R., Haraguchi, M., Calore, N.M., Cavaliere, M.J. and Sesso, A. (2000) Mitochondrial metabolism impairment in muscle fibres of rats chronically intoxicated with *Senna occidentalis* seeds. *Experimental Toxicologic Pathology* 52, 357–364.

Costagliola, A., Wojcik, S., Pagano, T.B., DeBiase, D., Russo, V., *et al.* (2016) Age-related changes in skeletal muscle of cattle. *Veterinary Pathology* 53, 436–446.

Furlan, F.H., Zanata, C., Damasceno Edos, S., de Oliveira, L.P., da Silva, L.A., *et al.* (2014) Toxic myopathy and acute hepatic necrosis in cattle caused by ingestion of *Senna obtusifolia* (sicklepod; coffee senna) in Brazil. *Toxicon* 92, 24–30.

Grobet, L., Martin, L.J., Poncelet, D., Pirottin, D., Brouwers, B., *et al.* (1997) A deletion in the bovine myostatin gene causes the double-muscled phenotype in cattle. *Natural Genetics* 17, 71–74.

O'Toole, D. and Sundgeroth, K.S. (2016) Histophilosis as a natural disease. *Current Topics in Microbiology and Immunology* 396, 15–48.

Useh, N.M., Nok, A.J. and Esievo, K.A. (2003) Pathogenesis and pathology of blackleg in ruminants: the role of toxins and neuraminidase. A short review. *Veterinary Quarterly* 25, 155–159.

Vangeel, L., Houf, K., Geldhof, P., De Preter, K., Vercruysse, J., *et al.* (2013) Different *Sarcocystis* spp. are present in bovine eosinophilic myositis. *Veterinary Parasitology* 197, 543–548.

Vashishtha, V.M., John, T.J. and Kumar, A. (2009) Clinical and pathological features of acute toxicity due to *Cassia occidentalis* in vertebrates. *Indian Journal of Medical Research* 130, 23–30.

Wouda, W., Snoep, J.J. and Dubey, J.P. (2006) Eosinophilic myositis due to *Sarcocystis hominis* in a beef cow. *Journal of Comparative Pathology* 135, 249–253.

SUGGESTED READING FOR SKELETAL SYSTEM

Agerholm, J.S., Arnberg, J. and Andersen, O. (2004) Familial chondrodysplasia in Holstein calves. *Journal of Veterinary Diagnostic Investigation* 16, 293–298.

Cavanagh, J.A., Tammen, I., Windsor, P.A., Bateman, J.F., Savarirayan, R., *et al.* (2007) Bulldog dwarfism in Dexter cattle is caused by mutations in ACAN. *Mammalian Genome* 18, 808–814.

Craig, L.E., Dittmer, K.E. and Thompson, K.G. (2016) Bones and joints. In: Grant Maxie, M. (ed.) *Jubb, Kennedy and Palmer's Pathology of Domestic Animals*, 6th edn. Elsevier, St Louis, Missouri, Chapter 2, pp. 16–163.

Firth, E.C., Kersies, A.W., Dik, K.J. and Hagens, F.M. (1987) Haematogenous osteomyelitis in cattle. *Veterinary Record* 120, 148–152.

Gyan, L.A., Paetsch, C.D., Jelinski, M.D. and Allen, A.L. (2015) The lesions of toe tip necrosis in southern Alberta feedlot cattle provide insight into the pathogenesis of the disease. *Canadian Veterinary Journal* 56, 1134–1139.

Jelinski, M., Fenton, K., Perett, T. and Paetsch, Ch. (2016) Epidemiology of toe tip necrosis syndrome (TTNS) of North American feedlot cattle. *Canadian Veterinary Journal* 57, 829–834.

Trostle, S.S., Nicoll, R.G., Forrest, L.J., Markel, M. and Nordlund, K. (1998) Bovine osteochondrosis. *Compendium on Continuing Education for the Practicing Veterinarian* 20, 856–863.

Valero, G., Alley, M.R., Badcoe, L.M., Manktelow, B.W., Merrall, M. and Lawes, G.S. (1990) Chondrodystrophy in calves associated with manganese deficiency. *New Zealand Veterinary Journal* 38, 161–167.

White, P.J. and Windsor, P.A. (2012) Congenital chondrodystrophy of unknown origin in beef herds. *Veterinary Journal* 193, 336–343.

CHAPTER 9

Diseases of the Endocrine System

9.1 Pituitary Gland
- 9.1.1 Anatomic location and retrieval
- 9.1.2 Inflammation

9.2 Thyroid Gland
- 9.2.1 Goiter
- 9.2.2 Neoplasia

9.3 Adrenal Gland
- 9.3.1 Circulatory disturbance
- 9.3.2 Neoplasia
- 9.3.3 Miscellaneous
  - 9.3.3.1 Amyloidosis
  - 9.3.3.2 Citrus pulp toxicosis

INTRODUCTION

The chapter covers pathologic changes affecting the pituitary gland, thyroid gland, and adrenal gland. Parathyroid glands, the endocrine pancreas, and gonads are not included. The pathology of gonads is discussed in Chapter 10: Diseases of the Reproductive System. In general, endocrine disorders are rare during the lifespan of domestic ruminants, but, none the less, their combined examination should be part of a complete bovine necropsy. It should be mentioned that the bovine parathyroid glands are not located anatomically next to the thyroid glands. For need of their retrieval, anatomy textbooks should be consulted before starting the necropsy.

9.1 PITUITARY GLAND

9.1.1 Anatomic location and retrieval

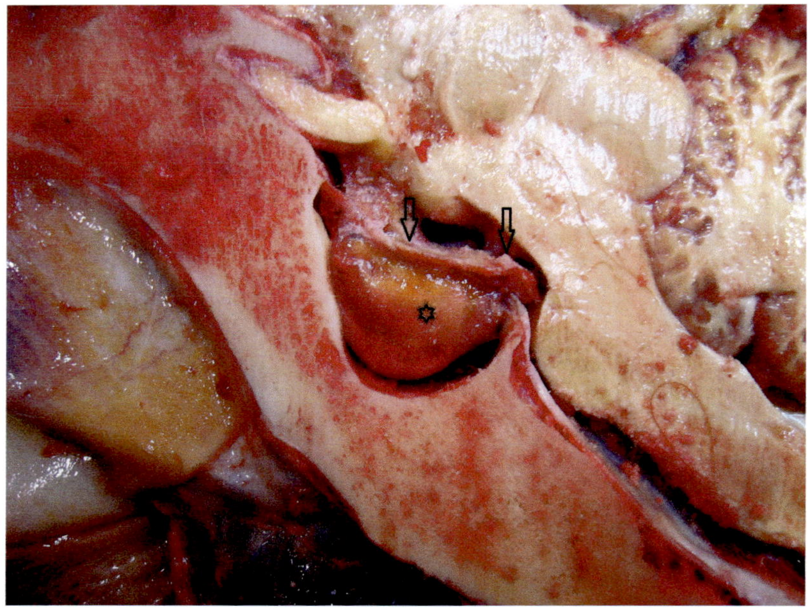

Fig. 9.1. Ox. Normal pituitary gland. Subdural location. The anatomic location of the bovine pituitary (asterisk) is beneath the dura mater membrane (arrows) and not immediately visible in the calvaria after removal of the brain.

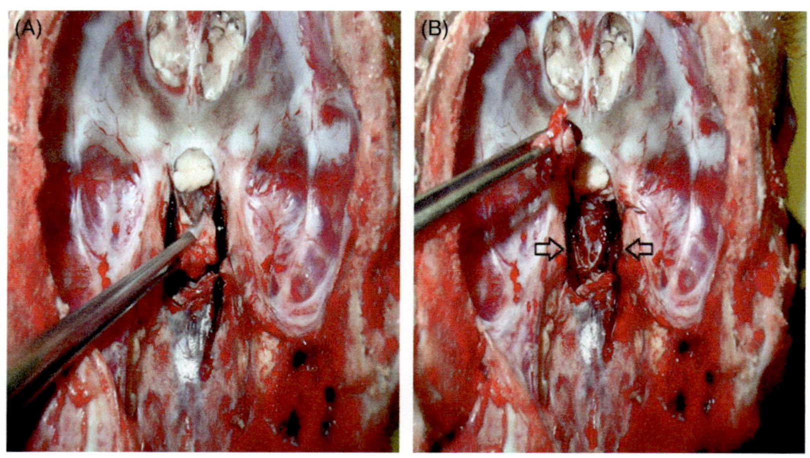

Fig. 9.2. Ox. Removal of pituitary gland. (A) For retrieval of the bovine pituitary, the dura should be cut with a scalpel caudal to the optic chiasm in a rectangular fashion, cut at the stalk, and lifted with forceps for removal. (B) When lifting the pituitary gland, the view is open to the carotid rete mirabile (arrows). The rete constitutes a rich vascular system that should be collected when attempting the microscopic diagnosis of malignant catarrhal fever vasculitis and transient bovine viral diarrhea virus (BVDV) vasculitis. For retrieval of the rete mirabile, see Fig. 2.27.

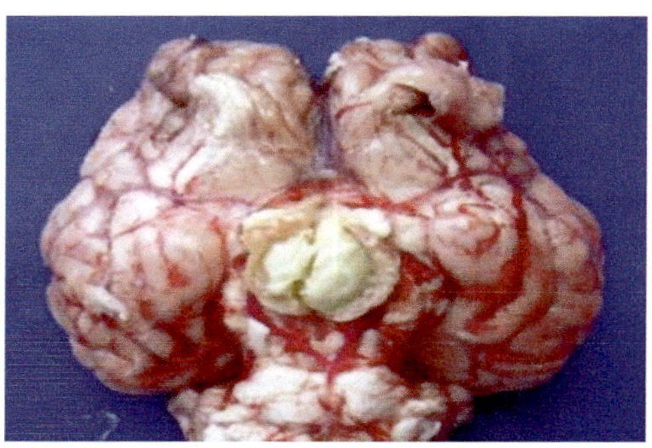

Fig. 9.3. Ox. Pituitary gland abscess. Bacterial in origin (most often *Trueperella pyogenes*, but on occasion *Streptococcus* spp.), a purulent exudate is seen to cover the pituitary. The inflammation may extend to the basisphenoid bone to cause osteomyelitis. The purulent inflammation may also spread intracranially to adjacent trigeminal and optic nerves. Traumatic horn lesions with subsequent sinusitis and basal meningoencephalitis are thought to be the pathway for pituitary inflammatory involvement. Hematogenous spread to the pituitary is a less likely alternative.

9.1.2 Inflammation

Clinical signs. Paresis, paralysis, only develop when adjacent nerves are affected.

9.2 THYROID GLAND

Anatomically, the thyroid glands are located laterally next to the cranial portion of the trachea. They have a dark brown, flattened, lobulated appearance.

9.2.1 Goiter

Introduction. Goiter (struma) is defined as a non-neoplastic, uniform enlargement of the thyroid gland associated with iodine deficiency, and an increase in serum thyroid-stimulating hormone (TSH) level. The main causes of iodine deficiency are endemic iodine-deficient water or soil, as is known for certain geographical mountainous regions in the world, and naturally occurring goitrogens such as kale, cabbage, rape, turnips, beans. Congenital goiter as the result of mutation of genes involved in thyroid hormone synthesis has been reported in African breeds of cattle. Neonatal goiter is presented in Chapter 1: Diseases of Neonates and Calves.

Clinical signs of hypothyroidism in goiter are usually absent (non-toxic).

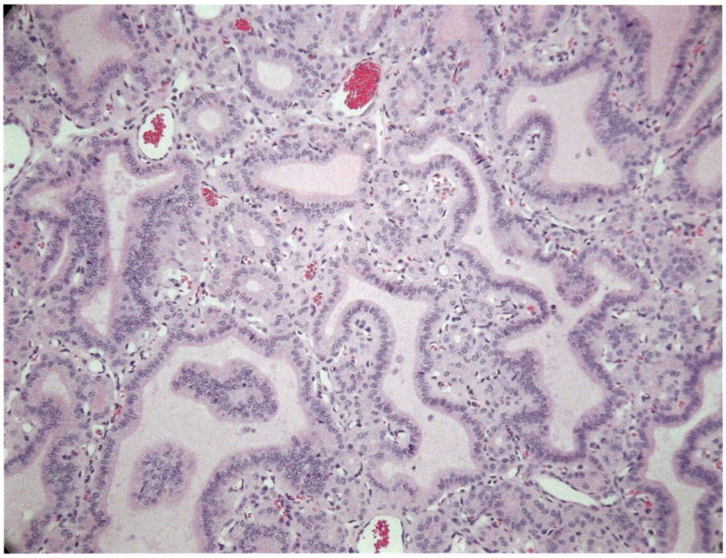

Fig. 9.5. Ox. Thyroid. Goiter. Hyperplasia of colloid follicles. Papillomatous proliferation of follicular epithelium results in colloid-rich, enlarged and multi-shaped follicles. The hyperplastic reaction is the structural compensatory response to iodine deficiency increasing the glandular parenchyma for hormone synthesis. The proliferative changes should not be confused with neoplasia (H&E).

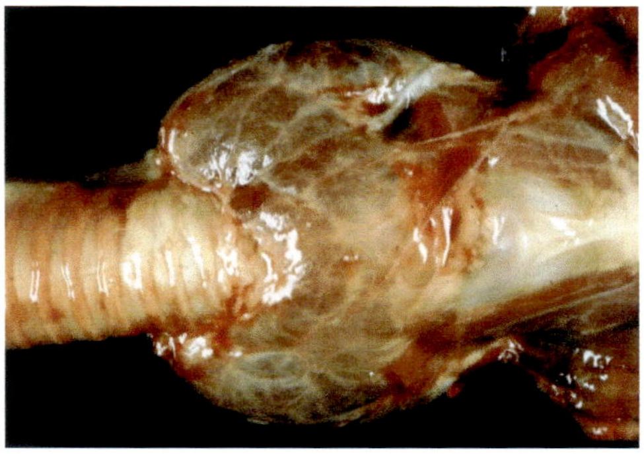

Fig. 9.4. Ox. Thyroid. Goiter. Thyroids including isthmus are diffusely enlarged and lobulated. Goiter can manifest itself as diffuse or in multinodular form at the gross level.

9.2.2 Neoplasia

Thyroid C cell carcinoma. Parafollicular 'C cells' of the thyroid have been reported to give rise to carcinoma in the aged bull, with a potential to metastasize. Also known as ultimobranchial tumors, they appear in bulls 6.5 years of age or older. Calcitonin and/or somatostatin can be demonstrated via immunohistochemistry, although serum calcium remains normal. Frequently, the affected bulls are reported to have ingested a calcium-rich diet in their forage or had been treated with vitamin D3 over a long period. Further, some of these bulls may have concurrent adrenal gland pheochromocytomas and pituitary acidophil adenomas. They are also predisposed to vertebral fractures and osteopetrosis.

9.3 ADRENAL GLAND

Bilateral adrenal glands are located cranial to the kidney and embedded in adipose tissue. Structurally, the adrenal gland is composed of the cortex and medulla, each responsible for different functions.

9.3.1 Circulatory disturbance

Hyperemia and hemorrhage are common sequelae to infectious diseases, particularly gram-negative sepsis (pneumonia, gastroenteritis). A syndrome resembling the human pediatric Waterhouse–Friderichsen syndrome occurs in calves with calf sepsis.

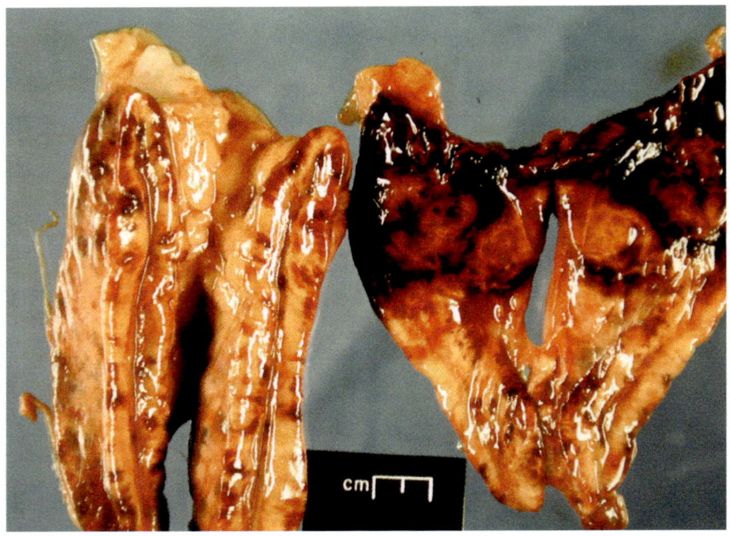

Fig. 9.6. Ox. Adrenal glands. Calf sepsis. Hemorrhage and necrosis. Multifocal and focally extensive fresh hemorrhage is present, mainly in the cortex. These changes can be seen in calves dying from endotoxic shock.

9.3.2 Neoplasia

These are infrequent incidental findings at necropsy.

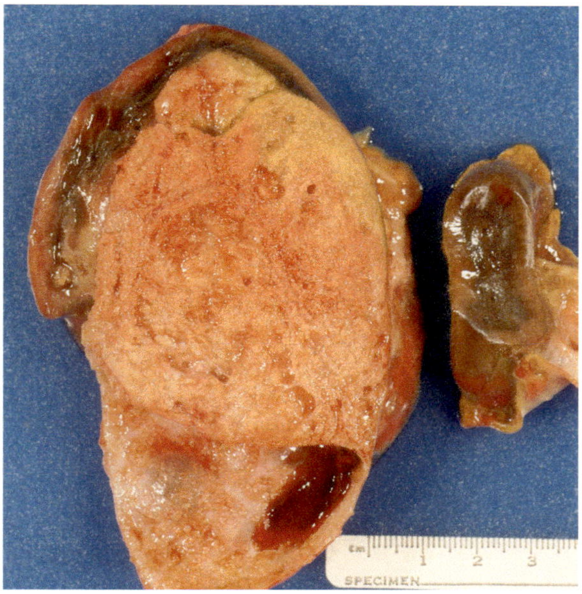

Fig. 9.9. Ox. Adrenal gland. Pheochromocytoma. A tan, bulging growth has obliterated the medulla and severely compressed the cortex. The normal adrenal gland on the right, surrounded by adipose tissue, demonstrates division into tan cortex and brown medulla. (Courtesy of Department of Veterinary Pathology, WCWM, University of Saskatchewan, Saskatoon, Canada.)

9.3.3 Miscellaneous

9.3.3.1 Amyloidosis

Reactive systemic amyloidosis of type AA in dairy cows following chronic inflammation can be encountered simultaneously in kidneys, liver, and spleen.

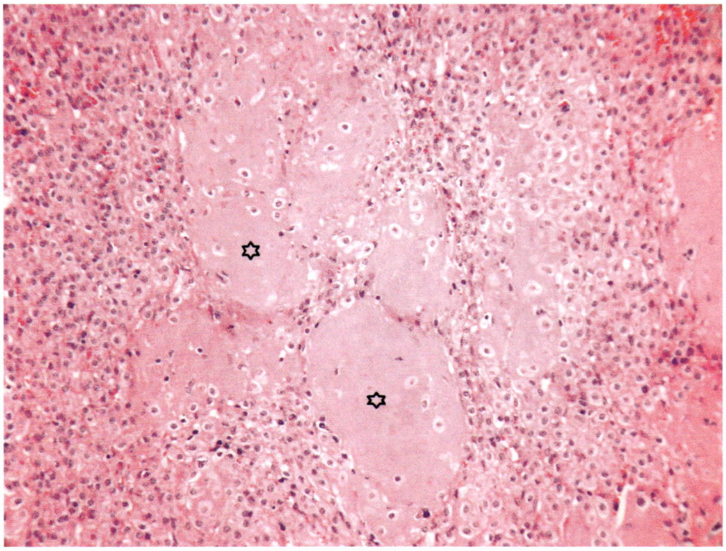

Fig. 9.10. Ox. Adrenal gland. Cortical amyloidosis. Pink homogeneous deposits (asterisks) have replaced cortical cells (H&E).

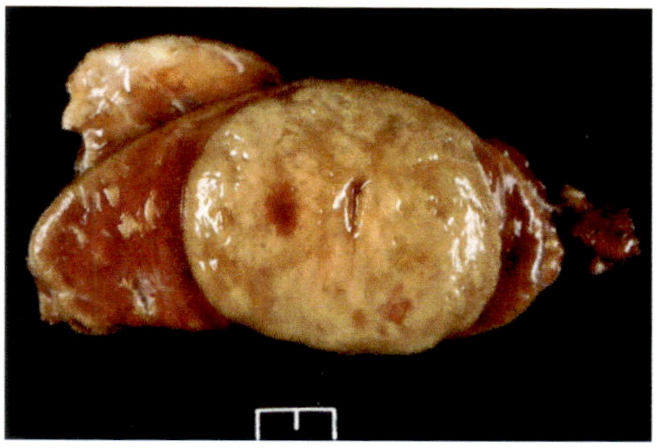

Fig. 9.7. Ox. Adrenal gland. Cortical adenoma. A circumscribed, uniform, yellow growth extends from the cortex into the medulla.

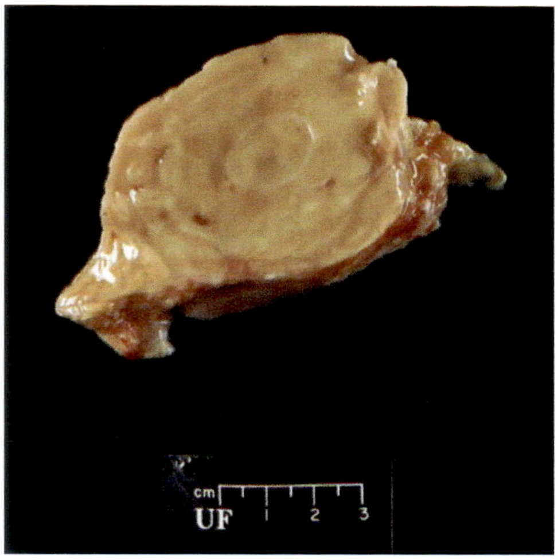

Fig. 9.8. Ox. Adrenal gland. Lymphosarcoma. A lamellate, tan growth has replaced the cortex and medulla.

9.3.3.2 Citrus pulp toxicosis

An energy-increasing carbohydrate by-product, citrus pulp, when excessively fed as supplement, has an adverse effect (granuloma formation, hypertrophic lymphadenopathy) on multiple organs such as adrenal glands, intestines, lymph nodes, liver, and kidneys. It has been suggested that the toxic principle is due to a type IV hypersensitivity stimulated by lectin. Citrus pulp may also contain citrinin, a mycotoxin.

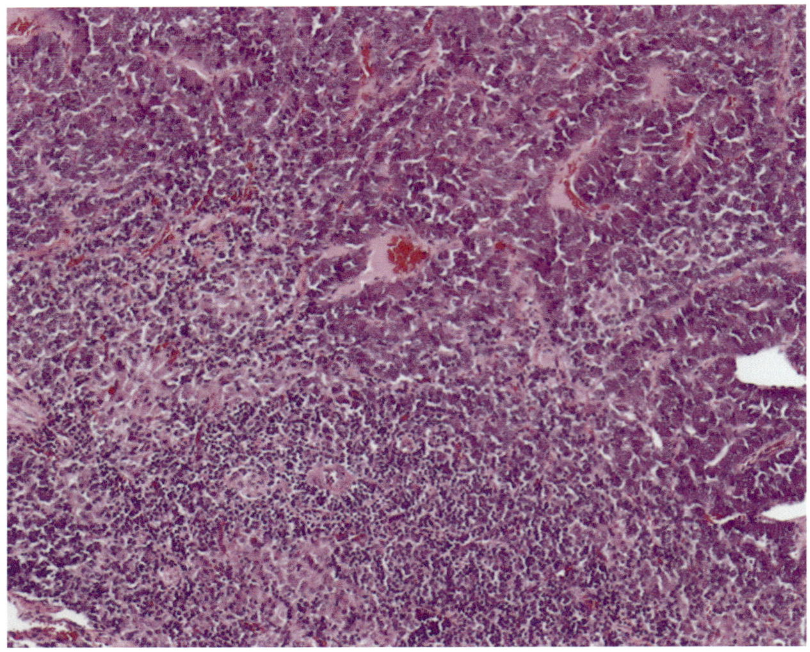

Fig. 9.11. Ox. Adrenal gland. Citrus pulp toxicosis. Lymphoplasmacytic adrenalitis. Clusters of lymphocytes intermixed with plasma cells infiltrate the architecture of the adrenal glands. At times, multinucleate giant cells may be interspersed. Grossly, the adrenal glands are bilaterally enlarged. Differential diagnosis should consider hairy vetch toxicosis (H&E). (Courtesy of Dr G. Saunders, Virginia Tech University, USA.)

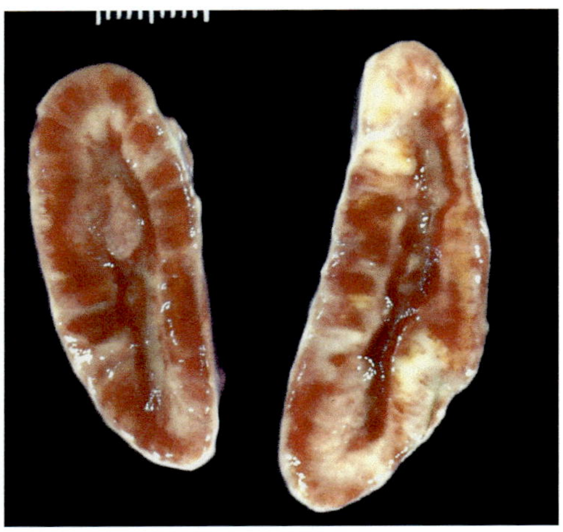

Fig. 9.12. Ox. Adrenal glands. Vetch poisoning. Granulomatous adrenalitis. (Courtesy of Dr R. Panciera, University of Oklahoma, USA.)

SUGGESTED READING

Geelhoed, G.W. (1996) 'Aging bull'. *Medical Hypotheses* 47, 471–479.

Johnson, R. and Jamison, K. (1884) Amyloidosis in six dairy cows. *Journal of the American Veterinary Medical Association* 184, 1538–1543.

Seimiya, Y., Ohshima, K., Ogasawara, N., Matsukida, Y. and Yuita, K. (1991) Epidemiological and pathological studies on congenital diffuse hyperplastic goiter in calves. *Journal* of *Veterinary Medical Science* 53, 989–994.

Seimiya, Y.M., Takakashi, M., Mizitani, K., Kimura, K. and Haritani, M. (2009) An aged bull with concurrent thyroid C cell carcinoma, adrenal pheochromocytoma and pituitary chromophobe adenoma. *Journal of Veterinary Medical Science* 71, 225–228.

CHAPTER 10

Diseases of the Reproductive System

Mark L. Anderson (contributed to Section 10.4.4 Abortion diseases)
California Animal Health & Food Safety Laboratory, School of Veterinary Medicine, University of California, USA

10.1 Testes and Accessory Sex Organs
- 10.1.1 Testes
  - 10.1.1.1 Normal testis
  - 10.1.1.2 Hypoplasia
  - 10.1.1.3 Necrosis, degeneration, and fibrosis
  - 10.1.1.4 Inflammation
  - 10.1.1.5 Neoplasia
  - 10.1.1.6 Miscellaneous
- 10.1.2 Epididymis
- 10.1.3 Seminal vesicle
- 10.1.4 External genitalia
  - 10.1.4.1 Penile abnormalities
  - 10.1.4.2 Penile hematoma
  - 10.1.4.3 Balanophosthitis
  - 10.1.4.4 Penile neoplasia

10.2 Intersexes
- 10.2.1 Gonadogenesis
- 10.2.2 Freemartinism

10.3 Non-gravid Female Reproductive System
- 10.3.1 Anomalies
  - 10.3.1.1 Segmental aplasia
  - 10.3.1.2 Uterus didelphys
- 10.3.2 Ovary
  - 10.3.2.1 Normal ovary *Bos taurus*
  - 10.3.2.2 Normal ovary *Bos indicus*
  - 10.3.2.3 Cysts
  - 10.3.2.4 Neoplasia
- 10.3.3 Uterine tubes (oviducts)
- 10.3.4 Uterus
  - 10.3.4.1 Inflammation
  - 10.3.4.2 Neoplasia
- 10.3.5 Cervix, vagina, vulva

10.4 Gravid Uterus
- 10.4.1 Cotyledonary placentation
- 10.4.2 Incidental findings on placental membranes
- 10.4.3 Disturbances of pregnancy
- 10.4.4 Abortion diseases
  - 10.4.4.1 Pathogenic principles of infectious abortions
  - 10.4.4.2 Viral abortions
  - 10.4.4.3 Bacterial abortions
  - 10.4.4.4 Mycotic abortions
  - 10.4.4.5 Protozoal abortions
  - 10.4.4.6 Miscellaneous

10.5 Fetal Malformations
- 10.5.1 Arthrogryposis
- 10.5.2 Schistosomus reflexus

10.6 Prolonged Gestation

INTRODUCTION

Reproductive health is paramount to the economic success of livestock management. Maintaining a steady fertility rate of sexually mature male and female animals requires multiple tasks to balance effective production of calves and milk for dairy cattle. Regular health and fertility examination of breeding bulls guarantees the desired sexual performance and expected semen quality. Disease control and observance of a high nutritional plane have a stabilizing effect on the ovarian cycle and conception rate. Diseases of the reproductive system of an individual animal may not attract immediate veterinary attention because generally they are not life threatening. They become important for attention if they interfere with commercial breeding practices or result in explosive abortion outbreaks.

Veterinary reproductive medicine has made significant progress in enhancing fertility through *in vitro* fertilization and semen analysis to assess sperm dysfunction. Selective chromosomal sexing has become a tool to produce preferred female offspring. Hormonal manipulation has been introduced for cycle synchronization. Embryo transfer techniques have been devised for global breeding concepts. Pharmacologic agents and surgical procedures have been developed to enhance reproductive health. Micromanipulation of oocytes has helped to improve pregnancy rates. Cryopreservation of embryos has helped to preserve embryos not transferred in a given cycle. All of these manipulations have the potential to produce pathologic conditions in reproductive organs that require veterinary attention.

The chapter summarizes disorders of the male, non-pregnant female and pregnant female reproductive systems, highlighting pathologic processes that affect individual components of the organ system. A major proportion of case examples will be dedicated to the causes of abortion diseases.

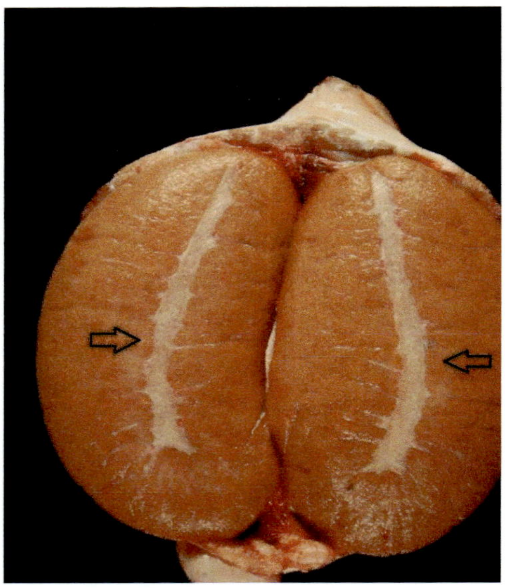

Fig. 10.1. Ox. Normal testis. The surface of a transverse section through a normal testis in a sexually mature bull should be moist, pigmented, and bulging. In the center, it normally reveals a white mediastinum testis (arrows) containing collagen, blood vessels including lymphatics, and nerves. This scaffolding structure should not be confused with testicular fibrosis.

10.1 TESTES AND ACCESSORY SEX ORGANS

10.1.1 Testes

10.1.1.1 Normal testis

Introduction. The testis performs two major complementary functions: the production of sperm and the secretion of steroid hormones. Testicular descent into the scrotum is necessary for optimal testicular hormonal and sperm production. For undisturbed spermatogenesis, the pampiniform plexus thermoregulates the blood entering the scrotal sac to a temperature 2–4°C lower than the body temperature.

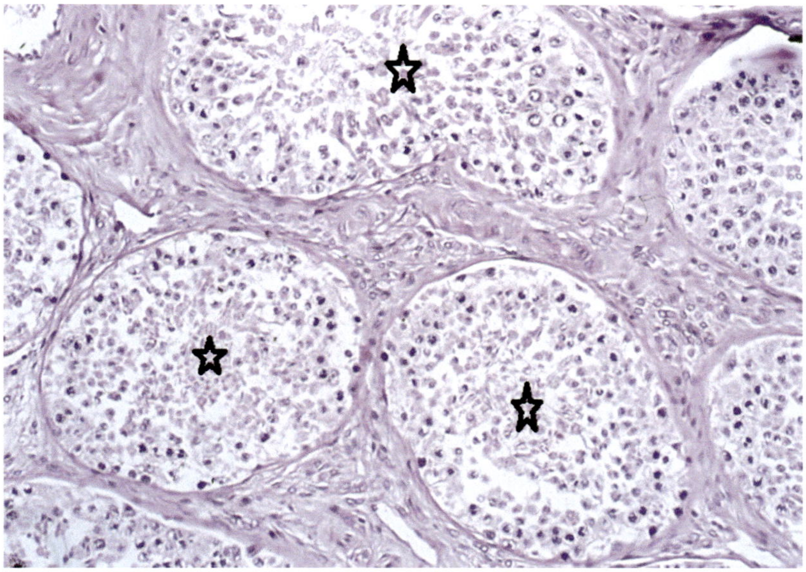

Fig. 10.2. Ox. Seminiferous tubules. Spermatogenesis. The histologic unit of the testis is the seminiferous tubule (asterisks). It is composed of several germ cell layers in maturation, Sertoli cells, the basement membrane, and myoid cells. The Sertoli cells, with tight junctions, basement membranes, and myoid cells represent the 'blood–testis' immunoregulatory barrier, preventing the recognition of sperm antigens as foreign by the animal's immune system. The interstitium is located between the seminiferous tubules. It contains the interstitial cells (Leydig's cells), connective tissue, nerves, and blood vessels. Spermatogenesis is controlled by hormones, nutritional factors, temperature, and photoperiod (H&E).

10.1.1.2 Hypoplasia

Testicular hypoplasia manifests itself at puberty. Breed (Swedish Highland), intersexuality, chromosome abnormalities, cryptorchidism, bovine viral diarrhea virus (BVDV), and nutrition are some factors responsible for the condition.

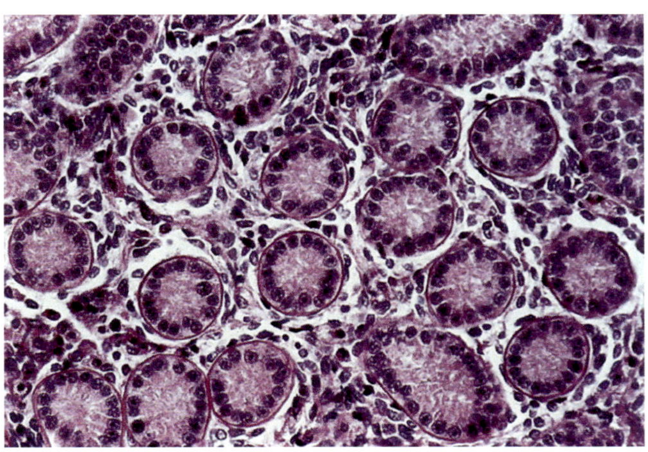

Fig. 10.4. Ox. Testis. Hypoplasia. Microscopically, seminiferous tubules are uniformly reduced in size. They are only lined by Sertoli cells (H&E). (Courtesy of Dr J.M. King and Section of Anatomic Pathology, Cornell University, USA.)

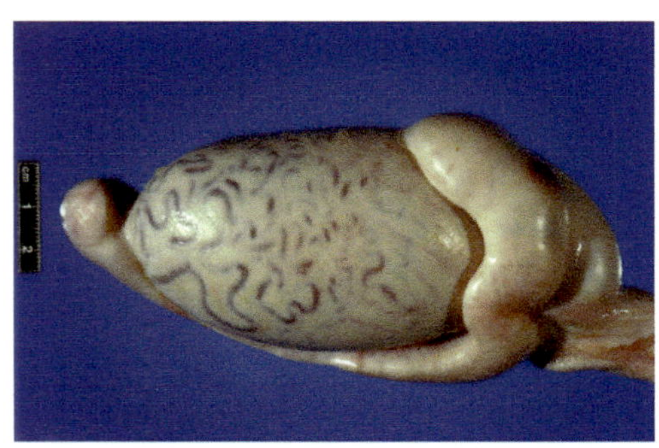

Fig. 10.3. Ox. Testis. Hypoplasia. The overall size of the testis is reduced when compared with the epididymis. (Courtesy of Dr J. Edwards, Texas A&M University, USA.)

10.1.1.3 Necrosis, degeneration, and fibrosis

The testicular germ cell epithelium is very sensitive to adverse influences. Causes for degeneration include trauma, torsion, elevated temperature, frostbite, systemic infections, nutritional deficiencies, toxins, hormonal disturbances, ischemia, and age. Testicular degeneration will develop into fibrosis and atrophy.

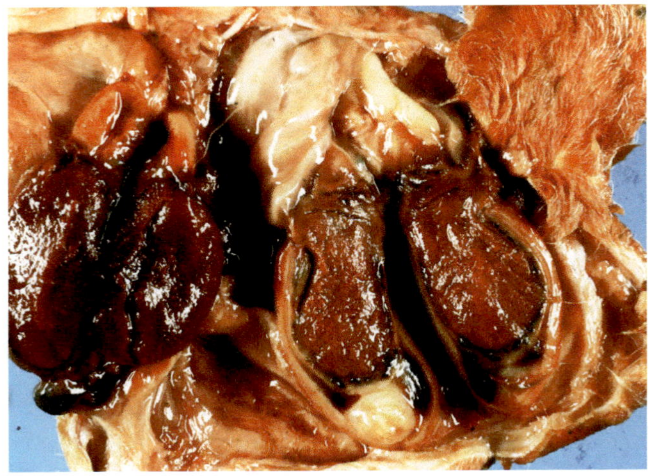

Fig. 10.5. Ox. Testis. Necrosis. Both testes are hemorrhagic and necrotic from elastrator application.

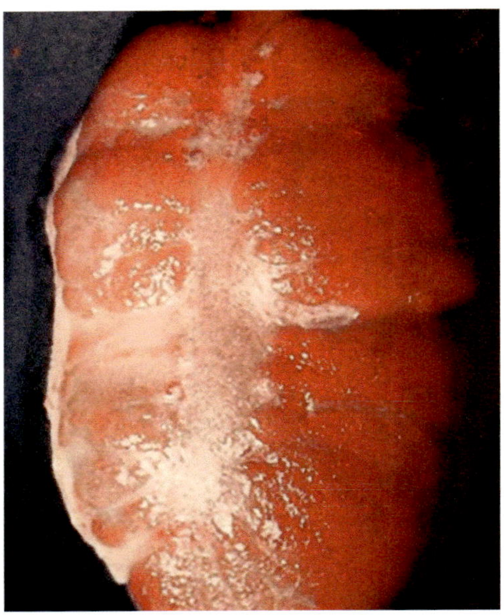

Fig. 10.6. Ox. Testis. Fibrosis. Wide bands of fibrous tissue project perpendicularly from the mediastinum testis. In older bulls, ventral wedge-shaped fibrosis suggests vascular impairment (ischemia).

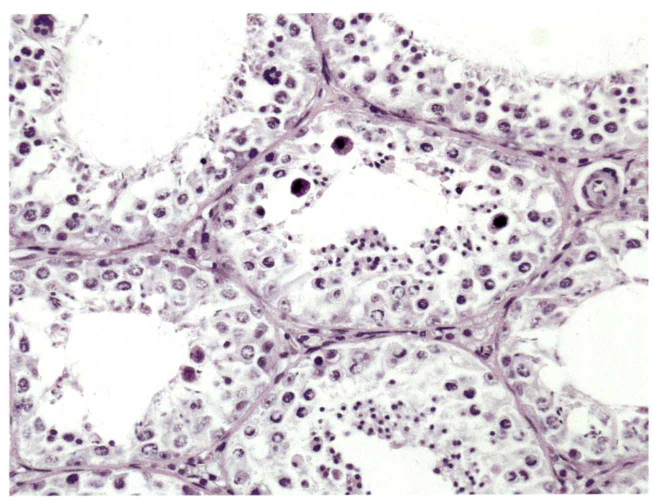

Fig. 10.7. Ox. Testis. Germ-cell degeneration and necrosis. Microscopically, seminiferous tubules show vacuolation, dissolution, chromatin clumping, giant cell formation, karyorrhexis, and karyolysis (H&E).

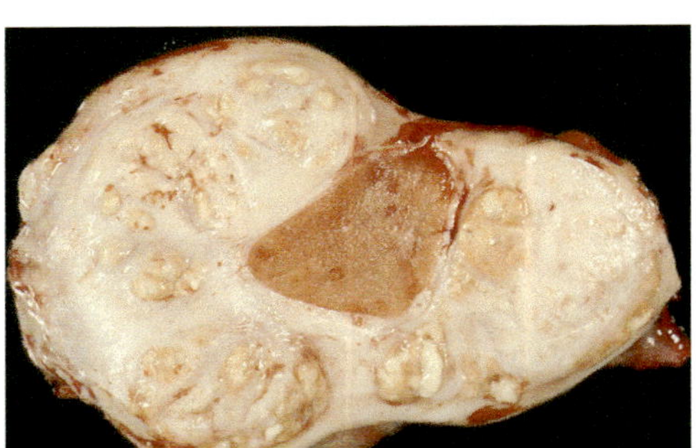

Fig. 10.8. Ox. Testis. Chronic periorchitis. Marked pyogranulomatous tissue envelops the testis. Undetermined bacterial origin. (Courtesy of Department of Pathology, Western College of Veterinary Medicine, WCVM, University of Saskatchewan, Saskatoon, Canada.)

10.1.1.4 Inflammation

Orchitis may start as periorchitis from inflammation of the tunica vaginalis cavity gradually spreading to the testes. Preceding peritonitis is usually the portal of entry. Hematogenous or ascending routes are other portals of entry for inflammation. Orchitis may be unilateral or bilateral. Trauma and bacteria including *Brucella abortus*, *Trueperella pyogenes*, *Escherichia coli*, and *Histophilus* spp., are possible pathogens. Orchitis is often accompanied by epididymitis.

10.1.1.5 Neoplasia

There are two histogenetic lines of primary testicular tumors: gonadal-stromal and germ cells. Gonadal-stromal tumors are: interstitial endocrine (Leydig) cell tumors and endocrine Sertoli (sustentacular) cell tumors. Germ cell tumors are: seminoma, teratoma, and embryonal carcinoma. Mesenchymal tumors such as mesothelioma are occasionally found to be associated with the tunica albuginea.

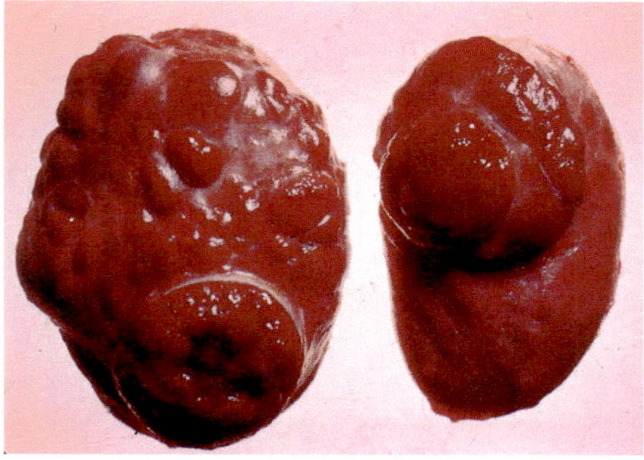

Fig. 10.9. Ox. Testis. Bilateral interstitial (Leydig) cell tumor. Multiple brown nodules, some of which are encapsulated, bulge at cut section. Some of the smaller nodules suggest interstitial cell hyperplasia. (Courtesy of Dr J.M. King and Section of Anatomic Pathology, Cornell University, USA.)

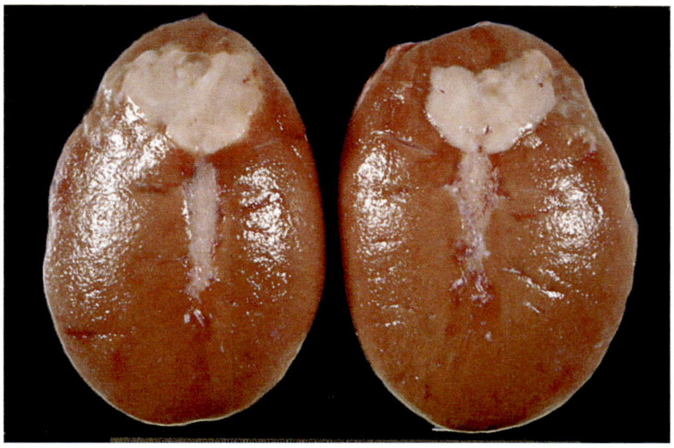

Fig. 10.10. Ox. Testis. Sertoli cell tumor. These are white, circumscribed, and firm on touch.

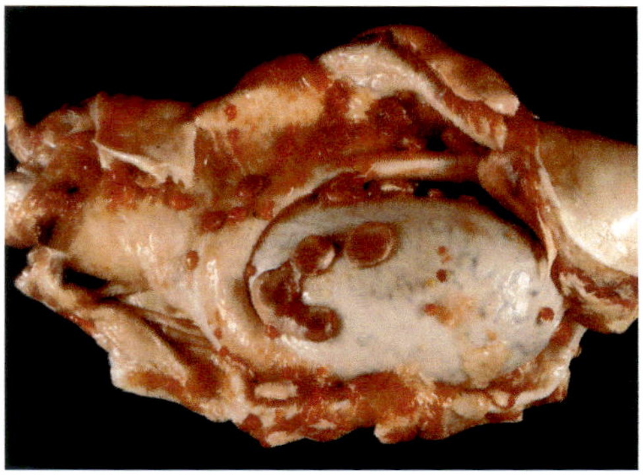

Fig. 10.11. Ox. Testis. Mesothelioma. Multiple plaque-like nodules seed the tunica albuginea and tunica vaginalis. The neoplasm arises from the serosal surface of the tunics.

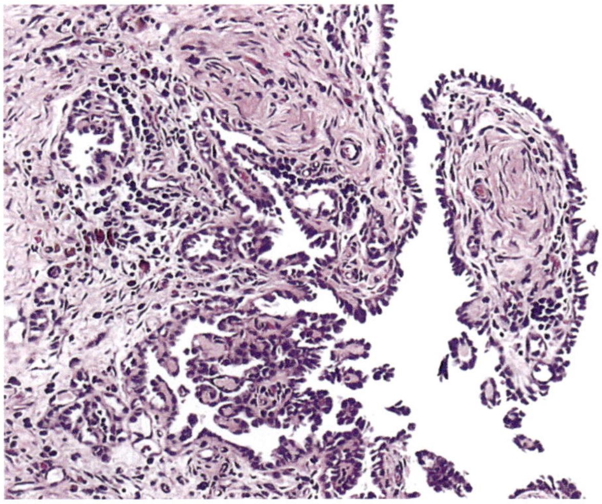

Fig. 10.12. Ox. Testis. Mesothelioma. The microscopic appearance is characterized by arborizing, cuboidal cells resting on a collagenous stroma (H&E).

10.1.1.6 Miscellaneous

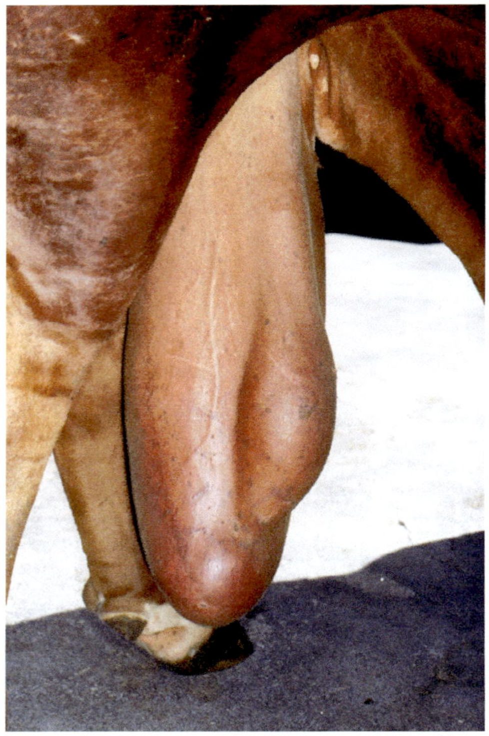

Fig. 10.13. Ox. Scrotum. Hematocele. The rupture of a vessel in the pampiniform plexus of one of the testes may result in severe bleeding (hematoma) into the scrotum, causing unilateral scrotal sac distension (scrotomegaly). Hydrocele or inguinal herniation should be considered in the differential diagnosis. Secondary degenerative changes should be expected in the opposite testicle. (Courtesy of Dr P. Chenoweth, University of Queensland, Australia.)

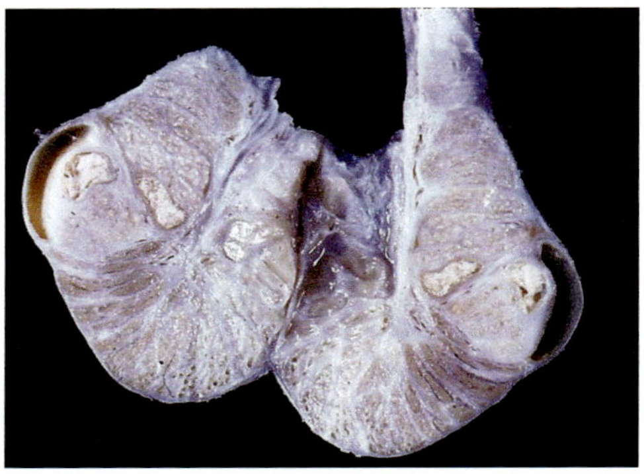

Fig. 10.14. Ox. Epididymis. Sperm granulomas. Multiple, mineralized, small and mid-sized foci are spread throughout the head of the epididymis. This non-infectious inflammation is the result of blindly ending efferent tubules entrapping sperm. The released mycolic acid from dead sperm initiates a granulomatous response similar to that of mycobacteriosis. (Courtesy of Dr J.M. King and Section of Anatomic Pathology, Cornell University, USA.)

10.1.2 Epididymis

The epididymis is closely attached to the testis. Anatomically, it is composed of head, body, and tail. Segmental aplasia, sperm granulomas, and bacterial infections, notably from *Brucella abortus*, are pathologic conditions involving the bovine epididymis.

10.1.3 Seminal vesicle

In areas where brucellosis has been eradicated, *T. pyogenes* is a frequent cause of seminal vesicle adenitis in young bulls. Other pathogens implicated are *Chlamydophila* spp., *Mycoplasma* spp., *Ureaplasma diversum*, *Histophilus somni*, *Streptococcus* spp., and *Staphylococcus* spp. Seminal vesicles can be found by opening the pelvic cavity.

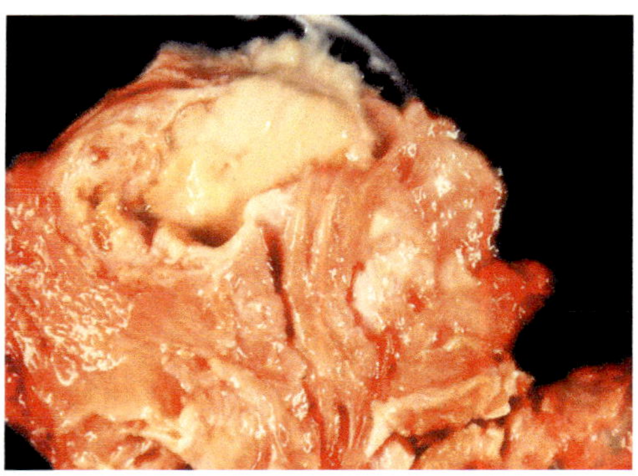

Fig. 10.15. Ox. Seminal vesicular gland. Purulent adenitis. Pockets of pus have caused enlargement, loss of lobulation, and adhesions.

10.1.4 External genitalia

10.1.4.1 Penile abnormalities

Persistent frenulum. Other penile abnormalities of the bovine penis include deviation, duplication (diphallus), hypoplasia.

10.1.4.2 Penile hematoma

Painful swelling below the skin surrounding the penis results from trauma to the corpus cavernosum or bleeding of the tunica albuginea. Infection of the hematoma is a clinical complication. Fracture of the penis should be considered as a differential diagnosis.

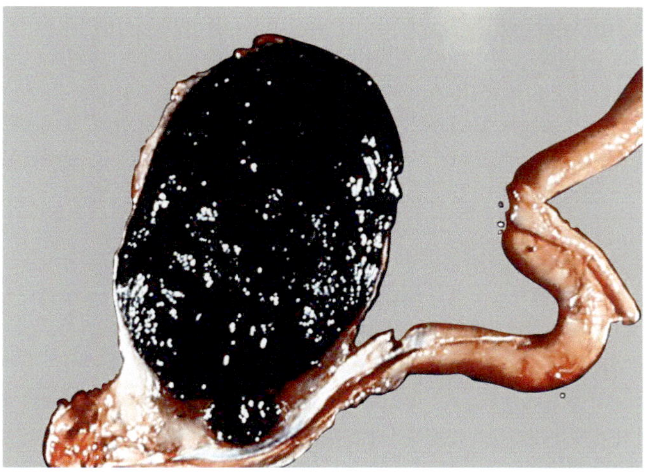

Fig. 10.18. Ox. Corpus cavernosum. Hematoma. Rupture of the vessel-rich corpus is one of the causes of penile and peripenile hematoma. (Reprinted with permission from *Color Atlas of Reproductive Pathology of Domestic Animals*, Buergelt, Fig. 6-10, p. 74, © Elsevier, 1997.)

10.1.4.3 Balanoposthitis

Inflammation of the penis is defined as phallitis, that of the glans penis as balanitis. It may occur together, with inflammation of the prepuce defined as posthitis, to develop balanoposthitis.

10.1.4.4 Penile neoplasia

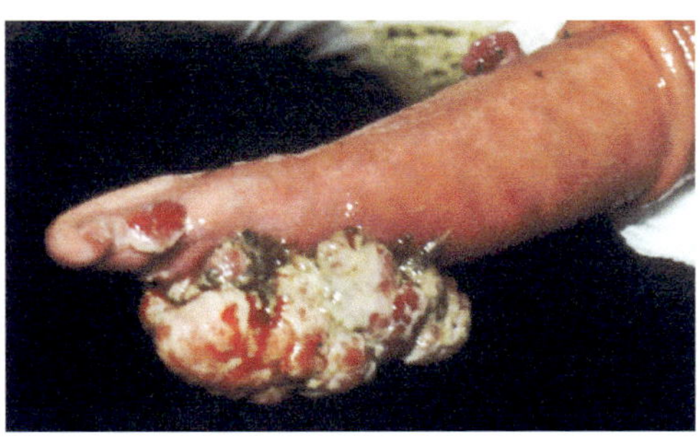

Fig. 10.20. Ox. Penis. Fibropapilloma. Caused by the bovine papilloma type 1 virus, the tumor develops in young, sexually mature bulls. The growths may become quite extensive, interfering with coitus. The condition is self-limiting. (Courtesy of Dr P. Chenoweth, University of Queensland, Australia.)

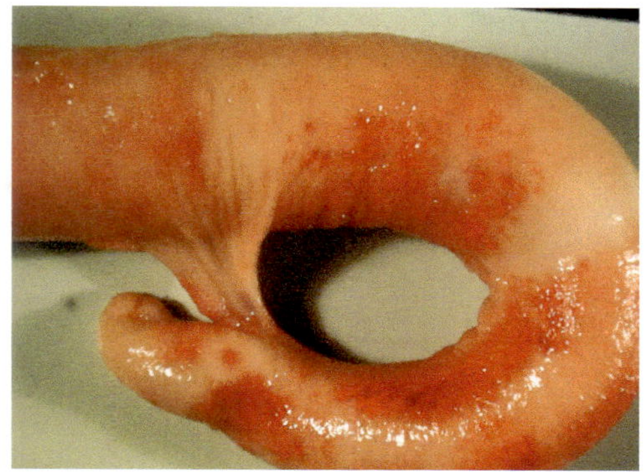

Fig. 10.16. Ox. Penis. Persistent frenulum. Results from failure of the prepuce to separate from the penis. If persisting beyond puberty, the condition will interfere with copulation. (Reprinted with permission from *Color Atlas of Reproductive Pathology of Domestic Animals*, Buergelt, Fig. 6-3, p. 72, © Elsevier, 1997.)

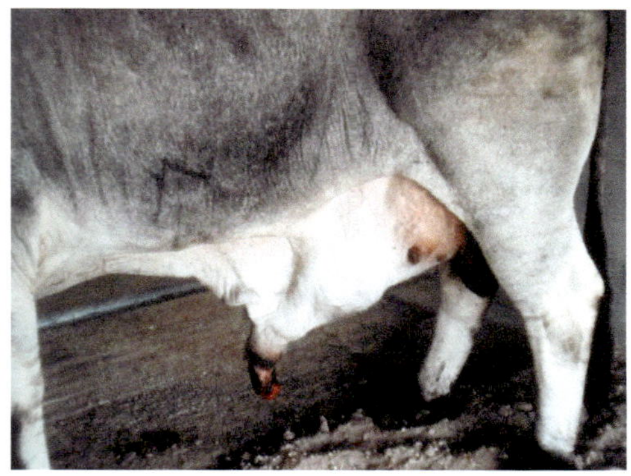

Fig. 10.17. Ox. Penis. Hematoma. Peripenile subcutaneous swelling is evident. (Reprinted with permission from *Color Atlas of Reproductive Pathology of Domestic Animals*, Buergelt, Fig. 6-9, p. 73, © Elsevier, 1997.)

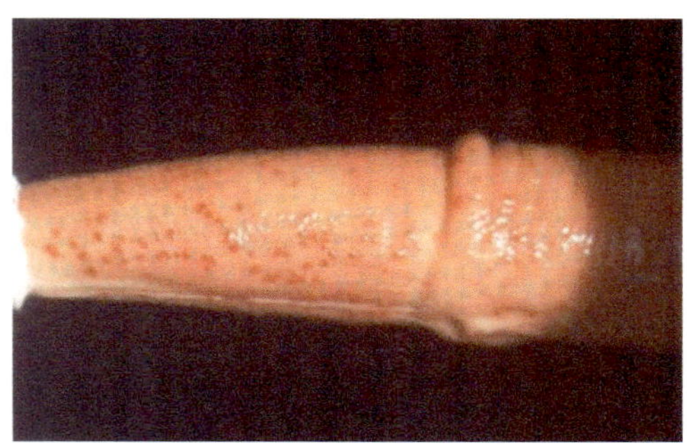

Fig. 10.19. Ox. Penis. Balanitis. Genital bovine herpesvirus type 1. Petechiae occupy the glans penis. These can progress to vesicles, pustules, and ulcers.

10.2 INTERSEXES

Introduction. An intersex is defined as a sterile animal in which the morphologic diagnosis of gender is ambiguous because characteristic morphologic elements of both sexes are present. Variations in sex characteristics may include chromosomes, gonads, and genitals. These different features may include genital ambiguity, and combinations of chromosomal genotypes and sexual phenotype other than XY-male and XX-female. Intersexes were previously referred to as hermaphrodites.

10.2.1 Gonadogenesis

Differentiation of the male and female reproductive tract occurs early in embryogenesis. The process of gender differentiation is driven mainly by the fetal testis actively secreting Muellerian-inhibiting substance (MIS) and fetal testosterone. The female role is largely passive in gender differentiation. Chromosomal sex determines gonadal sex, which determines phenotypic sex.

10.2.2 Freemartinism

Freemartinism occurs in 90% of female bovine dizygotic twins. A freemartin is defined as an intersex, which is genetically female but also has male characteristics (seminal vesicles). The condition occurs when a female twin calf is born to a male twin. The female calf is sterile. It typically shows juvenile ovaries and internal genitalia as a heifer. A shortened vagina ends blindly. The cervix is absent, and the clitoris is enlarged. During early gestation, placental anastomosis allows fetal testosterone produced by the male twin to cross into the placental circulation of the female, suppressing the female genital system and allowing male vestiges (seminal vesicles) to develop. There is some evidence that primordial germ cells and hematopoietic stem cells are exchanged in the conjoined fetal circulations as well. There is evidence that some male co-twins are affected by sterility.

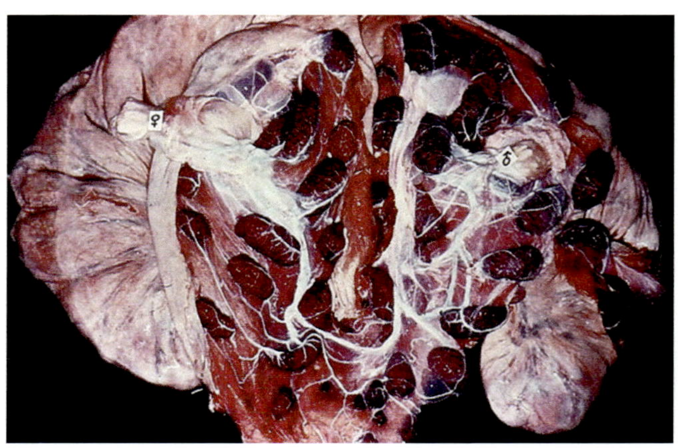

Fig. 10.21. Ox. Freemartinism. Placental anastomosis. Placental membranes of female and male co-twins. (Courtesy of Dr J.M. King and Section of Anatomic Pathology, Cornell University, USA.)

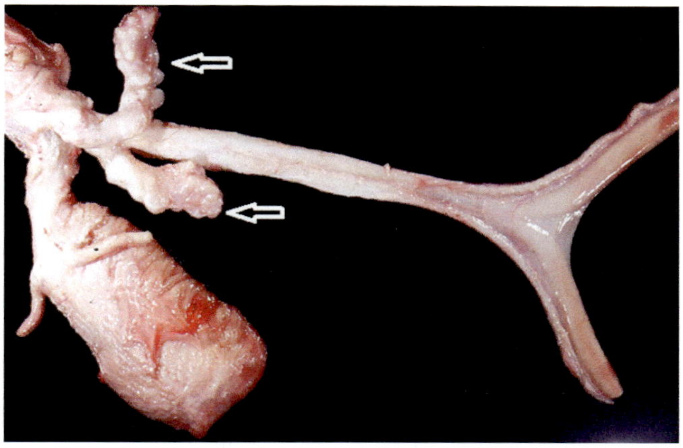

Fig. 10.22. Ox. Genital tract. Freemartin heifer. Uterine horns and body of uterus are hypoplastic. Seminal vesicles (arrows) are located caudal to the uterus. (Courtesy of Dr J.M. King and Section of Anatomic Pathology, Cornell University, USA.)

10.3 NON-GRAVID FEMALE REPRODUCTIVE SYSTEM

Introduction. A healthy, mature female reproductive tract is the prerequisite for successful breeding and pregnancy. Good management and feeding practice influence the ovarian cycle and conception rates.

10.3.1 Anomalies

These include ovarian hypoplasia, segmental aplasia of uterine horns, and duplication of vagina, cervix, and uterus fundus (uterus didelphys).

10.3.1.1 Segmental aplasia

The condition affects the paramesonephric (Muellerian) duct system in which portions of the uterine horns are missing and segments end blindly. The anomaly occurs in White Shorthorn cattle with some frequency and is caused by a recessive gene linked to the one responsible for the white coat color ('White Heifer Disease').

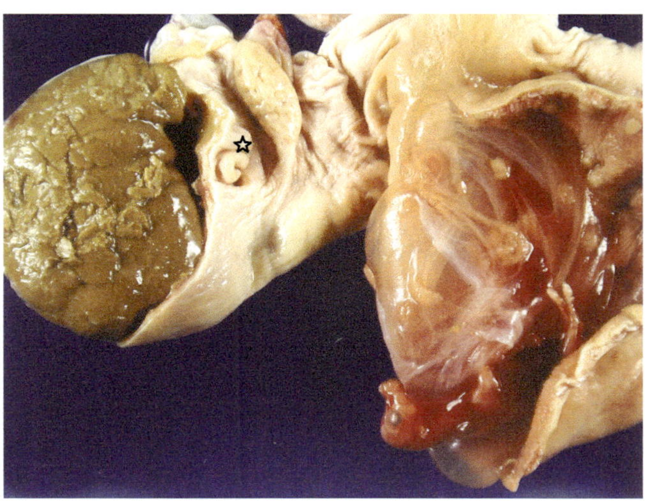

Fig. 10.23. Ox. Uterine horn. Segmental aplasia. The horn on the left (asterisk) ends blindly and is distended by an entrapped, inspissated, brown uterine concretion called *hysterolith*. The horn on the right is continuous and carries a conceptus.

10.3.1.2 *Uterus didelphys*

Failure of proper fusion of the caudal segments of the paired paramesonephric (Muellerian) ducts results in duplication of the uterine body and cervix.

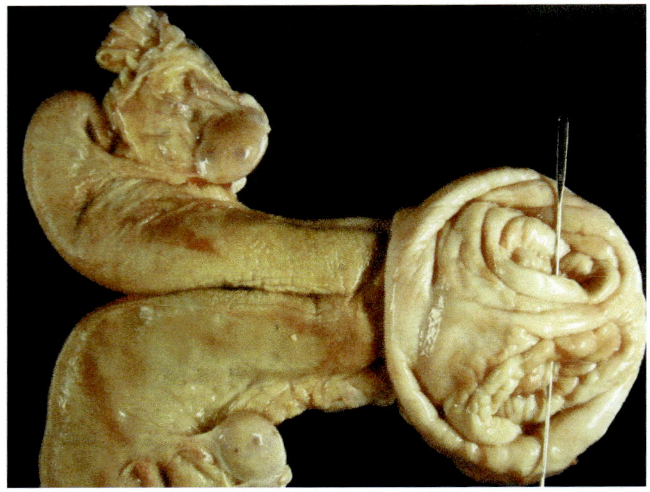

Fig. 10.24. Ox. Uterus didelphys. Duplication of the external os is indicated by the probe. (Reprinted with permission from *Color Atlas of Reproductive Pathology of Domestic Animals*, Buergelt, Fig. 7-7, p. 85, © Elsevier, 1997.)

10.3.2 Ovary

Introduction. The ovary fulfills two functions: production of mature eggs for fertilization, and synthesis of hormones for the regulation of the non-pregnant and gravid uterus. Unlike the testis, the ovary is relatively resistant to adverse injury from infectious agents, toxins, nutrient deprivation, or immune derangement. It is susceptible to radiation, chemotherapeutic agents, and endocrine disorders. Developmental anomalies (hypoplasia) and inflammation (oophoritis) are rare events in the cow's ovary.

10.3.2.1 *Normal ovary* Bos taurus

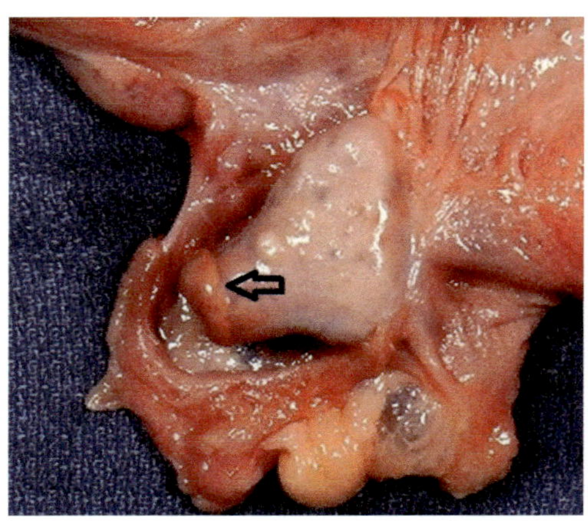

Fig. 10.25. Ox. Normal ovary and adnexa. A corpus luteum (arrow) at one pole and several ovulation scars on the ovarian surface are visible. (Courtesy of Dr M. Drost, Drost Project, University of Florida, USA.)

10.3.2.2 *Normal ovary* Bos indicus

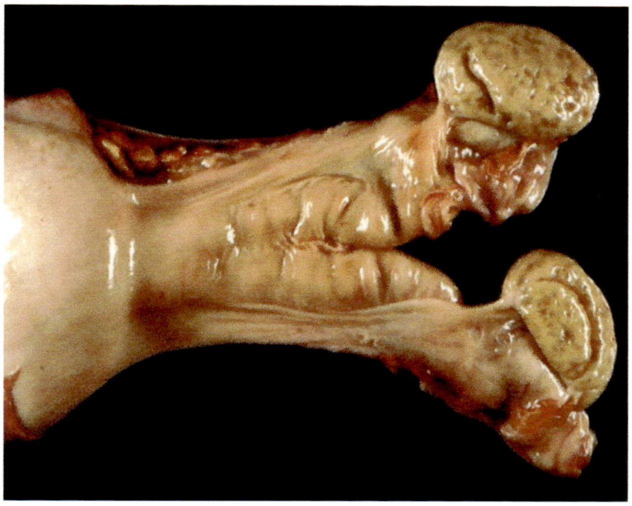

Fig. 10.26. Ox. 'Pancake' ovary. Normal appearance of ovulating ovaries in *Bos indicus* breeds.

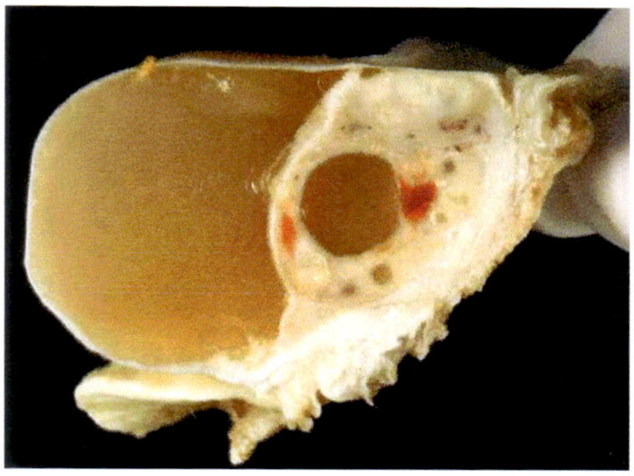

Fig. 10.27. Ox. Ovary. Paraovarian cyst. A large cyst with a thin wall and gelled proteinaceous fluid is located next to the ovary containing a Graafian follicle. Other examples of cysts that form outside the ovary are bursal cysts and tubo-ovarian cysts, both acquired. (Courtesy of Dr J. Roberts, Auburn University, USA.)

10.3.2.3 *Cysts*

Ovarian cysts are divided, depending on location, into intraovarian and paraovarian cysts. Paraovarian cysts originate from the remnants of mesonephric tubular and duct structures. Histologic examination of the cyst wall is needed for appropriate classification.

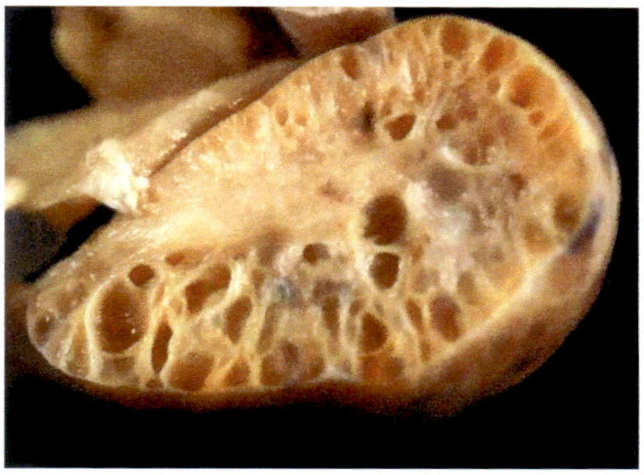

Fig. 10.28. Ox. Ovary. Polycystic ovary. The ovary contains multiple thin-walled, medium-sized cysts. These develop from insufficiency of luteinizing hormone (LH) function. (Courtesy of Dr J. Roberts, Auburn University, USA.)

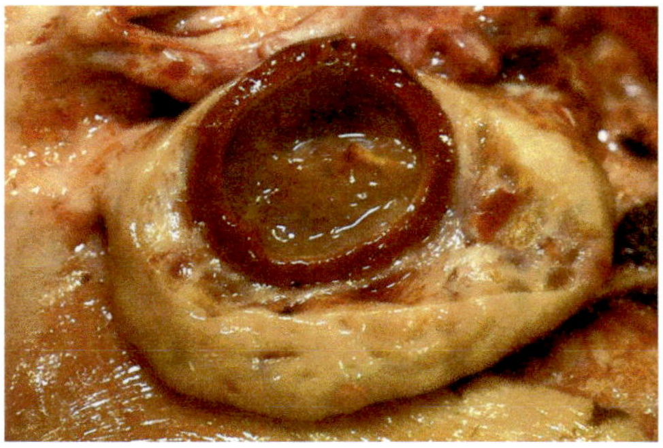

Fig. 10.30. Ox. Ovary. Cystic corpus luteum. A large cyst formed in the center of the corpus luteum. The cyst develops after ovulation. Differential diagnosis: anovulatory luteinized cyst. (Courtesy of Dr J. Roberts, Auburn University, USA.)

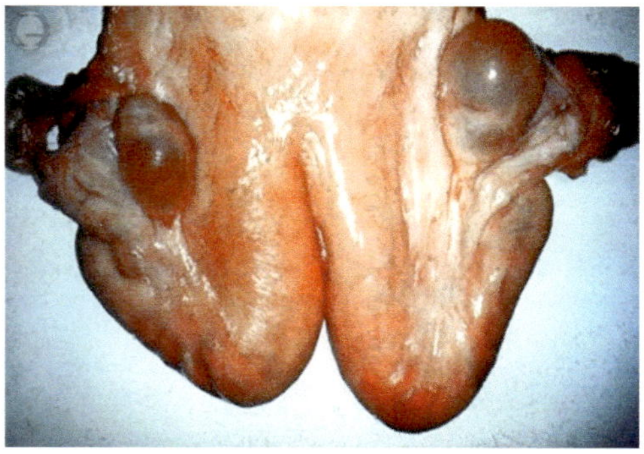

Fig. 10.29. Ox. Ovary. Cystic follicles. Each ovary contains an enlarged, fluid-distended Graafian follicle with a thin wall. Cystic follicles range from 2.5 cm or more in diameter, resulting in estrus irregularities, hydrometra (mucometra), and behavioral changes (nymphomania). (Courtesy of Dr M. Drost, Drost Project, University of Florida, USA.)

10.3.2.4 *Neoplasia*

Primary ovarian neoplasms are classified according to histogenesis into gonadal-stromal and germ-cell neoplasms. Gonadal-stromal neoplasms include granulosa cell/thecal cell tumors and arrhenoblastoma. Dysgerminomas and teratomas are of germ-cell origin. Multicentric lymphosarcoma is an example of a secondary ovarian tumor.

Granulosa cell tumor

Introduction. In cattle, this frequent ovarian tumor has a cystic or solid presentation. It is usually unilateral and benign. The tumor produces estrogens or androgens, and is associated with cystic endometrial hyperplasia of the uterus and signs of nymphomania.

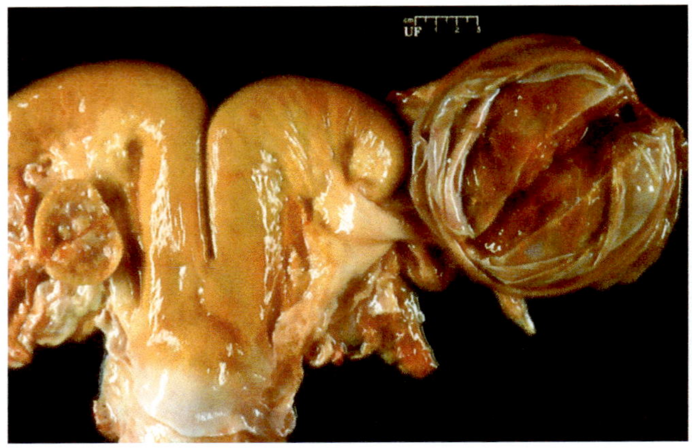

Fig. 10.31. Ox. Ovary. Granulosa cell tumor. An encapsulated, fleshy growth arises in the right ovary.

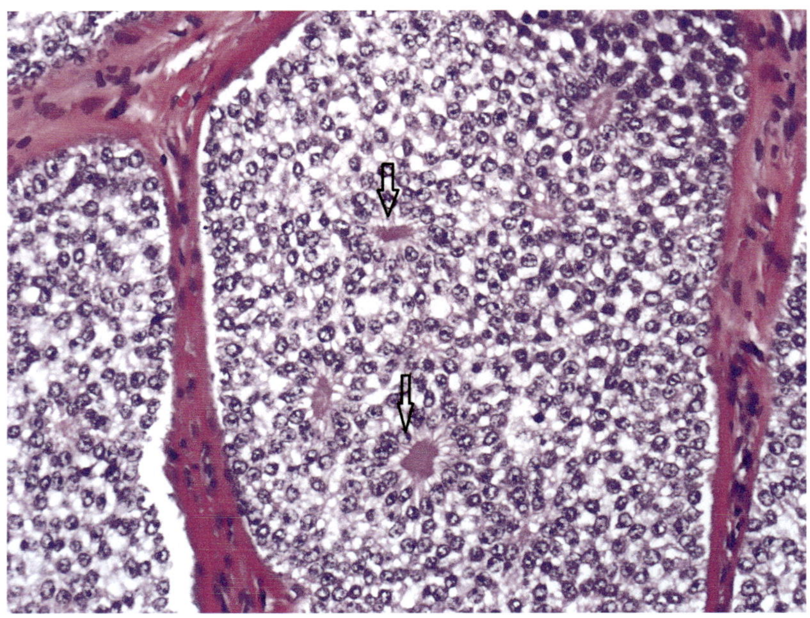

Fig. 10.32. Ox. Ovary. Granulosa cell tumor. The microscopic features of neoplastic granulosa cells are similar to the normal granulosa cells in a Graafian follicle. Round-to-oval, basophilic cells with a medium-sized, hypochromatic nucleus are arranged in sheets and surrounded by a collagen stroma. Mitotic figures are rare. Rosettes of granulosa cells with an eosinophilic body in the center (Call–Exner bodies) are interspersed (arrows). If the stroma is excessive, the neoplasm can transform into a thecoma (H&E).

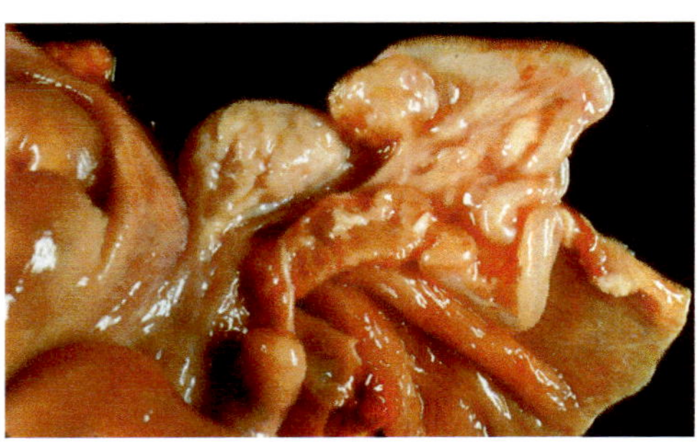

Fig. 10.33. Ox. Uterine tube. Hydrosalpinx. The convoluted oviduct is markedly distended by watery fluid. If the cause is inflammatory, infectious agents to consider are *Ureaplasma* spp., *Mycoplasma* spp., *Tritrichomonas* spp.

10.3.3 Uterine tubes (oviducts)

Introduction. The small uterine tubes become the site of fertilization, with the blastocyst remaining in the organ for several days until transported to the uterus. Disorders of uterine tubes include congenital malformation (aplasia) and occlusion secondary to inflammation (salpingitis).

10.3.4 Uterus

Introduction. The main function of the uterus is to provide a protective environment for the conceptus in case of pregnancy. Ovaries and uterus are interacting via hormones, bidirectionally regulating each segment. Locally produced uterine antibodies (opsonins) and intraendometrial immunoregulatory lymphocytes are effective in defending against pathogens. The cervix provides a physical barrier against external invaders. It is closed during the luteal phase of the cycle and open during the estrus period.

10.3.4.1 Inflammation

Inflammation of the uterus is associated with parturition or mating. The post-partum uterus is most susceptible to infection. Severe uterine tissue destruction allows rapid invasion by pathogens and the occurrence of sepsis. Post-coital infection includes venereal campylobacteriosis (*Campylobacter fetus* subsp. *venerealis*) and trichomoniasis (*Tritrichomonas foetus*).

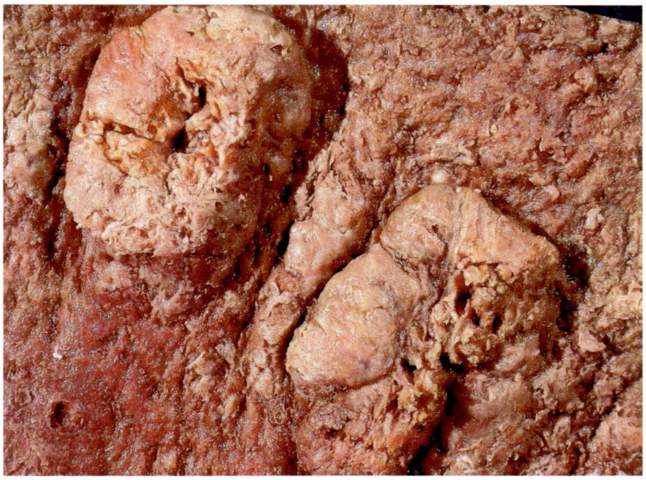

Fig. 10.34. Ox. Uterus. Fibrinous post-partum endometritis/metritis. Inflammation of the endometrium denotes endometritis. Metritis implies inflammatory involvement of the endometrium and myometrium. The severity of the condition is reflected by a massive accumulation of a necrofibrinous exudate. Placental retention can exacerbate the condition. *Trueperella pyogenes* was isolated. Other pathogens may include *Escherichia coli*, *Bacillus cereus*, and *Pseudomonas aeruginosa*.

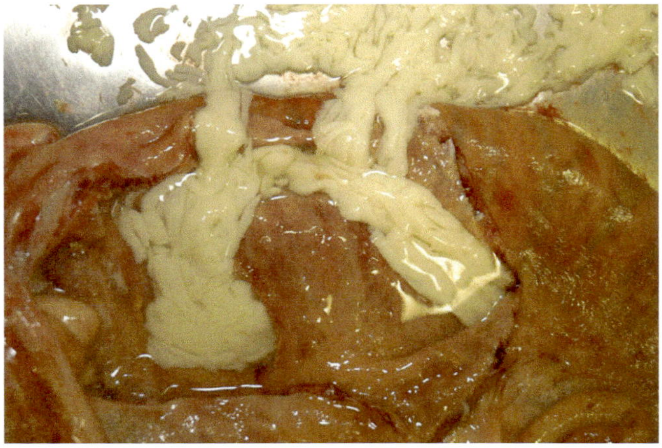

Fig. 10.35. Ox. Uterus. Pyometra. A purulent exudate covers a moist and thickened endometrium. *Tritrichomonas foetus* was isolated.

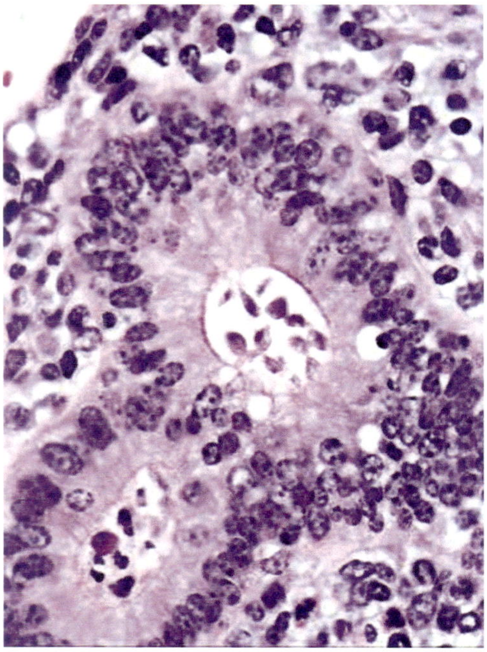

Fig. 10.36. Ox. Endometrium. Lymphoplasmacytic endometritis. Trichomoniasis. Flagellated protozoa are located in the lumen of the endometrial glands (H&E).

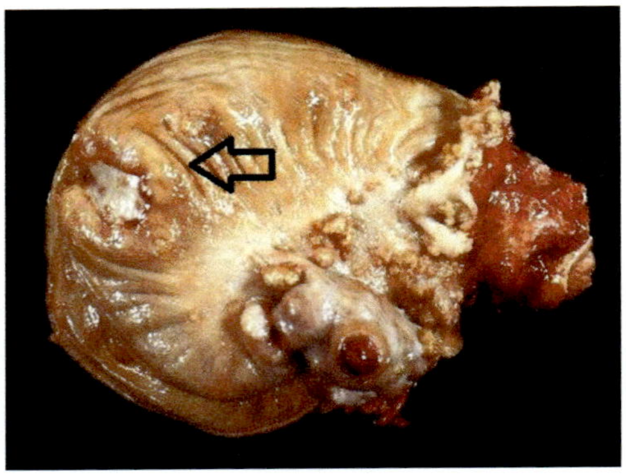

Fig. 10.37. Ox. Uterus. Carcinoma. A large umbilicated growth occupies the wall of the uterus (arrow). Serosal constriction bands are in the vicinity. Several smaller nodules seed the uterine serosa adjacent to the ovary.

10.3.4.2 Neoplasia

Primary tumors of the uterus are relatively rare in cattle. Both epithelial and mesenchymal tumors have been reported. Multicentric lymphosarcoma targets the uterus as one of the non-hematopoietic organs.

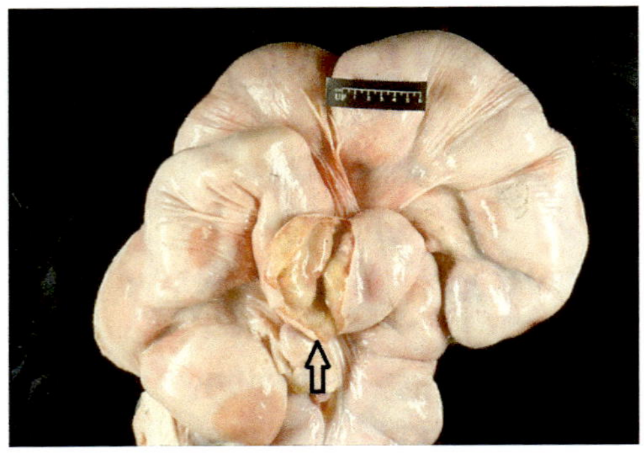

Fig. 10.38. Ox. Uterus. Lymphosarcoma. The wall of both uterine horns is thickened. A tan, glistening tissue is present in the uterine wall (arrow).

10.3.5 Cervix, vagina, vulva

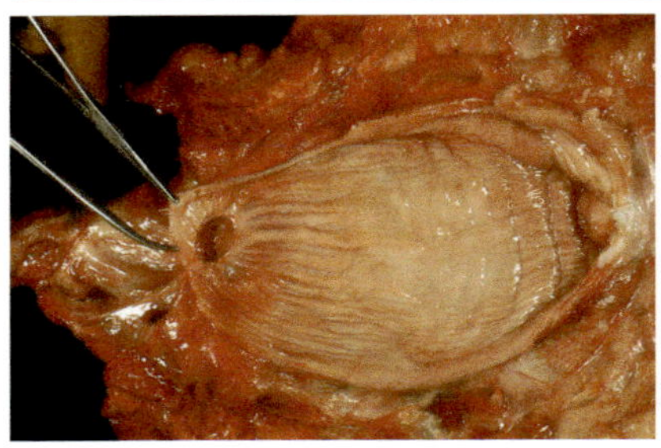

Fig. 10.39. Ox. Vagina. Persistent hymen. A membranous fold obstructs the external orifice of the vagina. (Courtesy of Department of Veterinary Pathology, WCVM, University of Saskatchewan, Saskatoon, Canada.)

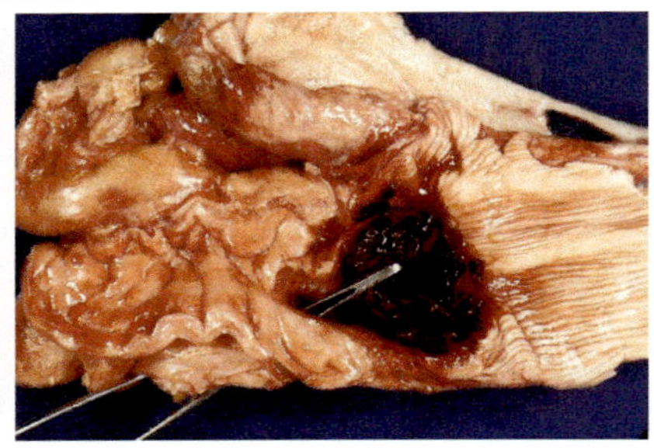

Fig. 10.40. Ox. Vagina. Laceration and hematoma. Traumatic lesion from penile penetration. Occurs when large bulls mount small heifers. Vagina is on the right, uterus on the left.

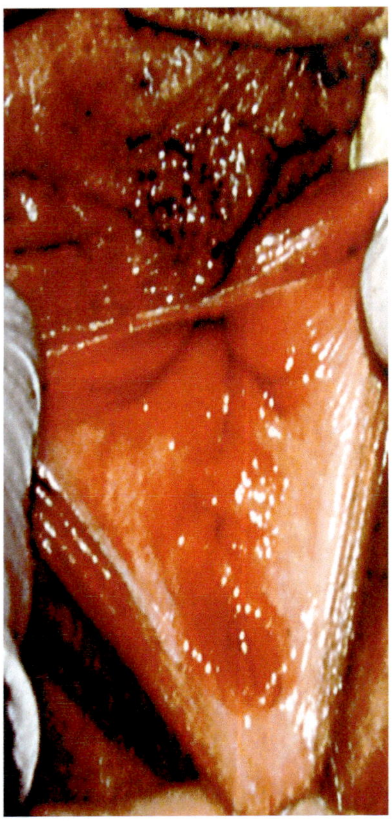

Fig. 10.41. Ox. Vulva. Granular vulvovaginitis. The vaginal–vulvar mucosa is characterized by hyperemia and granularity. The lesion is the result of infection with *Ureaplasma diversum*. The condition must be differentiated from infectious pustular vulvovaginitis (IPV), the venereal form of bovine herpesvirus-1.

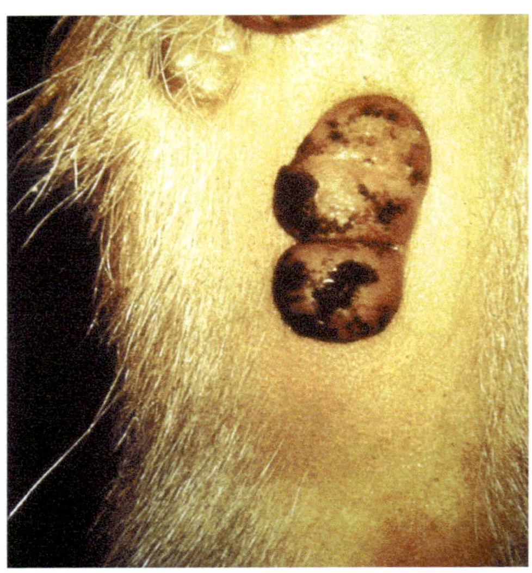

Fig. 10.42. Ox. Perineum. Fibropapilloma. Viral in origin. The growth affects the skin of the perineum next to the external genitalia (see Chapter 12: Diseases of the Integument).

10.4 GRAVID UTERUS

Introduction. Pregnancy adds, next to the developing conceptus, another organ dimension for discussion: the placenta and concept of placentation. This section introduces bovine placentation, contains incidental findings on placental membranes that may be confused with pathologic changes, presents examples of pregnancy disorders, defines embryonic and fetal death, and discusses infectious abortion diseases, fetal malformations, and prolonged gestation.

Placental membranes surrounding the fetus are the chorioallantois and amnioallantois, both fused membranes. They are separated by cavities containing defined amounts of fluid. The umbilicus forms the attachment of the fetus to the fetal membranes.

As a temporary organ, the placenta is functionally diverse. It protects the developing conceptus and facilitates exchange of nutrients. It produces enzymes, prostaglandins, cytokines, and transient hormones, all responsible for the maintenance of pregnancy.

10.4.1 Cotyledonary placentation

Based on anatomic appearance, bovine placentation is classified as epitheliochorial cotyledonary, with *cotyledons* of the chorioallantois and uterine *caruncles* as the maternal counterpart forming the attachment site known as the placentome.

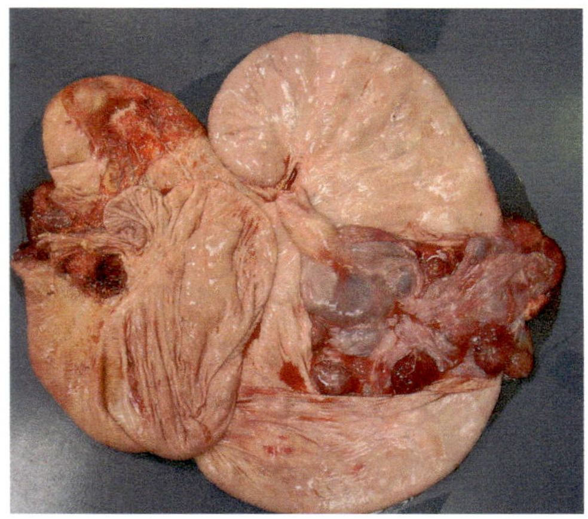

Fig. 10.43. Ox. Uterus. Placentation. *In situ* presentation of placental attachment sites (placentomes).

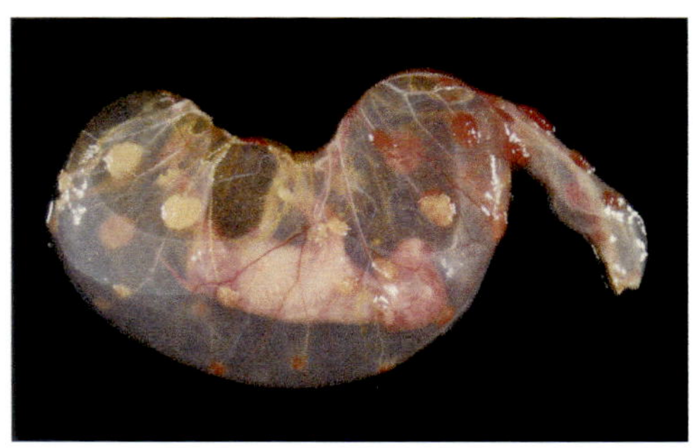

Fig. 10.44. Ox. Fetus *in situ*. Placental attachment sites distributed as button-like structures along both uterine horns. The fetus is enveloped by fluid-filled, transparent placental membranes.

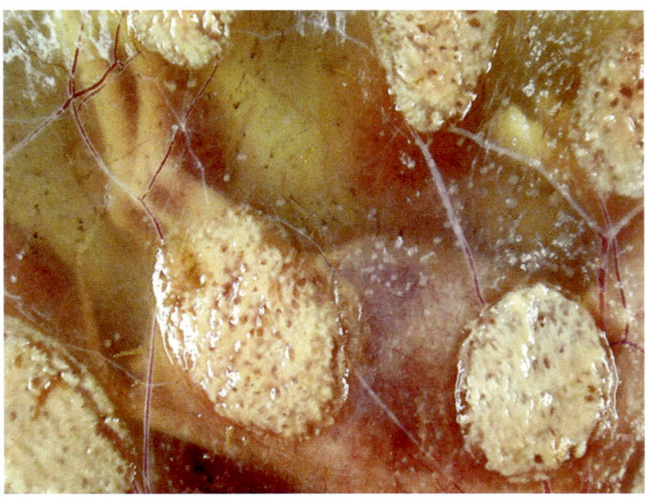

Fig. 10.45. Ox. Uterus. Placental cotyledons. Button-like structures on the chorionic side are cotyledons, the fetal interface interdigitating with maternal caruncles. The space between cotyledons is referred to as intercotyledonary. The small, white granules in the intercotyledonary spaces are calcium deposits, discussed under Fig. 10.46.

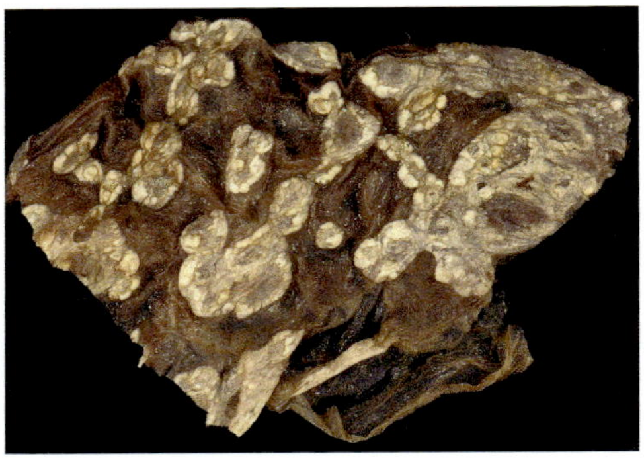

Fig. 10.47. Ox. Amnion. Epithelial plaques. Representing metaplastic keratinized squamous epithelium, the white elevated structures on the fetal side of the amnion should not be confused with mycotic placentitis. They vary in size and are incidental findings. Cause unknown.

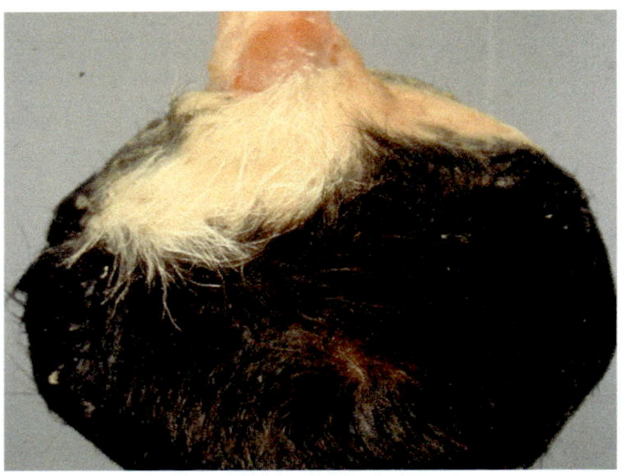

Fig. 10.49. Ox. Amorphous globosus. A round, solid structure covered by black and white hair and attached to the placenta is typically passed with the placental membranes after parturition of a healthy calf. On the cut section, the ovoid structure frequently reveals connective, adipose, muscle and osseous tissues. An amorphous globosus is thought to be the result of embryonic maldevelopment of a second fetus recognized in pregnancy with dizygotic twins (incomplete twin). Differential diagnoses include placental teratoma or mummified fetus.

10.4.2 Incidental findings on placental membranes

These should not be confused with pathologic changes.

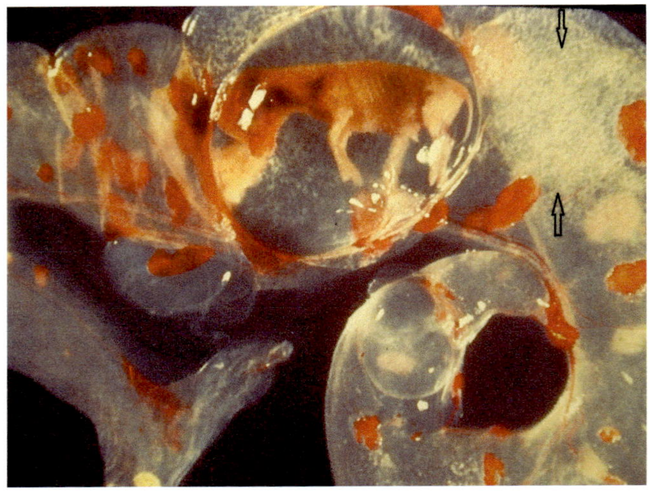

Fig. 10.46. Ox. Chorion. Calcium deposits. Conceptus. Dense, white granules (arrows) on the chorionic interface between cotyledons are calcium deposits distributed along capillaries. The deposits represent a physiologic process when they form between day 60 and 4 months of gestation, and create a depot to be incorporated into the rapidly developing skeletal system of the fetus.

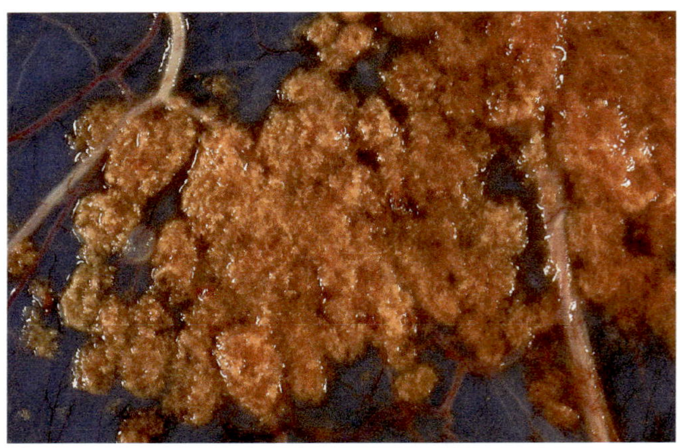

Fig. 10.48. Ox. Chorion. Adventitial placentation. A common finding in older cows, accessory cotyledons have formed between cotyledons. Advanced cases of adventitial placentation may be associated with hydroallantois.

10.4.3 Disturbances of pregnancy

Pregnancy is a complex event. Multiple factors can interfere, beginning with the zygote and terminating with late gestation. In early embryonic death, the conceptus disintegrates and resorption takes place with delayed commencement of estrus. During the later phases of gestation, the conceptus dies *in utero* and is expelled (abortion). Both infectious and non-infectious causes are involved.

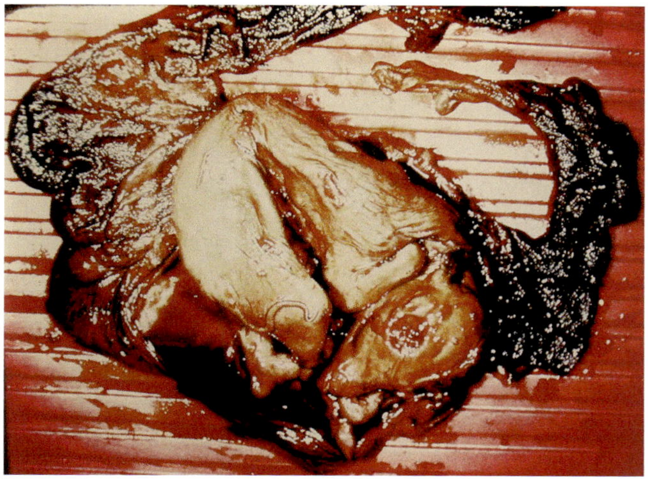

Fig. 10.50. Ox. Placenta. Fetal mummification. A dehydrated, desiccated fetus with sunken eye socket and yellow discoloration rests on a decomposed placenta. The process of mummification takes place for months. Bovine viral diarrhea virus (BVDV) and *Neospora caninum* have been associated with mummification.

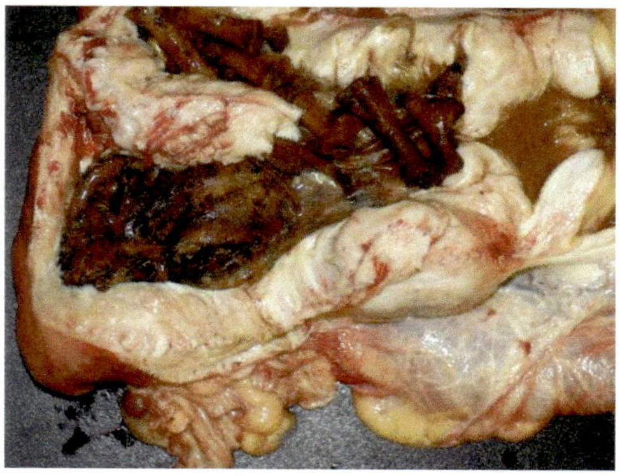

Fig. 10.51. Ox. Uterus. Fetal maceration. A composite of blood-tinged, putrefied, soft tissues and bones is contained in the uterus, with a thickened wall from chronic inflammation. When bacteria are present following fetal death *in utero*, the fetus will undergo bacterial degradation, leaving only bones behind after maceration. The infected uterine environment creates septic clinical signs in the affected cow. (Courtesy of Dr J. Roberts, University of Auburn, USA.)

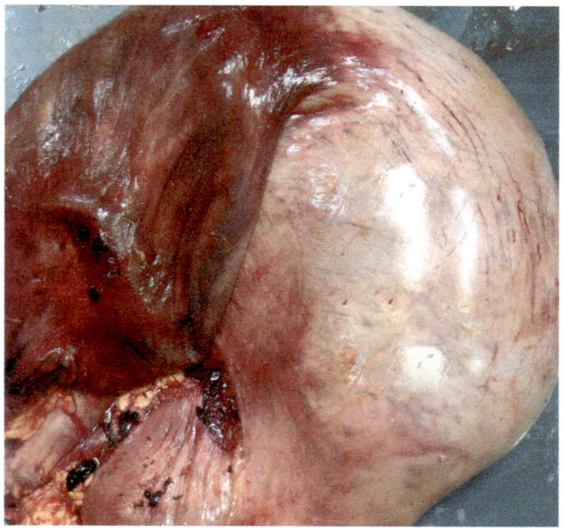

Fig. 10.52. Ox. Pregnant uterus. Tear. A major segment of the uterine wall is torn and associated with some hemorrhage. The wall of the uterus may subsequently rupture, interrupting gestation. Torsion of the uterus, leading to devitalization of the uterine wall, is another example of a compromised pregnancy.

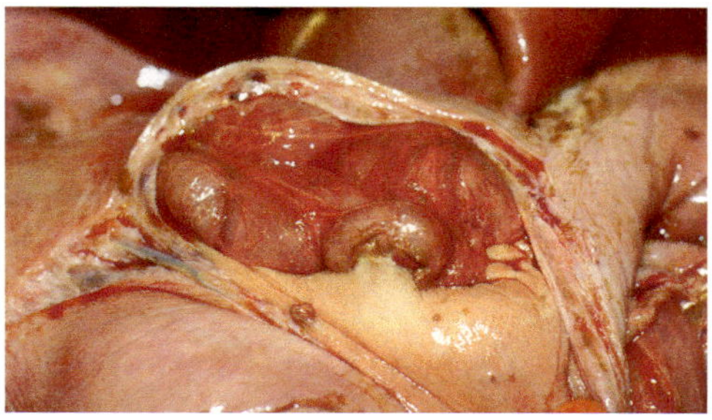

Fig. 10.53. Ox. Uterus. Placental retention. An edematous, brown/tan decomposed placenta rests within the uterus. The condition is associated with abnormalities of parturition such as dystocia, but also with vascular, nutritional (hyposelenosis) and hormonal factors. If retained for longer than 12 h post-partum, a devitalized placenta functions as growth medium for contaminating bacteria, to induce severe endometritis and metritis. (Courtesy of the Government of Alberta, Canada.)

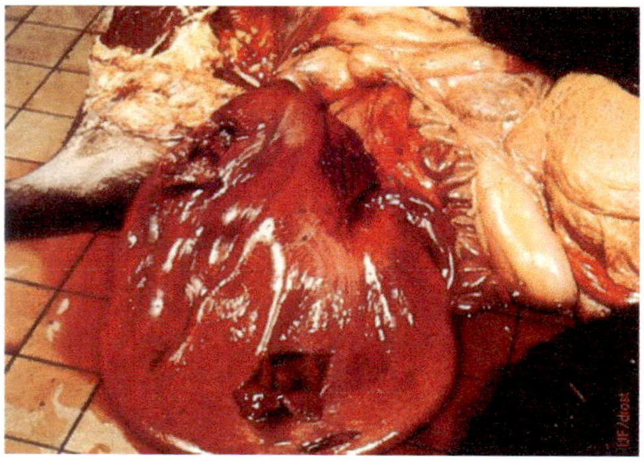

Fig. 10.54. Ox. Uterus. Torsion. A severely congested pregnant uterus twisted along its longitudinal axis. (Courtesy of Dr M. Drost, Drost Project, University of Florida, USA.)

10.4.4 Abortion diseases

Introduction. Abortion is defined as the expulsion of a dead fetus at any period of gestation. Dead fetuses expelled at term gestation are called stillbirths. Viable fetuses born alive before expected parturition are called premature.

The determination of the cause(s) of an abortion is notoriously difficult. When known, there are non-infectious and infectious factors to be differentiated with infectious agents more amenable for specific diagnosis.

Non-infectious causes in the cow are metabolites, toxins, plants, and trauma.

Infectious agents encompass viruses, bacteria, fungi, and protozoa. Infectious agents may contribute to up to 80% of bovine abortions, most being bacterial in origin.

10.4.4.1 Pathogenic principles of infectious abortions

In cattle, the hematogenous route is the most preferred for infectious agents to reach the placenta and fetus. Transcervical, ascending infection is less common. Additional routes of infection include venereal pathogens, contaminated semen, transferred embryos, and pre-existing infectious endometritis/metritis.

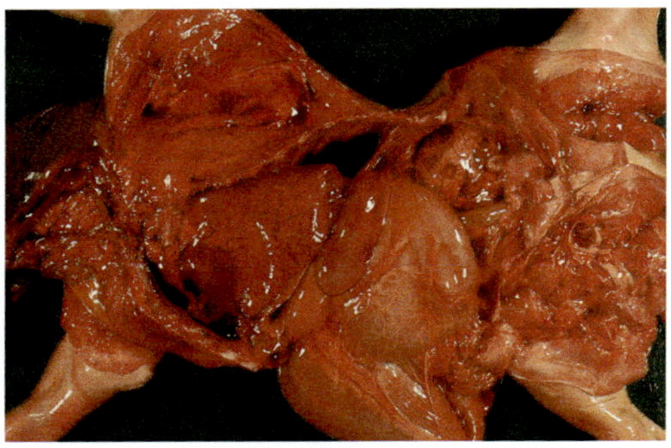

Fig. 10.55. Ox. Bovine herpesvirus type 1 (BHV-1) abortion. Whole body. Fetal autolysis. Abortion occurs in mid- to late-term gestation. The fetus dies *in utero* and stays there for 1 or 2 days before expulsion, causing autolysis. There are usually no gross changes except liver necrosis, reflected as subtle, light gray foci in more fresh cases.

Principal modalities of infection in which abortions may be expected are: (i) systemic infection (bacteremia) of the dam, as with salmonellosis; (ii) infection of the placentome, as with brucellosis and other abortigenic bacteria, fungi, and protozoa; and (iii) fetal invasion via the vascular route (usually leptospirosis, listeriosis, salmonellosis, campylobacteriosis) or amniotic fluid (some bacteria, fungi with fetuses having skin, eyelid, lung, and gastrointestinal tract (GIT) lesions), both originating from preceding placental infection.

10.4.4.2 Viral abortions

Viruses involved in bovine abortions are bovine herpesvirus type 1 (BHV-1), bovine viral diarrhea virus (BVDV), bluetongue virus (BT), and bunyavirus, including Schmallenberg virus.

Bovine herpesvirus type 1 (BHV-1)

Introduction. Up to 60% of unexposed, unvaccinated pregnant cows may abort (abortion storm). Abortions occur late in gestation. A lag period of several weeks may exist between natural exposure of the dam to the herpesvirus and subsequent abortion. Clinical signs of infection are usually absent in the dam. Abortion typically occurs several days after fetal death *in utero*.

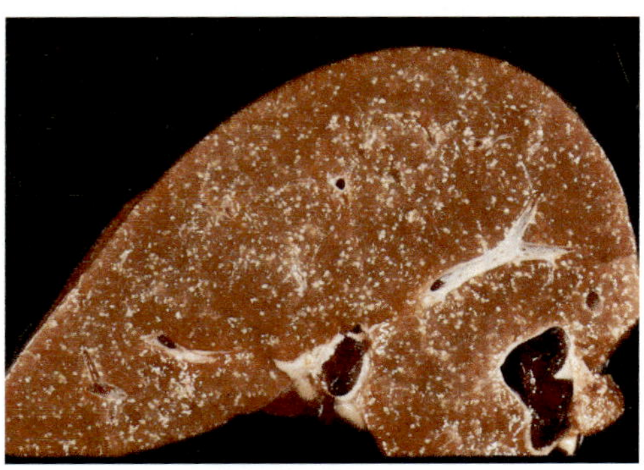

Fig. 10.56. Ox. Bovine herpesvirus type 1 (BHV-1) abortion. Liver. Multifocal necrosis. Atypically, multiple white foci of necrosis are disseminated throughout a well-preserved liver. The majority of cases have no gross foci of necrosis, and the diagnosis is made histologically.

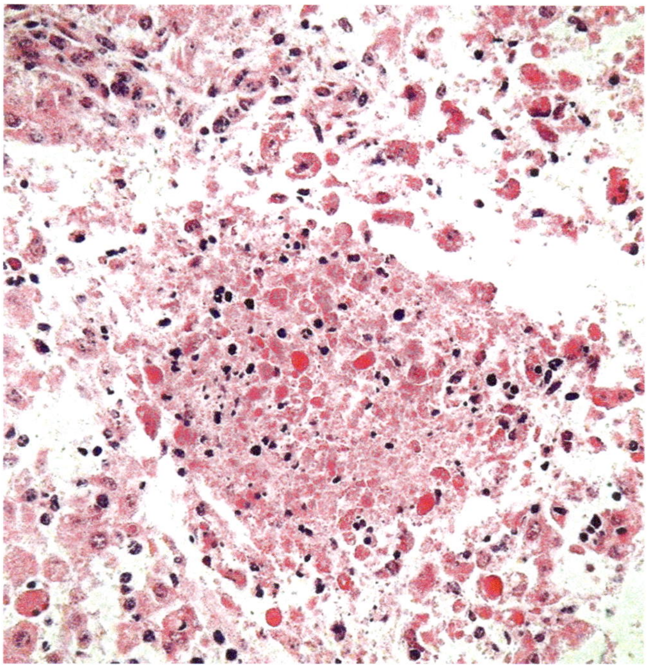

Fig. 10.57. Ox. Bovine herpesvirus type 1 (BVH-1) abortion. Liver. Focal necrosis. Karyorrhexis and karyolysis with chromatin stippling are evident in an autolytic liver. One may identify, with difficulty, intranuclear herpesvirus inclusion bodies in viable hepatocytes in the periphery of the necrotic focus (H&E).

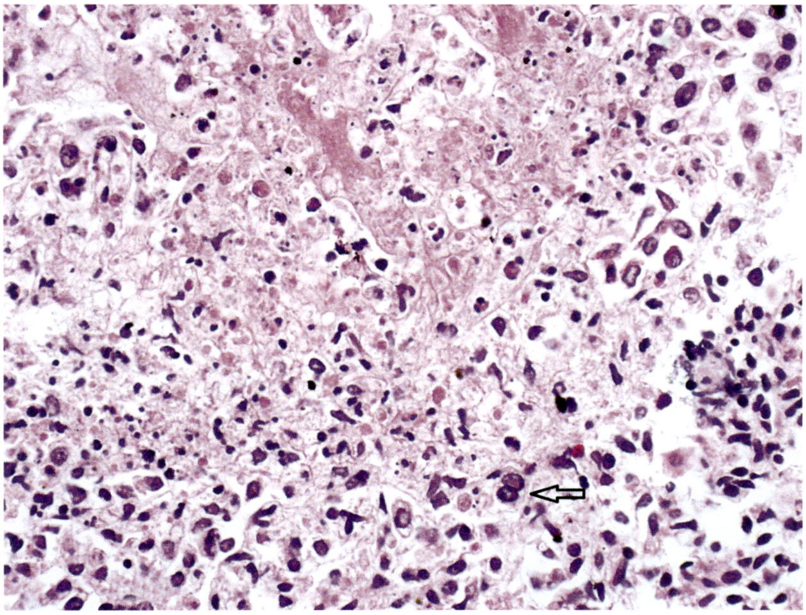

Fig. 10.58. Ox. Bovine herpesvirus type 1 (BHV-1) abortion. Lung. Necrosis. A pink, acellular focus of coagulative necrosis is surrounded by cellular debris. Some faint herpesvirus inclusions (arrow) are present in the periphery (H&E).

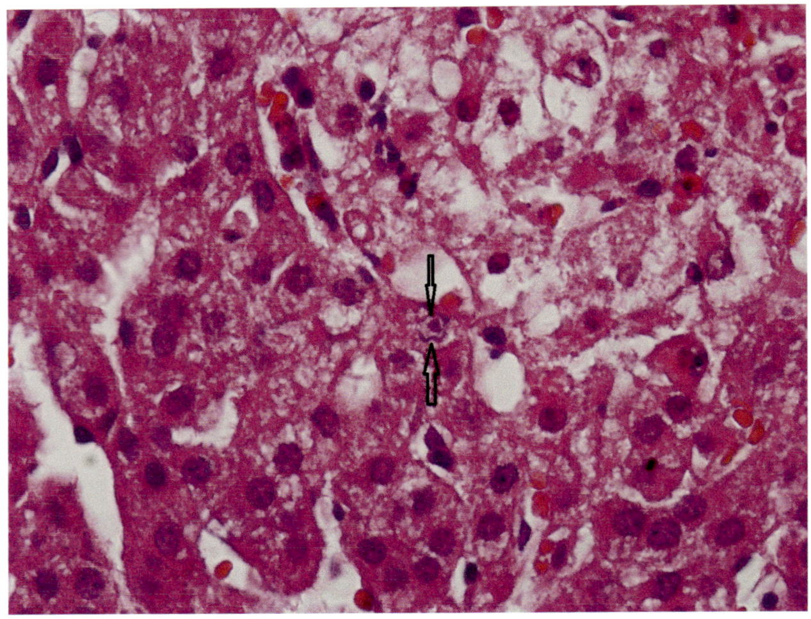

Fig. 10.59. Ox. Bovine herpesvirus type 1 (BHV-1) abortion. Adrenal gland. Intranuclear herpesvirus inclusion body in adrenal cortical cell (arrows). Adrenal glands should always be collected and examined for BHV-1 abortion diagnosis. The cortex of the adrenal gland is the most amenable tissue to search for herpesvirus intranuclear inclusion bodies.

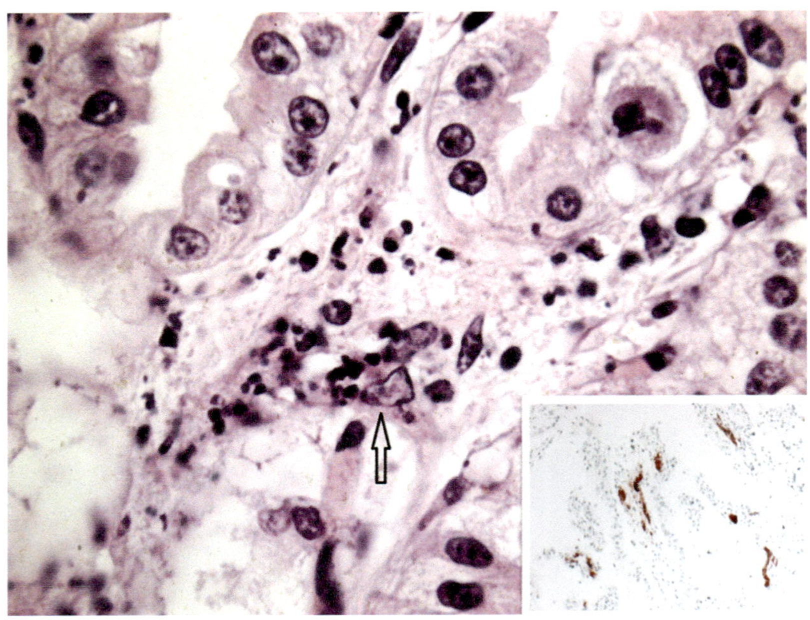

Fig. 10.60. Ox. Bovine herpesvirus type 1 (BHV-1) abortion. Placenta. Lymphoplasmacellular chorionitis. A few mononuclear inflammatory cells are located in the chorionic stroma. A viral intranuclear inclusion body is visible (arrow) (H&E). Inset: viral antigen is demonstrated in villi capillaries with indirect immunohistochemistry (IHC).

Bovine viral diarrhea virus (BVDV)

Introduction. Aborted fetuses vary in range of size and viability. Mummification is an alternative gross finding. Mid-gestational infection may result in the birth of weak calves with congenital malformations (cerebellar hypoplasia and other). (See Chapter 1: Diseases of Neonatcs and Calves.) Calves may be born small, with stunted growth, or premature. Calves may be born as persistently infected (PI) when exposed to the virus between 2 and 4 months of gestation. PI calves occur when the dam is exposed to BVDV-1, BVDV-2, or HoBi-like viruses (not identified in US herds).

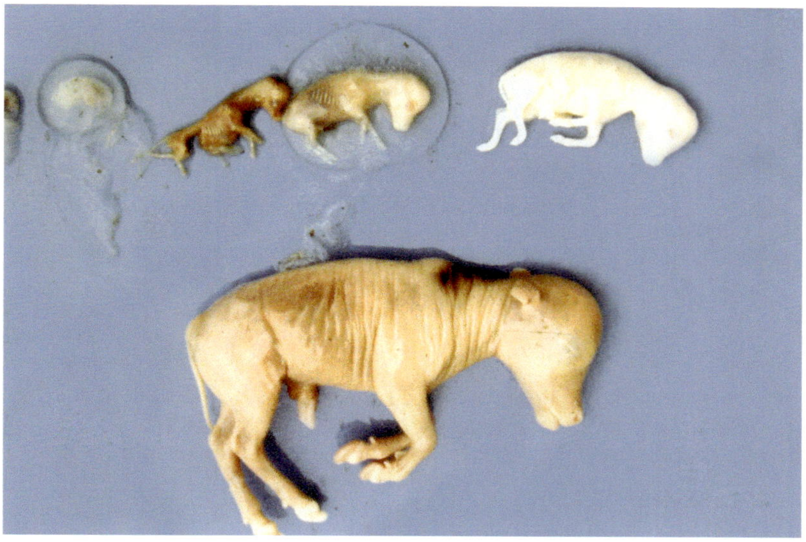

Fig. 10.61. Ox. Bovine viral diarrhea virus (BVDV) abortion. Fetuses. Early gestational aborted fetuses varying in size.

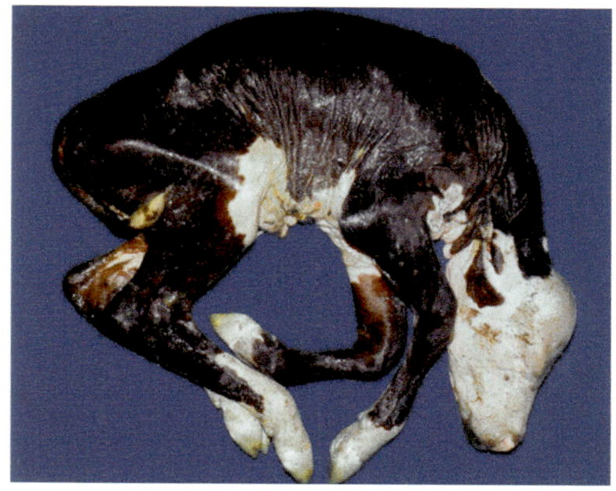

Fig. 10.62. Ox. Bovine viral diarrhea virus (BVDV). Term fetus. Small body presentation for gestational age.

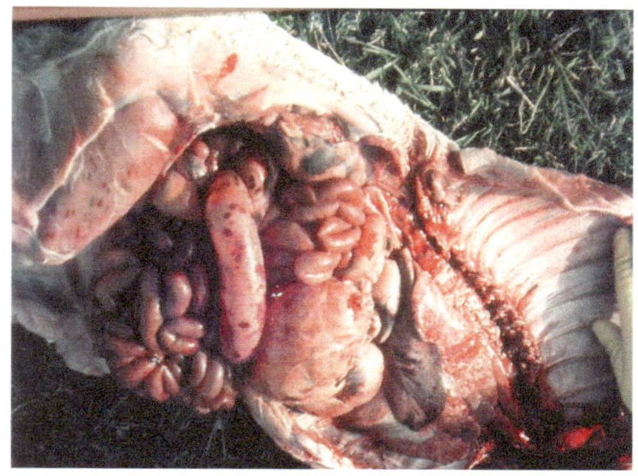

Fig. 10.63. Ox. Bovine viral diarrhea virus (BVDV) abortion. Abdominal cavity. Thrombocytopenic strain. Late-term aborted fetus with petechiae on serosal surfaces. Cytopathogenic BVD-1 subtype b or BVDV type 2 are isolated from these calves.

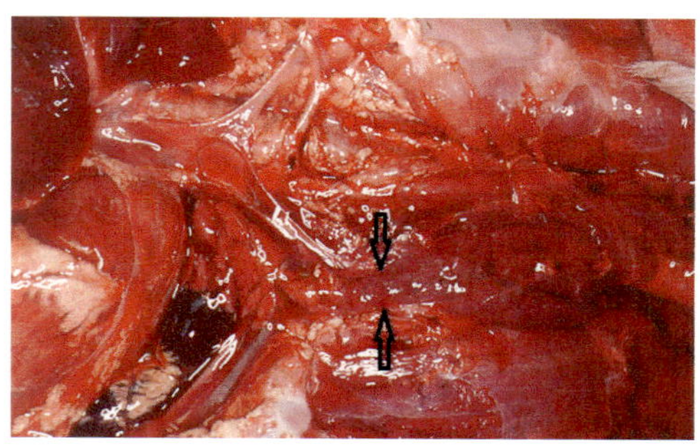

Fig. 10.64. Ox. Bovine viral diarrhea virus (BVDV) abortion. Thymus. Atrophy. Thymic tissue (arrows) is barely visible. Other gross findings may be cardiomegaly, liver congestion, and ascites.

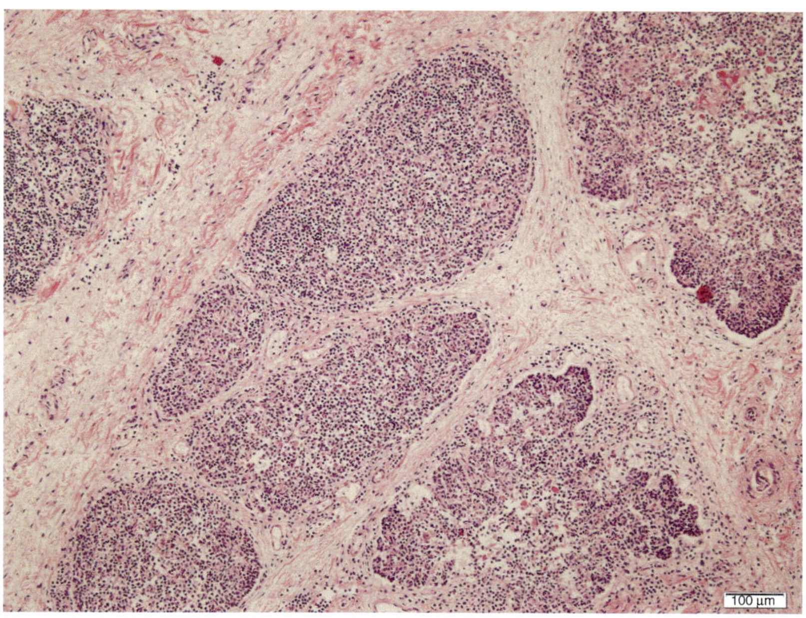

Fig. 10.65. Ox. Bovine viral diarrhea virus (BVDV) abortion. Thymus. Lymphoid depletion. Thymic lobules are poorly populated with lymphocytes, best evidenced in the cortex (H&E).

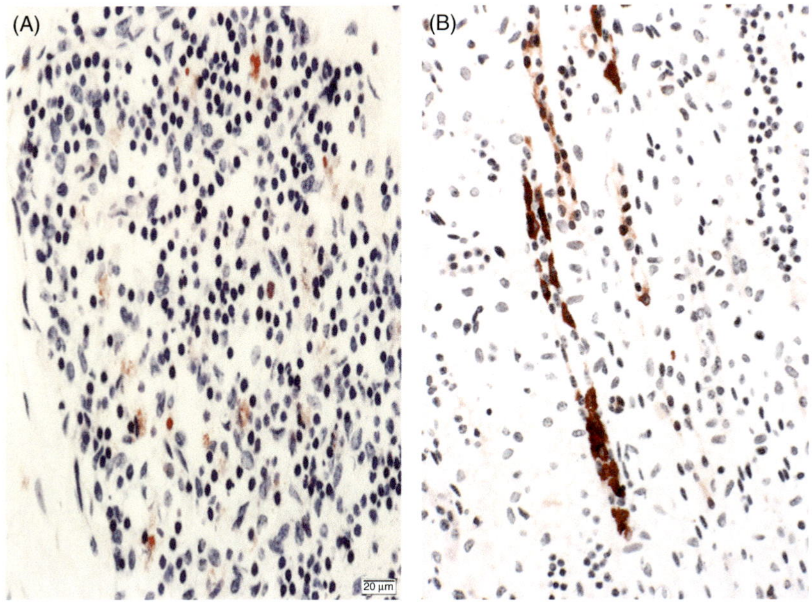

Fig. 10.66. Ox. Bovine viral diarrhea virus (BVDV) abortion. (A) Thymus. Viral antigen is demonstrated in lobular cells. (B) Kidney. Viral antigen is demonstrated in the cytoplasm of renal tubular cells (IHC).

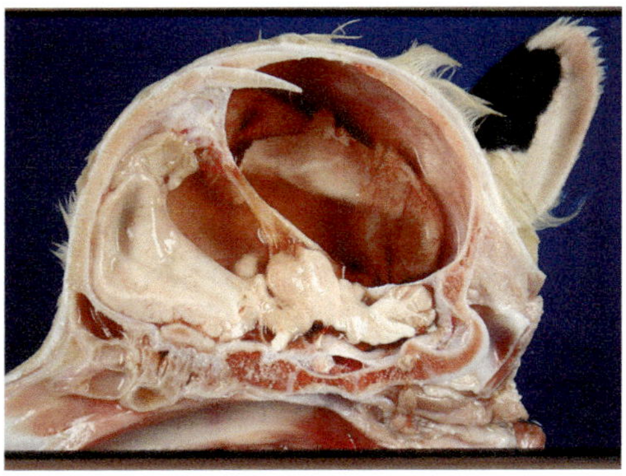

Fig. 10.67. Ox. Brain. Bluetongue virus (BT). Hydrocephalus. The brain parenchyma has been markedly compressed and replaced due to excessive fluid in ventricles, with only forebrain, corpus callosum, and cerebellum left. Meningeal membranes are folded.

Bluetongue virus (BT)

Introduction. Bluetongue virus is an Orbivirus transmitted by *Culicoides* midges. Though more detrimental to sheep fetuses regarding abortions, the virus targets the brain of calves 70–150 days into gestation. Calves will be born rather than aborted, with CNS lesions such as hydranencephaly, porencephaly, and hydrocephalus. (Also see Chapter 5: Diseases of the Gastrointestinal Tract.)

Schmallenberg virus (SBV)

Introduction. In 2011, a novel virus of the family Bunyaviridae, genus Orthobunyavirus, was identified on the continent of Europe following abortions of malformed calves, lambs, and goat kids. Malformations affected the CNS system, especially the brain, and musculoskeletal system (limbs). Intrauterine infection was thought to occur at gestation days 60–180. Involvement of biting midges in the transmission was postulated. **Clinical signs** in aborting dams were fever, drop in milk production, and diarrhea.

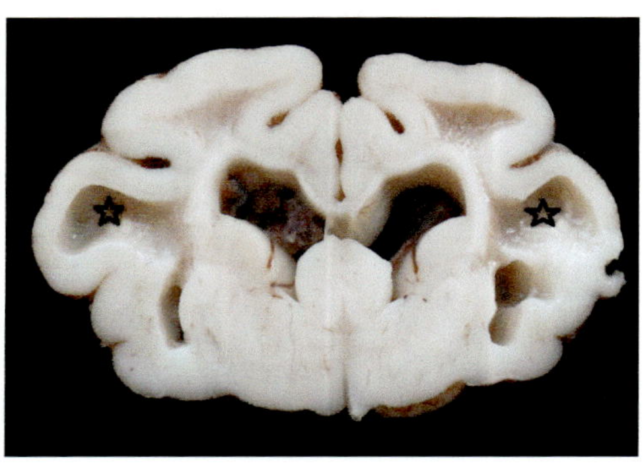

Fig. 10.69. Ox. Schmallenberg virus (SBV) abortion. Brain. Porencephaly. Coronal section of the brain exhibits multiple cavitations (asterisks) in the white matter substance. Additional malformations of the brain can include hydrocephalus, hydranencephaly, and cerebellar hypoplasia. (Courtesy of Dr M. Bruegmann, LAVES, LVI, Oldenburg, Germany.)

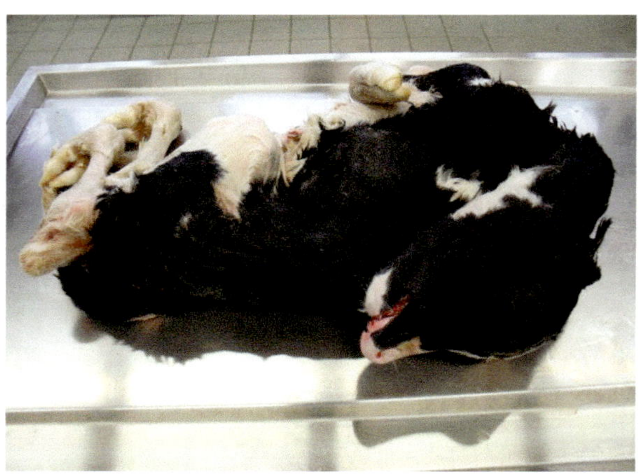

Fig. 10.68. Ox. Schmallenberg virus (SBV) abortion. Whole body. Arthrogryposis. Deformed angulation of limbs and torticollis. (Courtesy of Dr M. Bruegmann, LAVES, LVI, Oldenburg, Germany.)

Miscellaneous abortifacient viruses

These include parainfluenza 3 virus (P-3), bovine herpesvirus-4 and bovine herpesvirus -6, and bovine parvovirus infection.

10.4.4.3 Bacterial abortions

A variety of gram-positive and gram-negative bacterial pathogens are recognized as abortifacients. Most bacterial abortions are observed during the second and third trimester of gestation.

When present, gross lesions include an exudative chorionitis (placentitis), pneumonia, and fibrinous polyserositis in the thoracic or abdominal cavities. Histologic changes are frequently a severe fibrinonecrotic chorionitis containing clusters of bacterial colonies and neutrophilic bronchopneumonia.

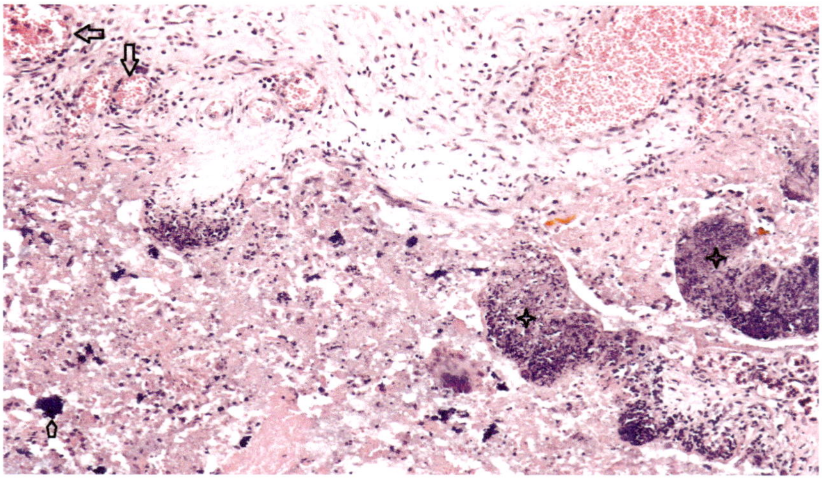

Fig. 10.70. Ox. Chorion. Fibrinonecrotic chorionitis. Prototype of bacterial placentitis. There is microscopic evidence of severe necrosis of villi intermixed with fibrin. Necrotic debris contains clusters of basophilic cellular debris, clumps of bacilli (asterisks), and dense basophilic aggregates of mineral deposits (short open arrow). Stromal blood vessels are rimmed by mild amounts of lymphocytes (open arrows). *Campylobacter* spp. were isolated in this case (H&E).

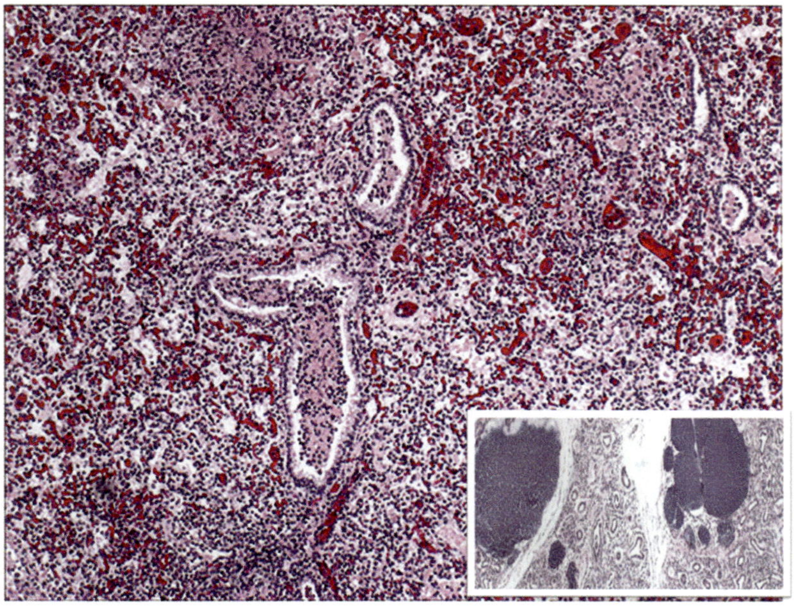

Fig. 10.71. Ox. Lung. Prototype fetal pneumonia. Purulent bronchopneumonia. Bronchioles are filled with neutrophils and fibrin. Alveoli are distended with neutrophils and lymphocytic aggregates. *Brucella abortus* was isolated in this case (H&E). Inset: demonstration of bacterial clusters in fetal bronchopneumonia (*Staphylococcus* spp.) (H&E).

Brucellosis

Introduction. *Brucella abortus* infection in cattle has been contained in many countries. In Northern America, however, the organisms, have a reservoir in the American bison (*Bison bison*). Infection occurs from contaminated aborted fetuses or placental tissue.

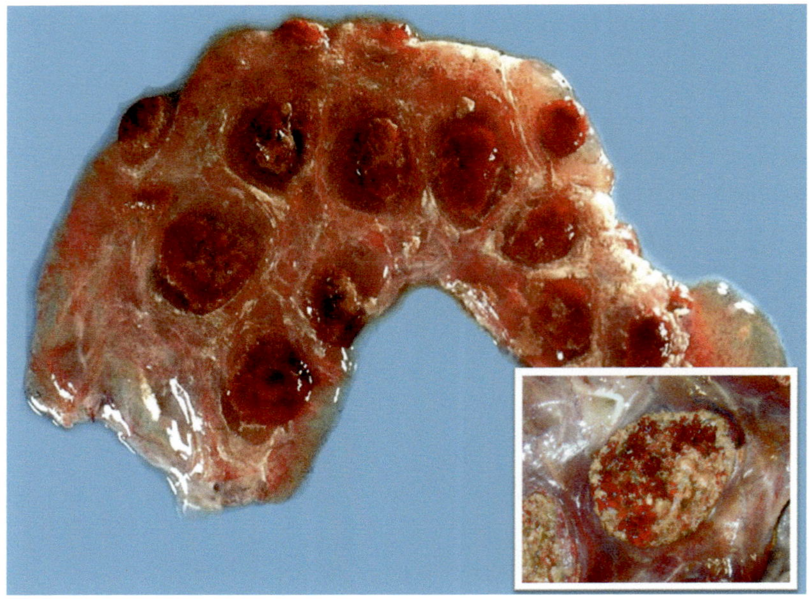

Fig. 10.72. Brucellosis. Chorion. Fibrinonecrotic chorionitis. Typically, the cotyledons, and in severe cases the intercotyledonary spaces, are thickened by fibrinonecrotic material and bloody exudates. (Courtesy of Dr J.M. King and Section of Anatomic Pathology, Cornell University, USA.) Inset: fibrinonecrotic chorionitis from bison. (Courtesy of Dr W. Layton, Bozeman, Montana, USA.)

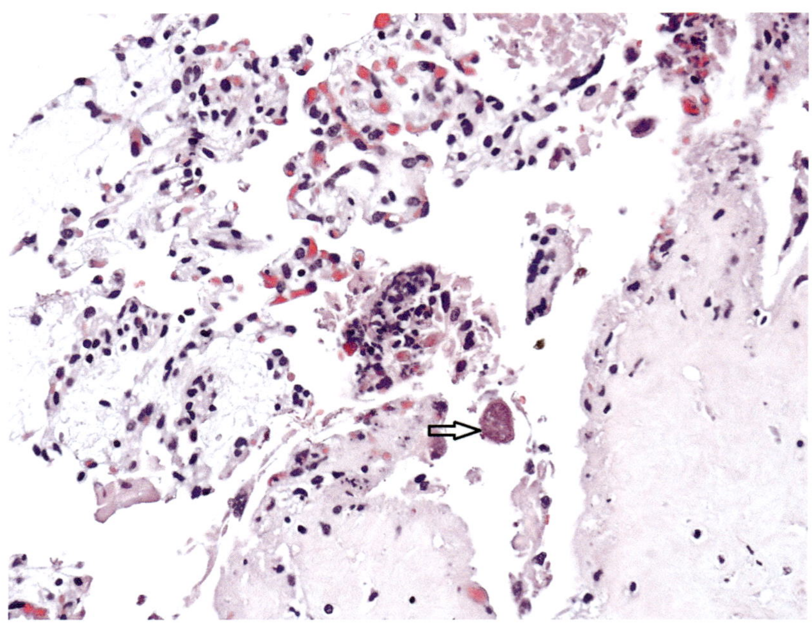

Fig. 10.73. Ox. Brucellosis. Chorion. Chronic placentitis. The placental trophoblast is invaded by *Brucella* bacteria (arrow). Bacteria replicate within trophoblastic cells. A vasculitis in the chorionic stroma is an additional microscopic feature in brucellosis, but can also be seen in other bacterial abortions such as *Chlamydophila abortus*, *Campylobacter* spp. (H&E).

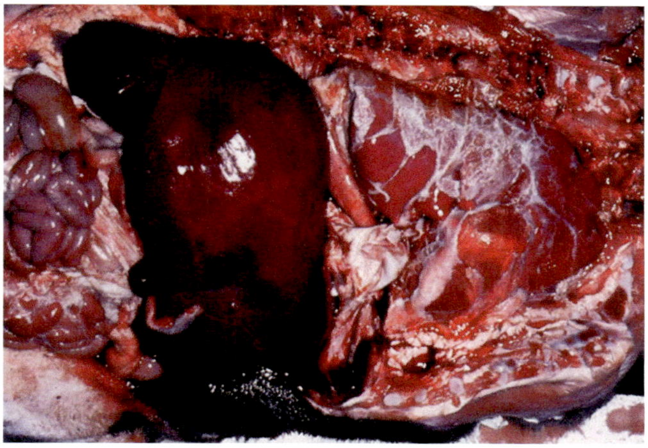

Fig. 10.74. Ox. Brucellosis. Lung. Fibrinous pleuritis. The pleura is covered by a film of white material. Such a lesion is also present in *Campylobacter* spp. abortion.

Leptospirosis

Introduction. Serovars involved in bovine abortions are *Leptospira interrogans* serovars *hardjo* and *pomona*. Serovar *hardjo* has now been incorporated into the genus *Leptospira borgpetersenii*. Infections result in abortions of midterm fetuses to term calves.

Clinical signs. Dams may exhibit icterus, anemia, and hemoglobinuria in acute infections.

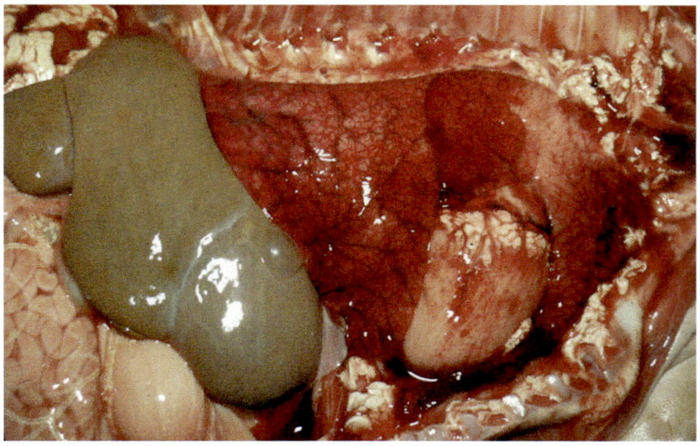

Fig. 10.75. Ox. Leptospirosis. Whole body. The liver exhibits a tan/green discoloration, suggesting bile retention.

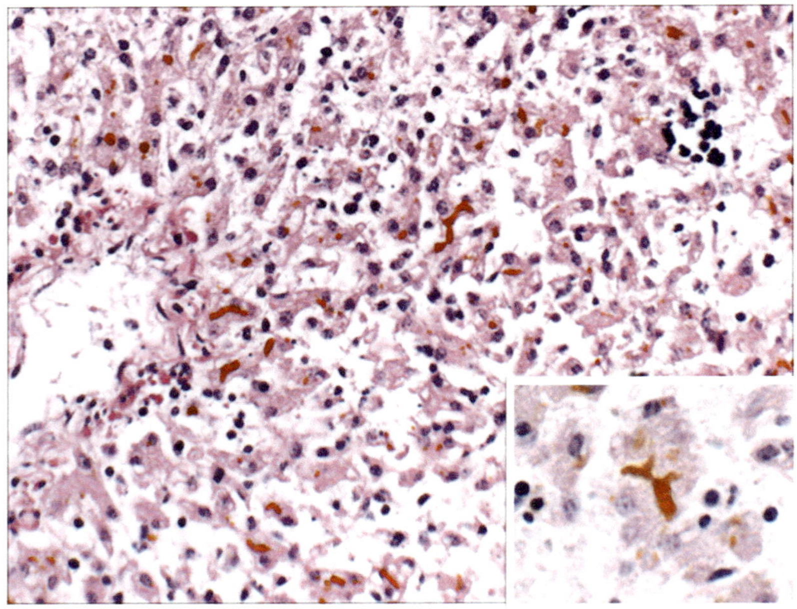

Fig. 10.76. Ox. Leptospirosis. Liver. Bile retention. Bile cananiculi contain bile plugs. Inset: higher magnification of bile retention (H&E).

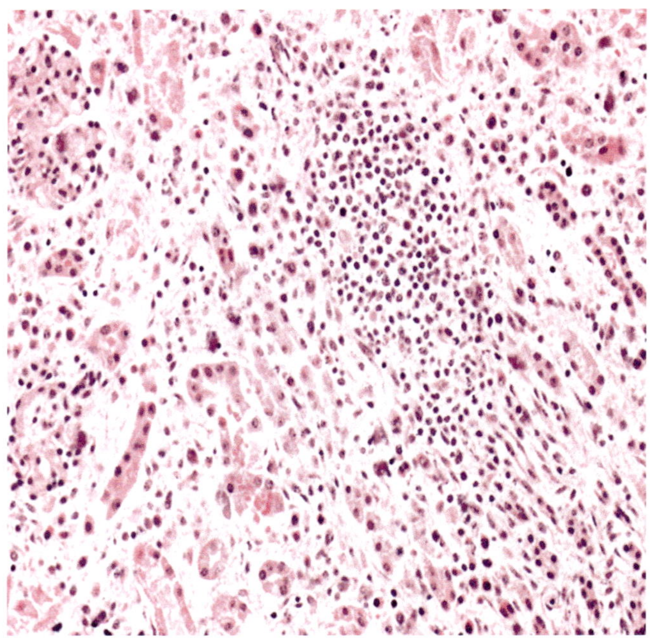

Fig. 10.77. Ox. Leptospirosis. Kidney. Interstitial nephritis. Microscopic features of tubulointerstitial lymphocytes are seen in the minority of bovine fetuses with leptospirosis, and are therefore non-diagnostic (H&E).

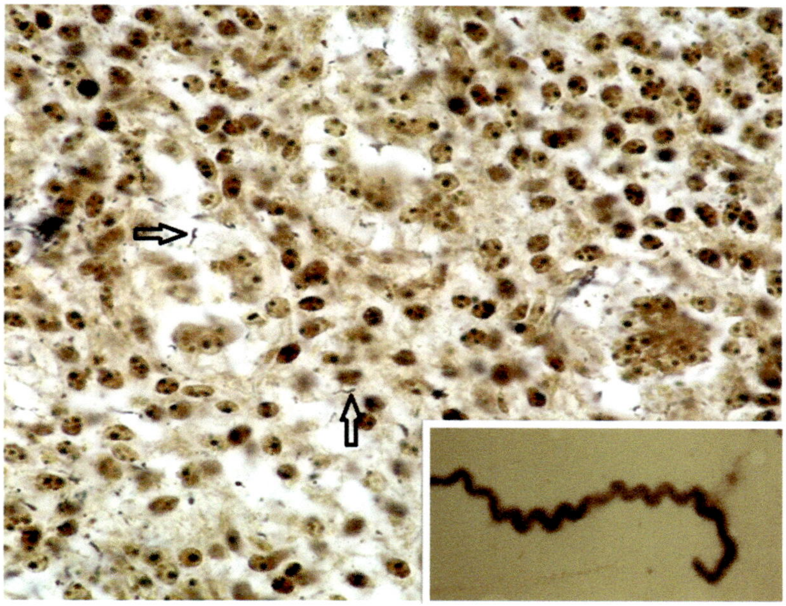

Fig. 10.78. Ox. Leptospirosis. Kidney. A silver stain demonstrates dark spirochetes in kidney samples (arrows). Inset: isolated silver-stained spirochetes (Warthin–Starry).

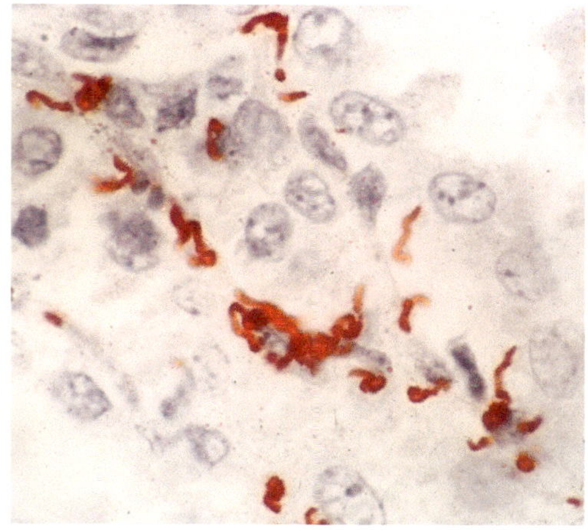

Fig. 10.79. Ox. Leptospirosis. Kidney. Demonstration of *Leptospira* spp. by indirect immunohistochemistry (IHC). Most diagnostic laboratories use kidney polymerase chain reaction (PCR) for leptospirosis testing. Fluorescent antibody testing of fetal kidney smears can be applied for the diagnosis, as also can darkfield microscopy of fetal fluids.

Listeriosis

Introduction. Caused by *Listeria monocytogenes* and *Listeria ivanovii*, abortions are usually sporadic and occur during the last trimester. Placental retention is encountered in the aborting dam.

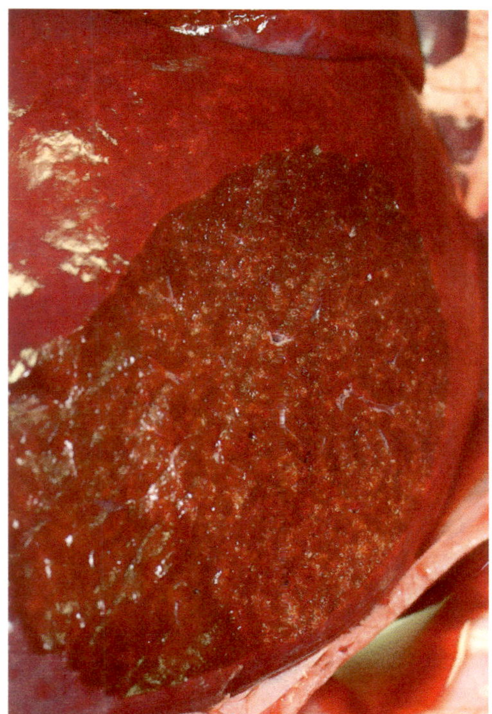

Fig. 10.80. Ox. Listeriosis. Liver. Necrotizing hepatitis. Small, white foci are visible through the capsule. Infectious bovine rhinotracheitis (IBR) should be suspected more often. (Reprinted with permission from *Kirkbride's Diagnosis of Abortion and Neonatal Loss in Animals*, 4th edn, Fig. 2.8, p. 28, © Wiley-Blackwell, 2012.)

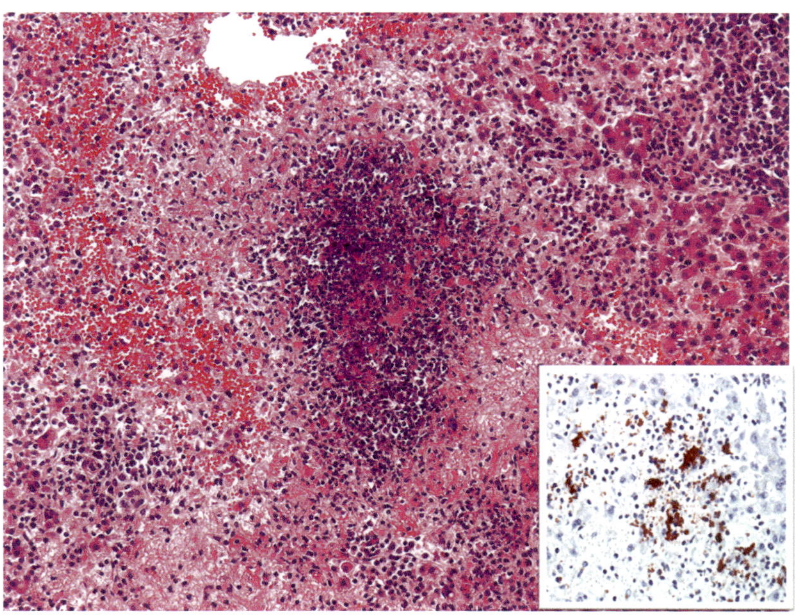

Fig. 10.81. Ox. Listeriosis. Liver. Necrotizing hepatitis. Foci of necrosis are scattered throughout liver (H&E). Inset: numerous bacilli are demonstrated by indirect immunohistochemistry (IHC).

Other histologic findings include suppurative placentitis.

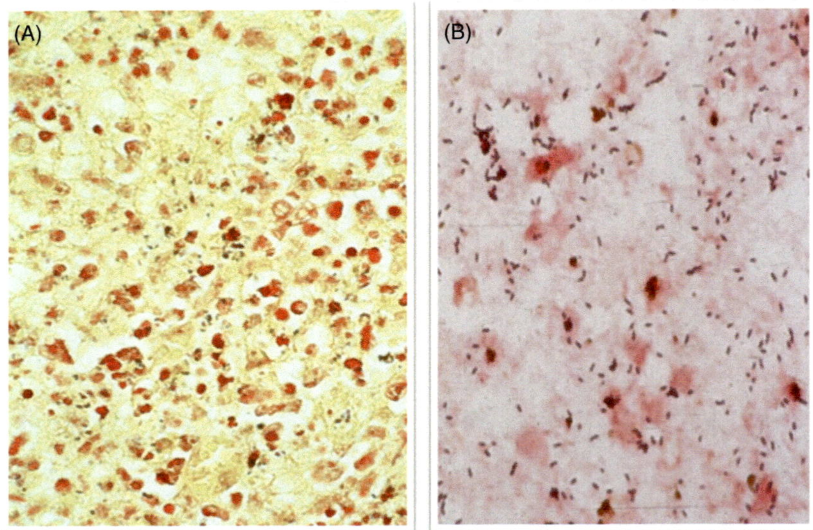

Fig. 10.82. Ox. Listeriosis. Liver. Diagnostic demonstration of bacilli. (A) A Gram stain reveals multiple positive rods between hepatocytes (Brown & Brenn). (B) A stained liver smear identifies multiple rods (Gram stain).

Intravascular multiplication of *Listeria* bacilli can be seen in histologic sections of lung and brain as well.

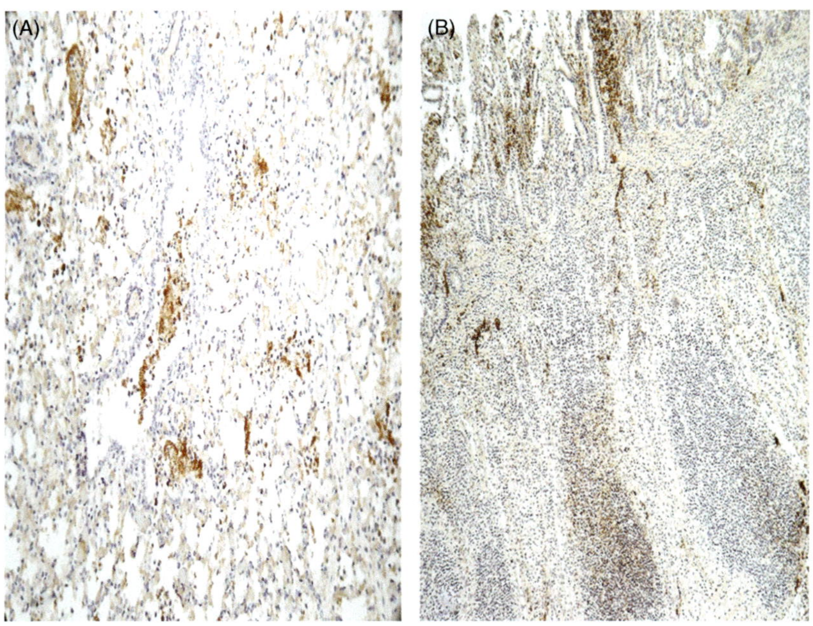

Fig. 10.83. Ox. Listeriosis. (A) Kidney. (B) Jejunum. Immunohistochemical distribution of *Listeria* spp. in kidney and intestine (IHC).

Ureaplasma diversum

Introduction. Abortions occur during the last trimester. There may be stillbirths, or calves are born weak. *Ureaplasma diversum* is a resident of the non-pregnant bovine reproductive tract (see Fig. 10.41), thus contamination of the aborted fetus and placenta has to be ruled out by culturing the fetal lung. PCR is another preferred diagnostic tool.

Grossly, the amnion is affected in ureaplasmosis, showing thickening, foci of hemorrhage, fibrin exudation, and fibrosis.

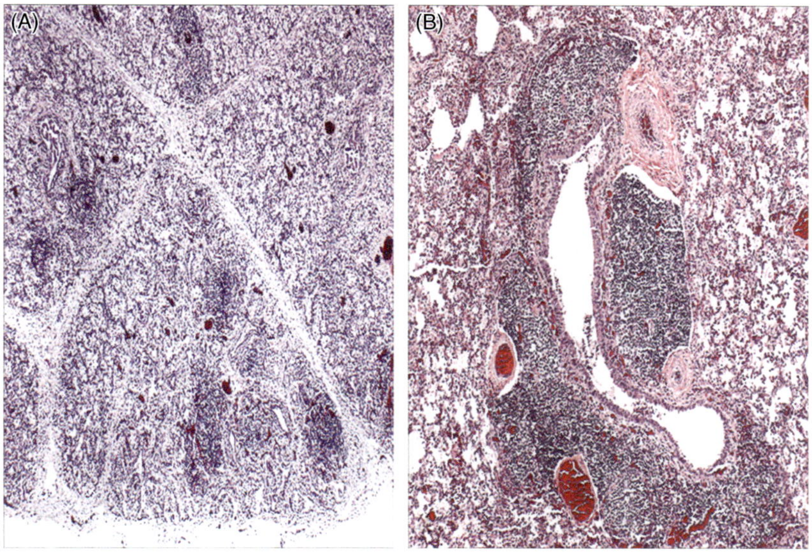

Fig. 10.84. Ox. Ureaplasmosis. Lung. Lymphocytic peribronchiolitis. (A) Aggregates of lymphocytes are scattered throughout the lung parenchyma. (B) On higher magnification, lymphocytic aggregates are closely associated with the wall of bronchioles (H&E).

Campylobacteriosis

Introduction. *Campylobacter* spp. involved in abortions are *Campylobacter fetus* subsp. *venerealis*, transmitted venereally, and *Campylobacter fetus* subsp. *fetus* and *Campylobacter jejuni*, transmitted from the intestinal tract. The latter causes abortion in late-term gestation.

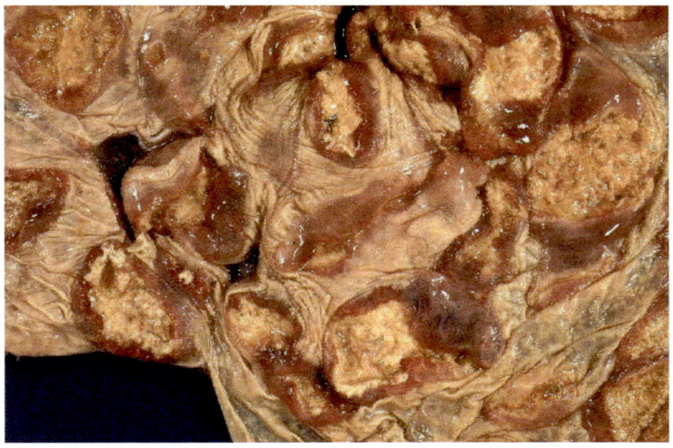

Fig. 10.85. Ox. Campylobacteriosis. Chorioallantois. Necrosuppurative chorionitis. Cotyledons are covered by a dry, necrotic exudate. The intercotyledonary areas are diffusely thickened and opaque. *Campylobacter jejuni* was isolated. Differential diagnosis: mycotic placentitis.

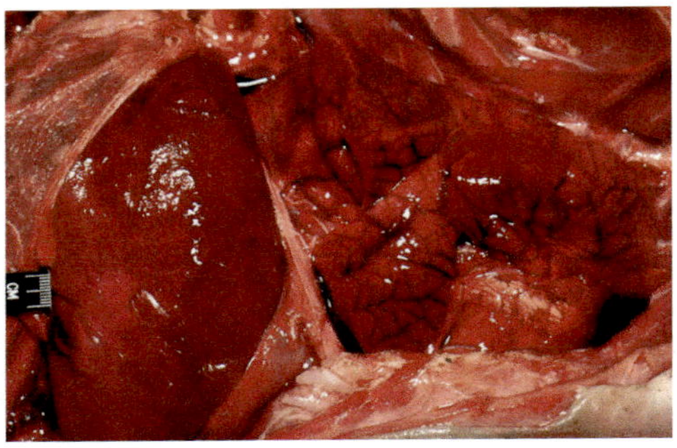

Fig. 10.87. Ox. Campylobacteriosis. Lung. Edema. The lungs are wet and prominent. The lobular interstitium is expanded by fluid.

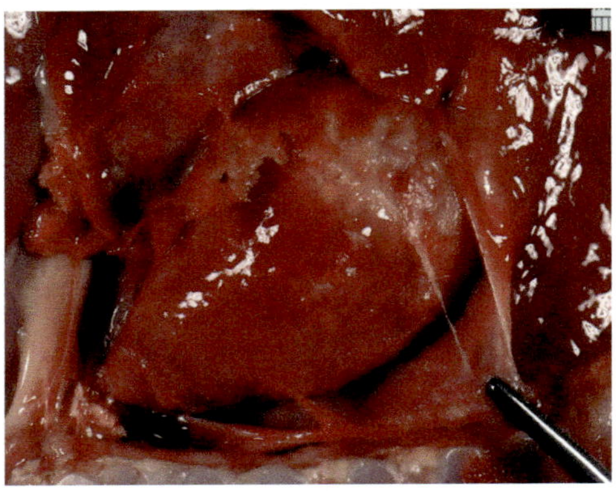

Fig. 10.88. Ox. Campylobacteriosis. Heart. Fibrinous pericarditis. Gross changes of the aborted fetus include fibrinous polyserositis of internal organs, especially the pericardial sac. (Reprinted with permission from *Kirkbride's Diagnosis of Abortion and Neonatal Loss in Animals*, 4th edn, Fig. 2.13, p. 34, © Wiley-Blackwell, 2012.)

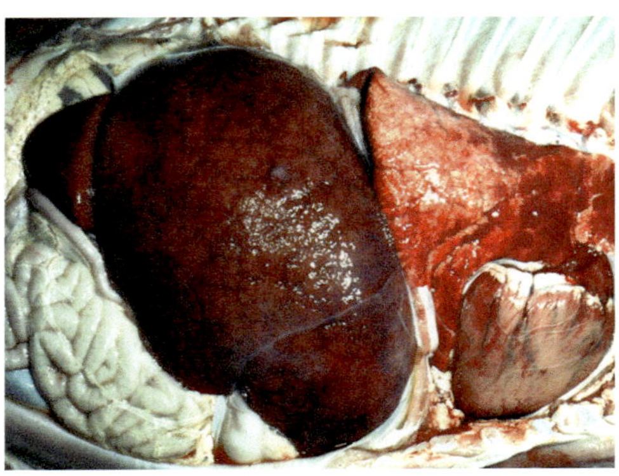

Fig. 10.90. Ox. Epizootic bovine abortion (EBA). Liver. Hepatomegaly. A cobblestone pattern of an enlarged liver is a distinctive morphologic feature in EBA. Other common gross findings are ascites and enlargement of the spleen and lymph nodes.

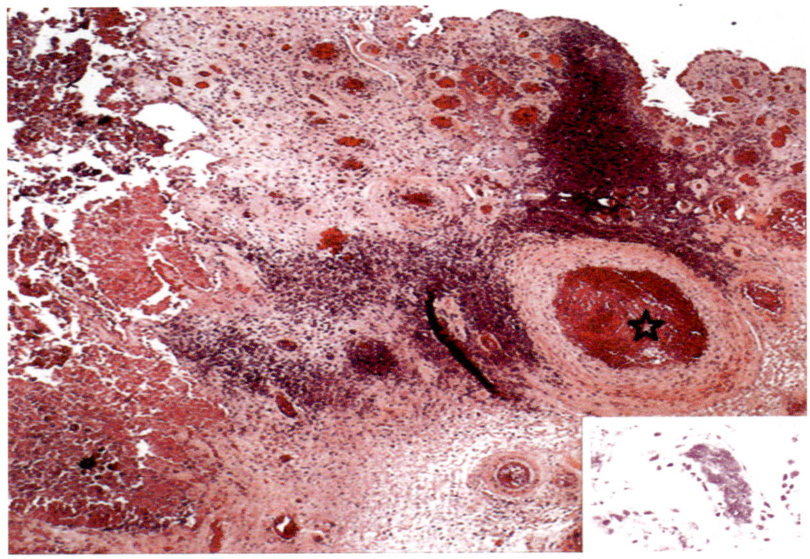

Fig. 10.86. Ox. Campylobacteriosis. Necrotizing chorionitis. Villi are distorted by the presence of a fibrinous exudate and a mixed inflammatory infiltrate. A medium-sized stromal artery (asterisk) is partially thrombosed (H&E). Inset: an arteriole showing clumps of *Campylobacter* bacilli (Brown and Brenn).

Epizootic bovine abortion (EBA)

Introduction. Known to be transmitted to pregnant cattle by ticks (*Pajaroello*), the infecting organism of the condition also known as foothill abortion has largely escaped identification. The bacterium has now been named *Pajaroellobacter abortibovis* and has been taxonomically placed in the order Myxococcales, suborder Sorangiineae, family *Polyangiaceae*. Diagnosis of the gram-negative bacterium can be achieved with a modified Gram and silver stain (Steiner) or indirect immunohistochemistry (IHC). Abortions occur to first-calf heifers or pregnant cows newly introduced to the foothills region on the west coast of the USA. Abortions occur during the last trimester, or calves are born weak or premature.

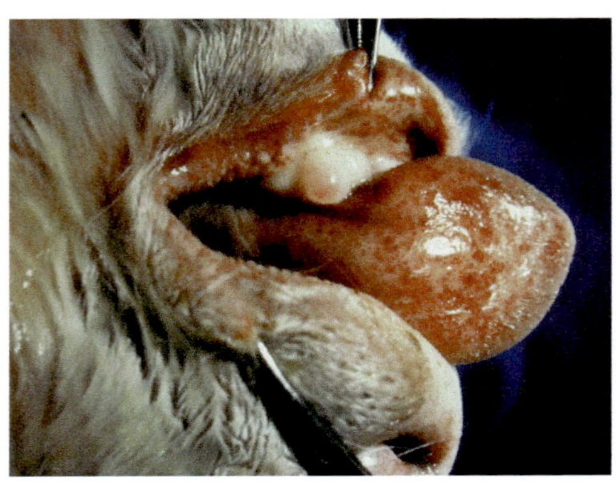

Fig. 10.89. Ox. Epizootic bovine abortion (EBA). Sublingual and oral mucosal petechial hemorrhage. Petechiae underneath the tongue are visible gross features for the diagnosis of EBA.

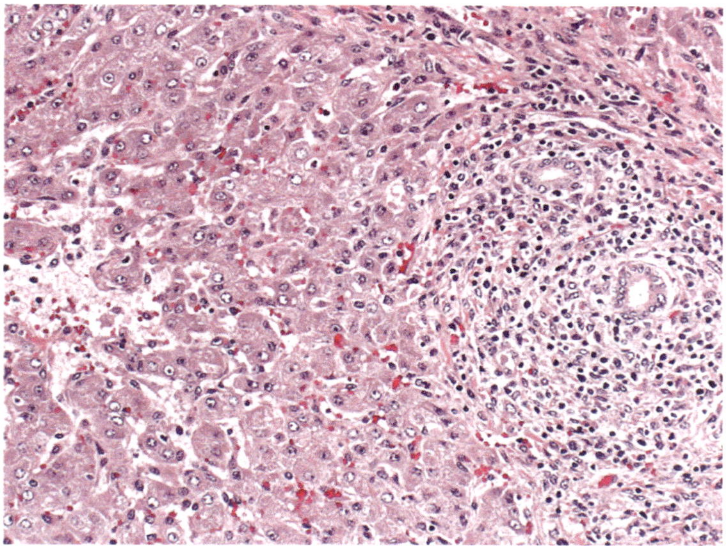

Fig. 10.91. Ox. Epizootic bovine abortion (EBA). Liver. Hepatitis. Portal triads are infiltrated by mononuclear cells, lymphocytes, and histiocytes (H&E).

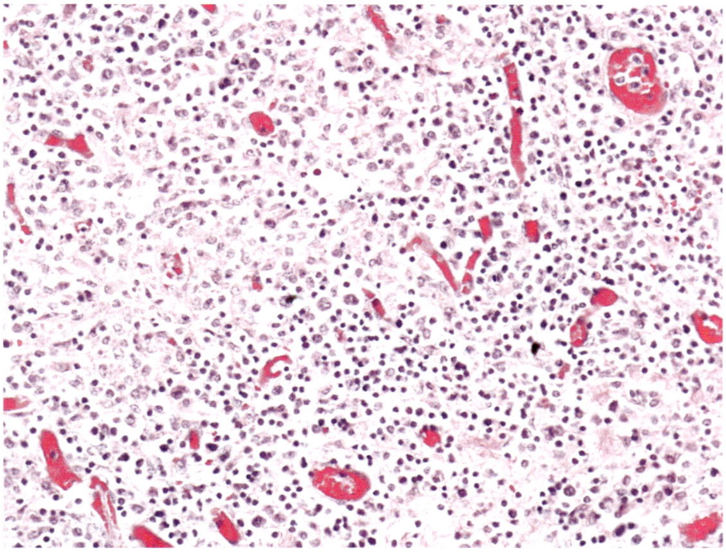

Fig. 10.92. Ox. Epizootic bovine abortion (EBA). Spleen. Histiocytic hyperplasia. Lymphoid hyperplasia and histiocytic infiltration of lymph nodes, and bone marrow are additional distinctive microscopic features in EBA (H&E).

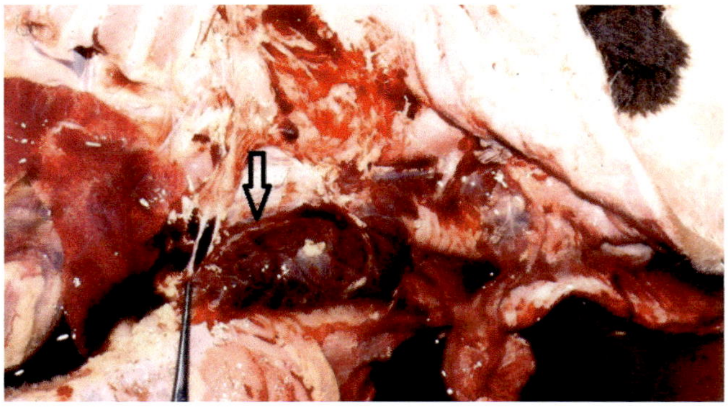

Fig. 10.93. Ox. Epizootic bovine abortion (EBA). Thymus. Hemorrhagic thymitis. The cervical portion of the thymus (arrow) is dark red, due to congestion and hemorrhage, with separation of the thymic lobules by serosanguinous fluid.

10.4.4.4 Mycotic abortions

Introduction. Fungal abortions are mainly encountered as sporadic events in cattle. *Aspergillus* spp. and Zygomycetes (*Absidia* spp., *Mucor* spp., *Rhizopus* spp.) are common isolates in the Western Hemisphere. Abortions occur late in pregnancy, and the placenta is often retained. Spread to the pregnant uterus is hematogenous.

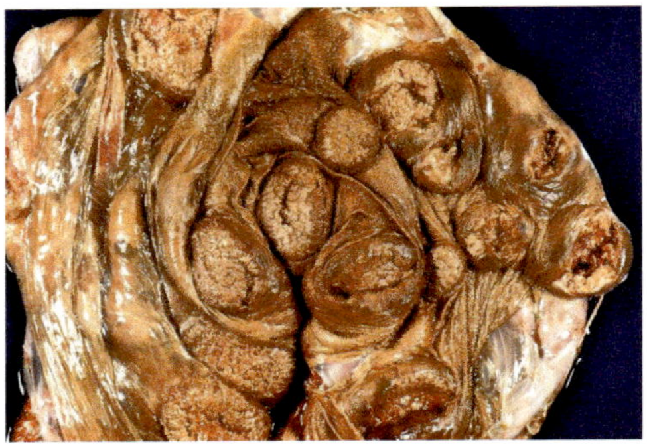

Fig. 10.94. Ox. Placenta. Mycosis. Necrosuppurative chorionitis. The placenta has a dry and thickened appearance. Cotyledons are covered by tissue debris.

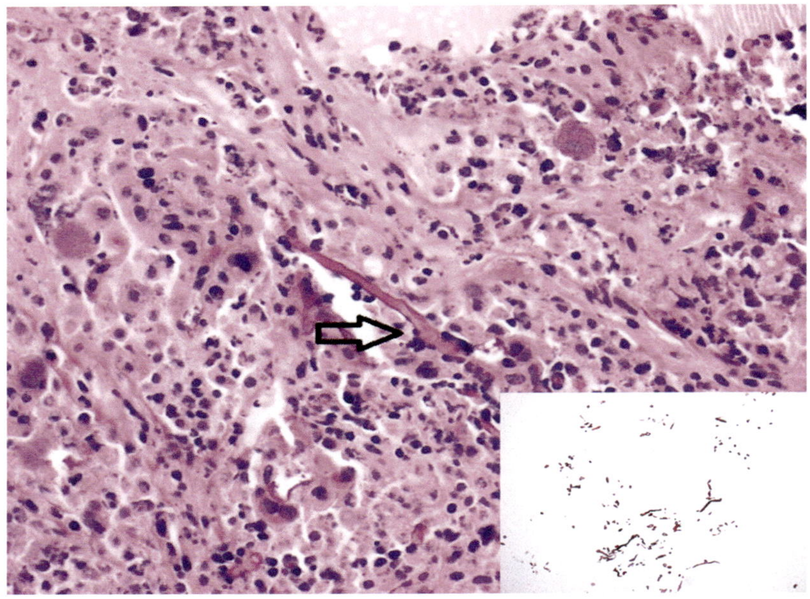

Fig. 10.95. Ox. Placenta. Mycotic placentitis. There is necrotic debris and a mixed cellular infiltrate on the chorionic surface. A fungal hypha (arrow) is located in the center of the image (periodic acid–Schiff). Inset: a special stain identifies a myriad of fungal hyphae. *Absidia* was recovered (silver stain).

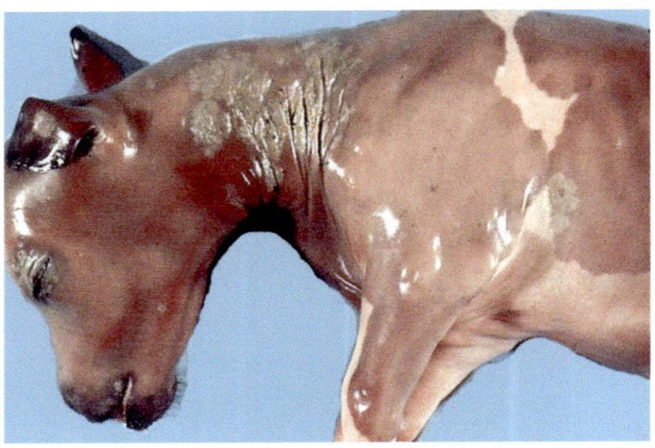

Fig. 10.96. Ox. Whole body. Aborted fetus. Fungal dermatitis. The skin over the neck is covered by greenish plaques. A stained smear taken from this area will demonstrate fungal organisms easily. (Courtesy of Dr J.M. King and Section of Anatomic Pathology, Cornell University, USA.)

10.4.4.5 Protozoal abortions

Introduction. *Tritrichomonas foetus* and *Neospora caninum* are the main pathogens to consider. *Toxoplasma gondii* and *Sarcocystis* spp. are rarely involved in bovine abortions. Unidentified apicomplexa protozoa have also been described.

Trichomoniasis

Introduction. *T. foetus* is transmitted through coitus. It causes pyometra in the non-pregnant cow. When infecting the pregnant animal, early embryonic death is the usual outcome. The protozoon can be observed in late-term abortions as well. Gross lesions are usually absent in aborted fetuses. Occasionally, a mild rumenitis can be encountered. Microscopic changes can be diagnosed in the placenta and lung.

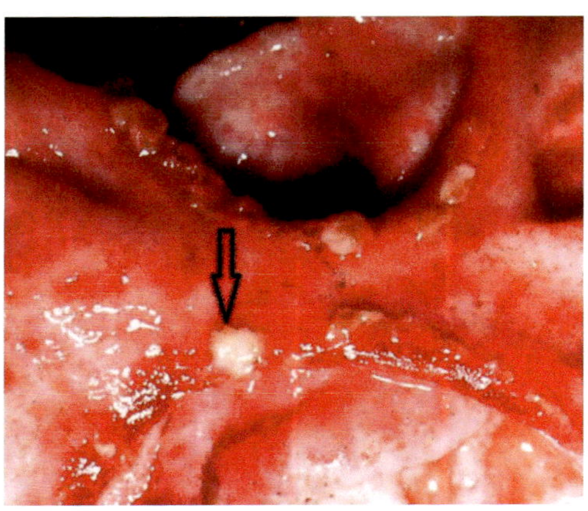

Fig. 10.97. Ox. Trichomoniasis. Rumen. Proliferative rumenitis. An elevated white plaque (arrow) occupies the mucosa. (Courtesy of Dr P. Blanchard, University of California, Davis, USA.)

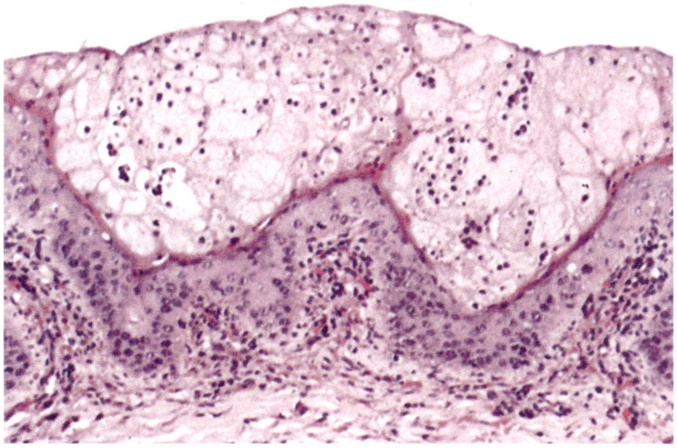

Fig. 10.98. Ox. Trichomoniasis. Rumen. Plaque. The focal mucosal elevation is composed of swollen and vacuolated, non-keratinized squamous cells that are infiltrated by lymphocytes. Lymphocytes also occupy the superficial lamina propria (H&E). (Courtesy of Dr P. Blanchard, University of California, Davis, USA.)

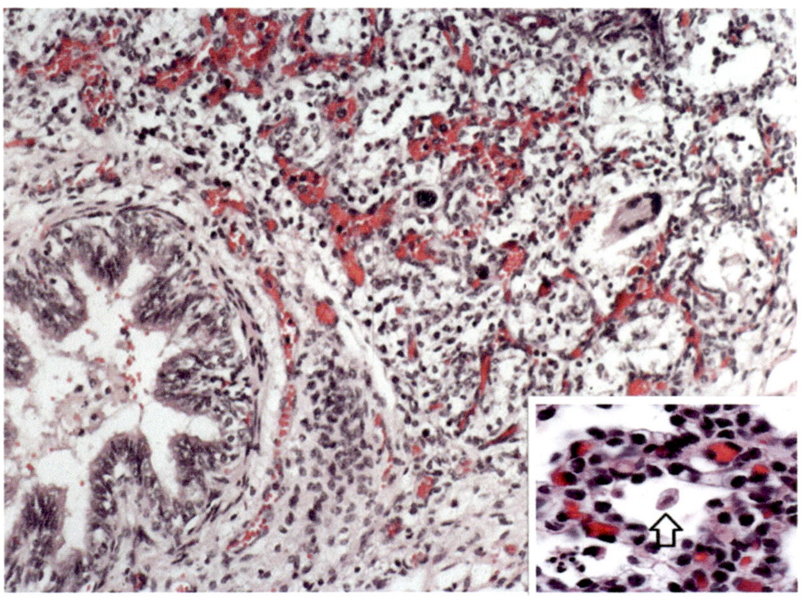

Fig. 10.99. Ox. Trichomoniasis. Lung. Giant cell pneumonia. Alveoli are infiltrated moderately by mononuclear cells. An occasional Langhans' giant cell is interspersed. This type of giant-cell pneumonia is not specific for the diagnosis of trichomoniasis (H&E). Inset: a trichomonad (arrow) is visualized in an alveolus (H&E).

Neosporiasis

Introduction. *Neospora caninum* has been recognized as a major cause of bovine abortions. The protozoon must be differentiated from *Toxoplasma gondii* and *Sarcocystis* spp. by IHC and/or PCR. Abortion from *N. caninum* occurs mainly during midterm gestation. The protozoon is transmitted by dogs (exogenous transmission) or coyotes (sylvatic transmission) serving as definitive hosts. Non-pregnant infected cows can be reservoirs for the parasite in a herd and transmit the protozoon to the calf during pregnancy. An infected aborting cow may show no clinical signs. Calves, when developing arthrogryposis, may be born alive. Mummification or fetal anasarca from *N. caninum* infection are rare additional findings.

Sarcocystis spp. and *T. gondii* are remote agents to consider in the differential diagnosis for protozoal-induced abortions in cattle.

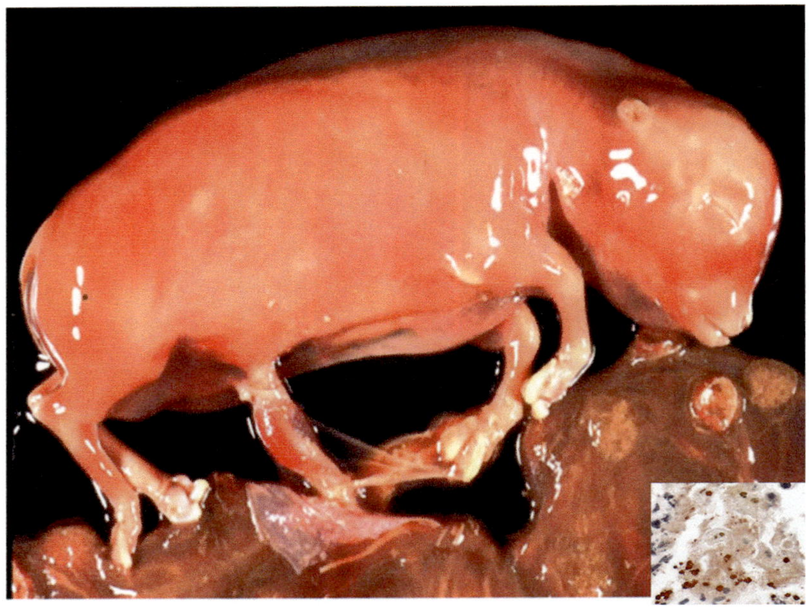

Fig. 10.100. Ox. Neosporiasis. Midterm abortion. Placenta. Placental edema. The chorioallantois membrane is thickened by watery fluid. Inset: demonstration of tachyzoites by indirect immunohistochemistry in placental stroma (IHC).

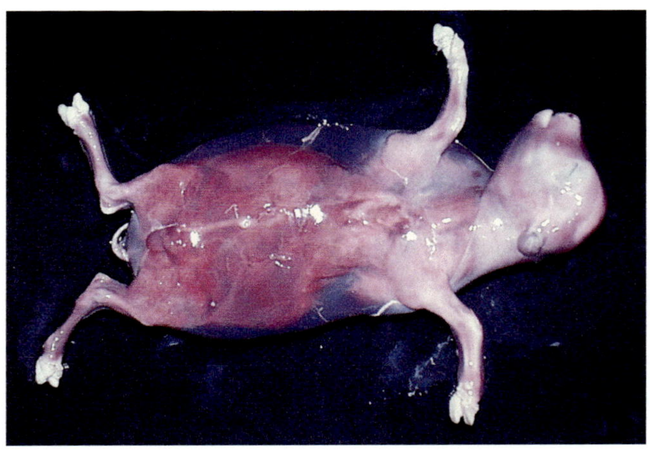

Fig. 10.101. Ox. Neosporiasis. Aborted midterm fetus. Anasarca. Watery fluid distends the subcutis.

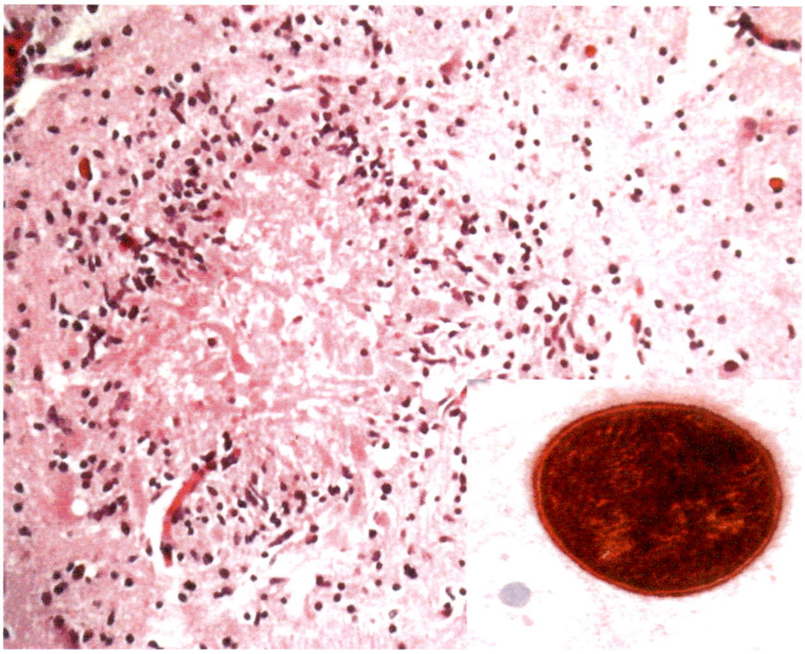

Fig. 10.102. Ox. Neosporiasis. Brain. Coagulative necrosis. A focus of coagulation necrosis in the neuropil is surrounded by mononuclear inflammatory cells. Glial cells are hyperplastic (H&E). Inset: an intensely stained tissue cyst is located in the cytoplasm of a neuron (IHC).

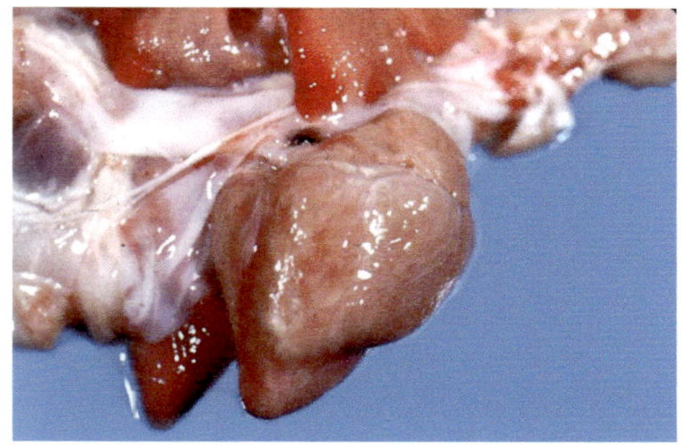

Fig. 10.103. Ox. Neosporiasis. Heart. Pallor. Pale white foci of inflammation are scattered throughout the myocardium. (Courtesy of Dr J.M. King and Section of Anatomic Pathology, Cornell University, USA.)

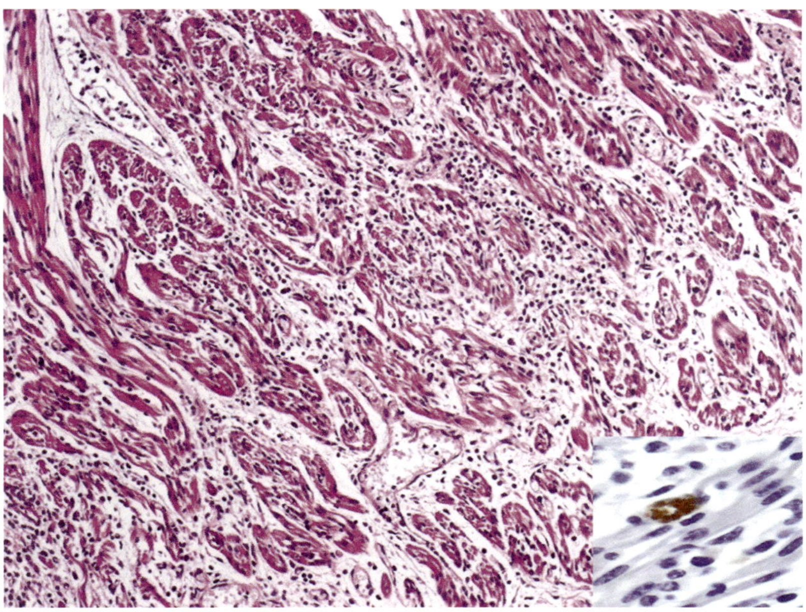

Fig. 10.104. Ox. Neosporiasis. Heart. Lymphocytic myocarditis. The myocardium is infiltrated by moderate numbers of mononuclear cells (H&E). Similar microscopic changes may be encountered in skeletal muscles. Inset: clusters of protozoa zoites positively stained by immunohistochemistry (IHC).

10.4.4.6 Miscellaneous

Sporadic abortion in cattle occurs by other abortigenic agents as well, albeit rare. These include *Yersinia pseudotuberculosis*, *Chlamydophila* spp., and *Coxiella burnetii* (Q-fever). Detection and differentiation of these infectious agents are achieved by special stains, immunohistochemical stains, and PCR.

10.5 FETAL MALFORMATIONS

Introduction. Bovine fetal anomalies are expressed in a variety of forms. Most are sporadic or congenital. Some of them are caused by teratogenic viruses, teratogenic protozoa (*N. caninum*), and teratogenic plants, inflicting non-lethal effects on the embryo or fetus but producing malformations of various organ systems. A few examples of neonatal malformations are presented in Chapter 1: Diseases of Neonate and Calves.

10.5.1 Arthrogryposis

One or more limbs may be affected. (See Fig.10.68.) The etiology is not always clear. Congenital, neurogenic, and myogenic etiology principles may be involved. Other causes include the consumption of toxic plants, and *in utero* viral infection with either bluetongue, Akabane and Schmallenberg virus. Regardless of the cause, the pathogenesis affects the neuronal innervation of muscles, interfering with fetal movement *in utero*, muscular dysfunction, stiff joints, and contracted limbs.

Arthrogryposis multiplex congenita (AMC) is a congenital disease with joint contracture in all limbs at birth. It occurs in Charolais calves, where it is due to a simple autosomal recessive trait. In affected animals, a cleft palate and hypoplastic patellae can occur simultaneously. In Angus calves, the condition is associated with three gene mutations, resulting in abnormal neuromotor development *in utero*.

10.5.2 Schistosomus reflexus

Defined as fetal malformation characterized by abdominal fissure and retroflexion of the vertebral column. The condition is incompatible with life.

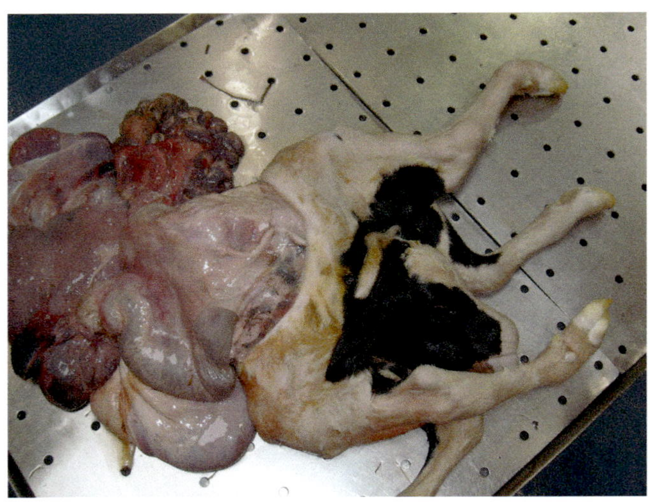

Fig. 10.105. Ox. Whole body. Neonate with abdominal evisceration, and vertebral column and hind limb retroflexion. (Courtesy Dr. P. Habecker, University of Pennsylvania, USA)

10.6 PROLONGED GESTATION

Introduction. An intact fetal pituitary–adrenal axis is required for the initiation of parturition in cattle. Prolonged gestation has been reported as a homozygous recessive genetic defect in Holstein and Guernsey cattle breeds. A constant morphologic feature in these animals with prolonged gestation is adenohypophyseal aplasia/hypoplasia.

Fact Sheet: Bovine Abortigenic Pathogens

Viruses
- Bluetongue virus (BT)
- Bovine herpesvirus type 1 (BHV-1)
- Bovine viral diarrhea virus (BVDV)
- Bunyavirus

Bacteria
- *Bacillus* spp.
- *Brucella abortus*
- *Campylobacter* spp.
- *Chlamydophila* spp.
- *Escherichia coli*
- *Leptospira* spp.
- *Listeria* spp.
- *Pajaroellobacter abortibovis* (order Myxococcales)
- *Pasteurella* spp.
- *Salmonella* spp.
- *Staphylococcus* spp.
- *Streptococcus* spp.
- *Trueperella pyogenes*
- *Ureaplasma diversum*
- *Yersinia pseudotuberculosis*

Protozoa
- *Neospora caninum*
- *Sarcocystis* spp.
- Tritrichomonas *foetus*
- *Toxoplasma gondii*

Fungi
- Aspergillus spp.
- *Candida* spp.
- *Mortierella wolfii*
- Zygomycetes: Mucor, Absidia, Rhizopus

Rickettsia
- *Coxiella burnetii*

Fact Sheet: Abortifacient Plants

Ponderosa pine tree (*Pinus ponderosa*) needles
Locoweed (*Oxytropis* spp. and *Astragalus* spp.)
Poison hemlock (*Conium maculatum*)
Broomweed (*Gutierrezia microcephala*)

Fact Sheet: Sample Submissions

Entire fetus
Placental membranes (cotyledons)
Blood from dam and fetus
Bodily fluids from fetus (abomasal fluid for bacteriology, thoracic fluid for immunology)

Fact Sheet: Tests for Abortion Diseases

- Conjunctival swab for fungi
- Fluorescent microscopy
- Histopathology on all other main organs and brain
- Immunohistochemistry
- Microbiology
- Molecular biology (PCR)
- Necropsy of fetus
- Placental impression smear
- Serology
- Toxicology
- Virology

SUGGESTED READING

Agerholm, J.S., Hewicke-Trautwein, M., Peperkamp, K. and Windsor, P.A. (2015) Virus-induced congenital malformations in cattle. *Acta Veterinaria Scandinavia* doi: 10.1186/s13028-015-0145-8.

Anderson, M.L. (2012) Disorders of cattle. In: Njaa, B.L. (ed.) *Kirkbride's Diagnosis of Abortion and Neonatal Loss in Animals.* Wiley-Blackwell, Chichester, UK, pp. 13–48.

Anderson, M.L., Kennedy, P.C., Blanchard, M.T., Barbaro, L., Chiu, P., *et al.* (2006) Histochemical and immunohistochemical evidence of a bacterium associated with lesions of epizootic abortion. *Journal of Veterinary Diagnostic Investigation* 18, 76–80.

Barr, B.C. and Anderson, M.L. (1993) Infectious diseases causing bovine abortion and fetal loss. *Veterinary Clinics of North America: Food Animal Practice* 9, 343–367.

Brooks, R.S., Blanchard, M.T., Clothier, K.A., Fish, S., Anderson, M. and Stott, J.L. (2016) Characterization of *Pajaroellobacter abortibovis*, the etiologic agent of epizootic bovine abortion. *Veterinary Microbiology* 192, 73–80.

Dubey, P., Buxton, D. and Wouda, W. (2006) Pathogenesis of bovine neosporosis. *Journal of Comparative Pathology* 134, 267–289.

Herder, V., Wohlsein, P., Peters, M., Hansmann, F. and Baumgaertner, W. (2012) Salient lesions in domestic ruminants infected with the emerging so-called Schmallenberg virus in Germany. *Veterinary Pathology* 49, 588–591.

King, D.P., Chen, C.L., Blanchard, M.T., Alridge, B.M., Anderson, M., *et al.* (2005) Molecular identification of a novel deltaproteobacterium as the etiologic agent of epizootic bovine abortion (foothill abortion). *Journal of Clinical Microbiology* 43, 604–609.

Miller, R., Chelmonska-Soyta, A., Smits, B., Foster, R. and Rosendal, S. (1994) *Ureaplasma diversum* as a cause of reproductive disease in cattle. *Veterinary Clinics of North America: Food Animal Practice* 10, 479–490.

Padula, A.M. (2005) The freemartin syndrome: an update. *Animal Reproduction Science* 87, 93–109.

Peperkamp, H.N., Luttikholt, S.J., Dijkman, R., Vos, J.H., Junker, K., *et al.* (2014) Ovine and bovine congenital abnormalities with intrauterine infection with Schmallenberg virus. *Veterinary Pathology*, 52, 1057–1066.

CHAPTER 11

Diseases of the Hematopoietic and Hemolymphatic System

Contributed by Jennifer L. Davies and Amy L. Warren
Department of Ecosystem and Public Health, Faculty of Veterinary Medicine, University of Calgary, Canada

11.1 The Hematopoietic and Hemolymphatic System
- 11.1.1 Thymus
- 11.1.2 Hemal nodes
- 11.1.3 Tonsils
- 11.1.4 Peyer's patches
- 11.1.5 Bone marrow
- 11.1.6 Reactive lymphoid hyperplasia

11.2 Congenital
- 11.2.1 Chediak–Higashi disease
- 11.2.2 Bovine leukocyte adhesion deficiency (BLAD)
- 11.2.3 Simmental hereditary thrombopathy
- 11.2.4 Congenital protoporphyria and porphyria

11.3 Degeneration
- 11.3.1 Serous atrophy of fat
- 11.3.2 Bone marrow infarction
- 11.3.3 Pigmentary changes of the lymph node
- 11.3.4 Lymph node infarction
- 11.3.5 Splenic infarction
- 11.3.6 Splenomegaly
- 11.3.7 Thymic atrophy

11.4 Inflammation
- 11.4.1 Infectious agents of anemia
  - 11.4.1.1 *Babesia*
  - 11.4.1.2 *Anaplasma*
  - 11.4.1.3 *Clostridium haemolyticum (novyi)*
  - 11.4.1.4 *Mycoplasma wenyonii*
  - 11.4.1.5 *Trypanosoma*
  - 11.4.1.6 *Theileria*
- 11.4.2 Bovine viral diarrhea virus (BVDV)
  - 11.4.2.1 Thrombocytopenic syndrome
  - 11.4.2.2 Peyer's patch necrosis/involution
- 11.4.3 Agents of lymphadenitis
  - 11.4.3.1 *Mycobacterium bovis*
  - 11.4.3.2 *Mycobacterium avium* subsp. *paratuberculosis*
  - 11.4.3.3 *Mycoplasma bovis*
- 11.4.4 *Bacillus anthracis*
- 11.4.5 Splenic abscesses

11.5 Toxic
- 11.5.1 Bracken fern toxicity
- 11.5.2 Oxidizing agents inducing hemolytic anemia
- 11.5.3 Moldy sweet clover (dicoumarol) poisoning
- 11.5.4 Nitrate poisoning

11.6 Neoplasia
- 11.6.1 Bovine leukemia virus (BLV)
- 11.6.2 Sporadic lymphoma
  - 11.6.2.1 Calf or juvenile form
  - 11.6.2.2 Thymic form
  - 11.6.2.3 Cutaneous form

11.1 THE HEMATOPOIETIC AND HEMOLYMPHATIC SYSTEM

Introduction. There are several peculiarities of the bovine hematopoietic and hemolymphatic system that can impact disease interpretation. Calves have a prominent cervical component to the thymus that can be mistaken for glandular or neoplastic tissue. Hemal nodes are similar structures to lymph nodes that are found along the great vessels, in the mediastinum, and in the mesentery of cattle. Functionally, they are believed to have a similar role to splenic tissue in the immune surveillance of the blood. Average erythrocyte diameter in cattle is 5–6 μm, which is small compared to other species, and this feature can result in falsely low red blood cell (RBC) counts if automated analyzers are not calibrated for cattle. Beef breeds have higher RBC counts than dairy breeds; bulls have higher RBC counts than cows; and non-lactating cows have higher counts than lactating cows. Adult cattle have one of the lowest neutrophil to lymphocyte (N:L) ratios at approximately 1.0. There is also, generally, a slower bone marrow response to early inflammation, with a delay in neutrophilia and left shift and a lower peak leukocytosis compared to other species. Bovine platelets are small, with a lifespan of 10 days in peripheral blood.

11.1.1 Thymus

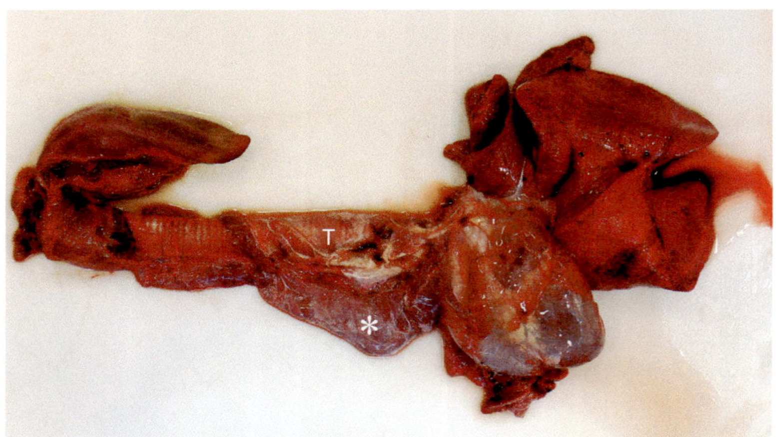

Fig. 11.1. Calf. Normal thymus. Full-term, non-viable neonate. In ruminants, the thymus is divided into cervical and thoracic lobes. The cervical lobe (asterisk) is large and extends along the trachea (T). In a young calf, thymic atrophy can be an important marker of underlying disease.

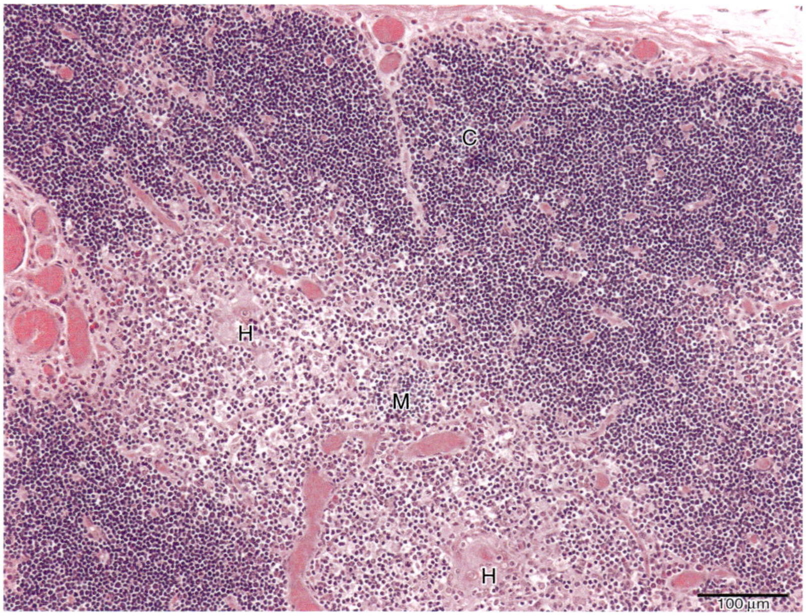

Fig. 11.2. Calf. Normal thymus. Full-term, non-viable neonate. The normal thymus is composed of incomplete lobules comprising an outer cortex (C) and an inner medulla (M). The cortex is characteristically deeply basophilic due to the large number of T-lymphocytes, while the medulla is comparatively more eosinophilic due to fewer numbers of thymocytes. Hassall's corpuscles (H) are characteristic of the medulla (H&E).

11.1.2 Hemal nodes

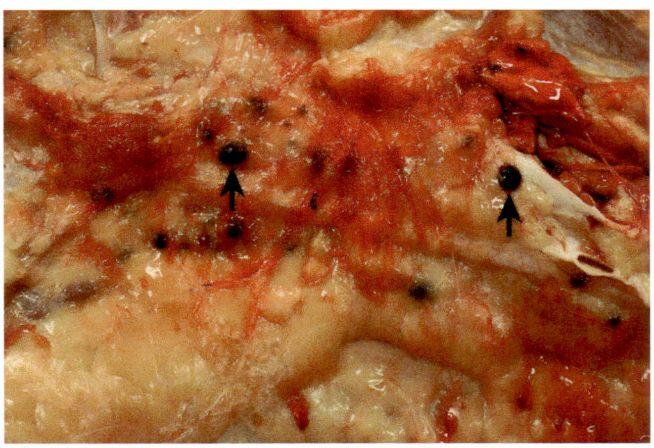

Fig. 11.3. Ox. Normal hemal nodes. Hemal nodes (arrows) are lymphoid structures with blood sinuses instead of lymph sinuses. There are very few diseases that specifically target the hemal nodes, though there are sporadic reports of hemal node enlargement associated with generalized lymphadenomegaly due to bovine leukemia virus (BLV) infection.

11.1.3 Tonsils

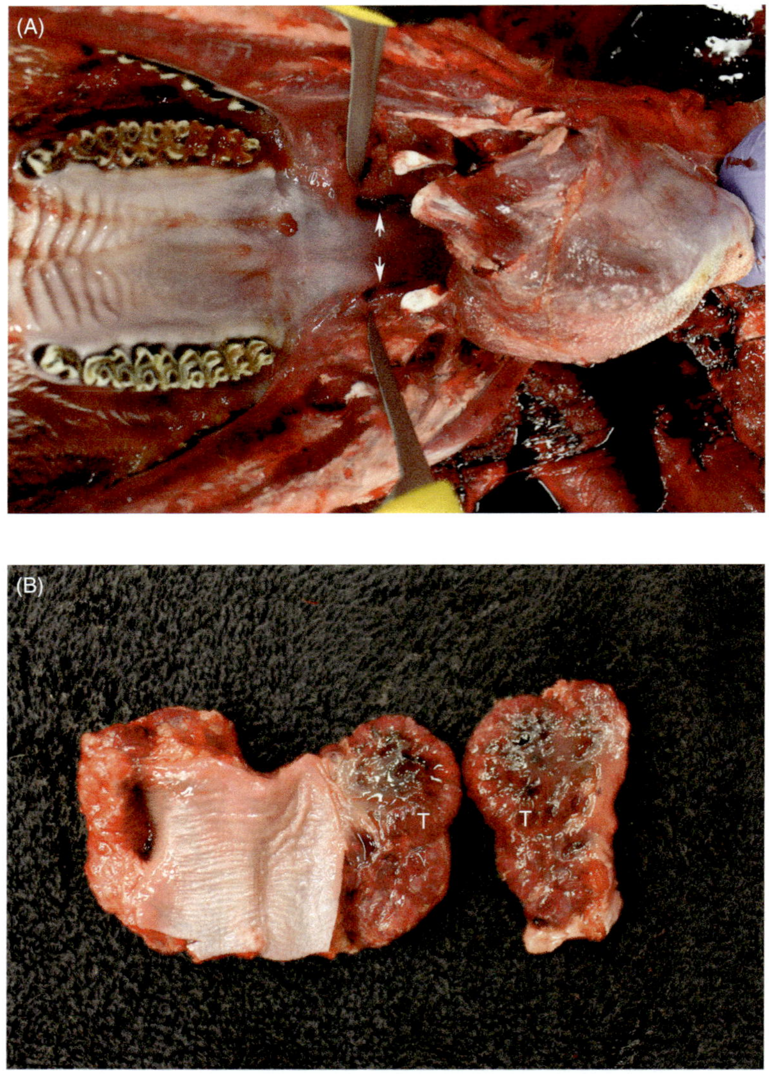

Fig. 11.4. Ox. Normal palatine tonsils. Tonsillar sinuses (A) and dissected tonsils (B). Tonsils in cattle are located in the mucosa of the oropharynx (palatine and lingual tonsils) and nasopharynx (pharyngeal and tubal tonsils) and are part of the mucosa-associated lymphoid tissue (MALT). Their placement is strategic as it allows for immunological surveillance of antigens that enter through the nasal and oral cavities. The palatine tonsils (T) are located in the lateral walls of the oropharynx. From the mucosal surface, only the tonsillar sinuses are visible (arrows) and the tonsil is revealed on dissection. Knowledge of the location of the palatine tonsils is essential, not only in routine post-mortem examination but also in the removal of specified risk material

11.1.4 Peyer's patches

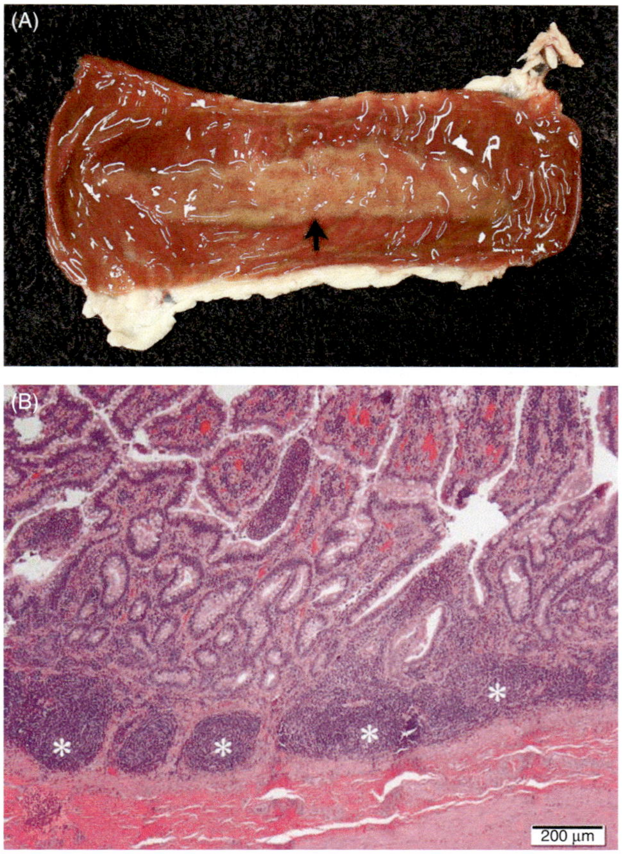

Fig. 11.5. Ox. Ileum. Normal Peyer's patch. Gross (A) and histology (B). In ruminants, continuous Peyer's patches are found along the antimesenteric border of the distal ileum. Grossly, they appear as oval to elongate thickenings of the intestinal wall (arrow). Microscopically, Peyer's patches appear as follicular aggregates of lymphocytes within the submucosa (asterisks). A number of viral and bacterial diseases specifically target this tissue or enter the body through this site (H&E).

11.1.5 Bone marrow

The normal hematopoietic cellularity of the bone marrow is dependent on age. In young animals, the bone marrow is hematopoietically active and extends into the medullary cavity, resulting in a diffusely red appearance. As an animal ages, the hematopoietically active tissue regresses to the epiphyseal spongy bone, and is gradually replaced by fat, resulting in yellow marrow.

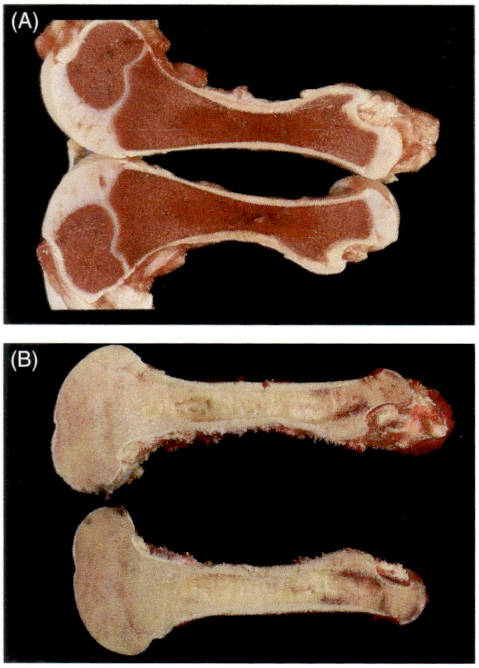

Fig. 11.6. Ox. Longitudinal sections of the femur. Normal calf (A) and adult bone marrow (B).

11.1.6 Reactive lymphoid hyperplasia

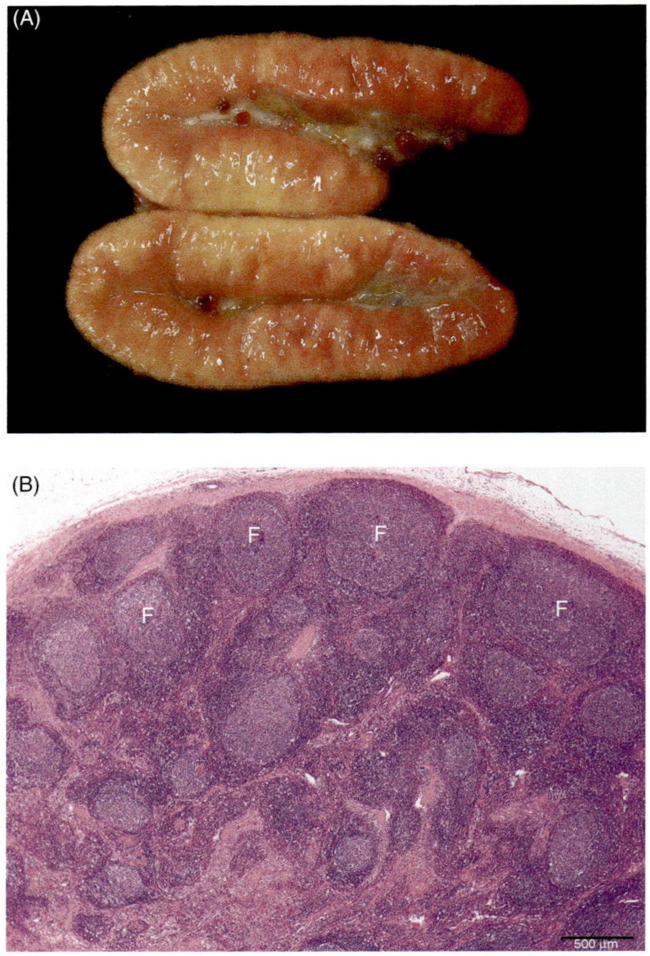

Fig. 11.7. Ox. Medial iliac lymph node. Gross (A) and histology (B). Reactive lymphoid hyperplasia. Reactive lymphoid hyperplasia is a generic response of the lymph node to a variety of inflammatory and infectious stimuli. Grossly, there is hyperplasia and expansion of the cortical and paracortical lymphoid tissue, with concurrent enlargement of the node. This can generally be differentiated from lymphoma by the anatomically confined expansion and the gross presence of lymphoid follicles. Histologically, there are increased numbers of follicles (F) with prominent germinal centers, expansion of the paracortex, sinus histiocytosis, and expansion of the medullary cords with plasma cells (H&E).

11.2 CONGENITAL

11.2.1 Chediak–Higashi disease

Introduction. Chediak–Higashi disease results from a mutation in the lysosomal trafficking regulator, CHS1, causing abnormal fusion of cytoplasmic lysosomes. This results in large, pleomorphic granules in the cytoplasm of leukocytes and almost all other granule-producing cells, as well as impaired granule function. As a consequence, the clinical manifestations include hypopigmentation or partial albinism (as a result of impaired melanin granule fusion), impaired immunological function, and impaired hemostasis due to platelet storage deficiency. Large eosinophilic granules can be seen in the cytoplasm of circulating neutrophils and eosinophils, renal tubular epithelial cells, and Kupffer cells that are peroxidase positive, Sudan black B positive and stain with periodic acid–Schiff (PAS). Chediak–Higashi disease has been reported in Hereford, Brangus, and Japanese Black cattle.

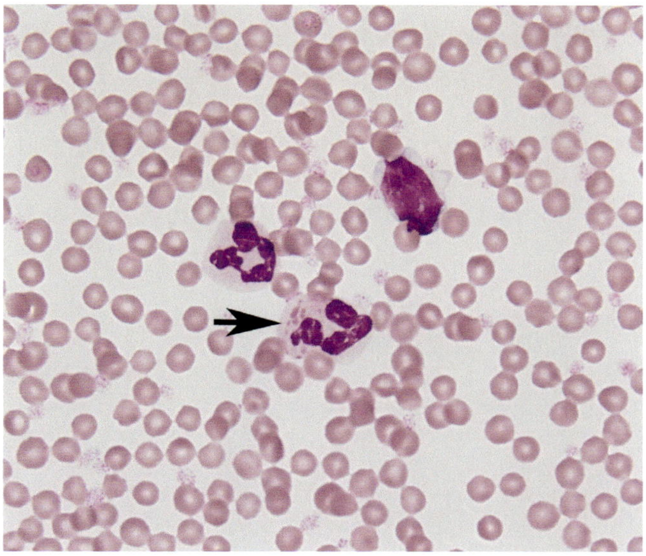

Fig. 11.8. Ox. Hereford. Blood smear. Chediak–Higashi disease. A proportion of circulating neutrophils (arrow) contain large cytoplasmic, pleomorphic, eosinophilic granules (Wright–Giemsa).

11.2.2 Bovine leukocyte adhesion deficiency (BLAD)

Introduction. Bovine leukocyte adhesion deficiency is a rare congenital, autosomal recessive immunodeficiency where leukocytes lack the cell surface receptors (due to a mutation in the CD18 gene) required for neutrophil migration and phagocytosis. This manifests as recurrent bacterial infections of the mucosa and gastrointestinal tract, pneumonia, oral ulceration, periodontal disease, and stunted growth. Cattle affected with BLAD also have a marked and persistent mature neutrophilia, hyperglobulinemia, lymphadenomegaly, and intermittent pyrexia.

11.2.3 Simmental hereditary thrombopathy

Introduction. Clinical findings include epistaxis, hematuria, superficial hematomas, and excessive bleeding secondary to injury or minor surgery. While platelet numbers are normal, there is impaired platelet aggregation. Studies suggest that mutations in the calcium diacylglycerol guanine nucleotide exchange factor I (CalDAG-GEFI) gene result in this thromboplastic phenotype.

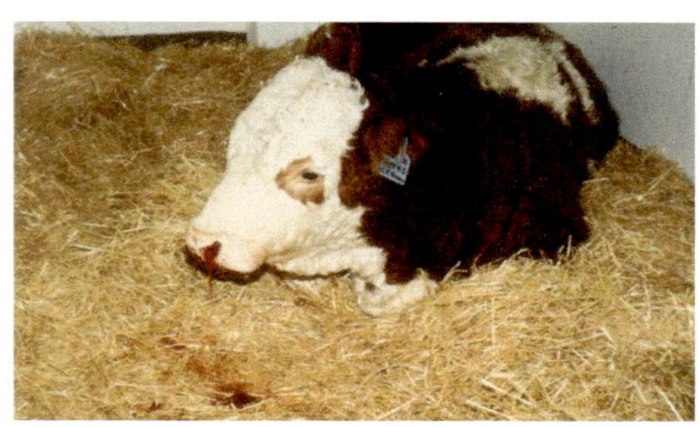

Fig. 11.9. Ox. Epistaxis in Simmental hereditary thrombopathy. Hemorrhagic diathesis in the Simmental cattle results from platelet dysfunction. (Courtesy of Dr G. Searcy, Western College of Veterinary Medicine, Canada.)

11.2.4 Congenital protoporphyria and porphyria

Introduction. Porphyrias are a group of diseases of abnormal porphyrin metabolism that result in the deposition of porphyrins in tissues, urine, feces, and skin. This manifests in cattle as photosensitization, red-brown discoloration of the teeth, bones and urine, and sometimes splenomegaly and hepatomegaly. Porphyrins are breakdown products of hemoglobin and other heme-containing enzymes. When not chelated to iron, porphyrins fluoresce under UV light and cause photosensitization in the skin. In cattle, there are two autosomal recessive porphyria disorders: bovine protoporphyria, affecting Limousin cattle, that results from reduced activity of the ferrochetalase enzyme; and congenital erythropoietic porphyria, reported in a number of cattle breeds including Shorthorns and Holsteins, that results from reduced activity of uroporphyringen III cosynthetase.

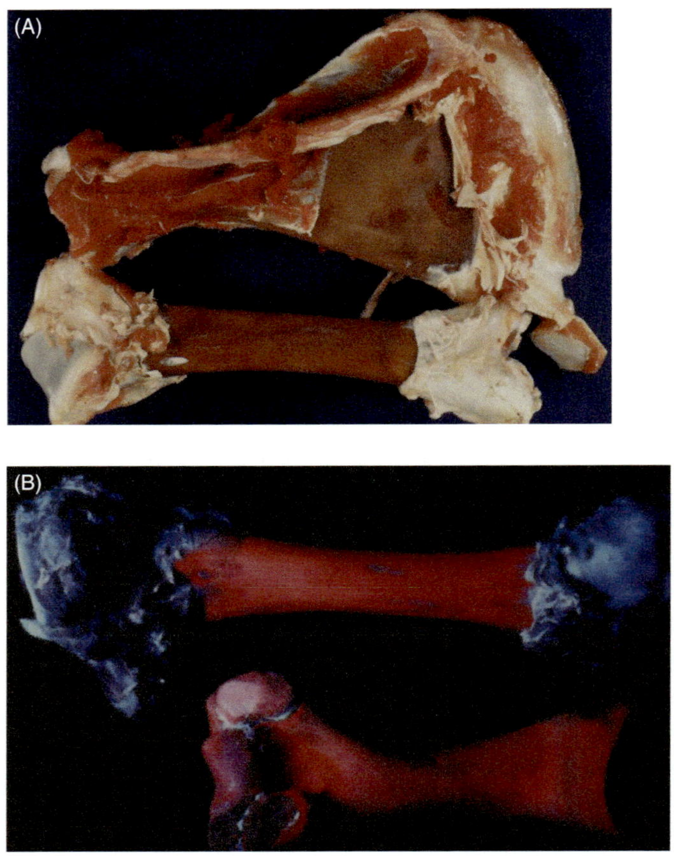

Fig. 11.10. Ox. Bones. Congenital porphyria (A); under UV light (B). Congenital porphyria results in the incorporation of porphyrins into the bone and teeth (pink tooth), leading to a red-brown discoloration of these tissues. In affected animals, the teeth, bones, and urine demonstrate characteristic cherry-red fluorescence when exposed to UV light (see Chapter 5: Diseases of the Gastrointestinal Tract).

11.3 DEGENERATION

11.3.1 Serous atrophy of fat

Introduction. During negative energy balance, the body uses fat stores in a sequential manner, first using the external fat, followed by internal thoracic and abdominal cavity fat, and then deep organ fat. Bone marrow fat is one of the last to be used.

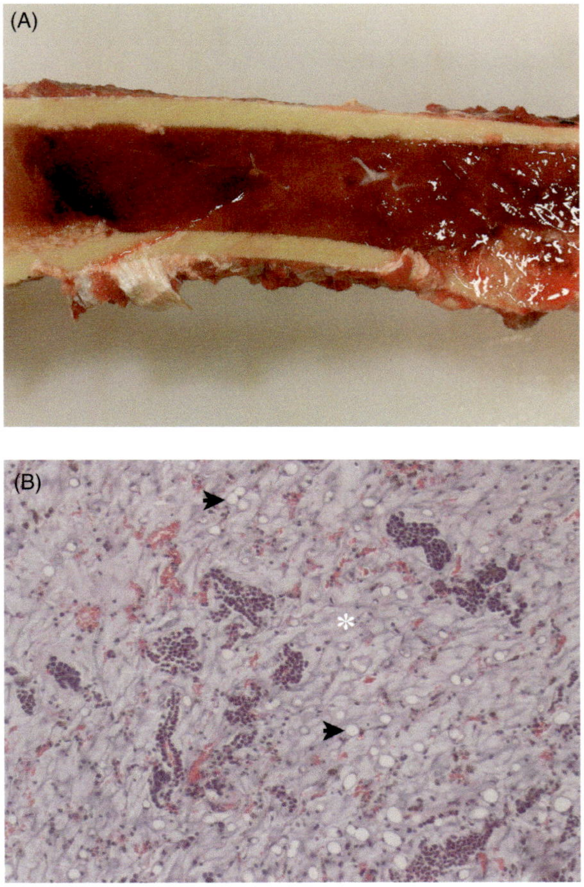

Fig. 11.11. Ox. Longitudinal section of the femur. Gross (A) and histology (B). Serous atrophy of bone marrow fat. Grossly, serous atrophy of fat is characterized by replacement of the adipose tissue with clear, gelatinous, yellow material. Microscopically, serous atrophy of fat is characterized by diminution of the adipocytes (arrows) and expansion of the interstitium by wispy, basophilic material consistent with mucopolysaccharides (asterisk). Mucopolysaccharide deposition can be highlighted by the use of an Alcian blue stain (H&E).

11.3.2 Bone marrow infarction

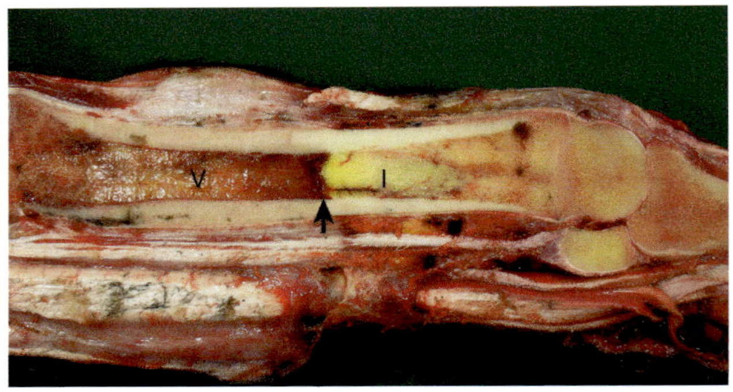

Fig. 11.12. Ox. Longitudinal section of the cannon bone. Bone marrow infarction in ergotism. Infarcted bone marrow (I) is differentiated from the viable marrow (V) by a well-demarcated area of pallor bordered by a hemorrhagic zone (arrow). In ergotism, bone marrow infarction is associated with the ingestion of toxic alkaloids, produced by the fungus *Claviceps purpurea*, resulting in peripheral arteriolar vasoconstriction, vascular thrombosis, and infarction of the extremities. (Also see Chapter 12: Diseases of the Integument and Chapter 13: Diseases of the Claw and Foot Skin.)

11.3.3 Pigmentary changes of the lymph node

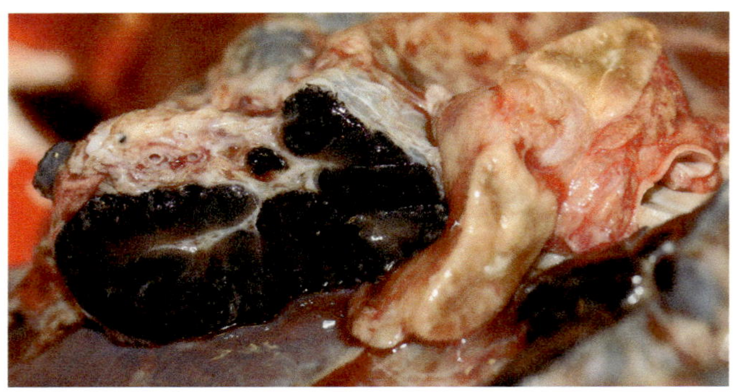

Fig. 11.13. Ox. Hepatic lymph node. Pigmentation in trematodiasis. Diffuse black discoloration of the hepatic lymph node can be seen in cattle with hepatic trematodiasis. While the jet black pigment is reminiscent of melanin, it likely represents iron-porphyrin pigment produced by the parasites (see Chapter 6: Diseases of the Hepatobiliary System and Pancreas).

11.3.4 Lymph node infarction

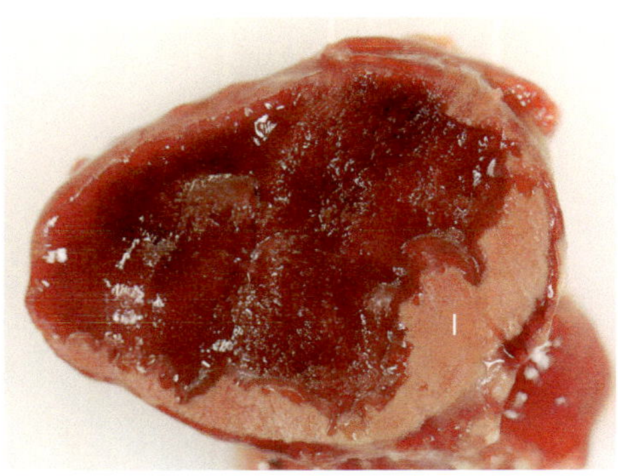

Fig. 11.14. Ox. Mesenteric lymph node. Infarction in salmonellosis. Lymph node infarction is characterized by a sharply demarcated zone of dull pallor in the cortex (I). Lymph node infarction is best described in cases of the calf form of sporadic bovine lymphoma, where neoplastic infiltration results in vascular obstruction.

11.3.5 Splenic infarction

Introduction. Embolism with splenic infarction is not uncommon and is often the result of a valvular endocarditis involving the left side of the heart. The resulting lesions are dependent on whether the emboli are sterile (infarct) or septic (abscess). Infarcts of the spleen are typically red, rather than pale, due to the expandable nature of the splenic parenchyma that does not allow for forcible removal of blood via necrosis-induced pressure.

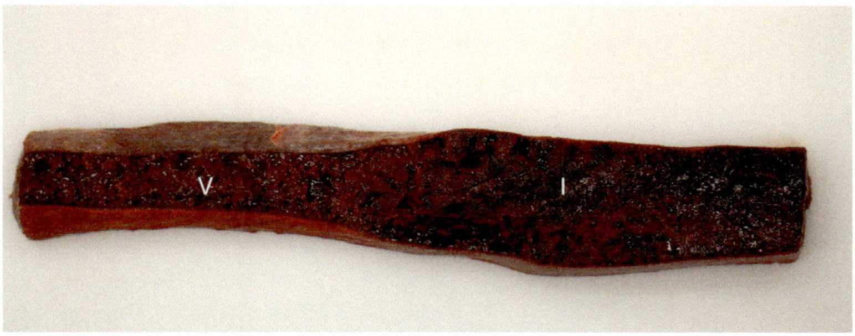

Fig. 11.15. Ox. Cross section of spleen. Infarction secondary to aortic valvular endocarditis. The splenic infarct (I) is differentiated from the viable parenchyma (V) by a well-delineated focus of swollen, firm, dark red, and lusterless tissue.

11.3.6 Splenomegaly

Introduction. Depending on the pathological process, splenic enlargement can be bloody in consistency (congestion or hyperemia) or firm (meaty) (cellular proliferation or infiltration). Differential diagnoses for a 'bloody' spleen include anthrax, other acute toxemias and septicemias, such as salmonellosis. Important differentials for the 'meaty' spleen include red blood cell parasites, such as *Anaplasma* and *Babesia*, and lymphoma.

11.3.7 Thymic atrophy

Introduction. Thymic involution is a normal physiologic process; however, there are a number of pathologic conditions that can result in premature involution and variable degrees of immunodeficiency. Thymic atrophy occurs in neonatal and aborted calves non-specifically in a variety of infectious agents, malnutrition, and secondary to high levels of endogenous corticosteroids. Grossly, there is diffuse thymic atrophy, and histologic lesions include lymphocytolysis, edema, and hemorrhage. In late stages of infection, there is thymic atrophy with little or no inflammation. In enzootic bovine abortion (EBA), there is additionally thymic petechiation and interlobular edema, and histiocytic thymitis histologically. In bovine viral diarrhea virus (BVDV), thymic lymphocyte loss can be so severe that there is almost complete collapse of the stromal tissue and hemorrhage.

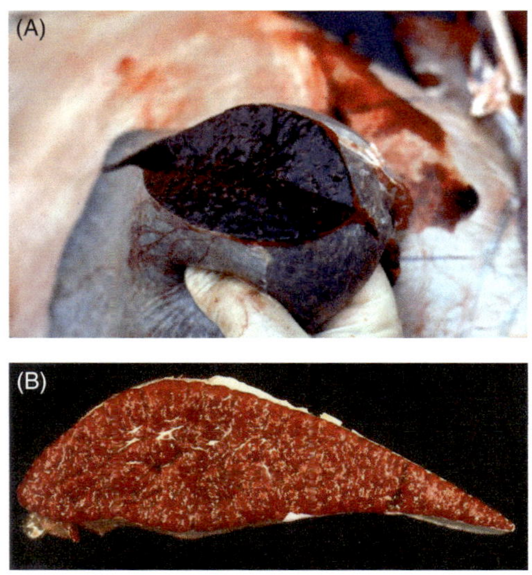

Fig. 11.16. Ox. Cross section of spleen. Congestion in anthrax 'bloody' spleen (A) and 'meaty' spleen in lymphosarcoma (B). In the 'bloody' spleen, splenic enlargement is due to congestion or hyperemia, and the spleen oozes blood on section. The 'meaty' spleen is the result of cellular proliferation of mononuclear cells and hematopoietic tissue, or diffuse neoplastic infiltration. The uniformly 'meaty' spleen is enlarged, firm, and on section, the splenic parenchyma is red and bulges.

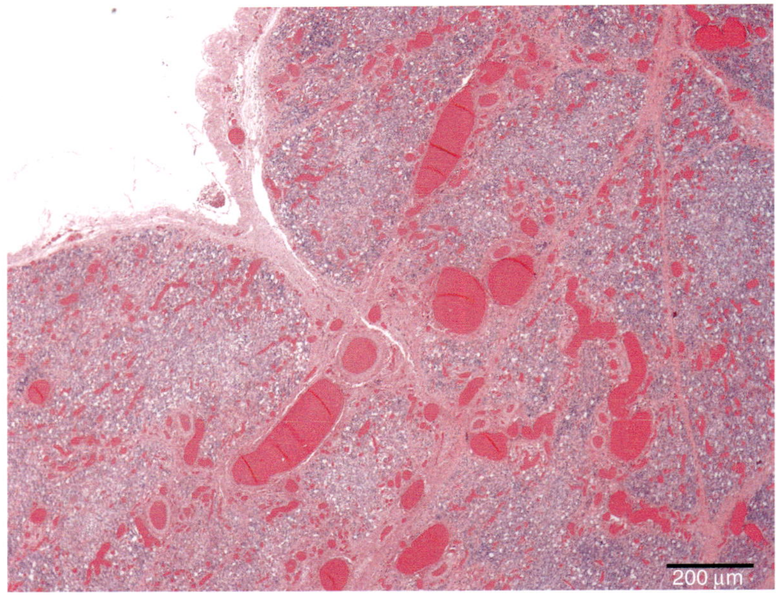

Fig. 11.17. Ox. Thymus from a 2-week-old calf. Salmonellosis. Thymic atrophy is characterized by reduced lobular size, cortical pallor (due to lymphocyte depletion), and a loss of demarcation between the cortex and medulla (H&E).

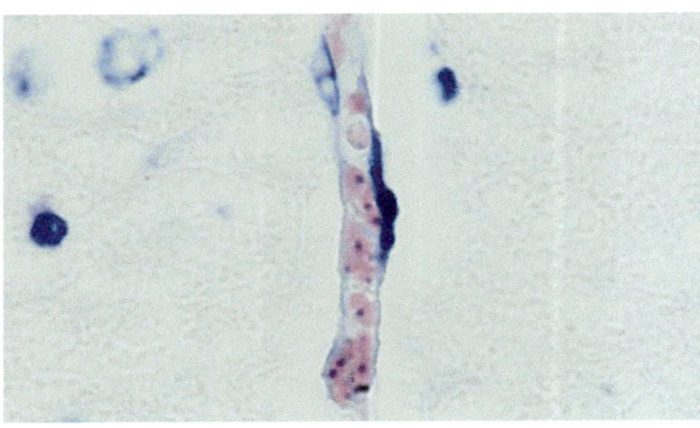

Fig. 11.18. Ox. Brain. Babesiosis. Within the cytoplasm of erythrocytes in the cerebral capillaries, there are small (1–3 μm), blue, round structures and rings (*Babesia* piroplasms). Grossly, brains with cerebral babesiosis are discolored 'cherry red', with prominent vasculature due to sludging of parasitized erythrocytes within vessels (Giemsa). (Courtesy of Dr O. Illanes, Ross University, St Kitts.) (Also see Chapter 2: Diseases of the Nervous System.)

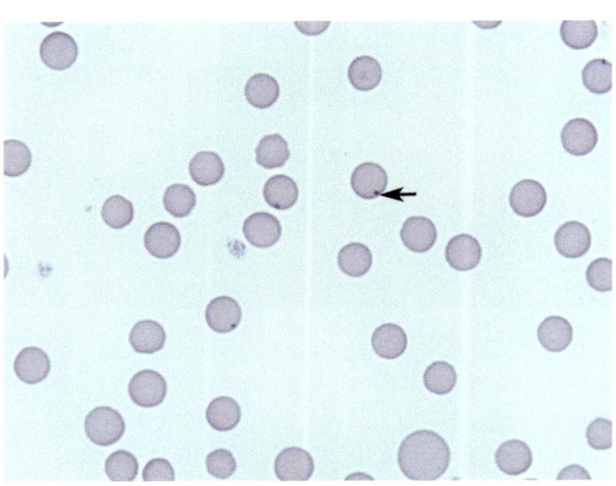

Fig. 11.19. Ox. Peripheral blood smear. Anaplasmosis. The erythrocyte density is decreased (anemia) and there are blue, round, 0.3–1.0 μm, homogeneously blue staining organisms at the periphery of the erythrocytic cytoplasm (arrow) (Wright–Giemsa). (Courtesy of Dr J. Webb, IDEXX, Canada.)

11.4 INFLAMMATION

11.4.1 Infectious agents of anemia

11.4.1.1 Babesia

Introduction. *Babesia* are intraerythrocytic protozoal parasites, and four species are recognized to infect cattle: *Babesia bovis*, *Babesia bigemina*, *Babesia divergans*, and *Babesia major*, with *B. bovis* and *B. bigemina* of the most pathologic and economic importance. Spread of *Babesia* is generally through a tick vector (*Boophilus* and *Rhipicephalus* spp.). Babesiosis (tick fever or red water) generally occurs in immuno-naïve, adult *Bos taurus* cattle, as cattle infected at a young age have only mild disease and develop long-term immunity, and *Bos indicus* cattle have natural resistance to ticks and *Babesia*. As replicating *Babesia* exit the erythrocyte, they cause cell rupture, intravascular hemolysis and anemia, with resultant hemoglobinemia and hemoglobinuria (red water). Cerebral babesiosis occurs when parasitized erythrocytes lodge in the cerebral vasculature, resulting in cerebral ischemia.

11.4.1.2 Anaplasma

Introduction. *Anaplasma marginale* and *Anaplasma centrale* are intraerythrocytic rickettsial parasites that cause hemolytic anemia in cattle, with *A. marginale* causing more severe disease. Like *Babesia*, infection of cattle prior to 1 year of age is often subclinical, and infected cattle become lifelong carriers. However, *de novo* infection of *A. marginale* in adulthood is often severe and fatal. Gross findings include pallor and watery blood (anemia), jaundice, and splenomegaly, consistent with extravascular hemolysis. Parasitized erythrocytes can be seen on peripheral blood smears or, at necropsy, on smears of the liver, spleen, kidney, or lung.

11.4.1.3 Clostridium *haemolyticum (novyi)*

Introduction. Bacillary hemoglobinuria is an acute hemolytic anemia caused by *Clostridium haemolyticum* (*novyi*) β-toxin (phospholipase C), which is released from subclinical hepatic infections during periods of hepatic anoxia. Typically, hepatic anoxia results from liver fluke migration, though other causes of hepatic necrosis may also trigger clostridial germination and β-toxin release. Gross findings of a focus of hepatic infarction, along with hemoglobinuria and anemia, are strongly suggestive of bacillary hemoglobinuria (see Chapter 6: Diseases of the Hepatobiliary System and Pancreas).

11.4.1.4 Mycoplasma wenyonii

Introduction. *Mycoplasma wenyonii* is a hemotropic, extracellular parasite of erythrocytes that rarely causes clinical disease other than in immunocompromised or splenectomized cattle. However, there are recent reports of udder and hindlimb edema, and lymphadenomegaly due to *M. wenyonii* infection in older, non-splenectomized cattle.

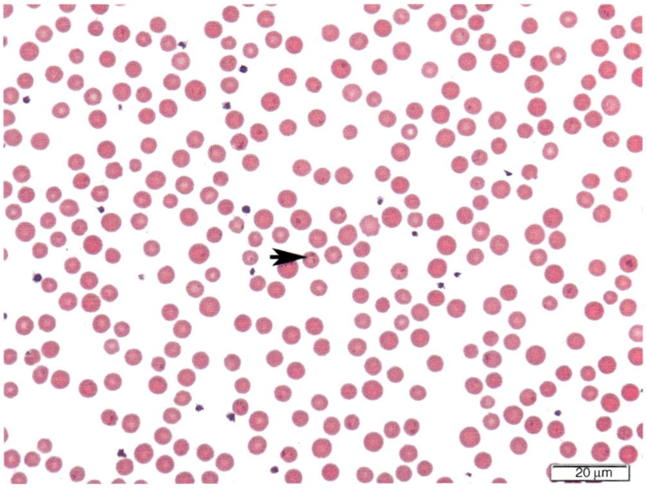

Fig. 11.20. Ox. Peripheral blood smear. *Mycoplasma wenyonii* infection. Within the cytoplasm of approximately 20% of erythrocytes, there are <1 µm diameter basophilic dots, chains and rings (arrow) (Wright–Giemsa).

11.4.1.5 Trypanosoma

Introduction. Trypanosomes are flagellated extracellular protozoal organisms that rarely cause clinical disease in cattle. *Trypanosoma theileri* is generally considered non-pathogenic in cattle, although African trypanosomes (*Trypanosoma congolense* and *Trypanosoma vivax*) can cause hemolytic anemia (see Chapter 2: Diseases of the Nervous System).

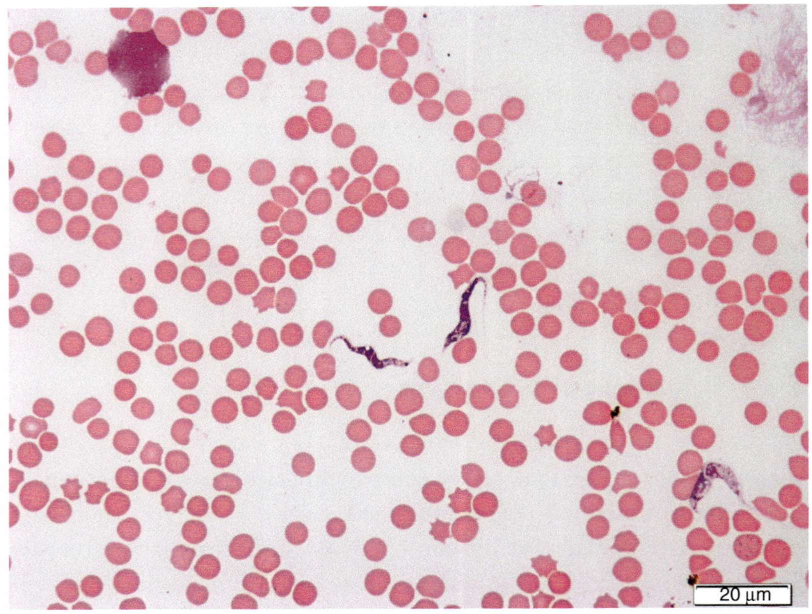

Fig. 11.21. Ox. Peripheral blood smear. Trypanosomiasis. Eighty to 100 µm long flagellated extracellular protozoa (*Trypanosoma theileri*) are present in the feathered margin of the smear.

11.4.1.6 Theileria

Introduction. A variety of *Theileria* organisms have been detected in cattle, many of which can cause severe anemia and lymphoproliferation. *Theileria* piroplasms are found in erythrocytes as pleomorphic forms, including round, comma, rod, piriform, and signet-ring shapes. *Theileria parva* causes East Coast fever in Africa and *Theileria annulata* causes tropical theileriosis in cattle. In North America, *Theileria buffeli* has been reported to cause hemolytic anemia in cattle.

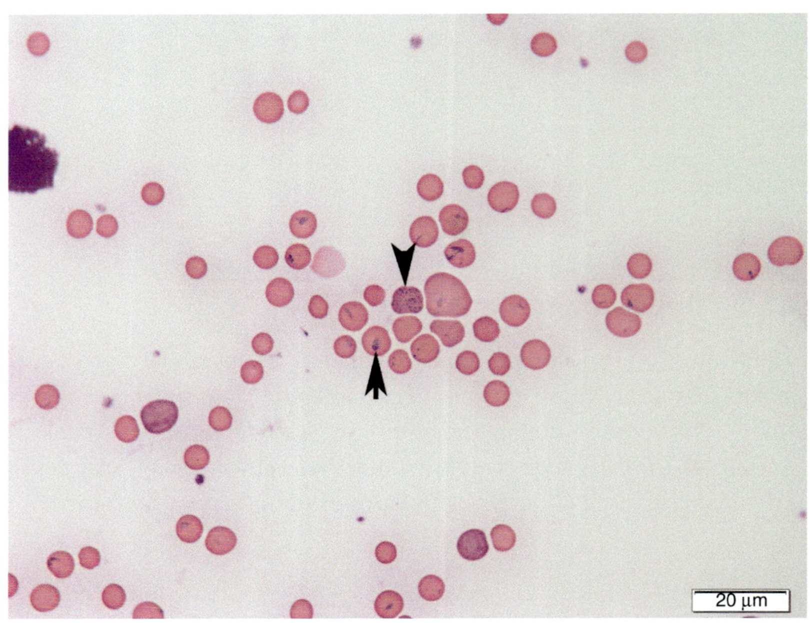

Fig. 11.22. Ox. Peripheral blood smear. *Theileria buffeli* infection. There is a marked reduction in erythrocyte density (anemia) and anisocytosis, polychromasia, and basophilic stippling (regeneration) (arrowhead). Within the cytoplasm of approximately 50% of erythrocytes, there are a variety of forms of basophilic staining *T. buffeli* piroplasms including round, rod, signet-ring, chains, and piriform shapes (arrow) (Wright–Giemsa). (Also see Chapter 2: Diseases of the Nervous System.)

11.4.2 Bovine viral diarrhea virus (BVDV)

11.4.2.1 Thrombocytopenic syndrome

Introduction. Bovine viral diarrhea virus (BVDV) is an RNA virus of the *Pestivirus* genus that is highly mutable and widespread within cattle populations. Since the early 1990s, virulent strains of non-cytopathic (NCP) BVDV type 2 (and, rarely, type 1b) have been associated with thrombocytopenic syndrome. Thrombocytopenia associated with BVDV type 2 infection is characterized clinically by fever and marked thrombocytopenia, manifesting as bloody diarrhea, epistaxis, petechial and ecchymotic hemorrhages, and bleeding from injection sites. Experimental studies suggest that decreased platelet production as a result of megakaryocyte infection and dysfunction may be the predominant mechanism leading to thrombocytopenia. (Also see Chapter 10: Diseases of the Reprodutive System.)

11.4.2.2 Peyer's patch necrosis/involution

Introduction. BVDV infects a wide variety of cell types, but has a tropism for cells of the acquired immune system, causing profound lymphoid depletion in the palatine tonsils, lymph nodes, thymus, and Peyer's patches, with lymphoid depletion in the Peyer's patches highly characteristic. In acute BVD, fibrin, blood, and necrotic debris coat Peyer's patches. This lesion is highly distinctive and rivaled only by lesions caused by rinderpest. In milder and more chronic infections, Peyer's patches are depressed and covered in a layer of catarrhal exudate. Microscopically, acute infections are characterized by lymphocytolysis accompanied by inflammation in the overlying mucosa. More chronic cases are characterized by herniation of the crypts into the involuted follicles. BVDV immunohistochemistry can be an invaluable tool in the diagnosis of BVD, especially in cases where only formalin-fixed tissues are available.

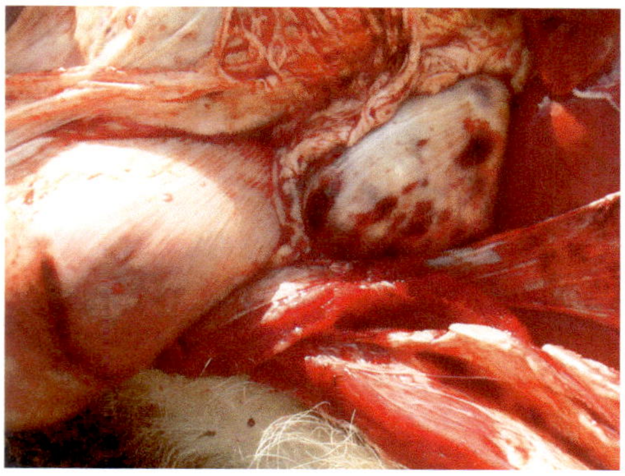

Fig. 11.23. Ox. Omasum. Thrombocytopenic syndrome. Bovine viral diarrhea virus (BVDV) type 2-associated thrombocytopenia can manifest as petechial and ecchymotic hemorrhages on mucosal and serosal surfaces. (Courtesy of Dr E. Janzen, University of Calgary, Canada.) (Also see Chapter 10: Diseases of the Reproductive System.)

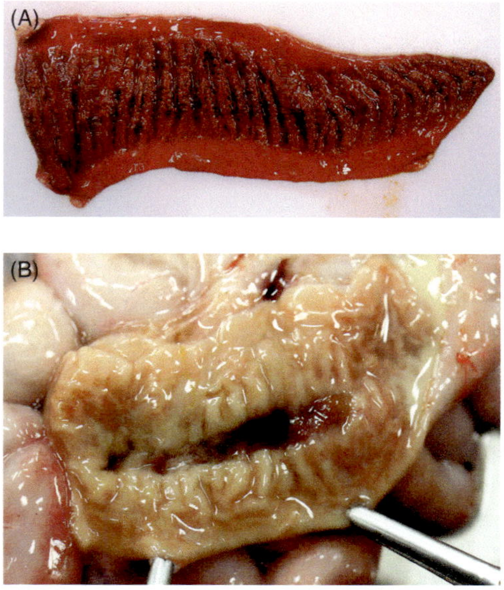

Fig. 11.24. Ox. Ileum. Peyer's patch necrosis in acute (A) and involution in chronic (B) bovine viral diarrhea virus (BVDV) infections. In acute infection, the Peyer's patches are covered by a layer of hemorrhage and fibrinonecrotic debris, producing an exaggerated appearance. In more long-standing infections, Peyer's patches are depressed and covered by mucus. (Courtesy of Dr C. Legge, University of Calgary, Canada.)

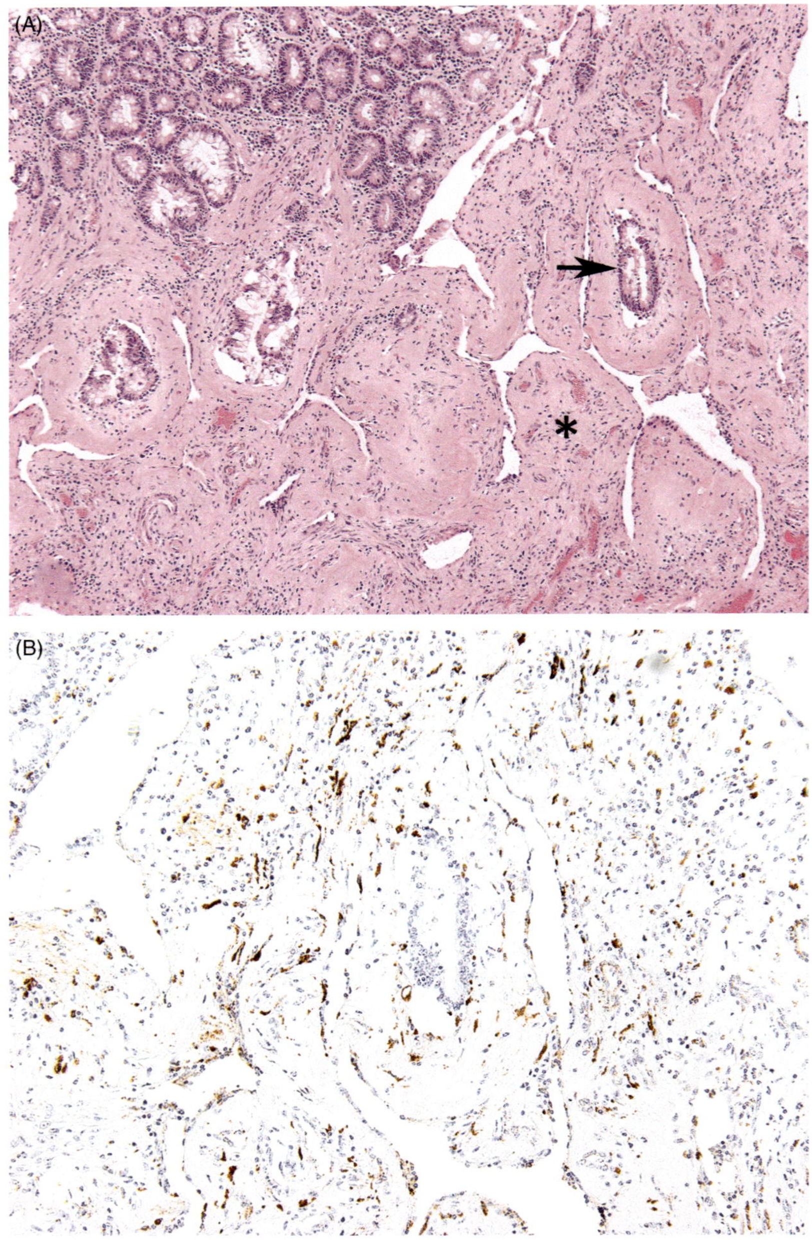

Fig. 11.25. Ox. Ileum. Involution of Peyer's patch in chronic bovine viral diarrhea virus (BVDV) infection. Histology (A) and BVDV indirect immunohistochemistry (B). The Peyer's patches (asterisk) are markedly depleted, with only stromal elements and adjacent lymphatic spaces remaining. There is also herniation of crypts into the involuted Peyer's patches (arrow). BVDV antigens are abundant within the stromal cells of the Peyer's patches and submucosa. While Peyer's patch involution is suggestive of BVDV infection, it can also be seen in other conditions such as chronic diseases leading to endogenous corticosteroid release, salmonellosis, and bovine coronavirus infection (H&E, IHC) (see Chapter 5: Diseases of the Gastrointestinal Tract).

11.4.3 Agents of lymphadenitis

Due to their location and function, inflammation of the lymph nodes is a frequent post-mortem finding.

Lymphadenitis is frequently regional and secondary to draining a site of inflammation and infection. As a result, the pathologic changes within the lymph node are often generic. However, there are certain infectious diseases in which the lymph nodes are affected characteristically.

11.4.3.1 Mycobacterium bovis

Introduction. Bovine tuberculosis, caused by *Mycobacterium bovis*, is characterized by the formation of caseating granulomas in the lungs, lymph nodes, and other organs. This organism has a broad host range and infection can spill over into humans, other domestic animals, and wildlife. Control programs have limited the occurrence of bovine tuberculosis in many developed countries, but wildlife reservoirs have complicated eradication programs. In cattle, lesions are most commonly seen in the retropharyngeal, bronchial, and mediastinal lymph nodes in respiratory infections. However, in generalized infections, lymph nodes throughout the body can be involved. Acid-fast stains reveal variable numbers of acid-fast bacilli within macrophage phagosomes, and free within the zone of necrosis in the center of granulomas. (Also see Chapter 3: Diseases of the Respiratory System.)

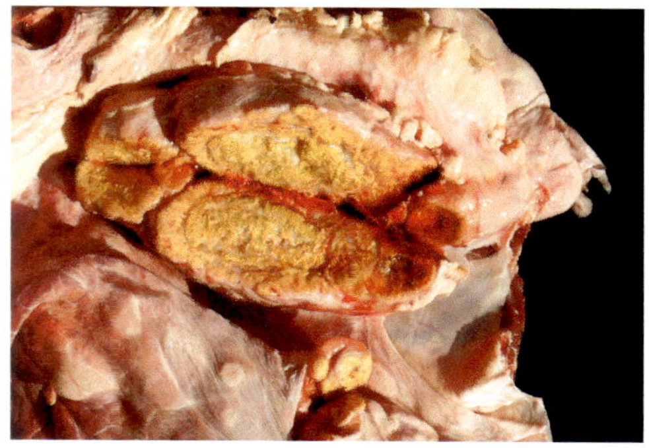

Fig. 11.26. Ox. Tracheobronchial lymph node. Bovine tuberculosis. The lymph nodal architecture has been replaced by dry, yellow, caseous material. Discrete nodules in the lung suggest the presence of tuberculosis in that organ. (Courtesy of Dr D. Driemeier, Universidade Federal do Rio Grande do Sul, Brazil.)

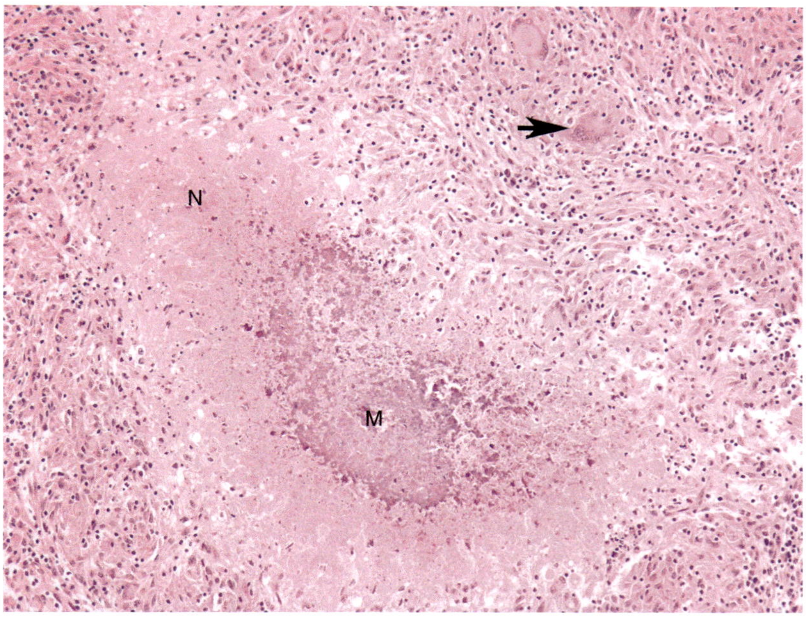

Fig. 11.27. Ox. Lymph node. Bovine tuberculosis. Histologically, the tubercle is characterized by a central eosinophilic area of caseous necrosis (N), often with dystrophic mineralization (M), surrounded by a rim of epithelioid macrophages and Langhans-type multinucleated giant cells (arrow) (H&E).

11.4.3.2 Mycobacterium avium *subsp.* paratuberculosis

Introduction. Paratuberculosis or Johne's disease, caused by *Mycobacterium avium* subspecies *paratuberculosis*, is an important enteric disease of cattle manifesting as transmural granulomatous enteritis, predominantly in the distal small intestine. While primarily thought of as an enteric disease, infection can produce characteristic lesions in the regional hemolymphatic system. Lymphangitis is common, and is recognized as thickened and dilated lymphatics traversing the intestinal serosa through the mesentery to the draining mesenteric lymph nodes. In some cases, lymphangitis may be the only gross finding, and is specific enough to lead to presumptive diagnosis of paratuberculosis. Microscopically, changes in the often enlarged mesenteric lymph nodes range from sinus histocytosis in the early stages to granulomatous lymphadenitis in the advanced stages of disease.

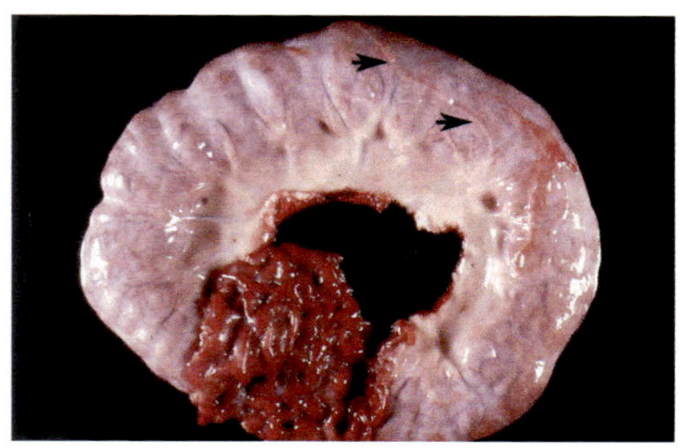

Fig. 11.28. Ox. Ileum. Granulomatous lymphangitis in paratuberculosis. Thickened and dilated lymphatics (lymphangiectasia and granulomatous lymphangitis) (arrows) traverse the serosal surface of the affected segments of small intestine.

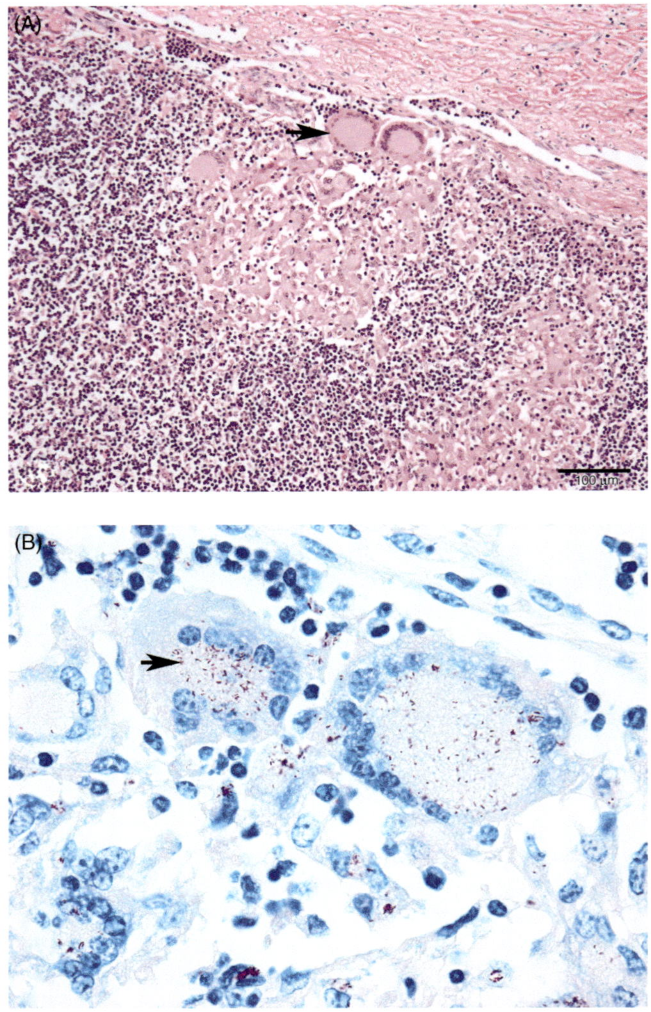

Fig. 11.29. Ox. Mesenteric lymph node. Granulomatous lymphadenitis in paratuberculosis. Histology (A) and acid-fast stain (B). Multifocal to coalescing granulomas are scattered within the cortex and are composed of epithelioid macrophages and Langhans-type, multinucleated giant cells (arrow). In cattle, the granulomas of paratuberculosis are non-caseating, in contrast to the caseating granulomas seen in bovine tuberculosis. Moderate numbers of small (1 μm × 2 μm), intracellular, acid-fast bacilli (arrow) are noted within the phagosomes of epithelioid macrophages and within multinucleated giant cells (H&E and Fite–Faraco stain) (see Chapter 5: Diseases of the Gastrointestinal Tract).

11.4.3.3 Mycoplasma bovis

Introduction. *Mycoplasma bovis* is an important cause of disease in cattle, with two principal manifestations: enzootic pneumonia in calves and chronic pneumonia and polyarthritis syndrome (CPPS) in feedlot cattle. CPPS has emerged as an important cause of morbidity and mortality in feedlot cattle. The classic lesions are of a caseonecrotic bronchopneumonia with potential hematogenous spread, resulting in arthritis and tenosynovitis. Similar areas of caseous necrosis are found uncommonly in the lymph nodes.

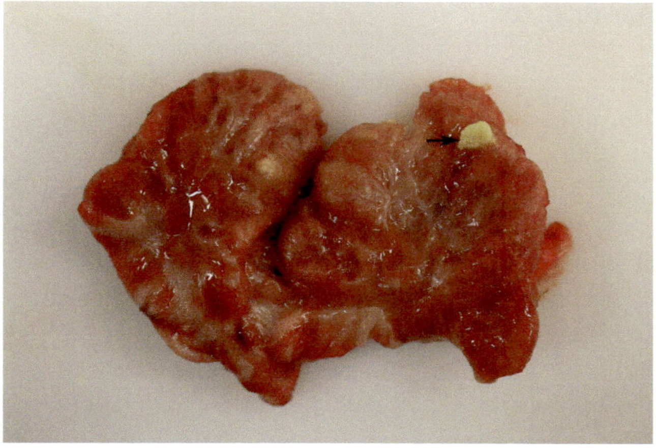

Fig. 11.31. Ox. Palatine tonsil. *Mycoplasma bovis.* Caseous tonsillitis. The upper respiratory tract appears to be the site of initial colonization of *M. bovis*. Experimental studies have found that the mucosa of both the palatine and pharyngeal tonsils are a major site of colonization following oral and transtracheal inoculation with multifocal foci of caseous necrosis (arrow) within the palatine tonsils. (Courtesy of Dr C. Legge, University of Calgary, Canada.)

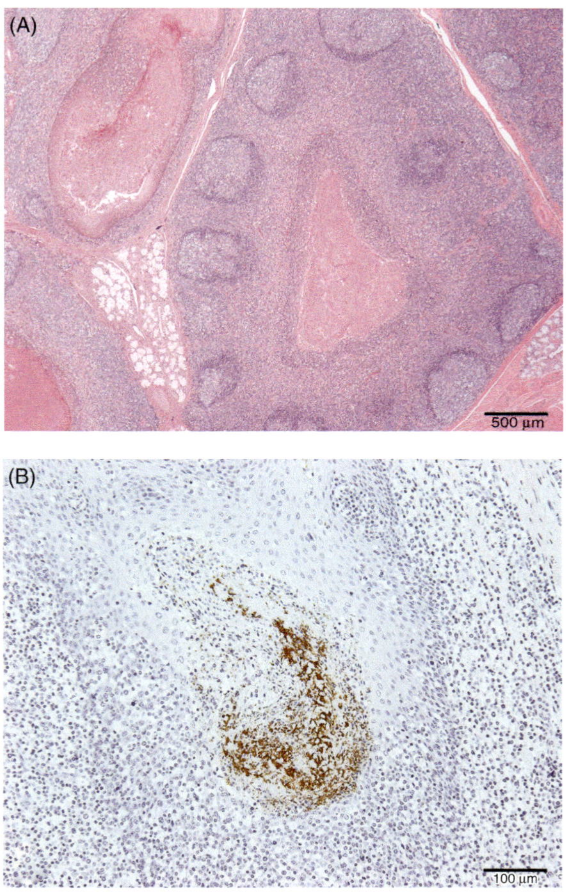

Fig. 11.32. Ox. Palatine Tonsil. *Mycoplasma bovis* tonsillitis. Histology (A) and *M. bovis* IHC (B). Histopathology reveals tonsillar crypts filled with a brightly eosinophilic coagulum admixed with nuclear debris (caseous necrosis) similar to the foci of necrosis typically observed in the lung. Immunohistochemical staining reveals abundant mycoplasmal antigen within the necrotic foci (H&E and IHC) (see Chapter 3: Diseases of the Respiratory System).

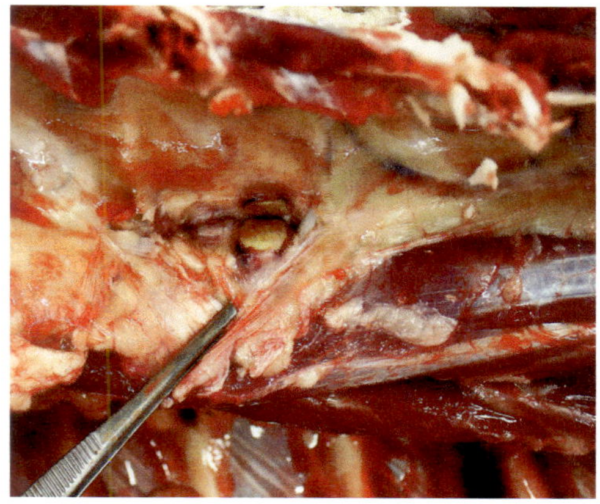

Fig. 11.30. Ox. Aortic lymph node. *Mycoplasma bovis* lymphadenitis. The normal lymph node architecture is effaced by caseous necrosis similar to the foci of caseous necrosis observed in the lungs.

11.4.4 *Bacillus anthracis*

Introduction. Anthrax is caused by *Bacillus anthracis*, a large, gram-positive, spore-forming bacterium with zoonotic potential. The presentation of anthrax depends on the host species, the bacterial strain, the dose, and the route of infection. Environmental conditions play a role in the number of environmental spores, and natural outbreaks are reported in instances of increased precipitation followed by hot, dry weather. In cattle, the likely route of infection is ingestion of contaminated soil, with percutaneous and inhalational transmission being of lesser importance. Ruminants are particularly susceptible to disease and the most common clinical form is peracute septicemia, with a clinical course lasting 1–2 h, with sudden death and no premonitory signs. Occasionally, animals will present with an acute form manifesting as extreme pyrexia, restlessness or depression, dyspnea, hemorrhagic or cyanotic mucous membranes, muscle tremors, and convulsions. Recent observations from a large outbreak in Canada also noted profuse ante-mortem hemorrhage from the nose and mouth of some infected cattle. Cutaneous anthrax in cattle is uncommon, and is the result of biting flies or contamination of open wounds. The clinical course is protracted. Typically, the lesions are described as edematous swellings over the shoulder, neck, and thorax, but a recent report describes necrotic skin lesions or 'eschars' similar to those described in human cutaneous anthrax. Pulmonary anthrax is described infrequently in cattle and is characterized by an acute course with a pronounced productive cough.

Suspected anthrax cases should not be necropsied as exposure to air causes the organism to sporulate and contaminate the environment. Rather, blood can be obtained from the ear, tail tip, or coronet and submitted for examination of typical organisms, culture, and PCR. Organisms can be destroyed in 48 h or less by putrefaction. Carcasses often have bloody fluids exuding from orifices, darkened blood that fails to clot, rapid putrefaction, hemorrhages, edematous connective tissues, and cavitary effusions. The most significant lesion is splenomegaly, and on section, the splenic parenchyma is soft and dark red to black and oozes blood. The splenic lesion is rarely absent and is the only lesion present in some cases.

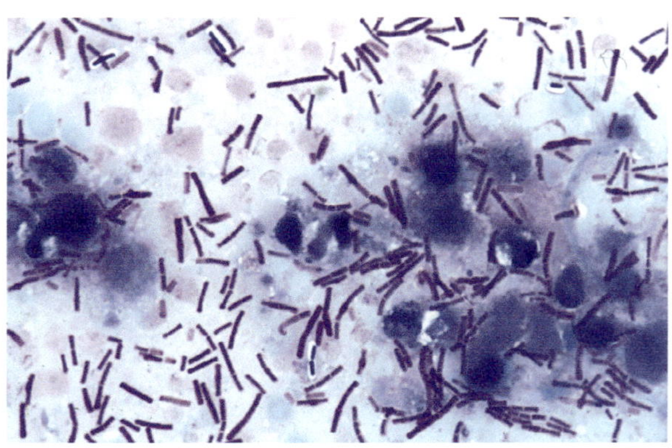

Fig. 11.33. Ox. Impression smear of the spleen. Anthrax. In the fulminating form is largely an intravascular disease and organisms are demonstrated easily in the peripheral blood and spleen. *Bacillus anthracis* are large, 1 × 6 µm bacilli, with truncated ends that occur in pairs or in short chains. They differ from putrefactive bacteria by their distinct capsule that stains pink with polychrome methylene blue (polychrome methylene blue). (Courtesy of Dr Musangu Ngeleka, Prairie Diagnostic Services, Canada.)

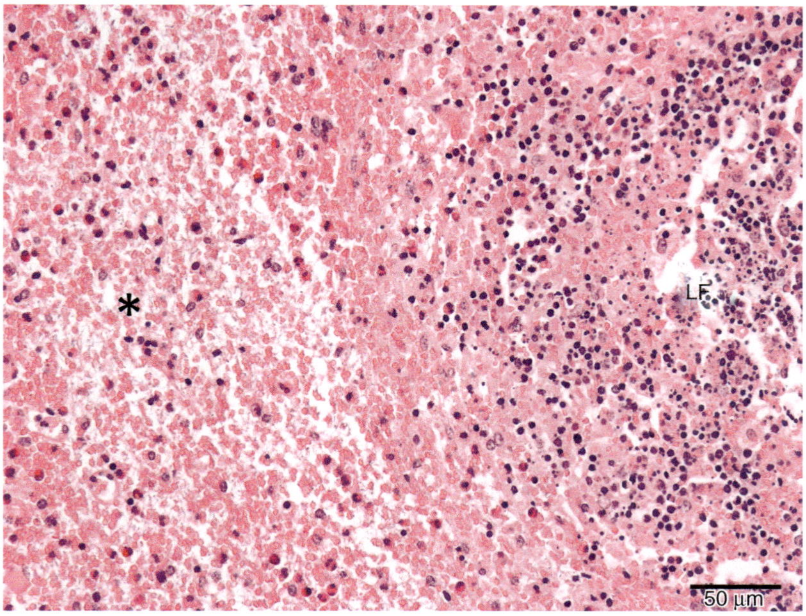

Fig. 11.35. Ox. Spleen. Anthrax. Congestion. There is marked congestion of the red pulp sinusoids (asterisk). Lymphoid follicles (LF) are hypocellular and there is marked lymphocytolysis, characterized by abundant pyknotic and karyorrhectic nuclear debris. Within the congested red pulp, there are innumerable 1 × 6 μm bacilli occurring individually or in short chains (H&E).

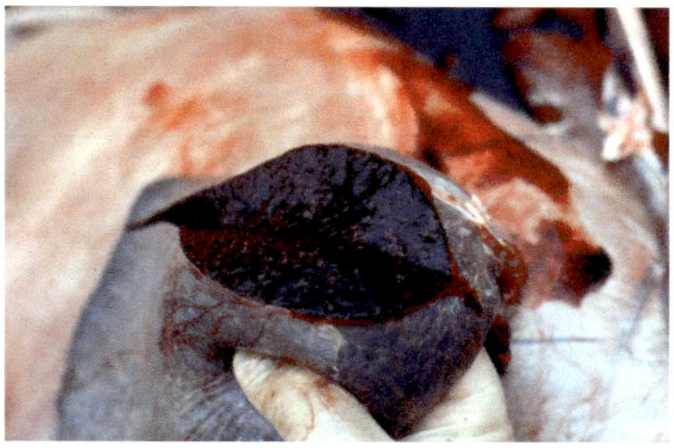

Fig. 11.34. Ox. Spleen. Anthrax. Splenomegaly. Splenic enlargement is the most distinctive lesion in anthrax, and on section, the spleen is soft and dark red to black (congestion). Finding splenomegaly in a bovine with a history of sudden death should always signal the potential for anthrax.

11.4.5 Splenic abscesses

Introduction. The monocyte–macrophage system of the spleen plays an important role in filtering blood-borne foreign material such as bacteria from circulation. Ineffectual killing of bacteria will allow the organism to proliferate, with the resultant formation of abscesses within the red pulp. In cattle, splenic abscesses can also result from direct extension of inflammation in traumatic reticuloperitonitis (hardware disease). Small nodules of lymphoid hyperplasia indicate chronic antigenic stimulation.

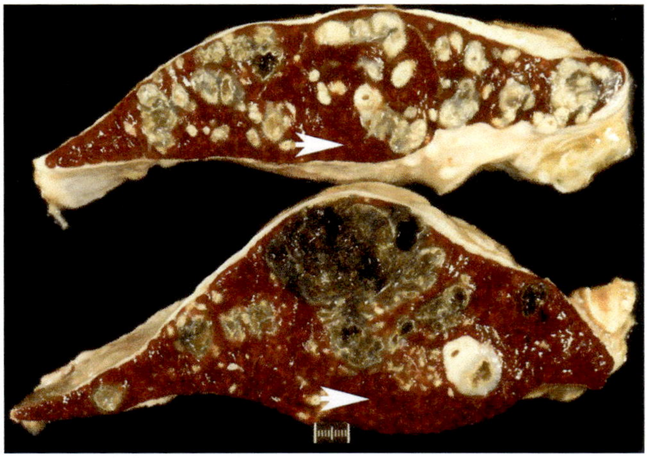

Fig. 11.36. Ox. Spleen. Abscesses. Multifocal to coalescing, variably sized, well-encapsulated nodules containing creamy, yellow to dark green exudate (arrows). Splenic abscesses are the result of bacteremia often due to pyogenic bacteria such as *Trueperella pyogenes*.

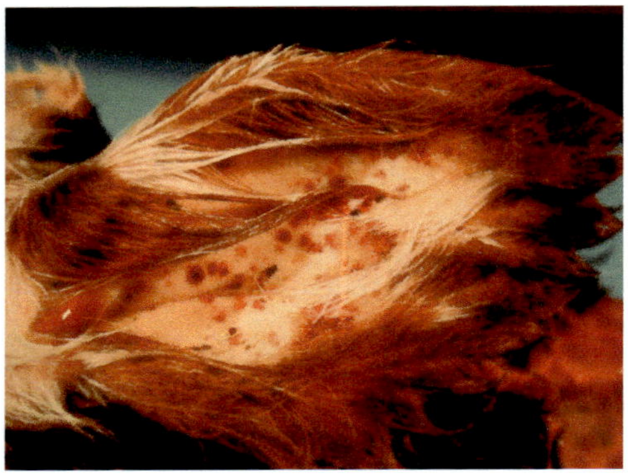

Fig. 11.37. Ox. Pinna. Bracken fern toxicity. Petechiae, Petechial and ecchymotic hemorrhages within the pinna are consistent with a defect in primary hemostasis due to thrombocytopenia. (See Chapter 7: Diseases of the Urinary System, and Chapter 16: The Pathology of Select Poisonous Plant-induced Diseases in Cattle.)

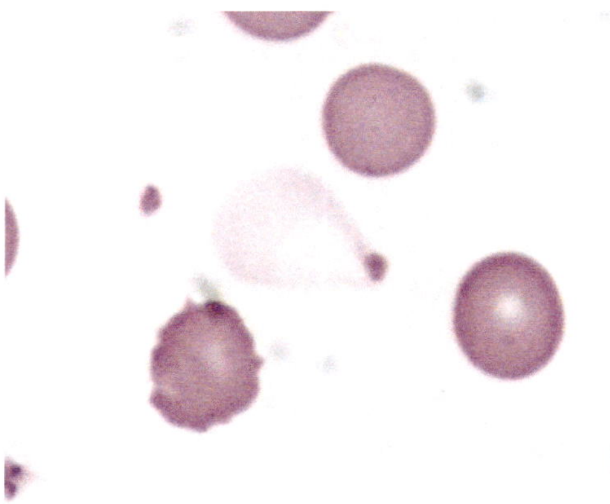

Fig. 11.38. Ox. Copper toxicity. Oxidation of hemoglobin in erythrocytes in copper toxicity results in the formation of Heinz bodies and lysis of the cell (ghost cell) (Wright–Giemsa).

11.5 TOXIC

11.5.1 Bracken fern toxicity

Bracken fern (*Pteridium aquilinum*) has a worldwide distribution, except for desert regions, and intoxication in cattle is most common in summer months when pastures have been overgrazed. In cattle, poisoning is associated with an acute syndrome of aplastic pancytopenia and a chronic syndrome characterized by the development of urinary tract neoplasms (enzootic hematuria). The acute syndrome reflects direct inhibition of pluripotent hematopoietic stem cells, resulting in thrombocytopenia, neutropenia, and non-regenerative anemia. The clinical signs and post-mortem findings include petechiae and bacteremia resulting from the thrombocytopenia and neutropenia, respectively. Histopathology of the bone marrow demonstrates marked hypocellularity, with either complete aplasia or only small islands of erythroid lineage remaining.

11.5.2 Oxidizing agents inducing hemolytic anemia

Introduction. Oxidative injury to erythrocytes occurs at a constant rate due to the formation of highly reactive oxygen species, including superoxide free radicals, hydrogen peroxide, and hydroxyl radicals. There are a number of enzymes in erythrocytes, including superoxide dismutase, glutathione reductase, and glutathione peroxidase, which protect, reduce, and reverse oxidative damage. Imbalances in this system (increased oxidation or removal of antioxidants) due to toxins results in oxidation of erythrocyte components, specifically hemoglobin (forming Heinz bodies), the erythrocytic cell membrane (forming eccentrocytes), and the ferrous (Fe^{2+}) ion to its ferric (Fe^{3+}) form (forming methemoglobin) (see Table 11.1). Both Heinz bodies and eccentrocytes are fragile and susceptible to lysis within the vasculature (resulting in intravascular hemolysis) and removal in the spleen (extravascular hemolysis).

Table 11.1. Oxidative agents causing hemolytic anemia in cattle.

Agent	Pathologic mechanism
Copper/selenium deficiency	Decrease in glutathione peroxidase enzyme (Se deficiency) and decrease in superoxide dismutase (Cu deficiency)
Copper toxicity	Direct oxidative damage to erythrocytes
Brassica plants	S-methylcysteine sulfoxide (SMCO) converted to propyl disulfides in the rumen cause direct oxidative damage to erythrocytes
Onions, garlic, and plants of *Allium* family	S-methylcysteine sulfoxide (SMCO) converted to propyl disulfides in the rumen cause direct oxidative damage to erythrocytes
Oak leaves and acorns	Tannic acid in immature leaves and acorns converted to pyrogallol, which oxidizes hemoglobin to methemoglobin and causes direct oxidative damage to erythrocytes

11.5.3 Moldy sweet clover (dicoumarol) poisoning

Introduction. Cattle ingesting moldly sweet clover silage or hay can develop a hemorrhagic diathesis. The disease is most commonly seen in the winter months, when cattle are fed stored hay or silage. Coumarol, a normal component of sweet clover, is converted to dicoumarol by some fungi. Dicoumarol competitively inhibits vitamin K epoxide reductase and impairs the synthesis of vitamin K-dependent coagulation factors, including factors II (prothrombin), VII, IX, and X. This results in dysfunction of the extrinsic, intrinsic, and common coagulation pathways, resulting in increased prothrombin time (PT) and activated partial thromboplastin time (APTT). Early in the course of disease, prolongation of PT may precede prolongation of APTT as factor VII has the shortest half-life of the vitamin K-dependent factors. These defects in secondary hemostasis are characterized by extensive hemorrhage into body cavities, joints, and subcutaneous tissues. While all ages of animal can be affected, aborted fetuses and young calves are more susceptible. Confirmation requires detection in feed, as there are no characteristic histopathologic lesions.

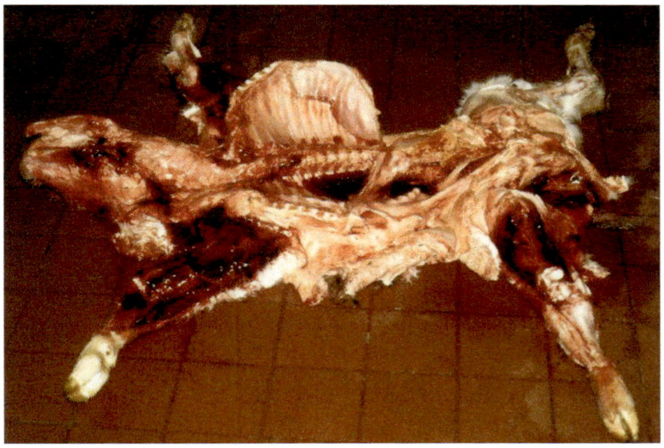

Fig. 11.39. Calf. Body. Dicoumarol toxicity. Hemorrhagic diathesis. There is extensive subcutaneous hemorrhage over the limbs, consistent with a defect in secondary hemostasis.

11.5.4 Nitrate poisoning

Introduction. The source of excess nitrates is variable and includes fertilizers, accumulation within certain plant species, and water. Nitrate is converted to nitrite in the rumen, and poisoning is associated with the formation of methemoglobin through the oxidation of ferrous to ferric ions in hemoglobin. Methemoglobinemia is associated with decreased oxygen transportation, and illness is recognized as dyspnea, weakness, stumbling gait, cyanosis, hypothermia, rapid and weak pulse, depression, convulsions, and death. In some outbreaks, the principal manifestation is abortions. Post-mortem changes include cyanosis of the mucous membranes, and brown discoloration of the blood and tissues as the result of methemoglobinemia. There are no characteristic histopathologic lesions.

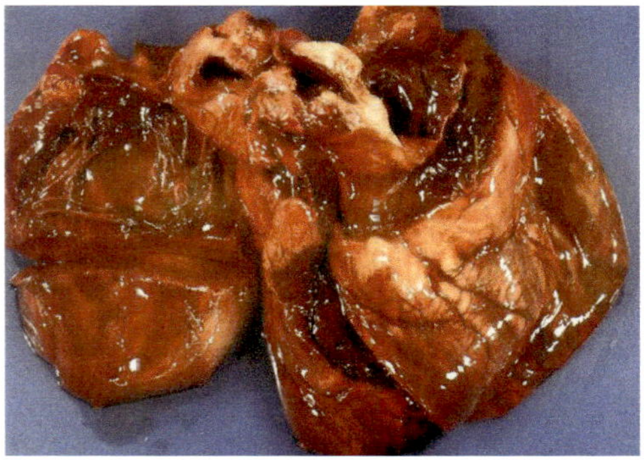

Fig. 11.40. Ox. Heart. Nitrate toxicity. Diapedesis. There is diffuse brown discoloration of the tissue as a result of methemoglobinemia.

11.6 NEOPLASIA

11.6.1 Bovine leukemia virus (BLV)

Introduction. Adult or enzootic lymphoma (lymphosarcoma), caused by bovine leukemia virus (BLV), is the most common neoplasm found in cattle. BLV infection is highly cell associated and typically infects immature B-cells that have undergone immunoglobulin gene rearrangement, but not hypermutation. Not all infected cattle develop lymphosarcoma, with approximately 30% developing persistent lymphocytosis (leukosis) and 3–4% developing B-cell lymphosarcoma. The susceptibility of cattle to infection is related to the BoLA haplotype, and transformation to lymphosarcoma is likely due to additional mutations in p53 tumor suppressor genes. Enzootic lymphoma occurs in cattle >4 years of age, with multiple body systems often affected. Tumors develop in a variety of locations, the most common being the lymph nodes, where cattle can present with exophthalmos due to retrobulbar lymph node enlargement, dysphagia due to pharyngeal node enlargement, or with palpable inguinal masses during rectal examination. Many animals have hepatic and splenic involvement. Myocardial infiltration of lymphosarcoma causes secondary heart failure. The submucosa of the abomasum and the uterus are other predilection sites, and cattle with abomasal lymphosarcoma present with abomasal ulceration, gastrointestinal hemorrhage, and weight loss. Finally, infiltration of lymphosarcoma into the peri-neural tissue of spinal nerves and the spinal cord can cause hindlimb lameness in cattle.

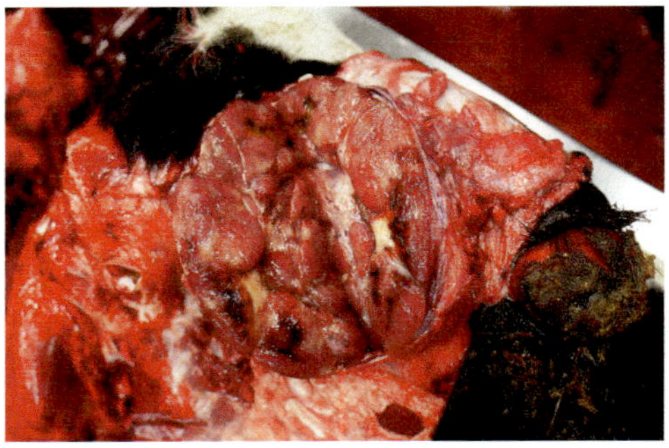

Fig. 11.42. Ox. Retrobulbar lymph nodes. Enzootic lymphoma. Involvement of the retrobulbar lymph nodes is common, and results in exophthalmos. Characteristically, lymphoma tissue is homogeneous, pale, bulges on section, and effaces the normal lymph node architecture (see Chapter 15: Diseases of Eye and Ear). (Courtesy of Dr C. Legge, University of Calgary, Canada).

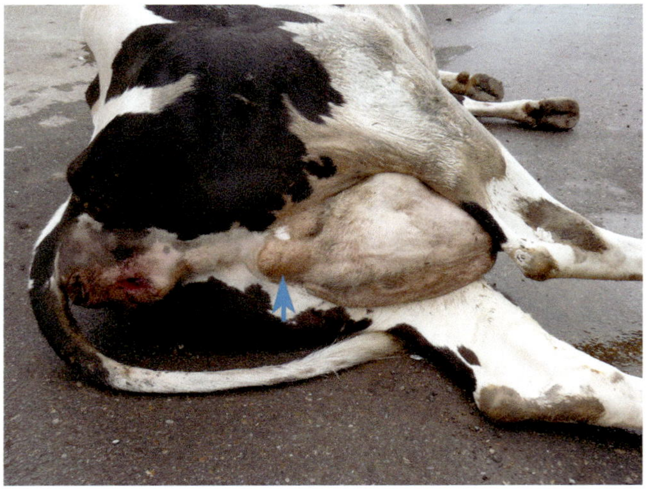

Fig. 11.41. Ox. Supramammary lymph nodes. Enzootic lymphoma. The most common presentation of enzootic lymphoma is enlargement of lymph nodes and is observed easily in the supramammary lymph nodes (arrow). (Courtesy of Dr C. Legge, University of Calgary, Canada.)

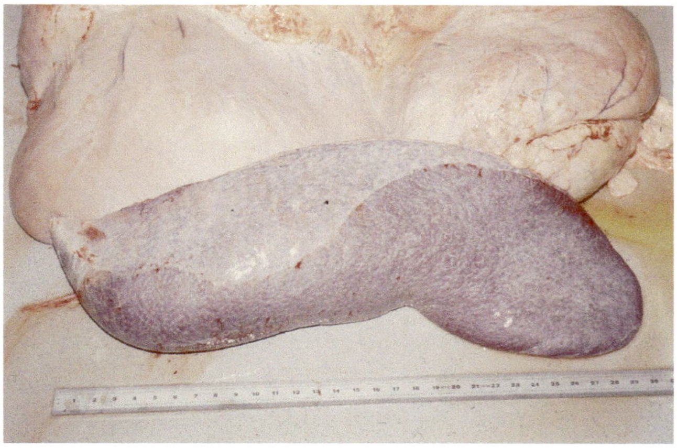

Fig. 11.43. Ox. Spleen. Splenomegaly. Enzootic lymphoma. There is diffuse enlargement due to infiltration of neoplastic lymphocytes. The spleen is firm and 'meaty'. Splenic rupture secondary to splenic lymphoma can cause rapid hemoabdomen and acute death.

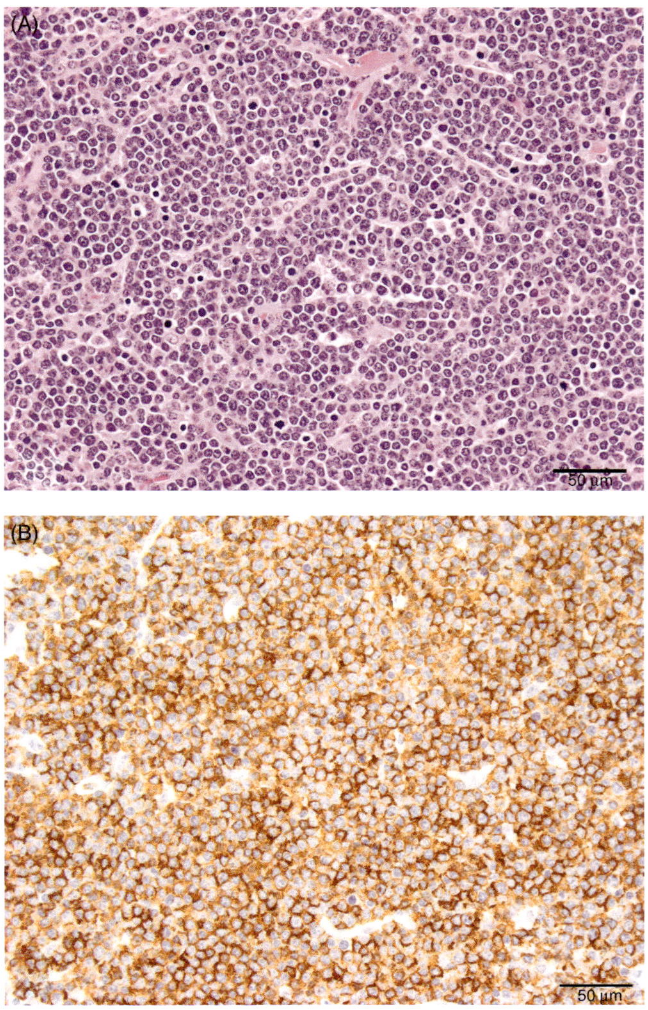

Fig. 11.46. Ox. Abomasum. Enzootic lymphoma. Histology (A) and CD20 IHC (B). Histopathology reveals a monomorphic population of large lymphocytes arranged in featureless sheets effacing the normal tissue architecture. Immunohistochemical staining for CD20 is strongly positive, indicating neoplastic lymphocytes of B-cell origin (H&E) (IHC).

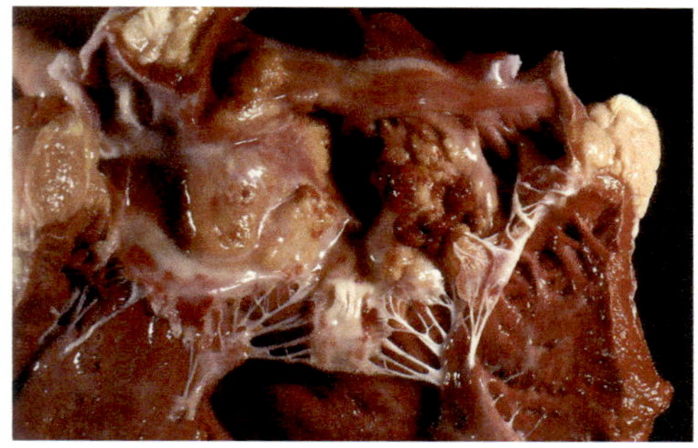

Fig. 11.44. Ox. Heart. Enzootic lymphoma. Cardiac involvement is often seen in bovine leukemia virus (BLV). Grossly, there are two presentations: a nodular form and a diffuse form. In the nodular form, lesions are most often seen in the atria and can be difficult to distinguish from epicardial fat. The diffuse form affects the ventricular myocardium more severely and can be difficult to distinguish from areas of myocardial necrosis. (Also see Chapter 4: Diseases of the Cardiovascular System.)

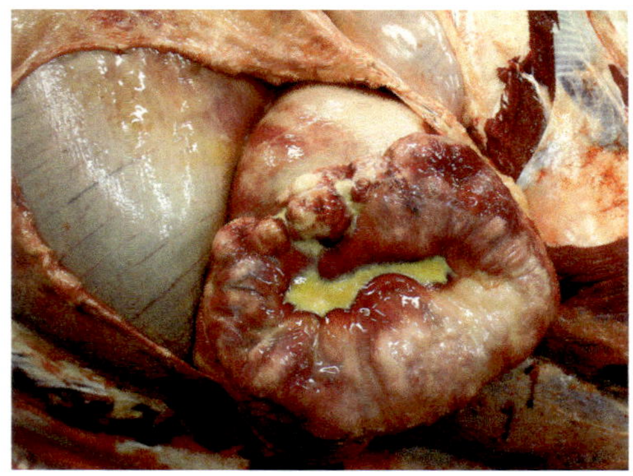

Fig. 11.45. Ox. Abomasum. Enzootic lymphoma. The wall of the abomasum is markedly expanded with lymphatic neoplasia. Involvement of the abomasum may eventually lead to ulceration and gastrointestinal hemorrhage. (Also see Chapter 5: Diseases of the Gastrointestinal Tract.) (Courtesy of Dr C. Legge, University of Calgary, Canada.)

11.6.2 Sporadic lymphoma

11.6.2.1 Calf or juvenile form

Calf lymphoma occurs early in life, <6 months old, and may be present from birth. There is diffuse lymphadenomegaly and frequent bone marrow involvement with secondary myelophthisis, bone marrow infarction, and lymphocytic leukemia.

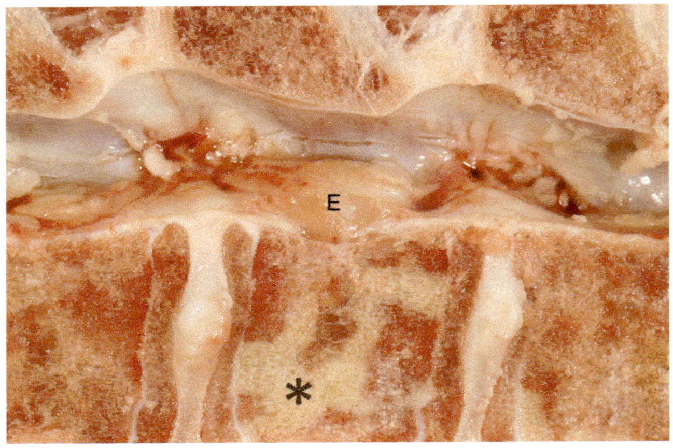

Fig. 11.47. Ox. Vertebral column. Calf lymphoma. Bone marrow infarction (asterisk) in the vertebrae and long bones is well described in the calf form of sporadic bovine lymphoma. Bone marrow infarction in bovine lymphosarcoma is likely the result of diminished bone marrow circulation due to neoplastic cells causing collapse of sinusoids or intravascular obstruction. There is extension of the neoplasm into the epidural space (E).

11.6.2.2 Thymic form

Thymic lymphoma in cattle generally occurs in younger, yearling cattle. Due to the cervical location of the thymus in cattle, there is often cervical enlargement, as well as brisket edema and esophageal compression that can cause secondary bloat or dysphagia. Like other thymic lymphomas, the lymphoma is usually T-cell in origin and positive on CD3 immunohistochemical staining.

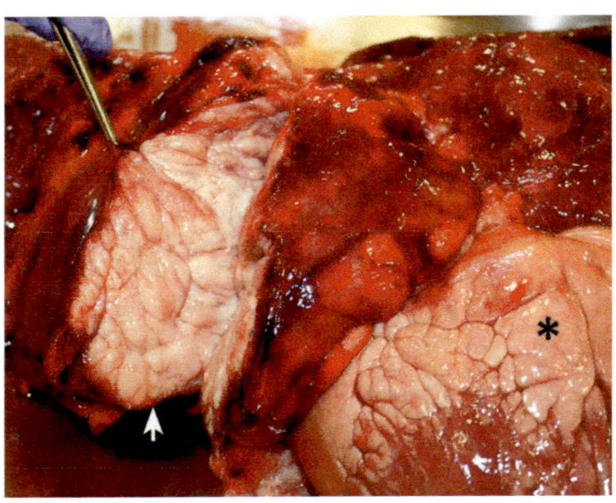

Fig. 11.49. Ox. Cranial mediastinum. Thymic lymphoma. Thymic enlargement. There is diffuse enlargement and effacement of the thymus with homogeneous, pale tissue that bulges slightly on section (arrow). Lymphoma is often described as having a lardaceous appearance; note the remarkable similarity between the tumor and the epicardial fat (asterisk).

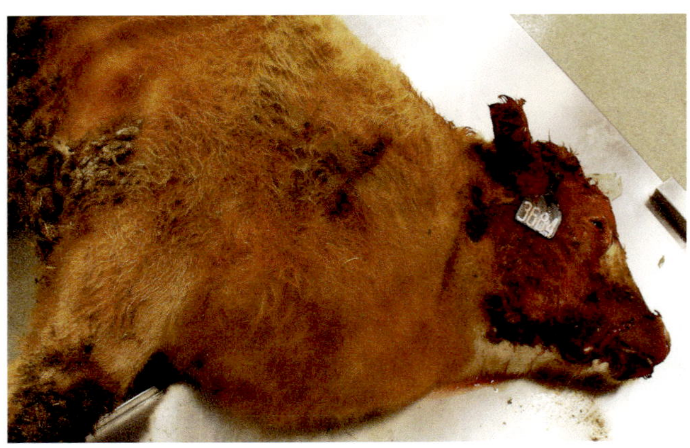

Fig. 11.48. Ox. Cervical lymph nodes. Thymic lymphoma. Lymphadenopathy. Thymic lymphoma in cattle can extend from the ramus of the mandible to the base of the heart, with constriction at the thoracic duct. (Courtesy of Dr C. Legge, University of Calgary, Canada.)

11.6.2.3 Cutaneous form

Cutaneous lymphoma in cattle is a more indolent form of lymphoma and presents as waxing and waning, plaque-like masses over the head, sides, and perineum. Similar to mycosis fungoides in humans, there is intense dermotropic infiltration, including focal epidermal invasion with formation of 'Pautrier's microabscesses' and, later, leukemia with 'Sezary' type cells. Late organ involvement is indistinguishable from enzootic lymphoma.

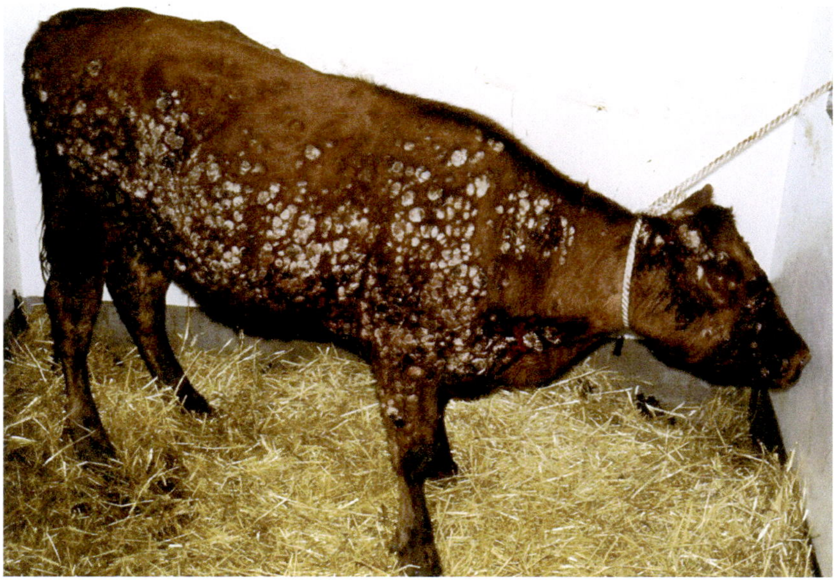

Fig. 11.50. Ox. Skin. Cutaneous lymphoma. Plaque-like masses are present over the head and sides of the animal, with secondary hair loss and ulceration (see Chapter 12: Diseases of the Integument).

SUGGESTED READING

Boudreaux, M.K., Schmutz, S.M. and French, P.S. (2007) Calcium diacylglycerol guanine nucleotide exchange factor I (CalDAG-GEFI) gene mutations in thrombopathic Simmental calf. *Veterinary Pathology* 44, 932–935.

Brodersen, B.W. (2014) Bovine viral diarrhea virus infections: manifestations of infection and recent advances in understanding pathogenesis and control. *Veterinary Pathology* 51, 453–464.

Fitzgerald, S.D. and Kaneene, J.B. (2012) Wildlife reservoirs of bovine tuberculosis worldwide: hosts, pathology, surveillance and control. *Veterinary Pathology* 50, 488–499.

Florins, A., Boxus, M., Vandermeers, F., Verlaeten, O., Bouzar, A.B., *et al.* (2008) Emphasis on cell turnover in two hosts infected by bovine leukemia virus: a rationale for host susceptibility to disease. *Veterinary Immunology and Immunopathology* 125, 1–7.

Himsworth, C.G. and Argue, C.K. (2009) Clinical impressions of anthrax from the 2006 outbreak in Saskatchewan. *Canadian Veterinary Journal* 50, 291–294.

Perez-Alenza, M.D., Blanco, J., Sardon, D., Sanchez Moreiro, M.A., Rodriguez-Bertos, A., *et al.* (2006) Clinico-pathological findings in cattle exposed to chronic bracken fern toxicity. *New Zealand Veterinary Journal* 54, 185–192.

Strugnell, B. and McAuliffe, L. (2012) *Mycoplasma wenyonii* infection in cattle. *In Practice* 34, 146–154.

Walz, P.H., Bell, T.G., Steficek, B.A., Kaiser, L., Maes, R.K. and Baker, J.C. (1999) Experimental model of type II bovine viral diarrhea virus-induced thrombocytopenia in neonatal calves. *Journal of Veterinary Diagnostic Investigation* 11, 505–514.

CHAPTER 12

Diseases of the Integument

12.1 Normal Skin

12.2 Congenital and Genetic Abnormalities
- 12.2.1 Hypotrichosis
- 12.2.2 Epitheliogenesis imperfecta
- 12.2.3 Cutaneous asthenia
- 12.2.4 Congenital ichthyosis
- 12.2.5 Familial acantholysis of Angus calves
- 12.2.6 Mechanobullous disease of Brangus calves
- 12.2.7 Epidermolysis bullosa

12.3 Idiopathic Diseases
- 12.3.1 Telogen defluxion, anagen defluxion and alopecia

12.4 Viral Diseases
- 12.4.1 Cutaneous papillomatosis ('warts')
- 12.4.2 Bovine viral diarrhea virus (BVDV)
- 12.4.3 Malignant catarrhal fever (MCF)
- 12.4.4 Bovine papular stomatitis (BPS)
- 12.4.5 Pseudocowpox
- 12.4.6 Pseudolumpy skin disease

12.5 Bacterial Diseases
- 12.5.1 Dermatophilosis ('streptothricosis', 'rain scald')
- 12.5.2 Tuberculosis (cutaneous mycobacteriosis)
- 12.5.3 Atypical cutaneous mycobacteriosis (non-tuberculoid)
- 12.5.4 Staphylococcal dermatitis
- 12.5.5 Actinomycosis ('lumpy jaw')
- 12.5.6 Actinobacillosis
- 12.5.7 Cutaneous cellulitis and abscesses

12.6 Protozoal Diseases

12.7 Parasitic Diseases
- 12.7.1 Pediculosis (lice)
- 12.7.2 Ectoparasitic mange
  - 12.7.2.1 Sarcoptic mange
  - 12.7.2.2 Chorioptic mange
- 12.7.3 Stephanofilariasis
- 12.7.4 Pelodera dermatitis (rhabditic dermatitis)
- 12.7.5 Hypodermosis (warbles, cattle grubs)

12.8 Mycoses (Fungal Infections)
- 12.8.1 Dermatophytosis ('ringworm')
- 12.8.2 Fungal granulomas

12.9 Neoplastic Conditions
- 12.9.1 Cutaneous lymphoma (lymphosarcoma)
- 12.9.2 Squamous cell carcinoma (SCC)
- 12.9.3 Mast cell tumor
- 12.9.4 Melanocytomas/melanomas
- 12.9.5 Juvenile bovine angiomatosis
- 12.9.6 Cutaneous lipomas
- 12.9.7 Fibromas, fibrosarcomas, and other spindle cell tumors
- 12.9.8 Congenital, disseminated, undifferentiated round cell tumor

12.10 Miscellaneous Conditions
- 12.10.1 Subcutaneous soft or fluctuant swellings
- 12.10.2 Distal extremity necrosis – dry gangrene
- 12.10.3 Allergic (type I hypersensitivity) dermatitis
- 12.10.4 Photosensitivity dermatitis
- 12.10.5 Thermal burns
- 12.10.6 Generalized idiopathic dermatitis
- 12.10.7 Cutaneous infarcts

INTRODUCTION

The skin is the largest organ system of the body and is readily visible for detailed clinical examination. The skin is critical to the good health and survival of bovine species. It has both haired and non-haired areas and, along with the hair, acts as an effective physical barrier to various infectious agents, as well as to various types of trauma. The general health of the animal is often reflected in the appearance of the bovine skin, a dry dull coat, exudates in or on the hair coat, or areas of hair loss, suggesting perhaps some internal visceral disease problem or malnutrition.

Bovine skin is thicker than most other species, especially over the dorsum of the trunk and lateral aspects of the limbs, but otherwise has the same microanatomical structures, including epidermis and dermis, with apocrine and sebaceous glands. The subcutis contains variable amounts of adipose tissue and collagenous tissue (fascia), and connects to the deeper fascial structures and muscle tissue. In cattle, the apocrine glands often extend deeper than in other species and are often quite dilated histologically, which is considered normal.

In general terms, bovine skin diseases are not as well studied as in many other species. They also do not have as many neoplastic entities as, for example, in dogs, cats or horses; nor do they have as many immunologic disease entities.

This chapter does not attempt to cover all skin diseases of cattle, especially some of the diseases seen outside of North America.

12.1 NORMAL SKIN

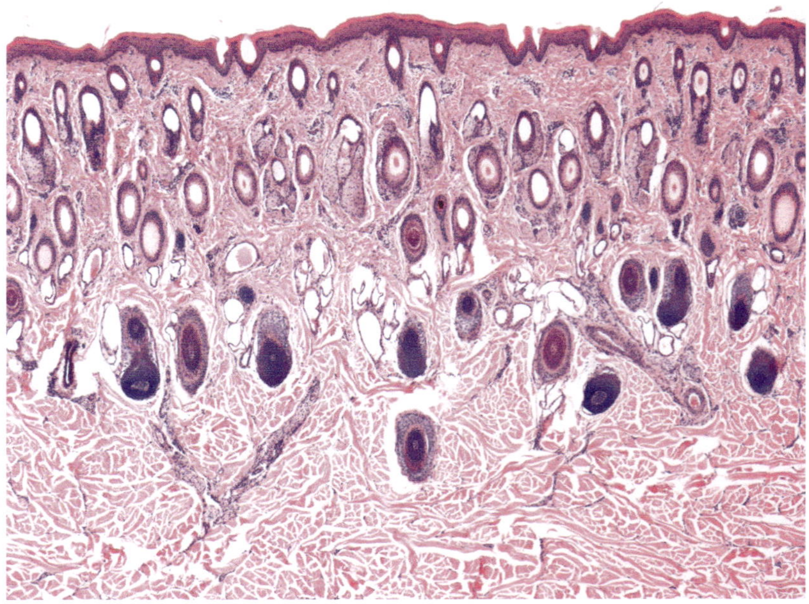

Fig. 12.1. Ox. Normal skin. Superficial dermis with hair follicles, apocrine and sebaceous glands. The deep dermis contains only blood vessels. The epidermis is thicker than in many other species, especially small animals (H&E).

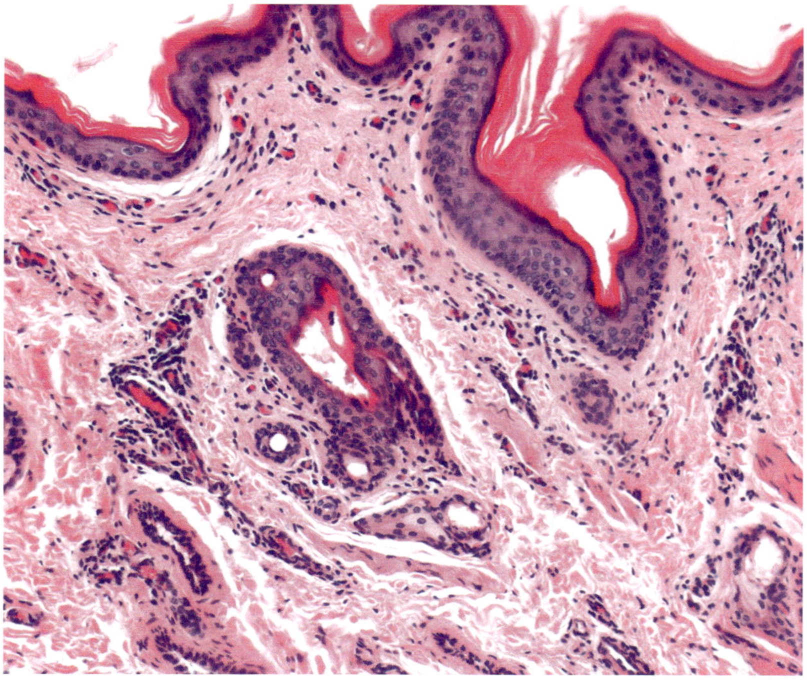

Fig. 12.2. Ox. Normal skin. Increased cellularity is considered normal in most ruminant species (H&E).

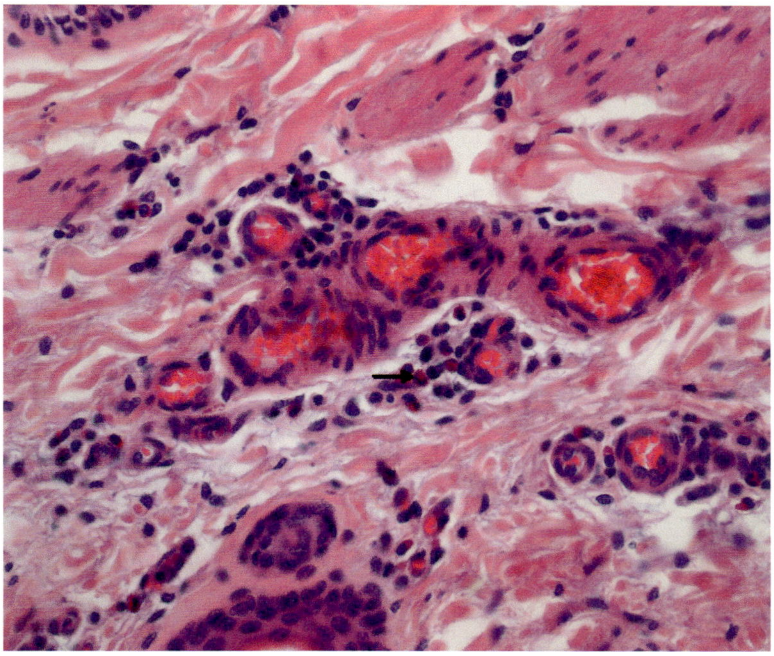

Fig. 12.3. Ox. Normal skin. Close-up of normal bovine skin to show increased cellularity in perivascular sites including variable numbers of eosinophils, also considered normal (arrow). Bovine eosinophils are not always easy to distinguish from neutrophils, so a Luna stain for eosinophils can be helpful. A periodic acid–Schiff (PAS) stain will usually stain neutrophil granules but not eosinophil granules. Numbers of eosinophils may vary with the presence of internal and no clinically visible external parasites, but this has not been studied closely (H&E).

12.2 CONGENITAL AND GENETIC ABNORMALITIES

12.2.1 Hypotrichosis

Introduction. This term means less than normal amount of hair and is usually seen at birth, whereas alopecia is loss of hair once present in normal amounts. At least 13 different types of hypotrichosis have been described in cattle, most of which are genetic. Some of the more important ones include lethal hypotrichosis in Holstein-Friesian and Japanese native cattle; simple autosomal recessive semi-hairlessness in polled and horned Hereford cattle; congenital anemia, dyskeratosis, and progressive alopecia in polled Herefords in Canada and the USA. Other breeds reporting hypotrichosis include Angus, Ayrshire, Brangus, Guernsey, Gelbvieh, Jersey, Anjou-Charolais, and Simmental crosses. Tardive hypotrichosis is a sex-linked condition in Holstein-Friesen females born normal but within a few months develop progressive hair loss. Although more common in piglets, congenital goiter calves are sometimes born with little to no hair (see Chapter 1: Diseases of Neonates and Calves), and bovine viral diarrhea virus (BVDV) infection *in utero* can result in partial hypotrichosis at birth as well.

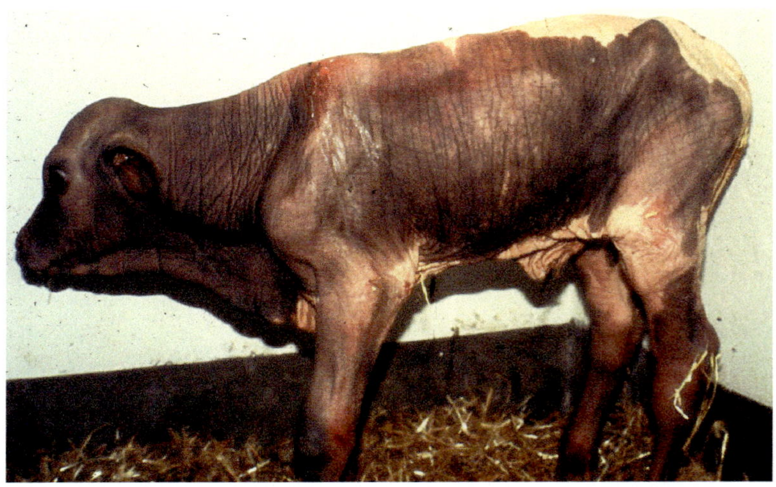

Fig. 12.4. Ox. Skin. Hypotrichosis. Newborn calf with severe hypotrichosis.

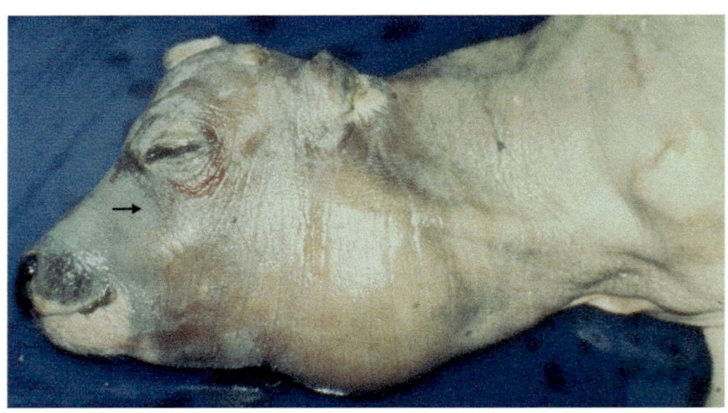

Fig. 12.5. Ox. Skin. Hypotrichosis. Full-term calf with goiter and hypotrichosis. Hair is seen on the tips of ears, and the gray patches on the head and face is surface hyperkeratosis (arrow).

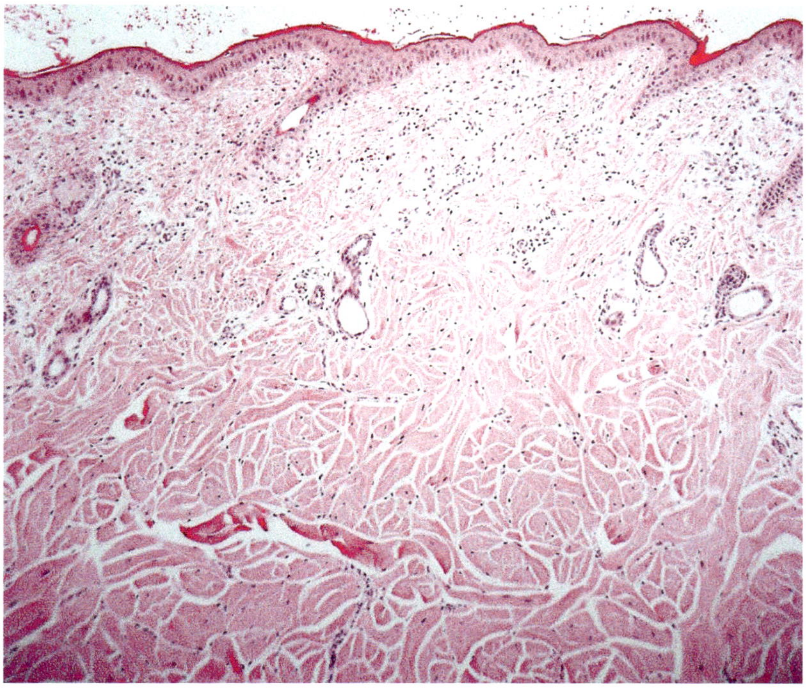

Fig. 12.6. Ox. Skin. Incomplete hypotrichosis. Full-term calf histologic picture of severe hypotrichosis showing lack of normal hair follicles, apocrine glands, and sebaceous glands (H&E).

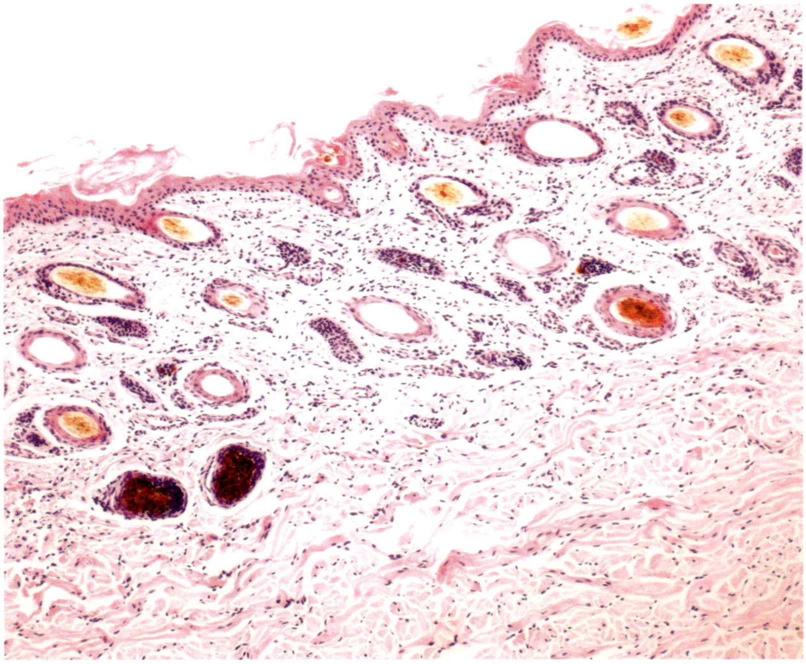

Fig. 12.7. Ox. Skin. Incomplete hypotrichosis. Case with irregular hair follicle bulbs: some follicles contain more normal-looking hair shafts, but apocrine and sebaceous glands are small or absent (H&E).

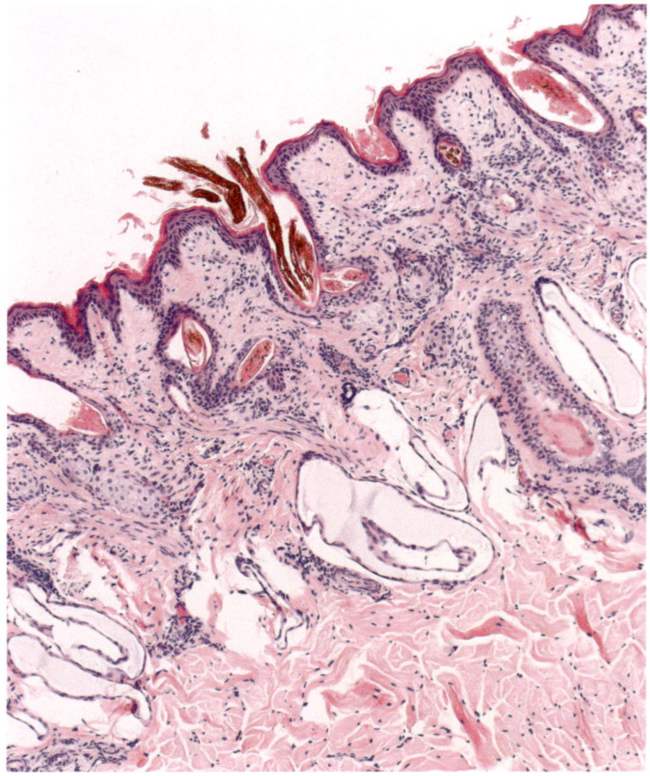

Fig. 12.8. Ox. Skin. Hypotrichosis. Case with no normal hair follicles, sebaceous and apocrine glands of unusual shapes, and a few hair shafts with variable thicknesses (H&E).

12.2.2 Epitheliogenesis imperfecta

Introduction. Epitheliogenesis imperfecta (aplasia cutis) has been reported in Holstein-Friesian, Hereford, Ayrshire, Jersey, Shorthorn, Aberdeen Angus, Dutch Black Pied, Swedish Red, Wagyu, and German Yellow Pied cattle. Calves are born with sharply demarcated areas of skin discontinuity, the areas being red, weeping, and most commonly affecting the limbs, sometimes lips and muzzle. Oral tissues can be involved with epithelial loss. Other defects such as cleft palate and polydactyly may be present. Secondary bacterial infections are common, and usually death occurs due to toxemia.

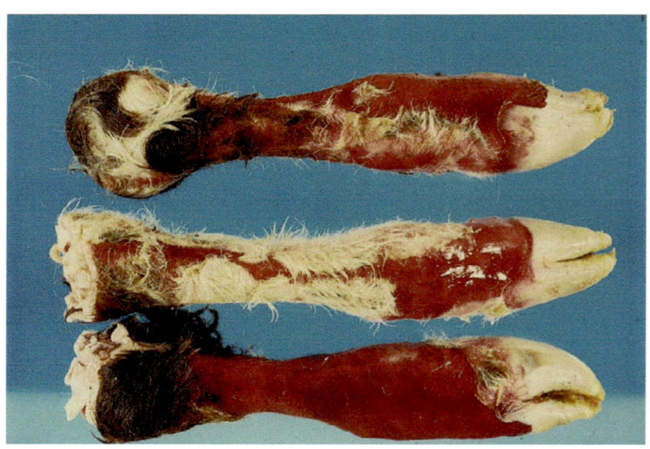

Fig. 12.9. Ox. Skin. Epitheliogenesis imperfecta. Three limbs from a newborn calf with large areas of absent epithelium.

12.2.3 Cutaneous asthenia

Introduction. Also known as collagen dysplasia, dermatosparaxis, Ehlers–Danlos syndrome, cutis laxis, and cutis hyperelastica. This is an inherited condition with hyperextensible skin, easily torn skin, and often coexisting joint laxity. Most cases are autosomal recessive and are reported in Simmental, Charolais, Holstein-Friesian, Hereford, Belgian Blue, and other crossbreeds. If healing occurs at all, the scars are thin. Subcutaneous edema sometimes occurs shortly after birth, especially of eyelids, dewlap, and distal limbs. If the skin has not separated, the diagnosis can be difficult or impossible to make by histopathology alone, and electron microscopic studies are needed. If there is suspect separation, the pathologist must receive full thickness biopsies (preferably incisional type) taken from areas of deep separation as well as normal skin sites even to attempt to make a diagnosis.

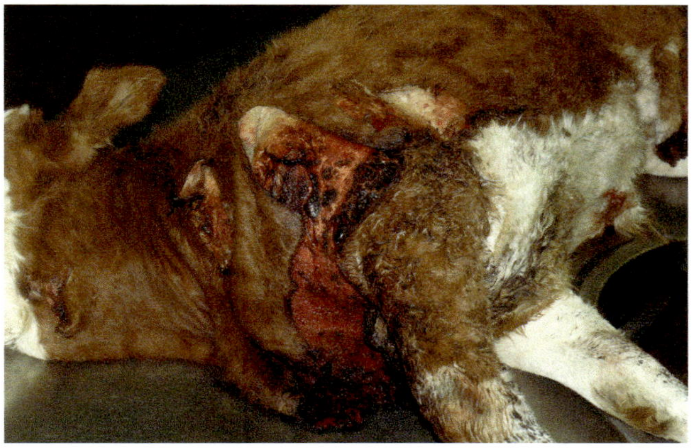

Fig. 12.10. Ox. Skin. Cutaneous asthenia. Simmental calf with extensive tearing of skin over shoulder and lateral neck regions. This region is particularly susceptible to minor trauma-induced tearing in a cutaneous asthenia case. The skin is torn easily with the fingers. The upper, freshly torn skin was done with bare fingers.

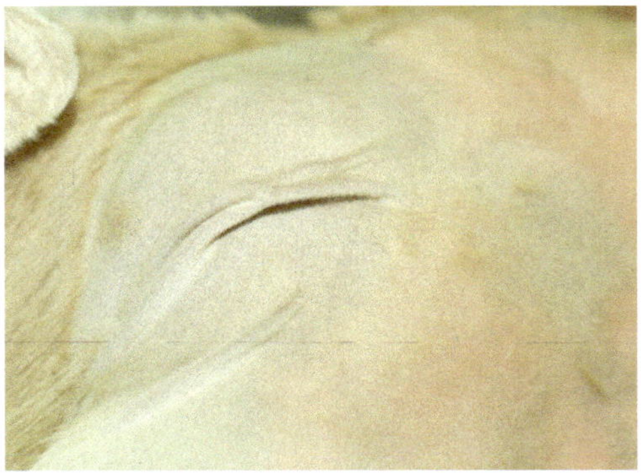

Fig. 12.11. Ox. Skin. Cutaneous asthenia. Charolais calf with cutaneous asthenia. Skin is easily thrown up into folds which persist and note the areas of cyanotic discoloration, due to separation of the deep dermal collagen cutting off normal blood supply.

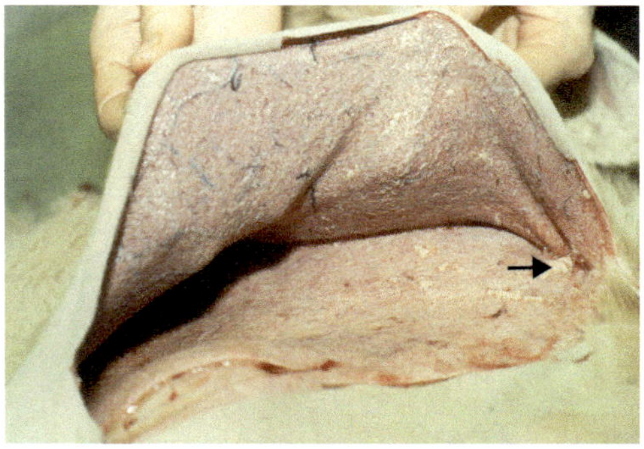

Fig. 12.12. Ox. Skin. Cutaneous asthenia. The same Charolais calf showing easily torn skin in the cyanotic areas, with separation having occurred through the deep (subadnexal) dermis. Note lack of any hemorrhage but small clumps of fibrin are present (arrow).

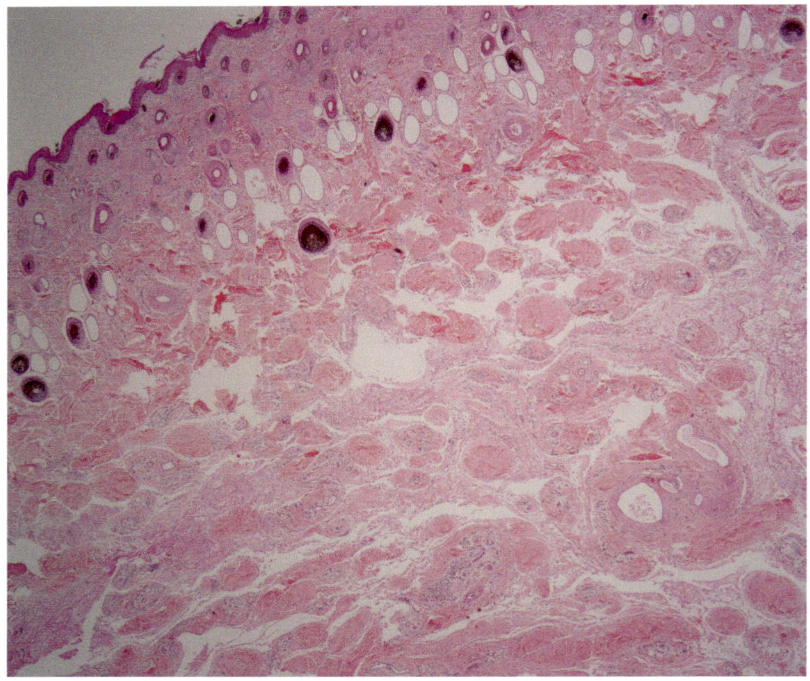

Fig. 12.13. Ox. Skin. Cutaneous asthenia. Histologic picture of a cutaneous asthenia calf with the deep dermis showing loose arrangement and clumping of collagen bundles, empty spaces between the collagen bundles, and the collagen fibers appear with abnormal shapes and sizes compared to the normal bovine skin presented in Fig. 12.1. A few areas of bright pink material are fibrin masses, and interstitial fibroblasts are far more numerous than normal. It is crucial when submitting samples for histopathology to choose skin adjacent to where separation has occurred, not just where it has separated, so the pathologist gets to view the full thickness skin (H&E).

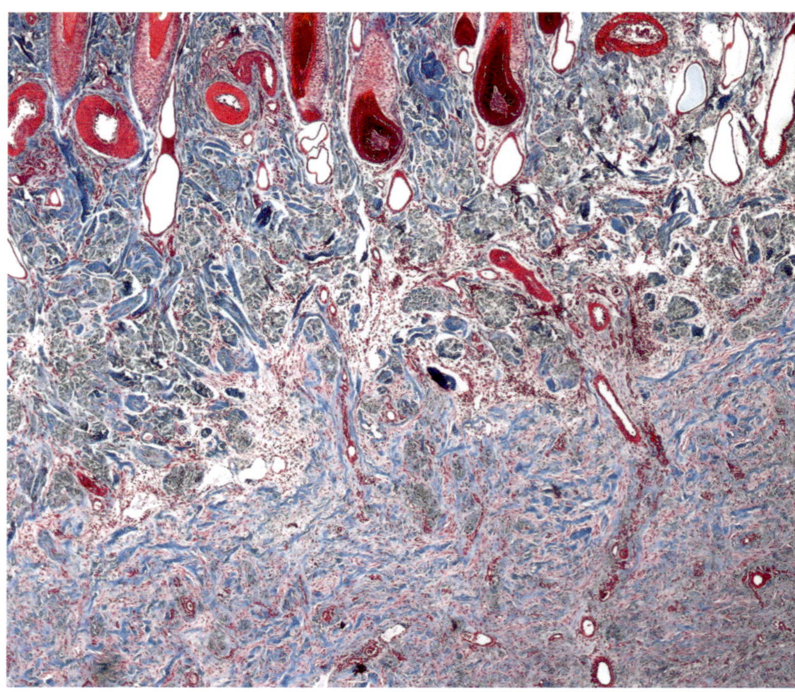

Fig. 12.14. Ox. Skin. In a special stain of the same case showing subadnexal loose arrangement of collagen, numerous interstitial fibroblasts and many collagen fibers stain green instead of the normal blue color. Sometimes, the abnormal fibers will show a red core as well (Masson's trichrome).

12.2.4 Congenital ichthyosis

Introduction. Defined as a rare keratinization defect problem, the most severe form known as ichthyosis fetalis, with diffuse, white, thick scale with deep fissures covering the whole body at birth (also known as Harlequin fetus). Hairs are present but not easily seen. Norwegian Red Polls, Friesians, and Brown Swiss are affected. Ichthyosis congenitalis, the other type, is less severe and occurs in Pinzgauer, Jersey, Chianina, and Holstein-Friesians. The latter breeds may be born with some lesions, but progressively develop more skin lesions later on. The condition is inherited as autosomal recessive.

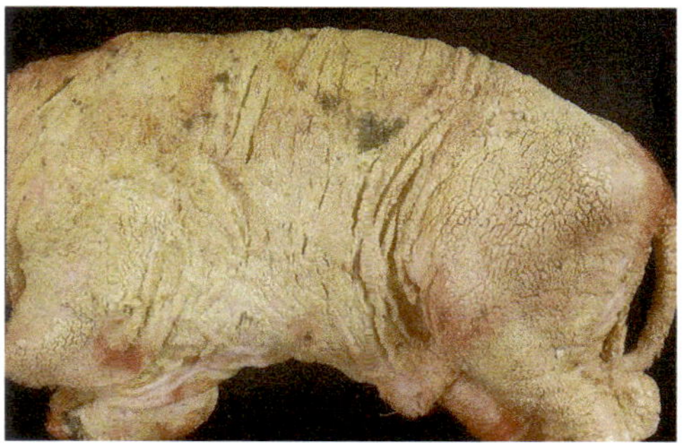

Fig. 12.15. Ox. Skin. Congenital ichthyosis. Newborn Charolais calf covered by thick white scales and horny epidermis with deep fissures. (Courtesy of Dr R. Postey, Manitoba Veterinary Diagnostic Laboratory, Canada.)

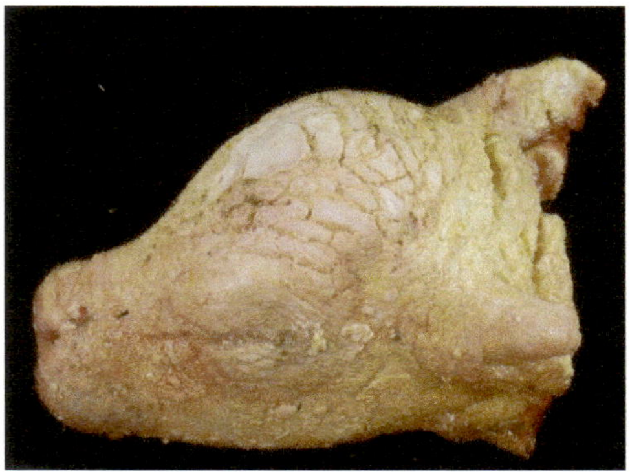

Fig. 12.16. Ox. Skin. Congenital ichthyosis. Newborn Charolais calf covered by thick white scales and horny epidermis with deep fissures. (Courtesy of Dr R. Postey, Manitoba Veterinary Diagnostic Laboratory, Canada.)

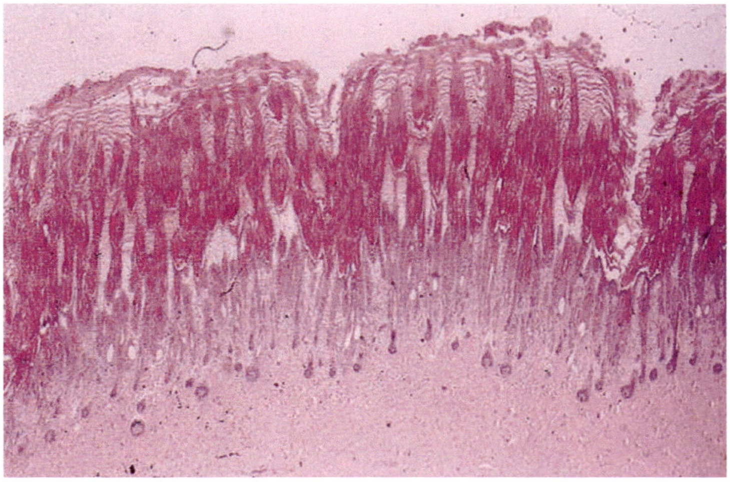

Fig. 12.17. Ox. Skin. Congenital ichthyosis. Same calf with laminated orthokeratotic hyperkeratosis arranged in frond projections, with hypergranulosis, keratohyalin granules abnormal in shape, size and number, and follicular hyperkeratosis (H&E). (Courtesy of Dr R. Postey, Manitoba Veterinary Diagnostic Laboratory, Canada.)

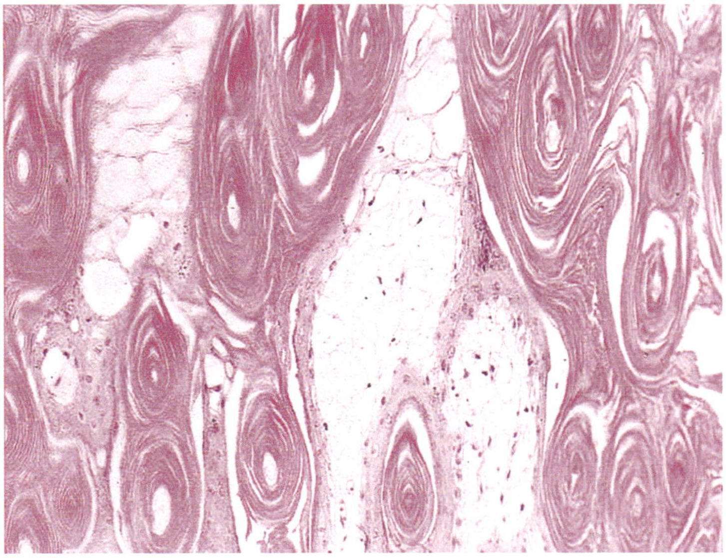

Fig. 12.18. Ox. Skin. Congenital ichthyosis. Higher magnification. Same calf with laminated orthokeratotic hyperkeratosis arranged in frond projections, with hypergranulosis, keratohyalin granules abnormal in shape, size and number, and follicular hyperkeratosis (H&E). (Courtesy of Dr R. Postey, Manitoba Veterinary Diagnostic Laboratory, Canada.)

12.2.5 Familial acantholysis of Angus calves

Introduction. A bullous and ulcerative dermatosis of Angus calves caused by a breakdown of intercellular adhesions due to anomalous development of desmosome–tonofilament complexes in epidermal and follicular basal and stratum spinosum cells. It is fatal and thought to be an autosomal recessive trait. Shedding of the epidermis and oral mucosa with ulceration occurs, especially in areas subject to trauma such as the carpus, metacarpophalangeal joints, phalanges, coronary borders, and with partial hoof separation. It is similar to epidermolysis bullosa but with the primary process being acantholysis.

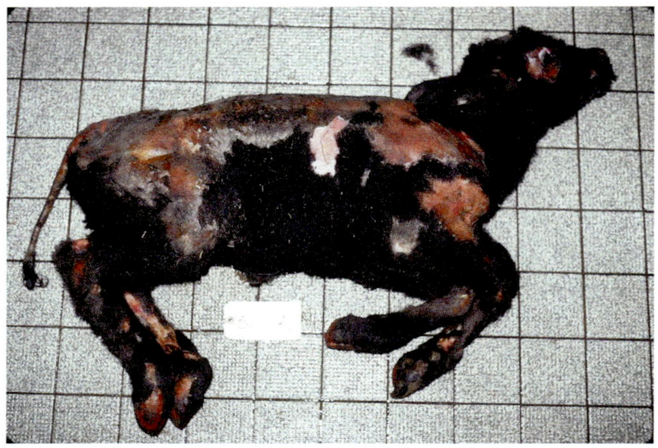

Fig. 12.19. Ox. Skin. Acantholysis. Small Angus calf with extensive trunk, limb, and periocular hair and epidermal loss. (Courtesy of Dr K. Thompson, Massey University, New Zealand.)

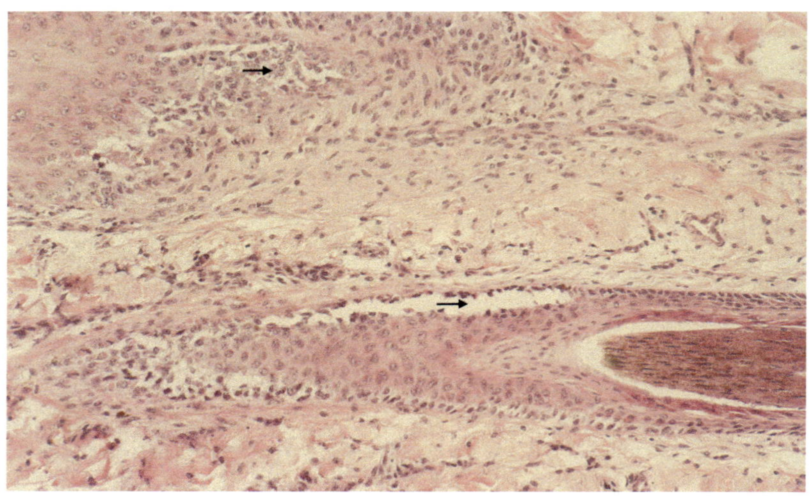

Fig. 12.20. Ox. Skin. Acantholysis. Histologic picture showing two hair follicles with acantholysis and with separation from the basal cells (arrows) (H&E). (Courtesy of Dr K. Thompson, Massey University, New Zealand.)

12.2.6 Mechanobullous disease of Brangus calves

Introduction. A few cases of this rare condition have been described. The condition is clinically identical to familiar acantholysis in Angus calves, but with no acantholysis occurring. The lesions instead are a result of sub-basement membrane ('sub-basilar') separation from the epidermis. The disorder is also different to epidermolysis bullosa in that no true lysis of the epidermis occurs.

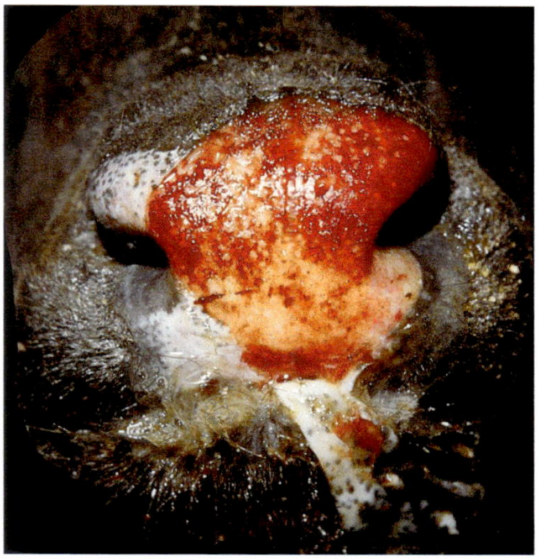

Fig. 12.21. Ox. Nose. Mechanobullous disease. Muzzle and nostrils of a Brangus calf with extensive ulceration/sloughing of the epidermis, exposing the weeping, hemorrhagic dermis/submucosa. (Courtesy of Dr K. Thompson, Massey University, New Zealand.)

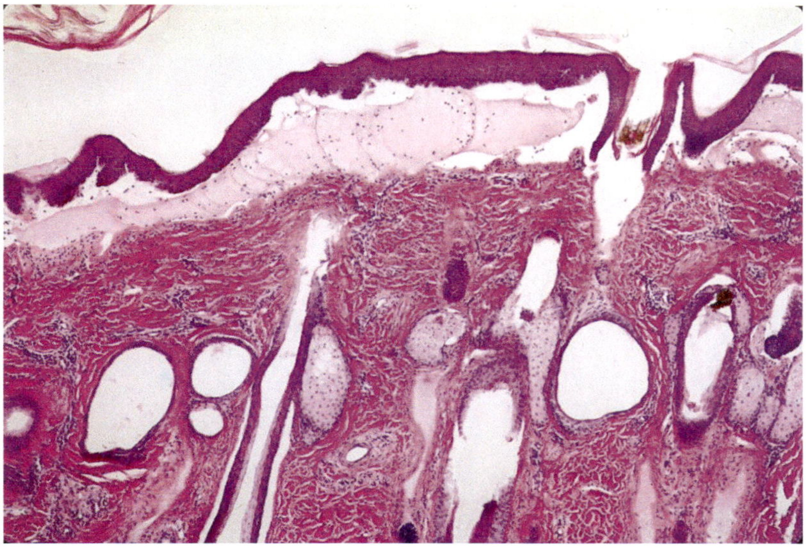

Fig. 12.22. Ox. Skin. Mechanobullous disease. Histologic picture of haired skin from a Brangus calf showing separation of the intact epidermis from the dermis, the bulla containing proteinaceous fluid and low numbers of inflammatory cells. No significant inflammatory changes are present in the dermis (H&E). (Courtesy of Dr K. Thompson, Massey University, New Zealand.)

12.2.7 Epidermolysis bullosa

Introduction. Another mechanobullous disease that in most cases has autosomal recessive traits (except in Simmental and crosses, where it is inherited as autosomal dominant with incomplete penetrance). The condition occurs in many breeds, including Holstein-Friesian, Ayrshire, Jersey, Shorthorn, Angus, Brangus, Dutch Black Pied, Swedish Red Pied, German Yellow Pied, Blonde d'Aquitaine, Charolais, Simmental, Red Breed of West Flanders, and Romagnola–Marchigiana crosses. Vesicles and bulla occur in sites easily traumatized. Sites of separation vary from basal cell zone to lamina lucida of basement membrane zone to superficial dermis. Occurs in very young calves and often proves fatal. Typical clinical signs coupled with histopathology and electron microscopy are needed to confirm the diagnosis. Lesions are most common in distal limbs, including hoof sloughing, in the oral cavity, pinna, muzzle, and pressure points. Depending on site of separation, the three types described in cattle include epidermolysis simplex, junctional epidermolysis bullosa, and dystrophic epidermolysis bullosa.

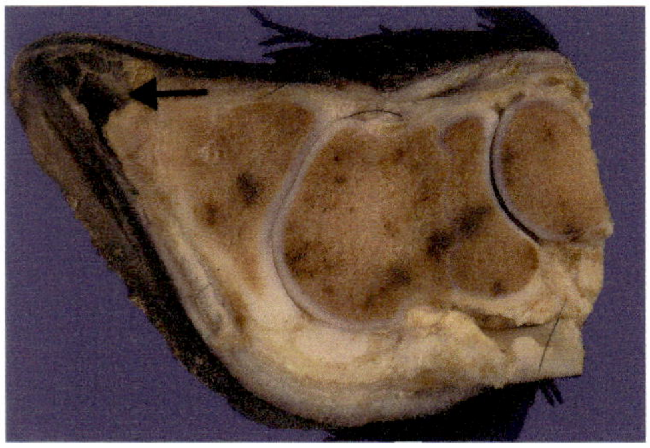

Fig. 12.23. Ox. Foot. Epidermolysis bullosa. Formalin-fixed sagittal section of a calf's hoof with separation of the cranial hoof wall from the corium in a Romagnola–Marchigiana cross calf (arrow).

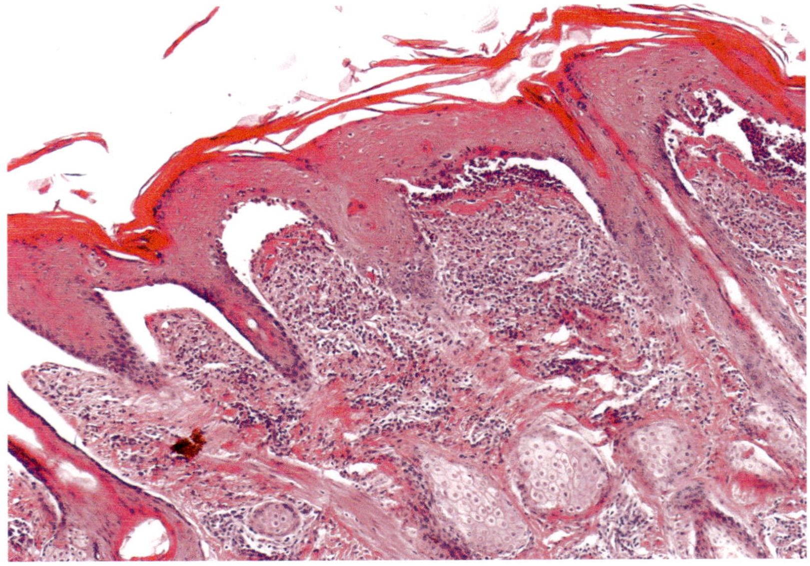

Fig. 12.24. Ox. Skin. Epidermolysis bullosa. Histologic example of undetermined type of epidermolysis bullosa in a Romagnola–Marchigiana cross calf, showing separation through or just beneath the basal lamina, with large numbers of inflammatory cells in the superficial dermis (H&E).

12.3 IDIOPATHIC DISEASES

12.3.1 Telogen defluxion, anagen defluxion and alopecia

Introduction. Telogen defluxion (effluvium) is the synchronized cessation of variable-sized areas or patches of hairs in growth phase (anagen), through catagen into resting or telogen phase, usually with hairs falling out or being rubbed out several weeks later, when new hairs then regrow. Stressors such as fever, illness, lactation, pregnancy, anaesthesia, or shock are usually responsible, but in many cases no stressors are obvious. Anagen defluxion (effluvium) is similar, but is rarer and the causes are more catastrophic events, such as more severe illness, with the hairs falling out within a week or 10 days. Both conditions result in patchy alopecia, sometimes symmetrical but not always. Alopecia is caused by both above conditions but, at least in western Canada, alopecia in often very valuable cattle, and especially bulls, commonly occurs in spring months. These latter cases are often multiple in a herd, and the animals are not sick or under any stress at all. The condition is referred to as idiopathic alopecia and the cause has not been determined. Rarely are external parasites demonstrated.

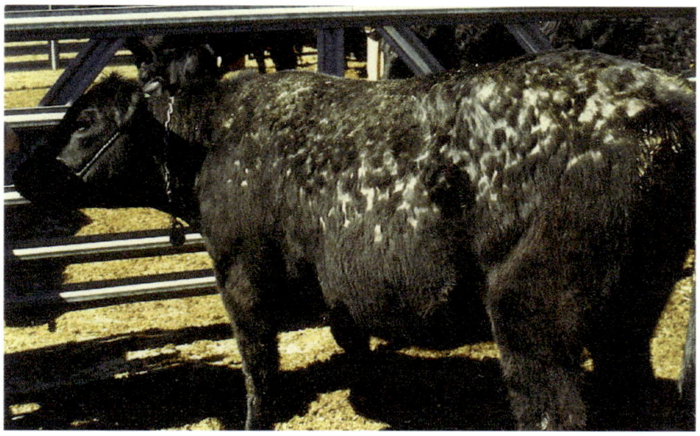

Fig. 12.25. Ox. Skin. Alopecia. Juvenile Angus with multifocal alopecia dorsolateral over the trunk. No known history of stressors in this case.

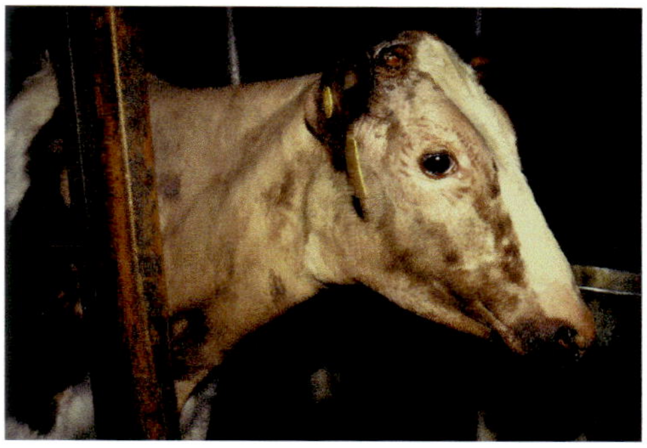

Fig. 12.26. Ox. Skin. Defluxion. Telogen or anagen defluxion in a Holstein-Friesian heifer following dehorning. Extensive alopecia of head, face, and neck regions. The timing after recent dehorning would suggest anagen defluxion.

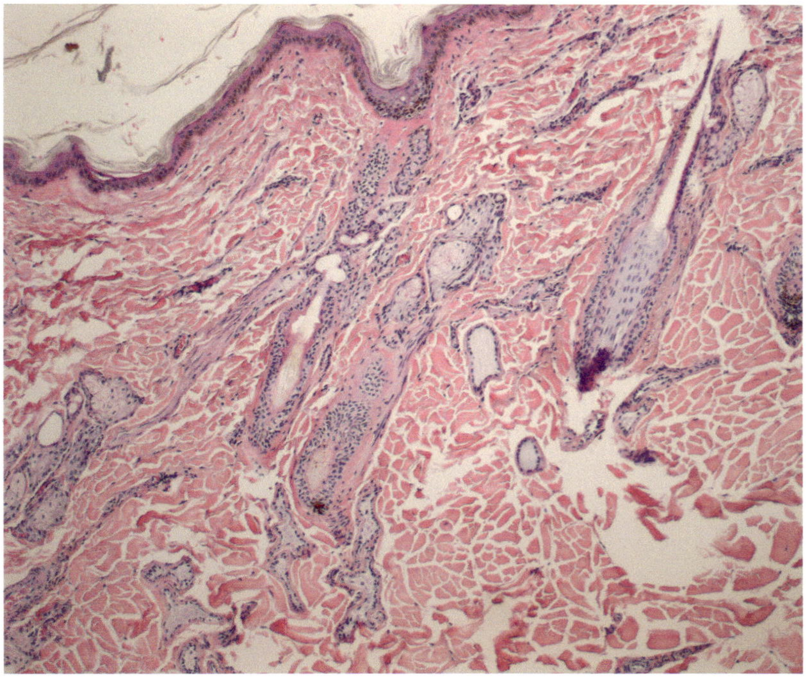

Fig. 12.27. Ox. Skin. Telogen defluxion. Histologic picture of telogen defluxion. Hair follicles present in resting phase (no hair bulbs visible), but hair shafts still present in two follicles (H&E).

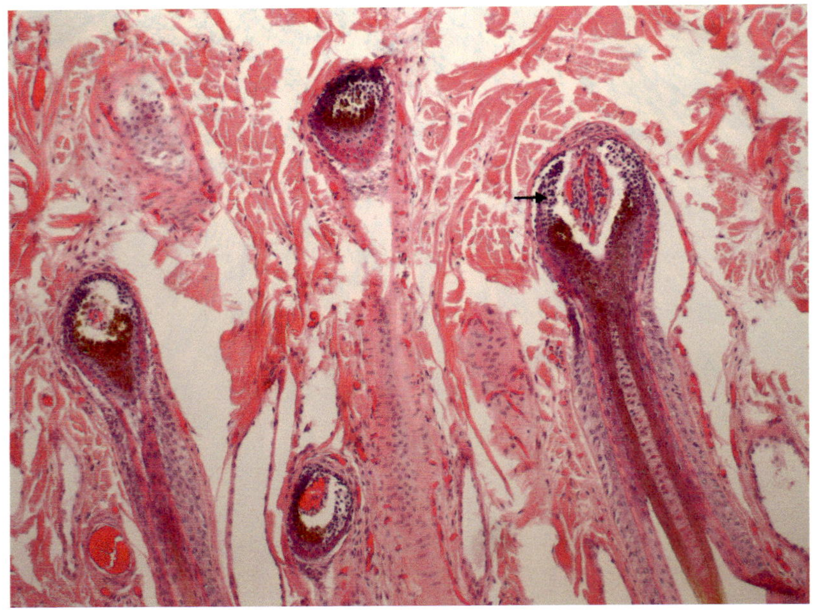

Fig. 12.28. Ox. Skin. Anagen defluxion. Skin from an animal with blackleg showing early stages of anagen defluxion. Note the pyknosis of hair bulb epithelial cells. If the animal had lived for a week or so, it would have probably lost abundant hair coat typical of anagen defluxion (arrow) (H&E).

12.4 VIRAL DISEASES

12.4.1 Cutaneous papillomatosis ('warts')

Introduction. Thirteen bovine papilloma viruses have been described, but only five so far that cause benign skin lesions in cattle. Bovine papilloma virus (BPV)-2 is by far the most common on haired skin, with other types occurring on teats, penis, rumen, and esophagus. The head, neck, dewlap, and shoulder are preferred sites, and are usually seen in animals younger than 2 years or in older cows severely immunosuppressed. Entry of the virus is usually through sites of minor injury, such as branding or even insect bites. The morphology of the five types are different in the various body sites.

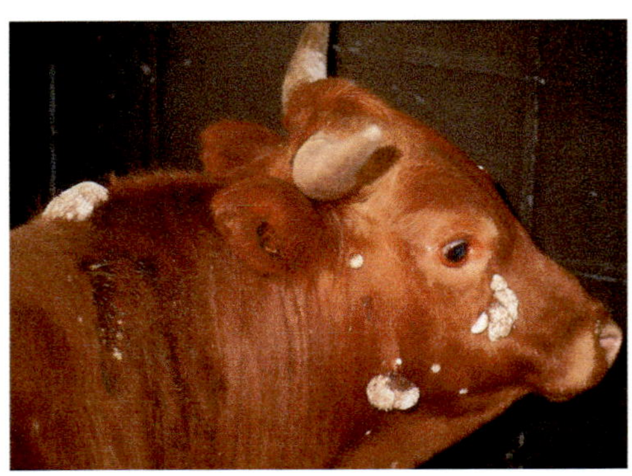

Fig. 12.29. Ox. Skin. Papilloma. Texas Longhorn steer with multiple various sized (one to multiple centimeters) papillomas on head and neck. The lesions are nodular, hyperkeratotic, cauliflower-like growths, but more plaque-like, flat lesions occasionally occur as well.

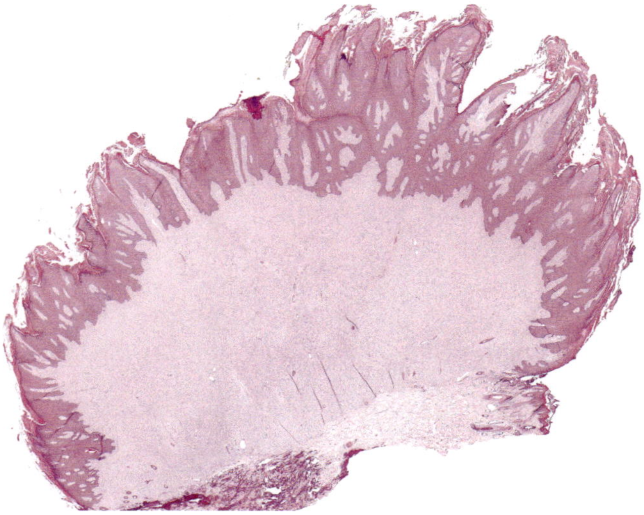

Fig. 12.30. Ox. Skin. Papilloma. Subgross histologic picture of a typical viral papilloma, which in the bovine are commonly called fibropapillomas due to the abundant connective tissue below the markedly papillated and hyperplastic epidermis. Surface hyperkeratosis is prominent (H&E).

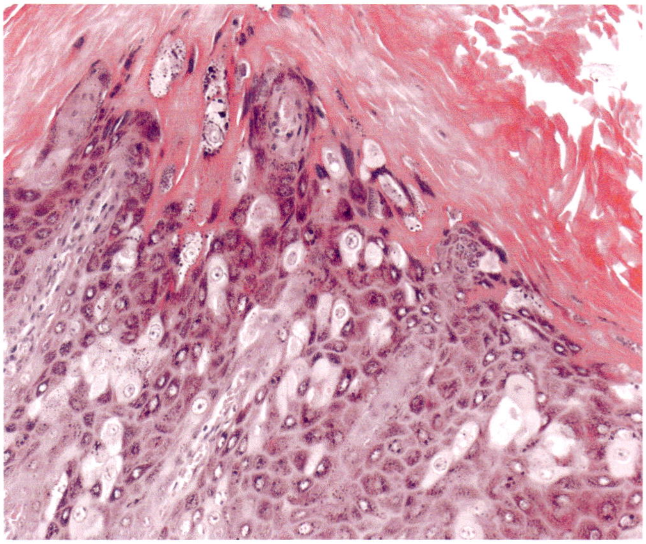

Fig. 12.31. Ox. Skin. Papilloma. High-power histologic picture of a bovine papilloma featuring multiple scattered keratinocytes with pale blue cytoplasm known as koilocytes. These are the cells where the nuclei will often stain positive for whole virus on immunohistochemistry. Excess keratohyaline (deeply basophilic) granules in surrounding keratinocytes is quite typical as well (H&E).

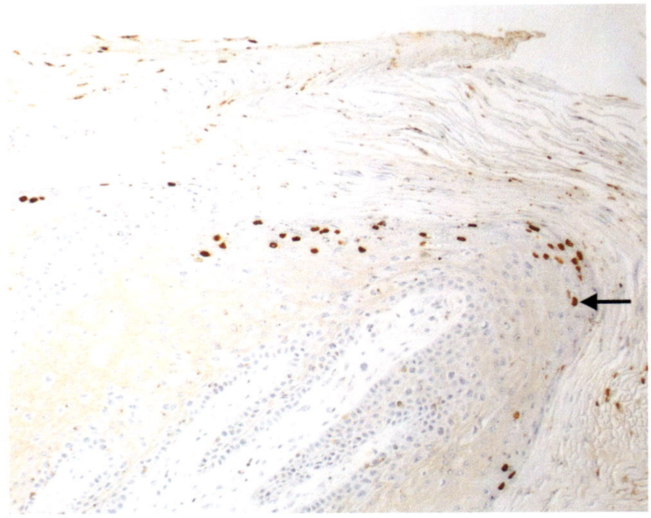

Fig. 12.32. Ox. Skin. Papilloma. Immunohistochemistry shows low numbers of keratinocyte nuclei staining positive for whole virus antigens (arrow). It is typical of papillomavirus in all species to stain only cells in the outer, more superficial epidermis where whole virus is being assembled. Unlike in some other species, intranuclear viral 'inclusion bodies' are usually not seen in the bovine species. Note the viral antigens are shed into the environment with the surface keratin flakes (IHC).

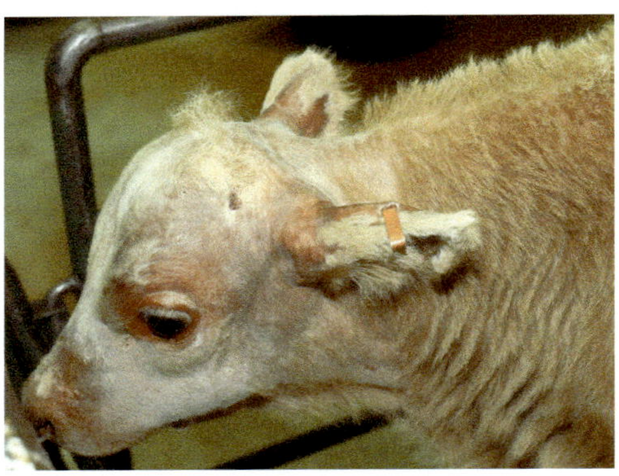

Fig. 12.33. Ox. Skin. Bovine viral diarrhea virus (BVDV). Alopecia. One-week-old calf born with extensive lack of hair of ears, head, neck, and nasal regions. A few small crusted and ulcerated lesions near the nasal region are visible.

12.4.2 Bovine viral diarrhea virus (BVDV)

Introduction. This pestivirus of the Flaviviridae family is a systemic disease, often having cutaneous manifestations. Fetuses infected *in utero* between days 100 and 150 gestation may be born with various defects, including hypotrichosis, alopecia, and curly hair coats. In animals that are persistently infected (PI) at birth and succumb to mucosal disease, skin lesions in especially chronic mucosal disease (MD) cases may, in addition to diarrhea, develop erosions, ulceration, and crusting of muzzle, lips, nostrils, coronet regions, interdigital spaces, teats, vulva, and prepuce. Some cases may also progress to scales, alopecia, and hyperkeratosis of the neck, ears, medial thigh, and perineal regions. Some acutely infected animals can also develop skin lesions, but this is less common than in PI individuals (see Chapter 5: Diseases of the Gastrointestinal Tract).

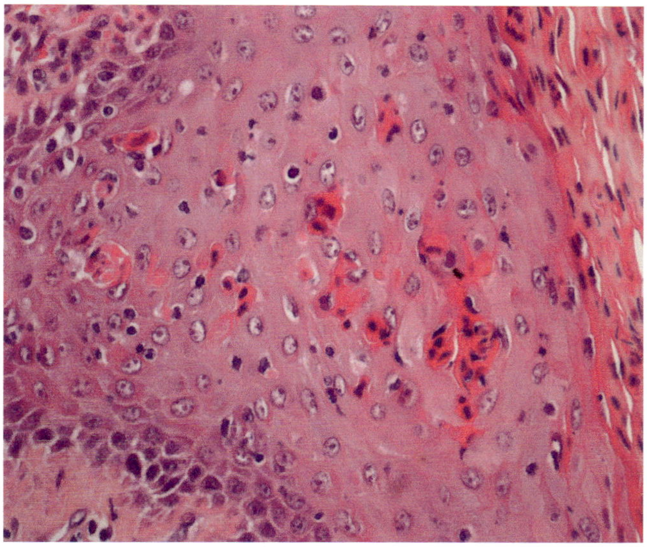

Fig. 12.35. Ox. Mouth. Bovine viral diarrhea virus (BVDV). Apoptosis. Oral epithelium of a persistently infected (PI) animal with mucosal disease showing typical apoptosis (single-cell necrosis) of numerous epithelial cells characteristic of several bovine viral infections. Epidermis of the skin would show similar histologic features (H&E).

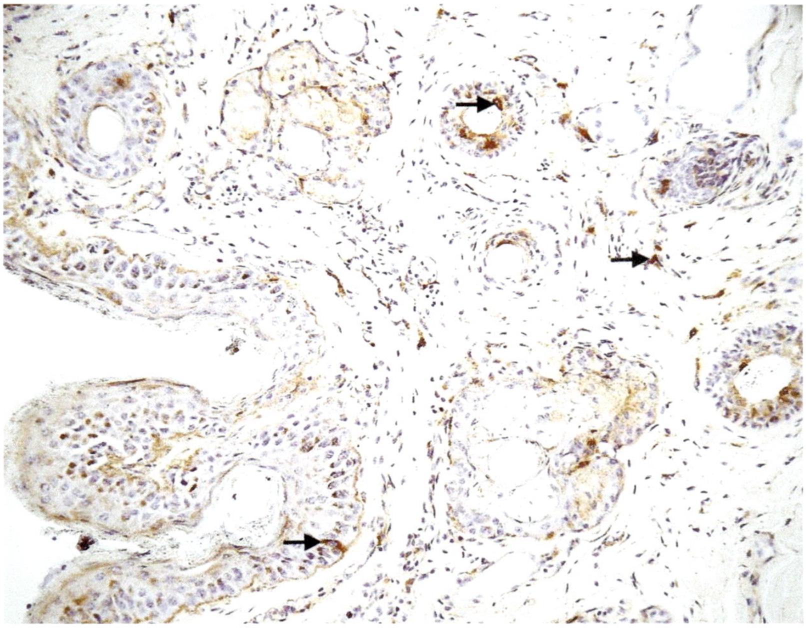

Fig. 12.36. Ox. Skin. Bovine viral diarrhea virus (BVDV). Immunohistochemistry performed on skin of a persistently infected (PI) individual showing abundant positive staining for virus in epidermal (bottom arrow) and follicular epithelial (top arrow) cells and numerous macrophages (arrow on right) scattered throughout the superficial and deep dermis. Skin from anywhere on the body will show this pattern, but ear notches are most commonly collected for this test. In acute stages of a transient infection, this reaction also can be demonstrated but is rare, with the subsequent image being more common (IHC) (see Chapter 5: Diseases of the Gastrointestinal Tract).

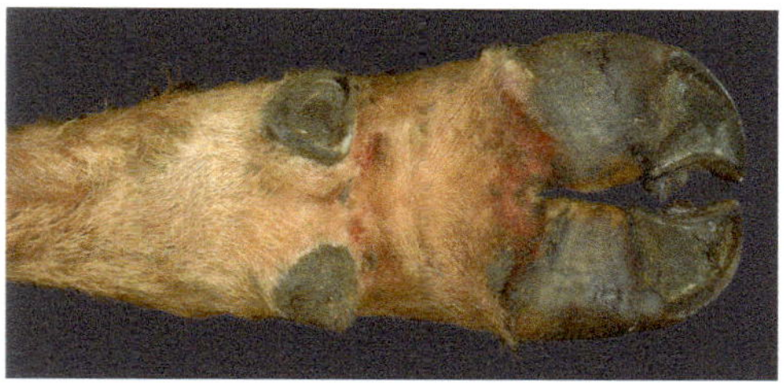

Fig. 12.34. Ox. Skin. Bovine viral diarrhea virus (BVDV). Dermatitis. Distal limb region of a feedlot animal with chronic mucosal disease showing interdigital and sub-dewclaw dermatitis with hyperemia and mild hair loss.

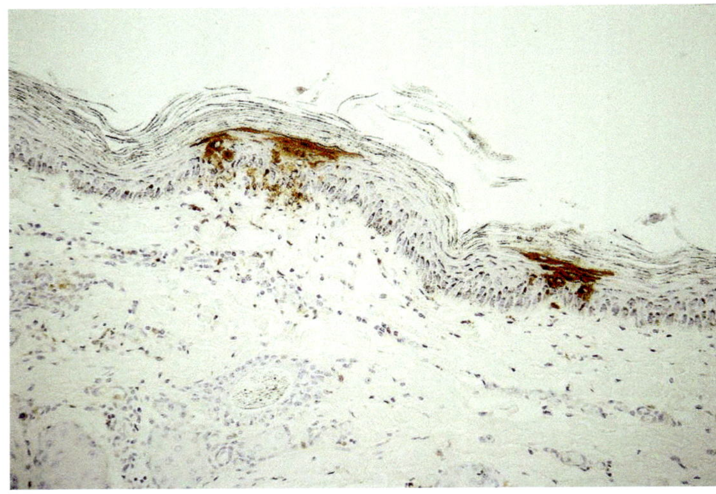

Fig. 12.37. Ox. Skin. Bovine viral diarrhea virus (BVDV). IHC of skin from a transiently infected animal showing only focal staining of epidermal keratinocytes. Some transiently infected animals will have no positive IHC staining, thus other tests, especially PCR, are needed to aid the diagnosis (IHC).

12.4.3 Malignant catarrhal fever (MCF)

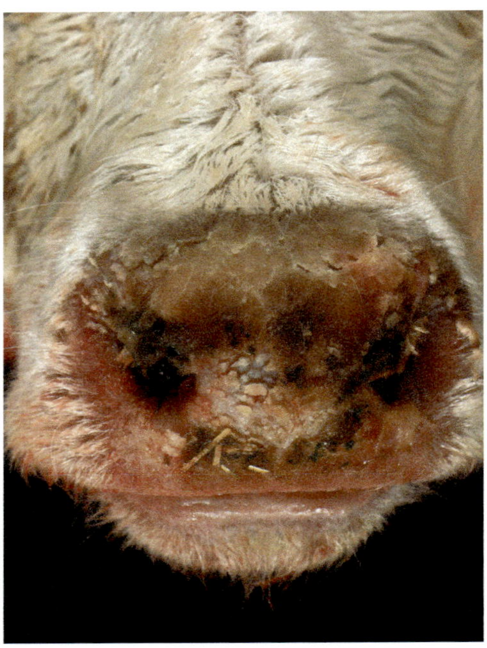

Fig. 12.38. Ox. Skin. Muzzle and nares. Malignant catarrhal fever (MCF). Case showing severe crusting, hyperemia, and necrosis.

Introduction. The multisystemic viral disease has a cutaneous manifestation. In cattle, the disease is caused by OVH-2, a gammaherpesvirus from close association with sheep, with the latter ruminant species not developing clinical disease. The condition is also called malignant head catarrh or snotsiekte. Most bovine cases are sporadic, but herd outbreaks have been reported. Deranged cytotoxic T-cells cause vasculitis, non-suppurative encephalitis, and epithelial cell necrosis in a variety of tissues, including skin (also refer to Chapter 2: Diseases of the Nervous System and Chapter 5: Diseases of the Gastrointestinal Tract). Lymph node hyperplasia is a prominent pathologic feature. The muzzle and nares are usually heavily crusted, but other cutaneous regions often involved include teats, udder, perineum, and inner thighs, with weeping and loss of hair. Hooves and/or horns may slough.

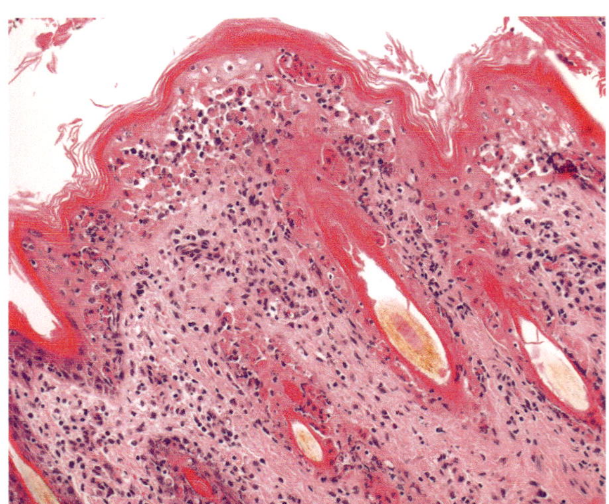

Fig. 12.39. Ox. Skin. Muzzle. Malignant catarrhal fever (MCF). Necrotizing dermatitis. Histologic picture of skin of the muzzle region of an MCF case showing extensive keratinocyte necrosis of both epidermis and hair follicles. Section taken of haired skin adjacent to non-haired muzzle (H&E).

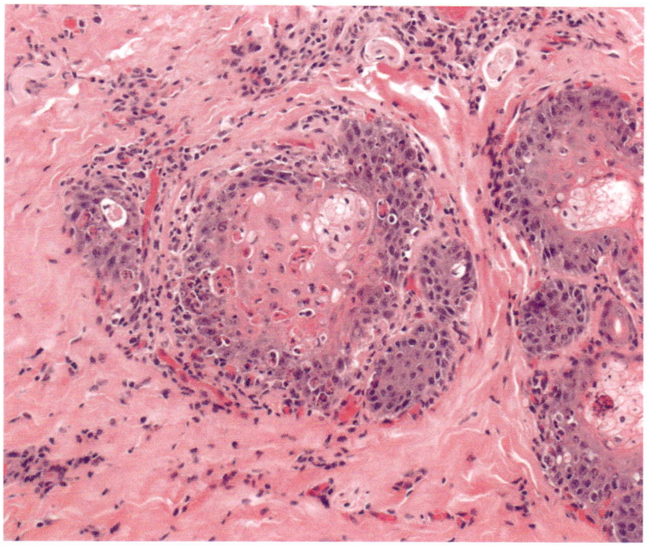

Fig. 12.40. Ox. Skin. Muzzle. Malignant catarrhal fever (MCF). Less severe single-cell necrosis typical of several other viral skin diseases, especially bovine viral diarrhea virus (BVDV) (H&E).

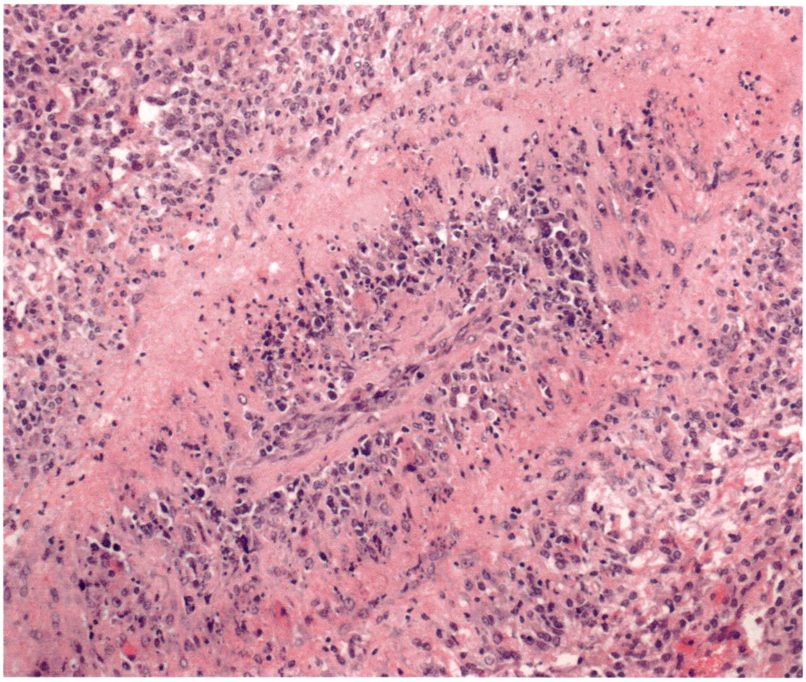

Fig. 12.41. Ox. Kidney. Malignant catarrhal fever (MCF). Lymphoplasmacytic vasculitis. Vasculitis as distinct as this is not as common in the skin with MCF (H&E).

12.4.4 Bovine papular stomatitis (BPS)

Introduction. This parapoxvirus (parapoxvirus bovis-1) is a zoonosis and is most commonly seen as oral cavity or esophageal lesions in cattle less than 1 year of age. Not uncommonly, however, muzzle, nostril, and lips are affected. Cows with affected calves suckling can develop teat and udder lesions. Occasionally, more chronic proliferative lesions can be noticed in other sites such as tail and perineum, especially representing immunosuppressed individuals (see Chapter 5: Diseases of the Gastrointestinal Tract).

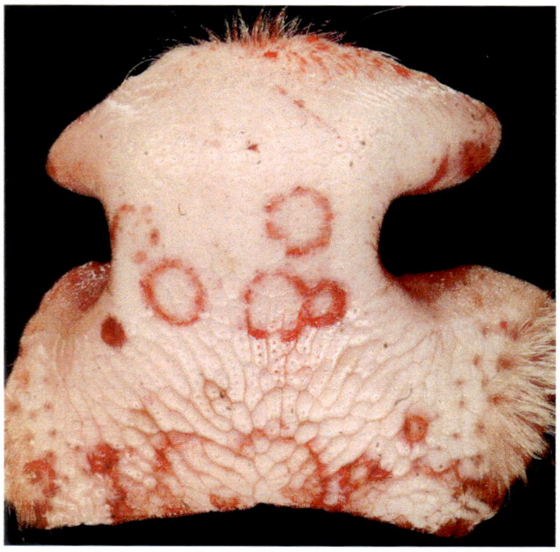

Fig. 12.42. Ox. Skin. Head. Bovine papular stomatitis (BPS). Hyperemia and erosions. Two cases showing circular erosive lesions, with hyperemia on the muzzle and nares.

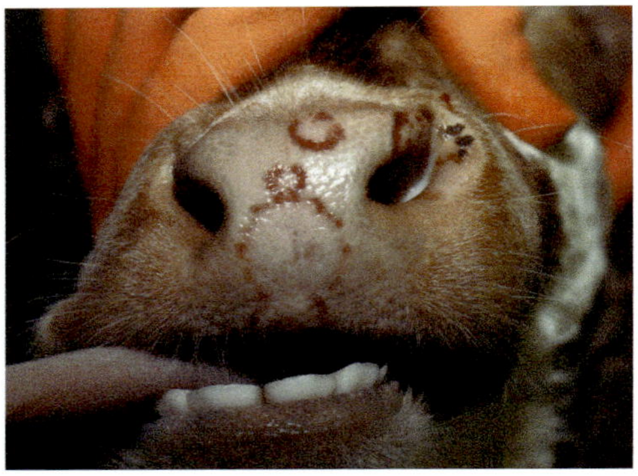

Fig. 12.43. Ox. Skin. Head. Bovine papular stomatitis (BPS). Hyperemia and erosions. Two cases showing circular erosive lesions, with hyperemia on the muzzle and nares.

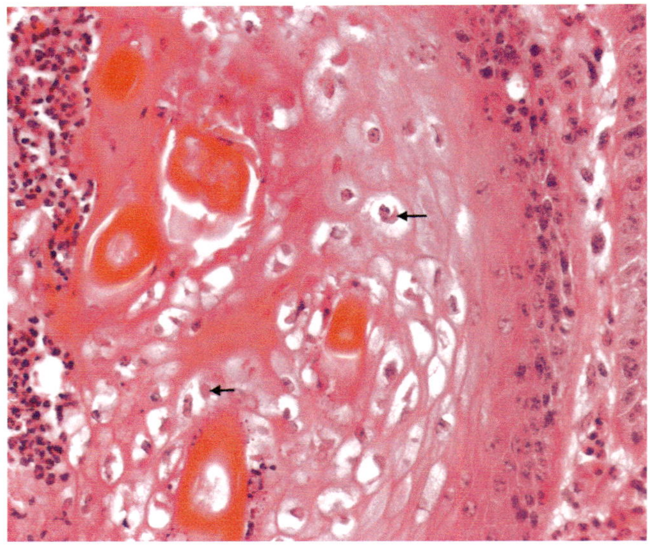

Fig. 12.44. Ox. Epidermis. Bovine papular stomatitis (BPS). Keratinocyte necrosis. Histologic section of epidermis showing multiple vacuolated keratinocytes with irregular intracytoplasmic basophilic viral inclusion bodies typical of a parapoxvirus (arrows). These inclusions occur in pseudocowpox as well, and PCR is needed to differentiate between these two parapoxviruses. To our knowledge, no IHC is available for parapoxviruses (H&E).

12.4.5 Pseudocowpox

Introduction. Representing another zoonotic parapoxvirus infection (parapoxvirus bovis-2), with lesions starting as umbilicated papules that later develop more proliferative changes. Histologically, BPS virus lesions on the teats look virtually identical, and PCR is required to differentiate the two viral infections. It would be very rare to have oral and muzzle pseudocowpox lesions, however.

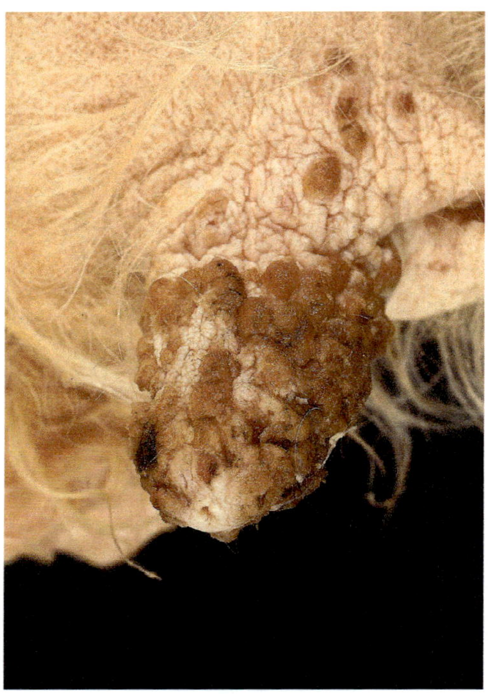

Fig. 12.45. Ox. Teat. Pseudocowpox. Proliferative dermatitis. Close-up of pseudocowpox lesions on a teat extending to the udder (see Chapter 14: Diseases of the Udder and Teats). Similar lesions occasionally occur on the perineum and the scrotum of males.

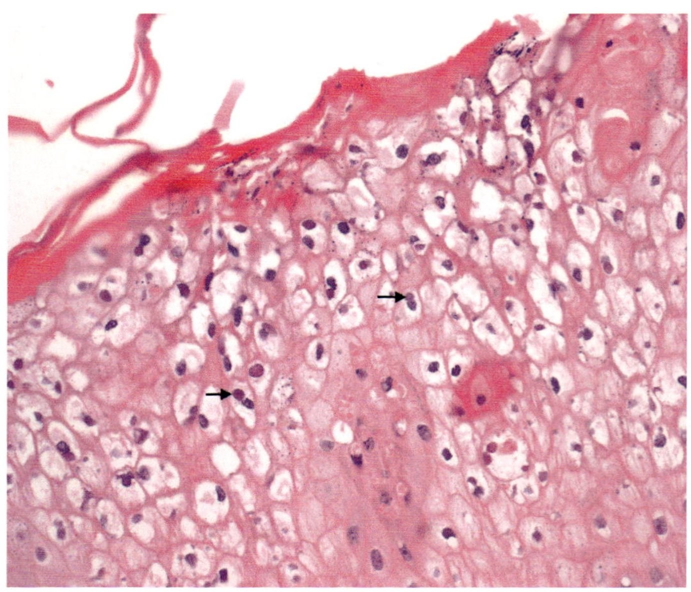

Fig. 12.46. Ox. Teat. Pseudocowpox. Cytoplasmic vacuolation. Keratinocytes are vacuolated, with intracytoplasmic inclusion bodies (arrows) present in some cells (H&E).

12.4.6 Pseudolumpy skin disease

Introduction. A generalized skin disease caused by bovine herpesvirus 2 (BHV-2), of the alphaherpesvirinae subfamily. It has also been called Allerton virus, to distinguish it from the cause of lumpy skin disease. The virus is closely related to herpes simplex 1 of humans. Lumpy skin disease is caused by a pox virus and does not occur in North or South America. A localized form of pseudolumpy skin disease occurs on the teats and udder, where it is known as ulcerative mammillitis. Disseminated circular, slightly raised, flat lesions develop suddenly over the whole body and progress to localized alopecia. The centers are slightly depressed where sloughing occurs. When the lesions heal, characteristically no scars remain. Cases tend to be sporadic, but multiple cases can occur in a herd. In Canada, adult cows are most commonly affected. The virus is isolated easily from the lesions.

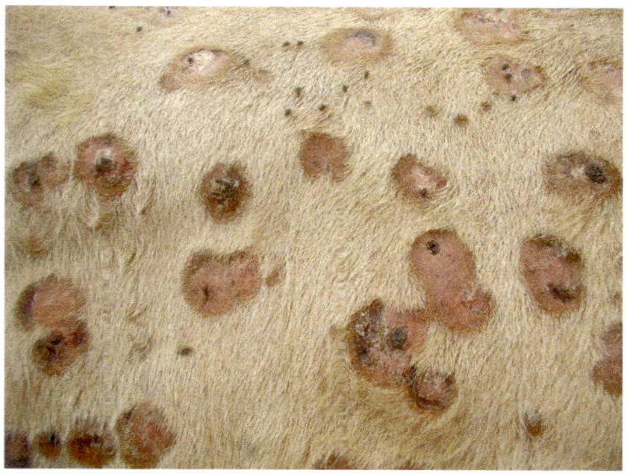

Fig. 12.48. Ox. Skin. Pseudolumpy skin disease. Proliferative, ulcerative dermatitis. Close-up showing the lesions in more detail.

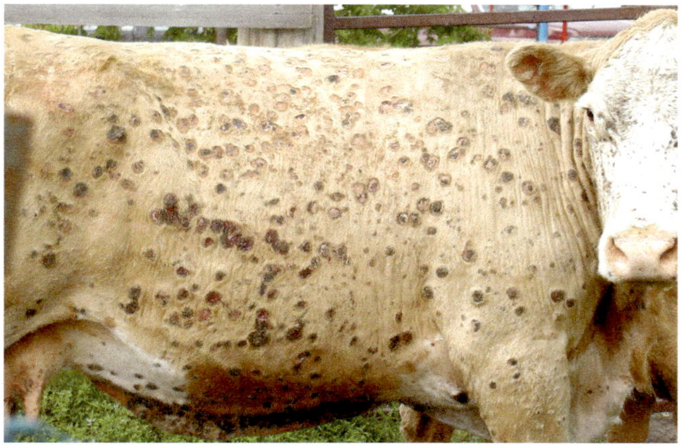

Fig. 12.47. Ox. Skin. Pseudolumpy skin disease. Proliferative, ulcerative dermatitis. Mature cow with numerous randomly scattered and coalescing areas of epidermal necrosis, with central depressed areas of crusting and alopecia.

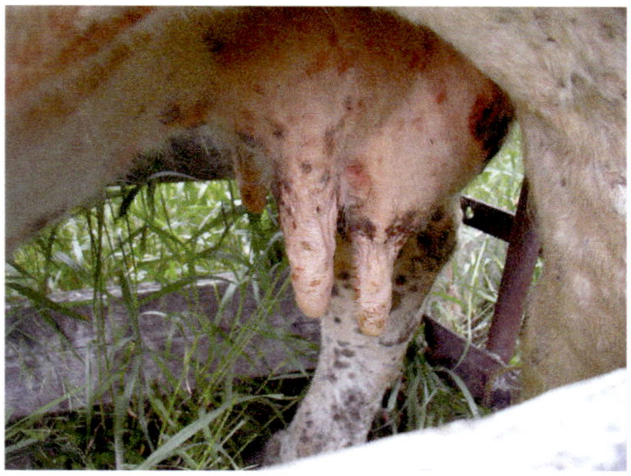

Fig. 12.49. Ox. Skin. Pseudolumpy skin disease. Proliferative, ulcerative dermatitis. Close-up of teats and udder showing involvement of those areas, but also of haired skin on the legs. Cases of ulcerative mammillitis usually do not involve other parts of the body.

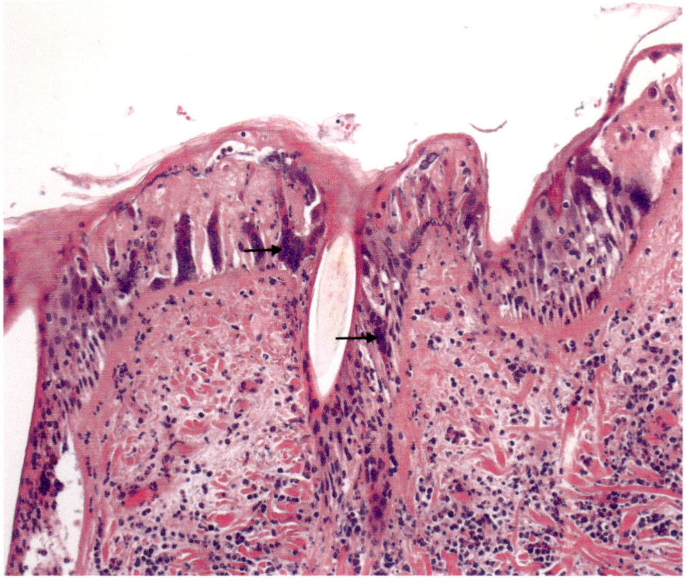

Fig. 12.50. Ox. Skin. Pseudolumpy skin disease. Keratinocyte necrosis. Histologic picture of epidermis, dermis, and hair follicles with necrosis of keratinocytes and formation of syncytial cells (arrows) typical of this disease. Intranuclear viral inclusion bodies can be identified. Increased mixed inflammatory cells occupy the superficial dermis (H&E).

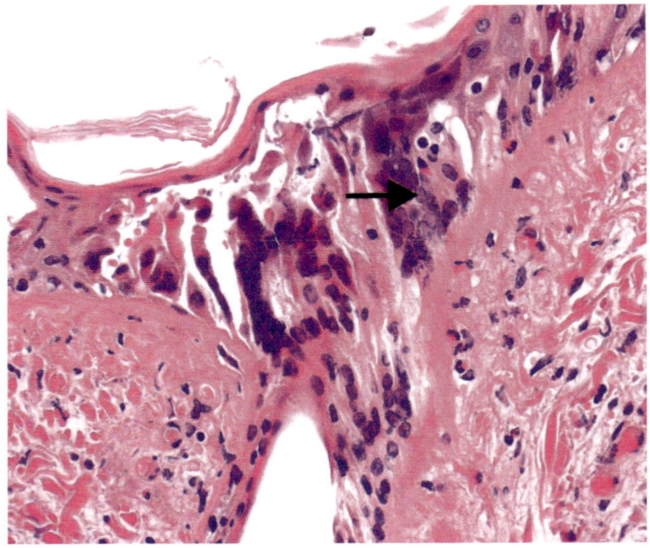

Fig. 12.51. Ox. Skin. Pseudolumpy skin disease. Intranuclear inclusion bodies. Higher-power histologic picture to show the intranuclear viral inclusion bodies (arrow) in both epidermal and follicular keratinocytes (H&E).

12.5 BACTERIAL DISEASES

12.5.1 Dermatophilosis ('streptothricosis', 'rain scald')

Introduction. A common bacterial skin disease caused by the Actinomycete *Dermatophilus congolensis*, a facultative anaerobic organism. It occurs in tropical and subtropical areas most commonly, but anywhere with heavy or steady rainfall and warm environmental conditions. Skin lesions can occur at any site on the body and at any age of the animal. Acute to chronic forms exist. Basically, the skin disease constitutes a superficial exudative dermatitis with heavy surface crust formation. The organisms stain gram-positive and typically have 'railroad track' morphology when they form spores in the outer hyperkeratotic epidermis.

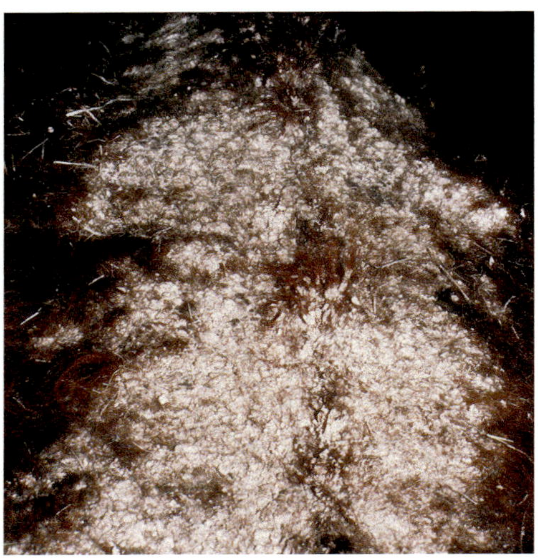

Fig. 12.52. Ox. Skin. Dermatophilosis. Exudative dermatitis. Thick, heavy white crusts overshadow the dorsal thorax and lumbar regions of a yearling animal.

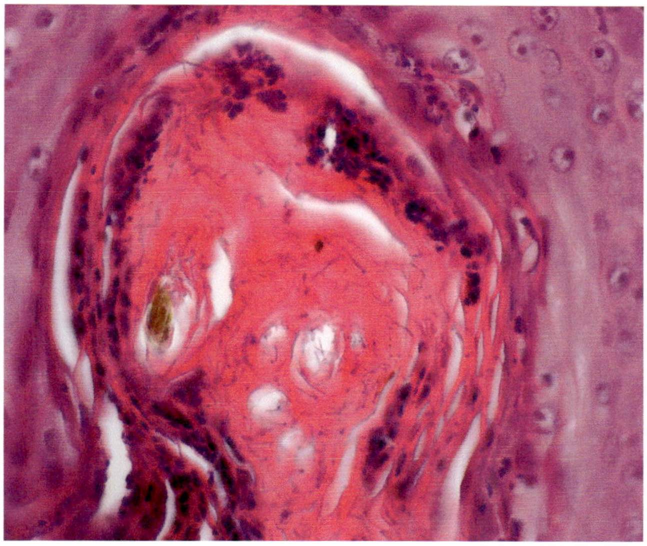

Fig. 12.56. Ox. Skin. Dermatophilosis. Hair follicle. Histologic picture of the superficial lumen of a hair follicle containing numerous elongated organisms typical of the disease. Formations of cross-striations representing the early stages of the organism forming spores are visible (H&E).

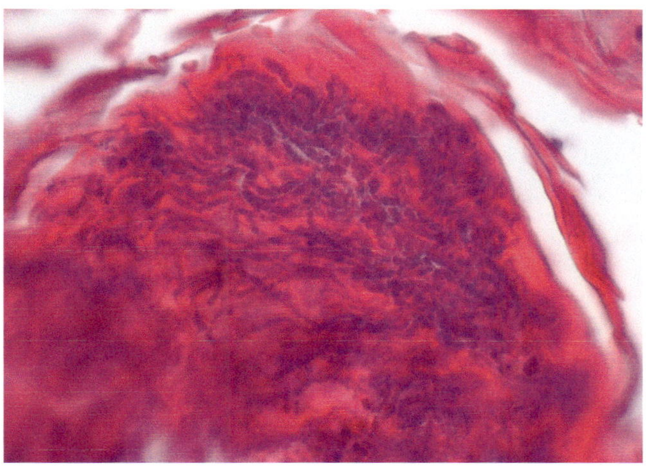

Fig. 12.57. Ox. Skin. Dermatophilosis. More superficial accumulation of keratin containing clusters of organisms with the typical 'railroad track' morphology of cross-striations. The organisms appear wider because they are forming spores (H&E). Gram or Giemsa stains should be used to better visualize bacteria.

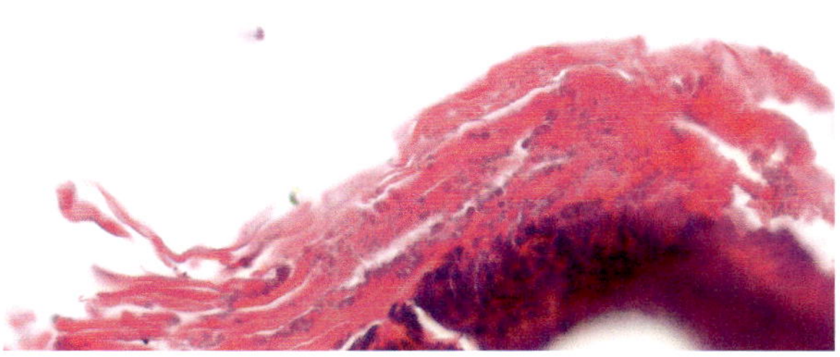

Fig. 12.58. Ox. Skin. Dermatophilosis. Outer mass of keratin containing the organism broken up into spores, not recognizable as filamentous bacteria at this stage (H&E).

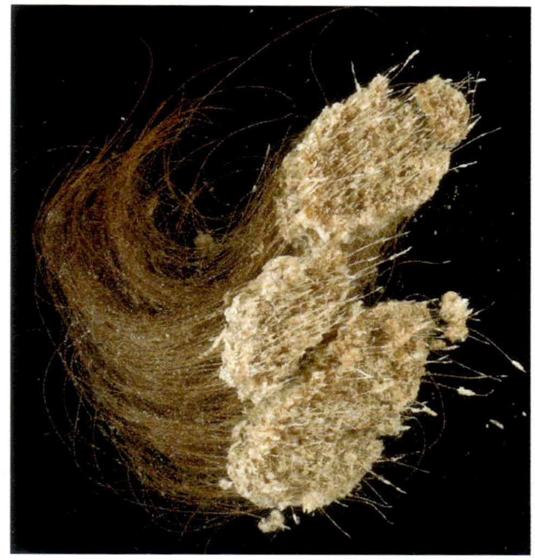

Fig. 12.53. Ox. Skin. Dermatophilosis. Dermal crust. A removed tuft of hair to show the attached thick, yellow-tan crust material consisting of keratin, neutrophils, and organisms.

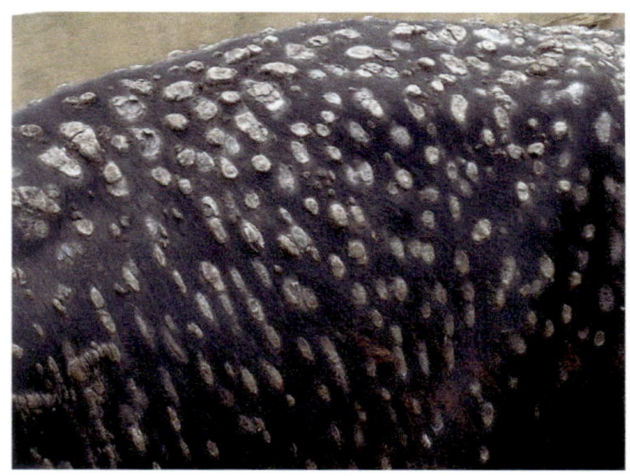

Fig. 12.54. Ox. Skin. Dermatophilosis. Pustular, erosive dermatitis. Chronic form of dermatophilosis with multifocal, raised, wart-like tan masses of dry hyperkeratotic material. Removed crusts show a denuded hair loss area. In more acute cases, ulceration and purulent material may be visible. (Courtesy of Dr A. Campbell, Whangarei, New Zealand.)

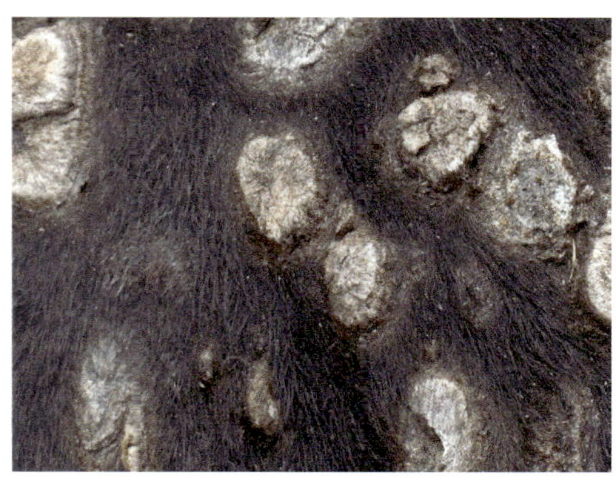

Fig. 12.55. Ox. Skin. Dermatophilosis. Pustular, erosive dermatitis. Higher power of the same chronic case with laminated keratin crusts and alopecia. (Courtesy of Dr A. Campbell, Whangarei, New Zealand.)

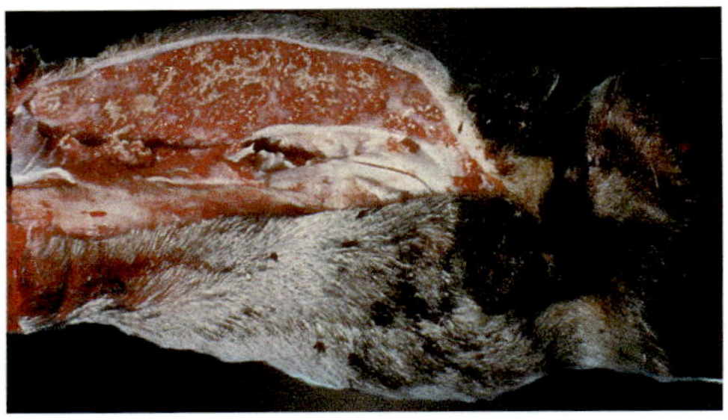

Fig. 12.59. Ox. Distal limb. Subcutaneous *Mycobacterium bovis* tuberculosis. Yellow, multifocal to coalescing caseous foci are separated by chronic fibrous tissue.

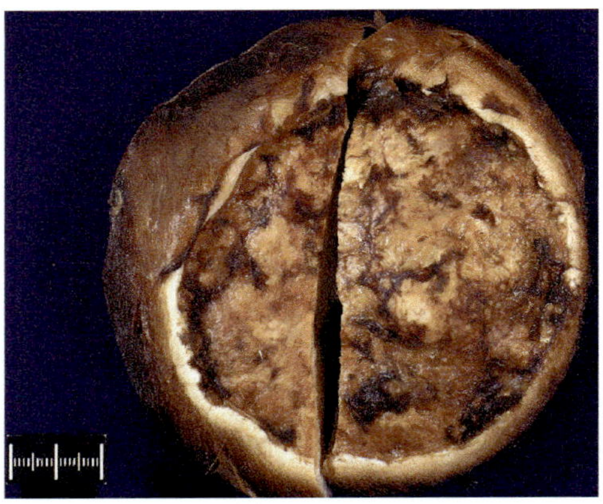

Fig. 12.60. Ox. Skin. Atypical mycobacteriosis. Granuloma. Large, non-tuberculoid, ulcerated granuloma on the lateral body wall of a steer.

12.5.2 Tuberculosis (cutaneous mycobacteriosis)

Introduction. Very rarely does *Mycobacterium bovis* cause visible nodular skin lesions, but swellings may be seen if there is subcutaneous tissue infection or peripheral lymph node involvement. Atypical or non-tuberculous mycobacterial infections due to contamination of skin wounds sometimes develop. *Mycobacterium kansasii*, *Mycobacterium ulcerans*, and *Mycobacterium avium* subsp. *avium* are isolates from many of these cases and are slow-growing, opportunistic organisms. The atypical infections cause ulcerative granulomas that are single and vary in size, or form chains if lymphatic invasion occurs.

12.5.3 Atypical cutaneous mycobacteriosis (non-tuberculoid)

Introduction. See above.

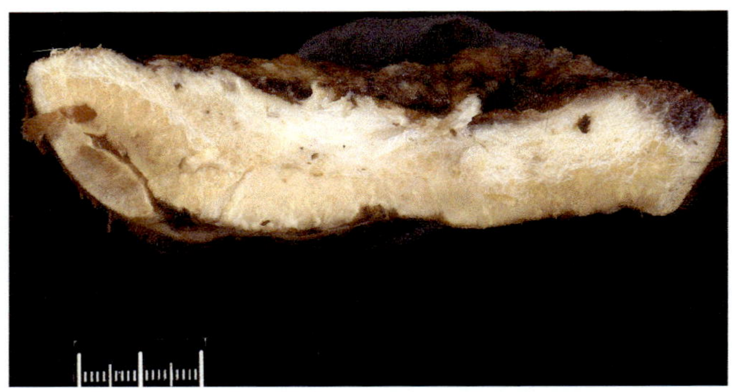

Fig. 12.61. Ox. Skin. Atypical mycobacteriosis. Granuloma. Cut surface showing white connective tissue and the tan granulomatous tissue.

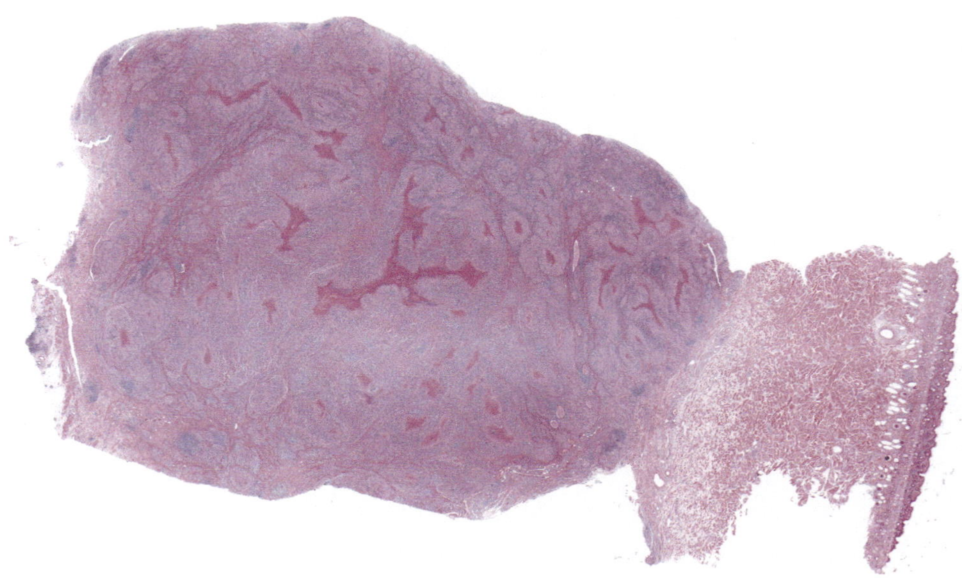

Fig. 12.62. Ox. Skin. Atypical mycobacteriosis. Granuloma. Subgross, with hypereosinophilic areas of necrosis and mixed mononuclear cells extending within the deep dermis below the hair follicles and adnexal glands. The basophilic areas are inflammatory cells with central eosinophilic foci of necrosis (H&E).

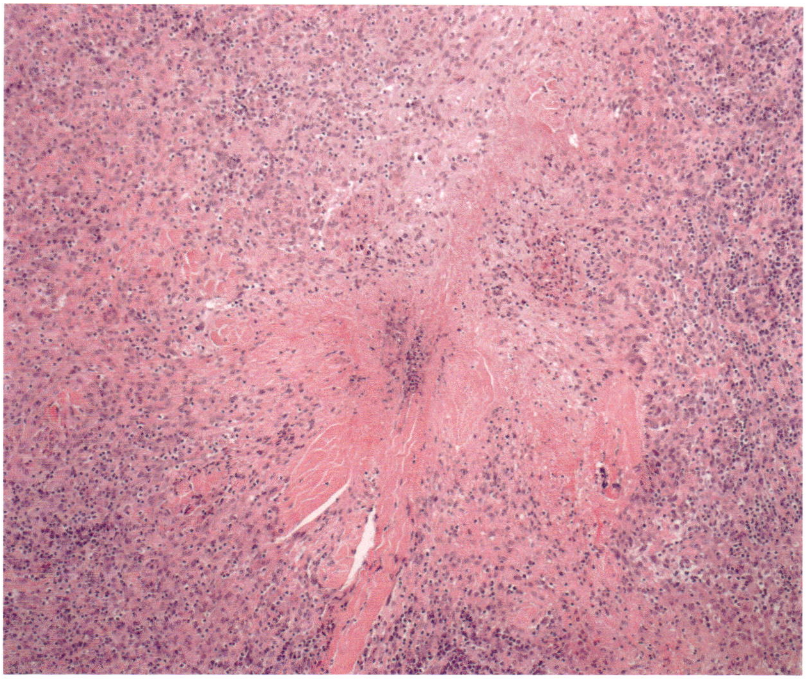

Fig. 12.63. Ox. Skin. Atypical mycobacteriosis. Granuloma. Histologic section with an area of coagulative necrosis surrounded by mixed mononuclear cells, being mainly histiocytic-type cells, lymphoid cells, and fibrocytes. Note the relative absence of giant cells in this particular section (H&E).

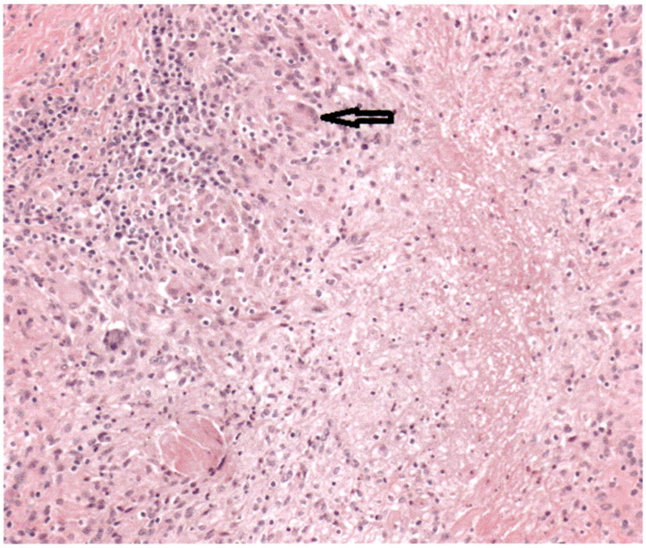

Fig. 12.64. Ox. Skin. Atypical mycobacteriosis. Initially, IHC was done. It appeared to be positive in focal areas, but the reaction was not conclusive. A Fite's stain was confirmative. Note the presence of several giant cells in this particular area (arrow) (H&E).

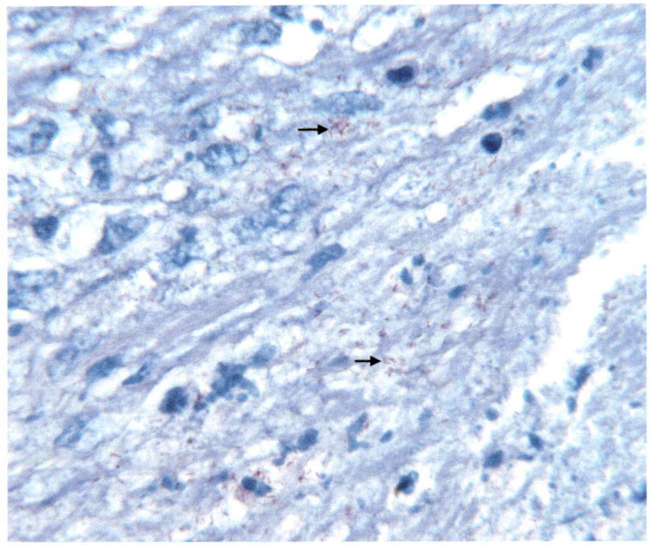

Fig. 12.65. Ox. Skin. Atypical mycobacteriosis. Fite's acid-fast stain identifies significant numbers of acid-fast rods typical of a *Mycobacterium* spp. (arrows) Cultures were not done on this lesion to characterize the species (Fite's acid fast).

12.5.4 Staphylococcal dermatitis

Introduction. *Staphylococcus aureus* and *Staphylococcus hyicus* are uncommon skin infections in cattle, except on the udder and teats, where *S. aureus* causes udder impetigo (see Chapter 14: Diseases of the Udder and Teats). *S. hyicus* is commonly isolated from the skin of cattle. In one study, it was found in 47 of 81 animals examined, without overt disease. Damage to the epidermis is the prerequisite for *S. hyicus* to invade, proliferate, and produce the exfoliative toxin responsible for the lesions. These can be multifocal initially, and then spread to become generalized.

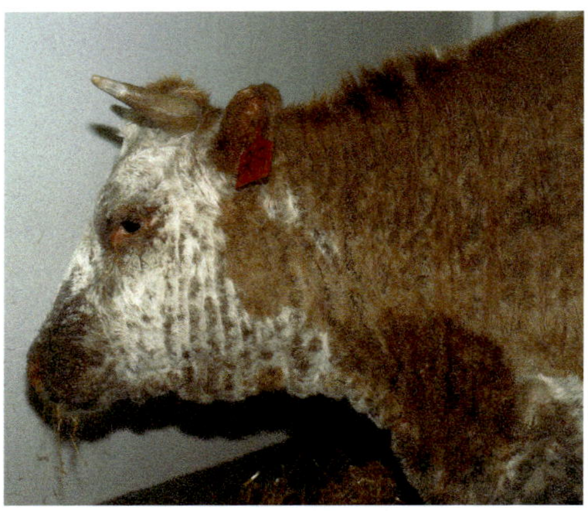

Fig. 12.66. Ox. Skin. Staphylococcal dermatitis. An adult cow with severe generalized *Staphylococcus hyicus* dermatitis, including folliculitis and furunculosis. Raised tufts of hair with extensive surface crusting are characteristic features. Cultures, histopathology and Gram stains easily identify this organism.

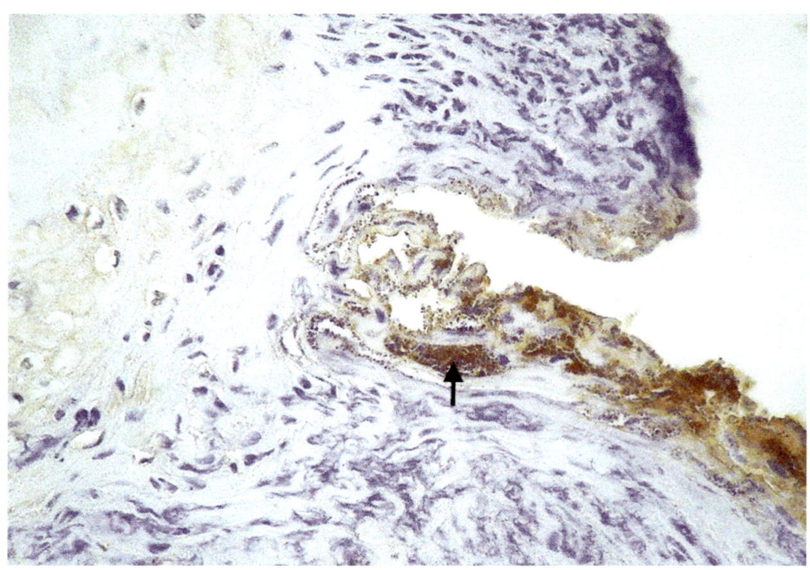

Fig. 12.67. Ox. Skin. Staphylococcal dermatitis. Immunohistochemistry (arrow) used by some laboratories to identify this organism as a *Staphylococcus* genus, but not as *Staphylococcus hyicus*. The procedure is useful if extensive antibiotic therapy interferes with bacterial isolation (IHC).

12.5.5 Actinomycosis ('lumpy jaw')

Introduction. *Actinomyces bovis* is a gram-positive, filamentous organism that causes a suppurative to pyogranulomatous osteomyelitis and overlying ulcerative skin infection, especially of the mandibular and maxillary regions. Entry of the organism is through some break in the oral mucosa, such as caused by plant awns or other causes of ulcers (foreign bodies, dental eruption). Abscesses, draining tracts and nodules occur on the skin, with white to yellow sand-like 'sulfur granules' usually seen grossly.

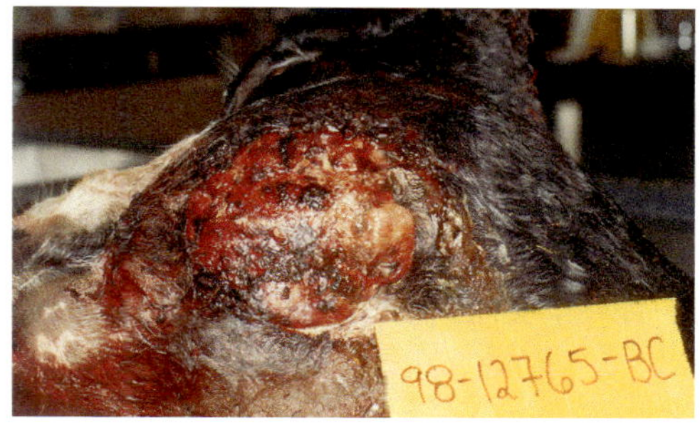

Fig. 12.68. Ox. Skin. Actinomycosis. Pyogranulomatous dermatitis. A large, pyogranulomatous connective tissue growth due to underlying *Actinomyces bovis* osteomyelitis has protruded through the ventral mandibular skin of this adult cow. (Also see Chapter 8: Diseases of the Musculoskeletal System).

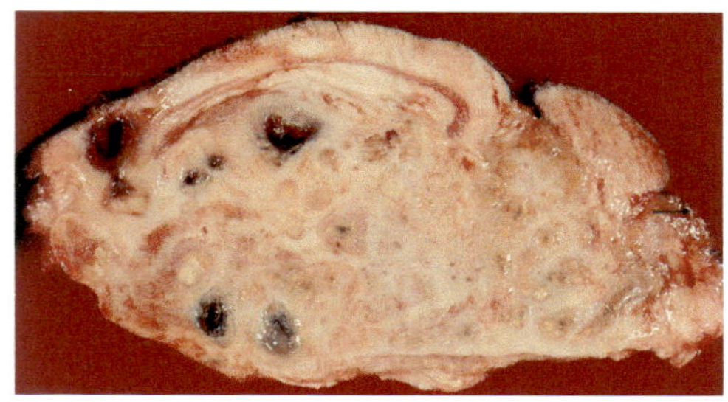

Fig. 12.69. Ox. Skin and bone. Actinomycosis. Pyogranulomatous inflammation. A cross section through the jawbone and overlying skin shows pockets of purulent material with bone and excessive connective tissue. Focally, skin ulceration has occurred. Sulfur granules are not visible in this view due to their small size.

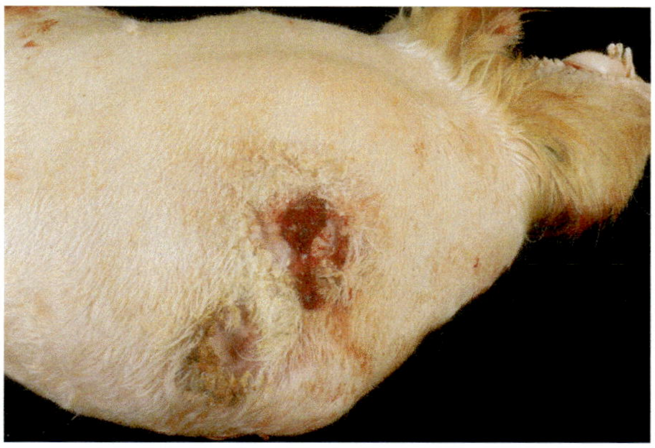

Fig. 12.70. Ox. Skin. Actinomycosis. Draining tracts. In this less severe case, draining tracts extend from the underlying osteomyelitis to the skin surface.

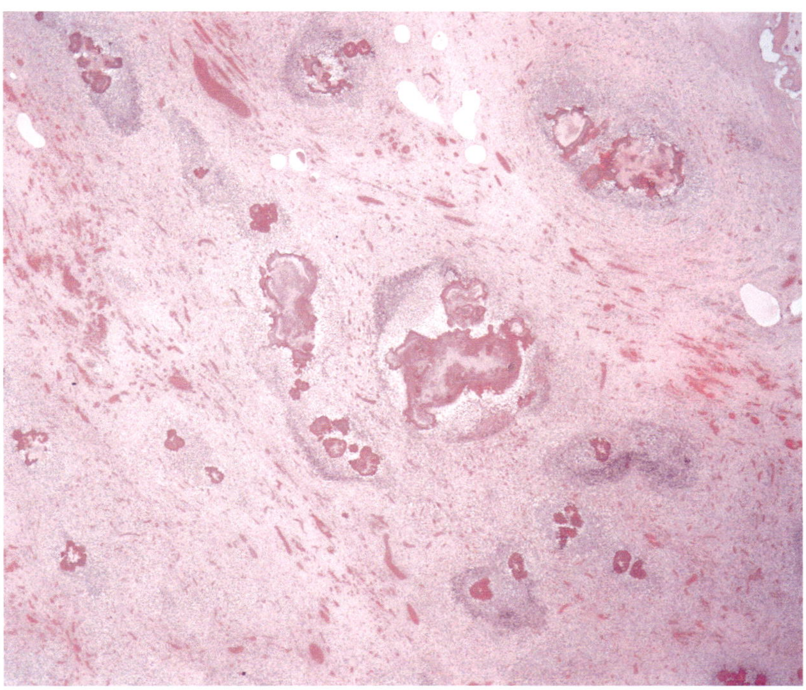

Fig. 12.71. Ox. Skin. Actinomycosis. Pyogranulomatous dermatitis. The low-power histologic section of a lumpy jaw case exhibits multifocal pyogranulomatous foci, with large numbers of neutrophils surrounding sulfur granules composed of clusters of the filamentous bacteria. These are embedded into hypereosinophilic, club-like Splendore–Hoeppli material. A Gram stain would show gram-positive organisms within these granules (H&E).

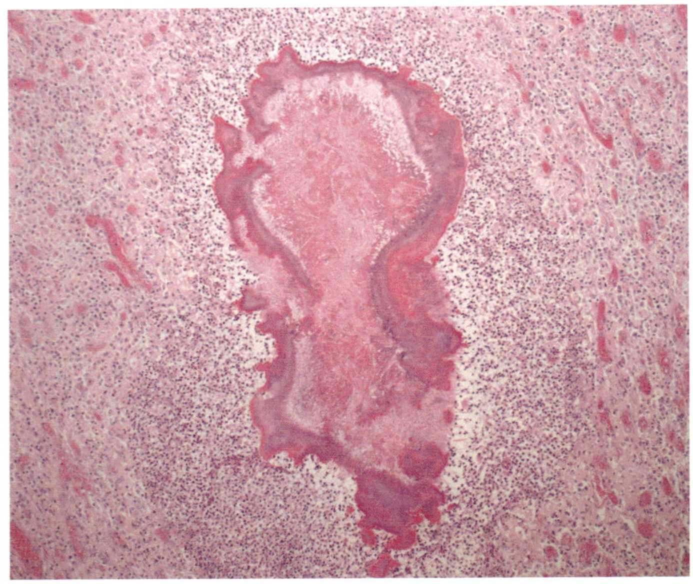

Fig. 12.72. Ox. Skin. Actinomycosis. Sulfur granules. The basophilic areas are clusters of organisms (H&E).

12.5.6 Actinobacillosis

Introduction. *Actinobacillus lignieresii* is a gram-negative coccobacillus that commonly causes pyogranulomatous glossitis ('wooden tongue'), but occasionally causes pyogranulomas in lymph nodes and skin. The organism breaks through skin or mucous membranes. Lesions around the head, neck, and face are most common. Sulfur granules similar to those in actinomycosis are characteristic gross findings and histologically tend to be smaller (often less than 1 mm diameter). (Also see Chapter 5: Diseases of the Gastrointestinal Tract.)

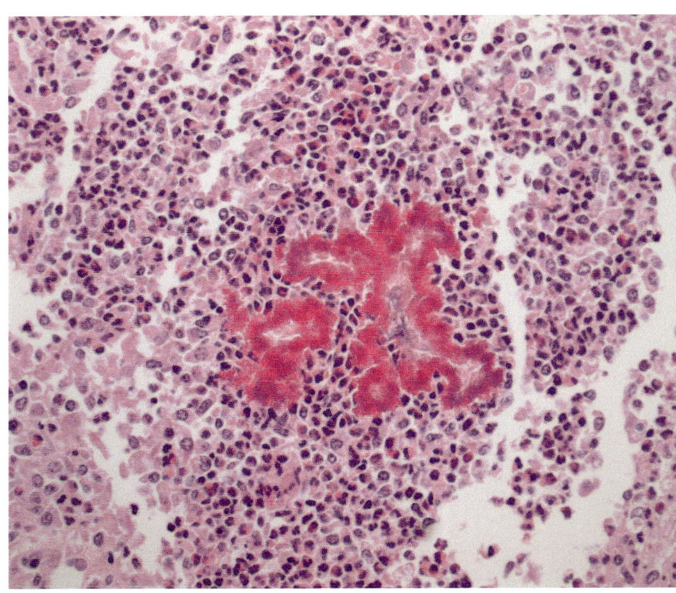

Fig. 12.73. Ox. Skin. Actinobacillosis. Sulfur granule. Histologic picture of a sulfur granule with an irregular central hypereosinophilic, club-shaped aggregate of Splendore–Hoeppli material surrounded by large numbers of neutrophils. The radiating clubs consist of immune complexes. The center of these granules contains colonies of bacteria requiring bacterial stains for identification, such as Gram, Giemsa or silver stains (H&E).

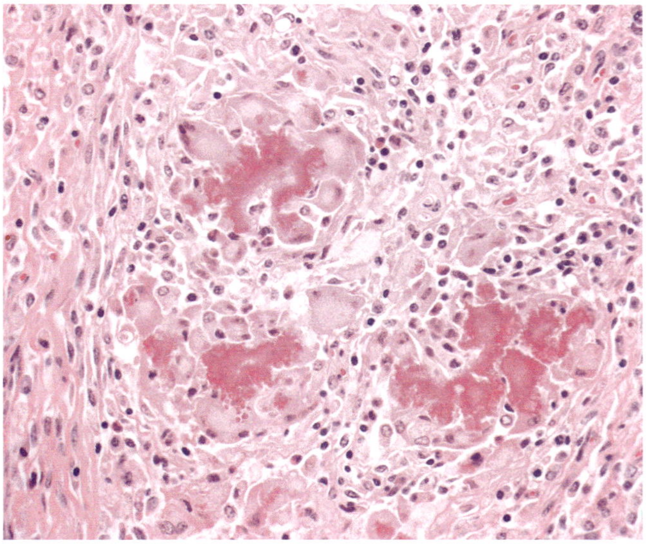

Fig. 12.74. Ox. Skin. Actinobacillosis. Sulfur granules. The granules are granulomas, with plenty of giant cells surrounding them. Lymphocytes, plasma cells, and macrophages are visible throughout the intervening connective tissue (H&E).

12.5.7 Cutaneous cellulitis and abscesses

Introduction. Cellulitis is defined as bacterial infection of the dermis and/or panniculus. A variety of aerobic and anaerobic bacteria can be involved, such as *Clostridium* spp., *Fusobacterium necrophorum*, *Bacteroides* spp., and *Trueperella pyogenes*, the latter especially causing abscesses. Infections occur secondary to wounds, spread through lymphatics or via fascial planes from other sites.

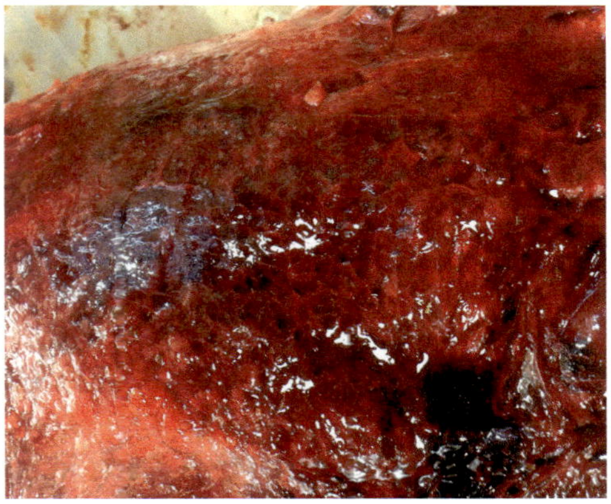

Fig. 12.75. Ox. Subcutis. Necrotizing cellulitis. Subcutaneous tissues of an animal with blackleg caused by *Clostridium chauvoei*. Edema and hemorrhage are extensive. Dry, hemorrhagic necrosis with emphysema of underlying muscle tissues are characteristic features (see Chapter 8: Diseases of the Musculoskeletal System). Malignant edema caused by *Clostridium septicum* is of similar appearance, with the edema of the subcutaneous tissue being even more severe. (Courtesy of Dr C. Knight, University of Calgary, Canada.)

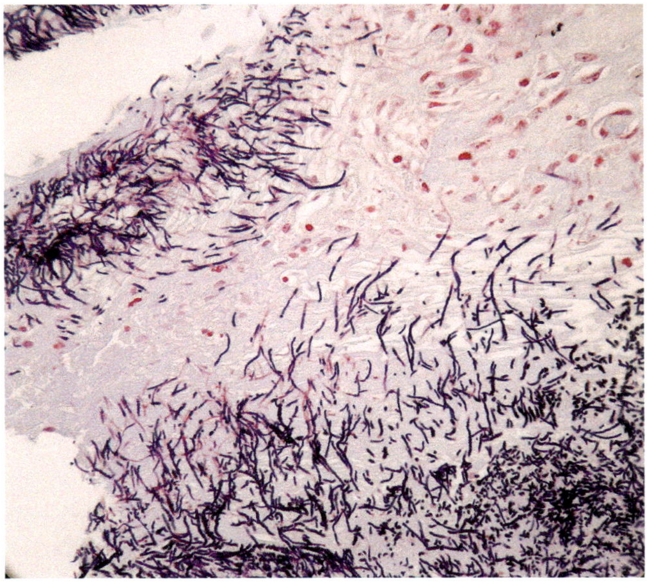

Fig. 12.76. Ox. Skin. Malignant edema. A Gram stain of skin from a case of malignant edema showing long rods of the gram-positive *Clostridium septicum* organisms (Brown and Brenn). (Also see Chapter 8: Diseases of the Musculoskeletal System.)

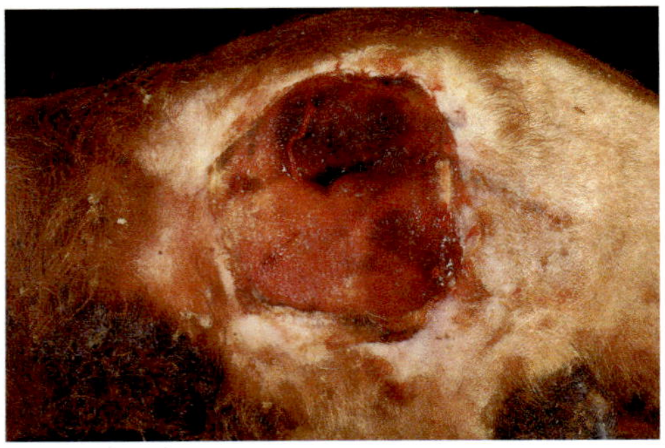

Fig. 12.77. Ox. Skin. Focal ulcerative gangrenous dermatitis and cellulitis. Skin of the distal limb of a feedlot animal with focal ulcerated inflammation. *Fusobacterium necrophorum* was isolated via anaerobic cultures.

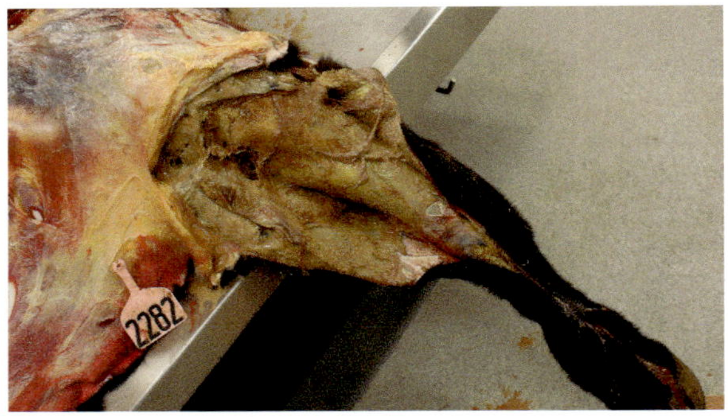

Fig. 12.78. Ox. Skin. Cellulitis and fasciitis. Pelvic limb of a feedlot animal with an ascending infection from a case of toe-tip necrosis. A variety of organisms can be isolated or demonstrated by special stains, including *Trueperella pyogenes*, *Fusobacterium necrophorum*, and *Bacteroides* spp.

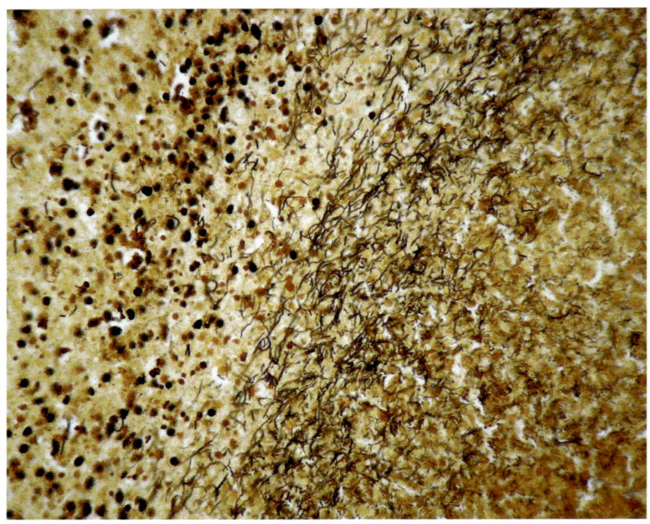

Fig. 12.79. Ox. Subcutis. Silver stain of a cellulitis case caused by *Fusobacterium necrophorum* demonstrating the typical filamentous organisms (Warthin–Faulkner).

12.6 PROTOZOAL DISEASES

Introduction. Only three genera of this infectious disease group cause skin disease in the bovine species – *Besnoitia* spp., *Leishmania* spp., and *Sarcosporidia* spp. *Besnoitia besnoiti* is not commonly seen in cattle in North America, being spread more in South America and on other continents (emerging in Europe). Caribou and reindeer in arctic regions of North America are often affected. All ruminant species are intermediate hosts, with feline species the definitive host. *Sarcosporidia* spp. are commonly encountered histologically in the muscle and heart myofibers of virtually all cattle. Occasionally, hair loss is reported in severe cases involving the rump, neck, and ears, with tail switch hair loss thought to be characteristic (see Chapter 8: Diseases of the Musculoskeletal System).

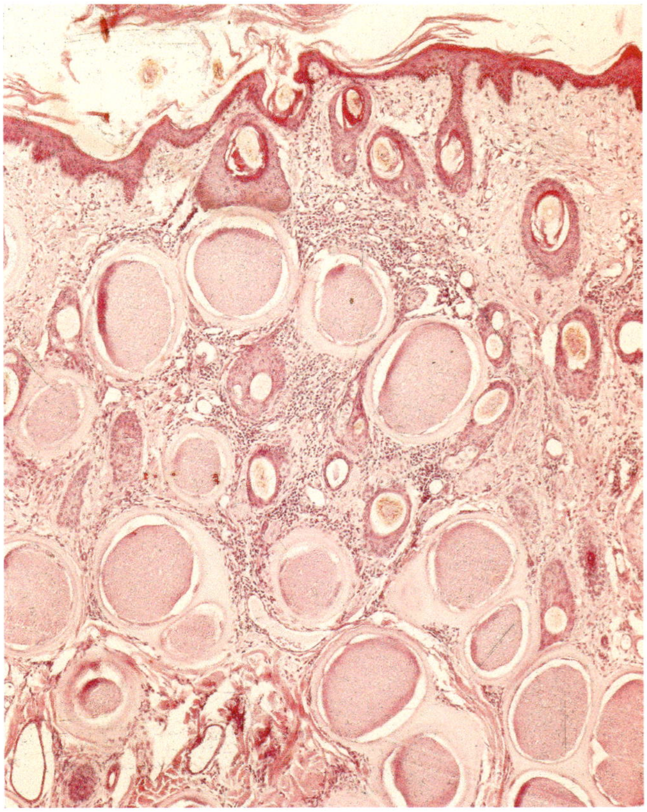

Fig. 12.80. Ox. Skin. Besnoitiosis. Proliferative dermatitis. A low-power histologic section of bovine skin with numerous large cysts typical of *Besnoitia* spp. The cysts have a thick, hyalinized connective tissue wall and are filled with clusters of bradyzoites (H&E). (See Chapter 15: Diseases of Eye and Ear.)

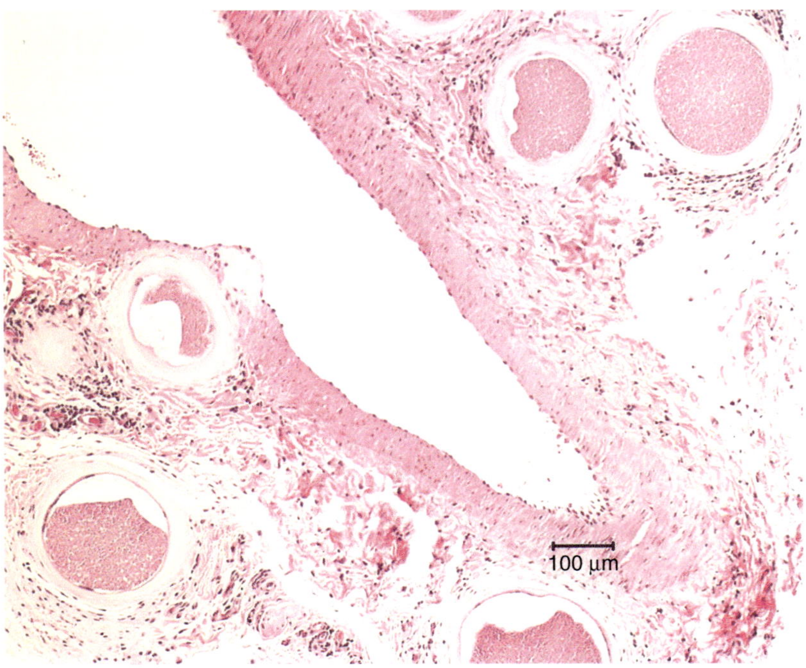

Fig. 12.81. Ox. Skin. Besnoitiosis. Multiple large *Besnoitia* cysts in a vessel wall and surrounding connective tissue with minimal lymphoid cell infiltrations (H&E).

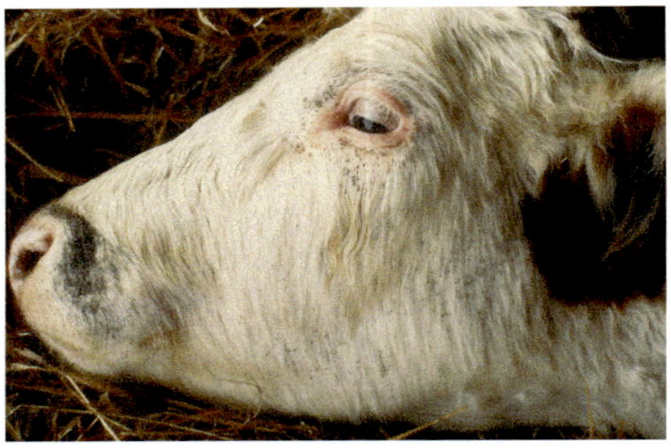

Fig. 12.82. Ox. Skin. Pediculosis. Head region of an adult animal with numerous lice visible periocular, around the muzzle region and lateral sides of the jaw. No other skin lesions present.

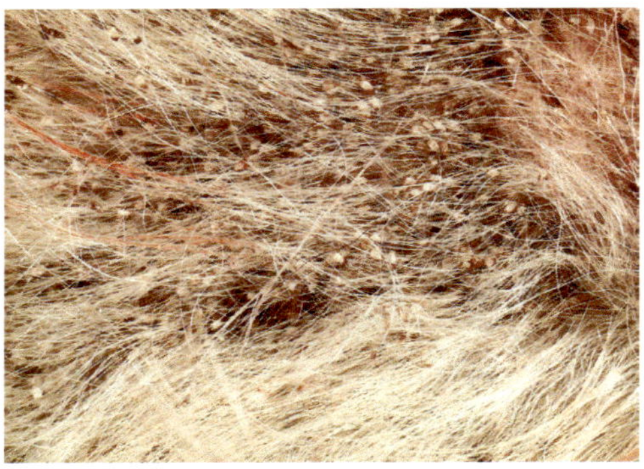

Fig. 12.83. Ox. Skin. Pediculosis. Numerous lice ova ('nits') attached to the hair of this animal.

12.7 PARASITIC DISEASES

12.7.1 Pediculosis (lice)

Introduction. Caused by two orders of lice: Mallophaga (biting lice) and Anoplura (sucking lice). These tend to be winter infestations and cause pruritis, with rubbing and subsequent hair loss only if infections are severe. Pour-on insecticides have controlled these infections to a large extent, but resistance to some treatment is being reported.

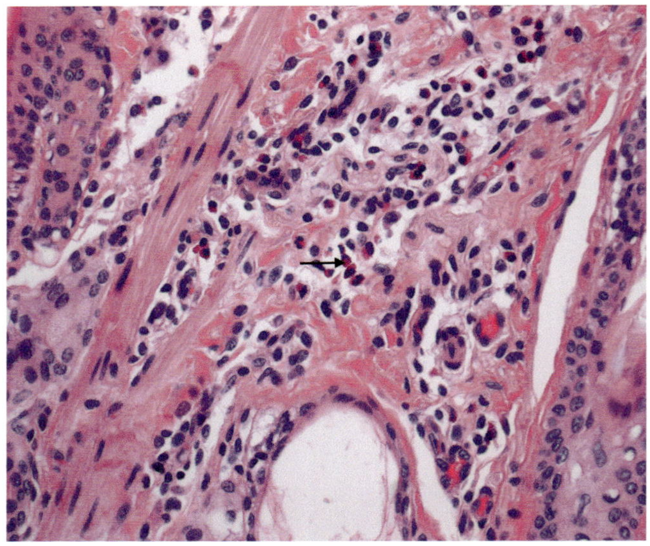

Fig. 12.84. Ox. Skin. Pediculosis. Dermatitis. Mixed cellular dermatitis including eosinophils (arrow) in a case of lice. It should be emphasized that eosinophils are so common in the skin of cattle that they are not at all a diagnostic feature (H&E).

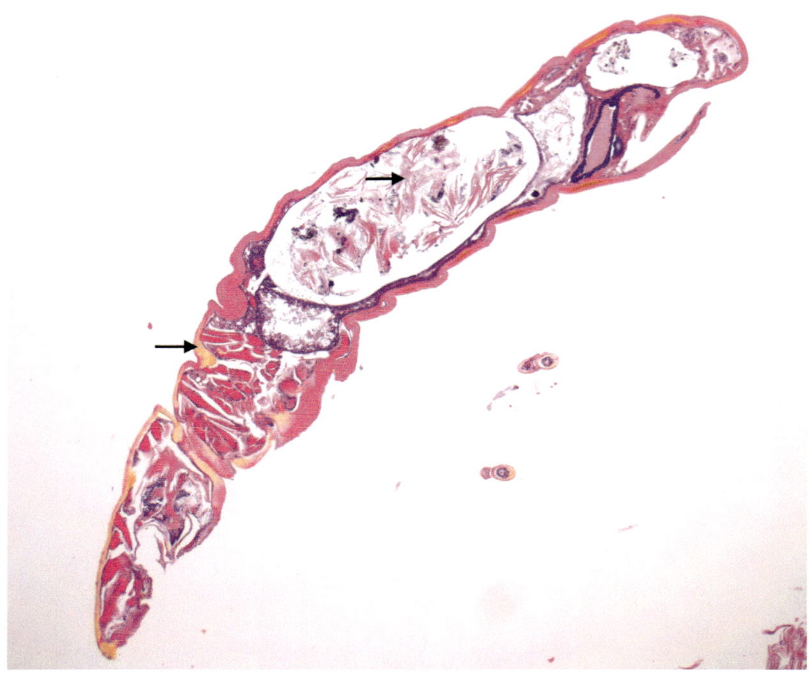

Fig. 12.85. Ox. Louse. Microscopic image of a louse showing the chitinous exoskeleton (top arrow). The presence of keratin squames and surface debris in the gut (bottom arrow) reveals this is a biting louse, probably *Damalinia bovis* (H&E).

12.7.2 Ectoparasitic mange

Introduction. Skin infection is not common, and cattle cases may acquire the disease from contact with mangy stray dogs, coyotes, or foxes, at least in North America. Transmission is both direct and indirect. Lesions begin as erythema and progress to severe crusting and alopecia, with pruritis being intense. Head, neck, and shoulder areas are most often affected.

12.7.2.1 Sarcoptic mange

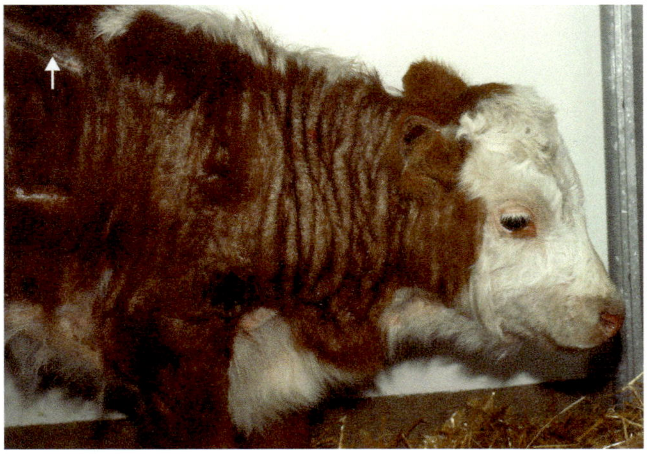

Fig. 12.86. Ox. Skin. Chronic dermatitis. A young calf with a severe confirmed case of sarcoptic mange (*Sarcoptes scabiei*). Extensive alopecia, with thickened skin and crusting. Linear excoriations (arrow) are due to severe pruritis, resulting in rubbing and scratching excessively.

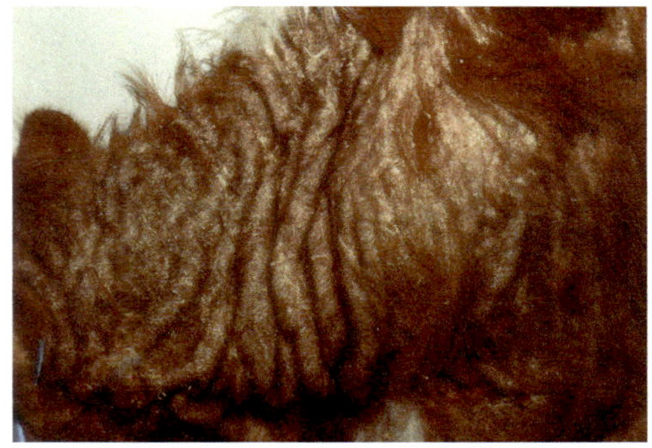

Fig. 12.87. Ox. Skin. Chronic dermatitis. Closer photograph of the same calf with severe lesions on the left side.

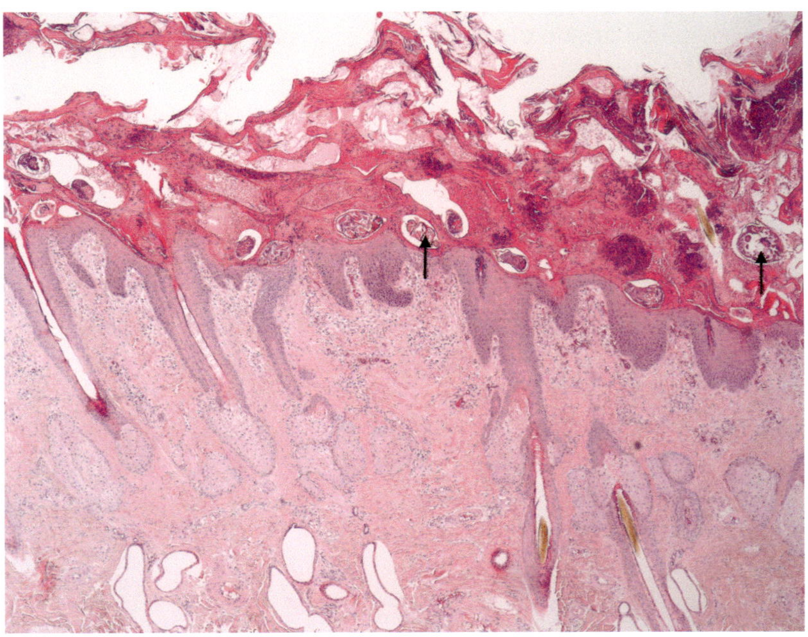

Fig. 12.88. Ox. Skin. Chronic dermatitis. Histologic picture showing marked epidermal hyperplasia, extensive surface parakeratotic hyperkeratosis, and serum exudation, with numerous mites residing on the epidermis or in the surface serocellular crusts (arrows) (H&E).

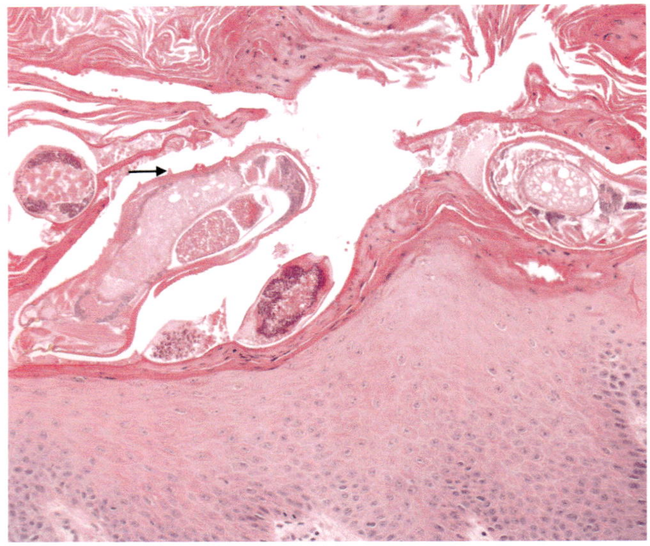

Fig. 12.89. Ox. Skin. Mites. Closer histologic view of several mites with typical cuticular spines (arrow). These spines occur in other species of mites as well, so alone they are not useful for differentiation. Morphologic features on skin scrapings are helpful to identify the mite species (H&E).

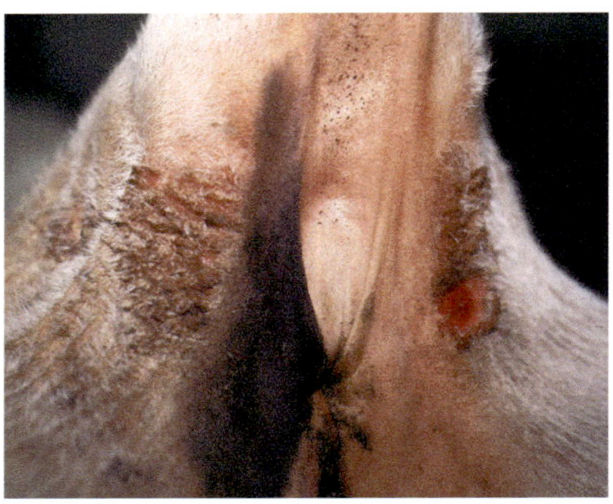

Fig. 12.90. Ox. Skin. Chronic dermatitis. A dairy cow with proximal tail and adjacent dorsal rump skin thickening and crusting due to chorioptic mange (*Chorioptes bovis*).

12.7.2.2 Chorioptic mange

Introduction. *Chorioptes bovis* is most commonly seen in dairy cows housed indoors in winter months, and the lesions are more common in the perianal, perineal, escutcheon, and inner thighs or caudal udder regions. Recent experience in western Canada identified multiple beef bulls with involvement of the caudal thigh regions and scrotum. Pour-on insecticides appear to render partial protection and have been used for many years. There are now reports of at least partial resistance to these parasiticides by many parasite species.

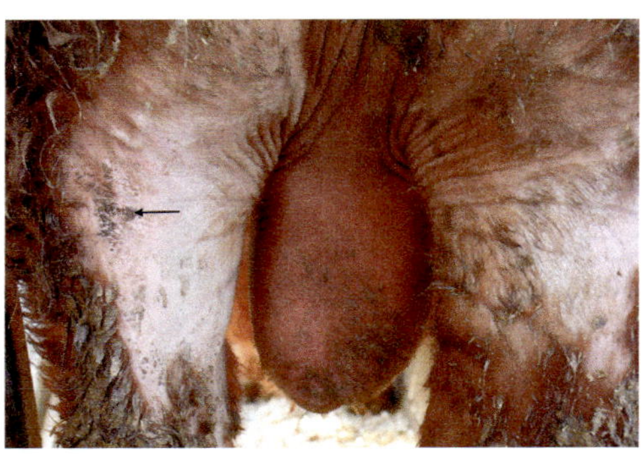

Fig. 12.92. Ox. Skin. Chronic dermatitis. Focal areas (arrow) of inner thigh of a yearling bull with localized crusting. Scrapings easily identified Chorioptes mites present in large numbers. (Courtesy of Dr M. Jelinski, Airdrie, Alberta, Canada.)

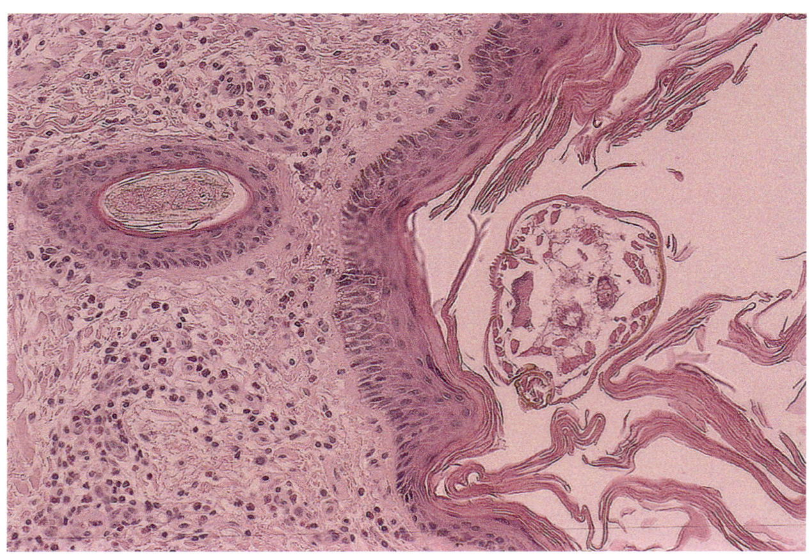

Fig. 12.91. Ox. Skin. Biopsy. Numerous Chorioptic mites are located on the skin surface, with spines on the mite cuticular surface like in the *Sarcoptes* spp. mites (H&E).

Other manges encountered are psoroptic mange (*Psoroptes ovis*) and demodectic mange.

12.7.3 Stephanofilariasis

Introduction. A very common localized skin condition caused by the nematode Stephanofilaria, of which there are many species. *Stephanofilaria stilesi* is most common, especially in western North America. *Haematobia* and *Musca* flies are the intermediate hosts. Localized areas of thickened skin with alopecia and variable crusting and weeping are most common along the ventral midline, but occasionally the udder and teats can be involved. The condition is most often seen in beef cattle on pasture.

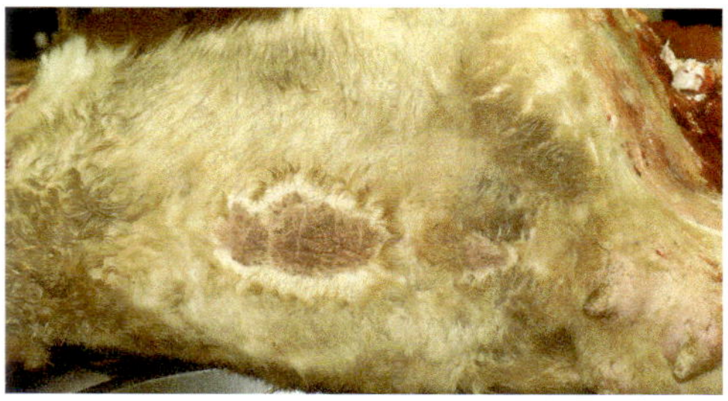

Fig. 12.93. Ox. Skin. Stephanofilariasis. Chronic dermatitis. A beef cow with two localized ventral midline lesions.

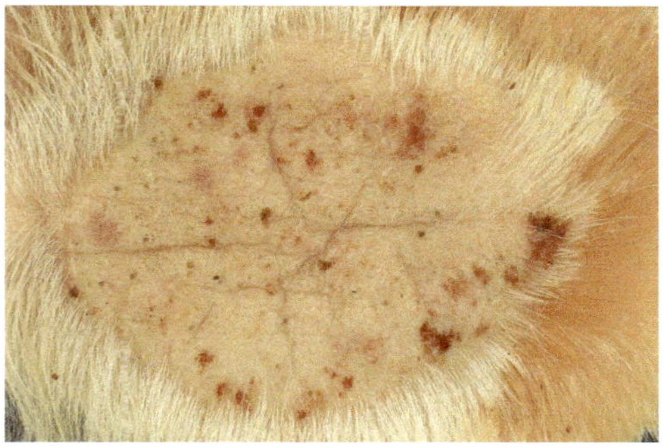

Fig. 12.94. Ox. Skin. Stephanofilariasis. Chronic dermatitis. Close-up of a case with alopecia and small foci of hemorrhagic crusts, erythema, and excoriations.

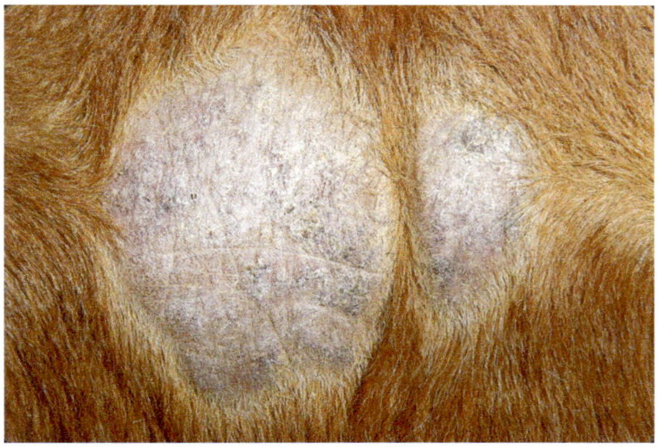

Fig. 12.95. Ox. Skin. Stephanofilariasis. Chronic dermatitis. A similar case, with discoloration possibly due to subcutaneous vascular congestion.

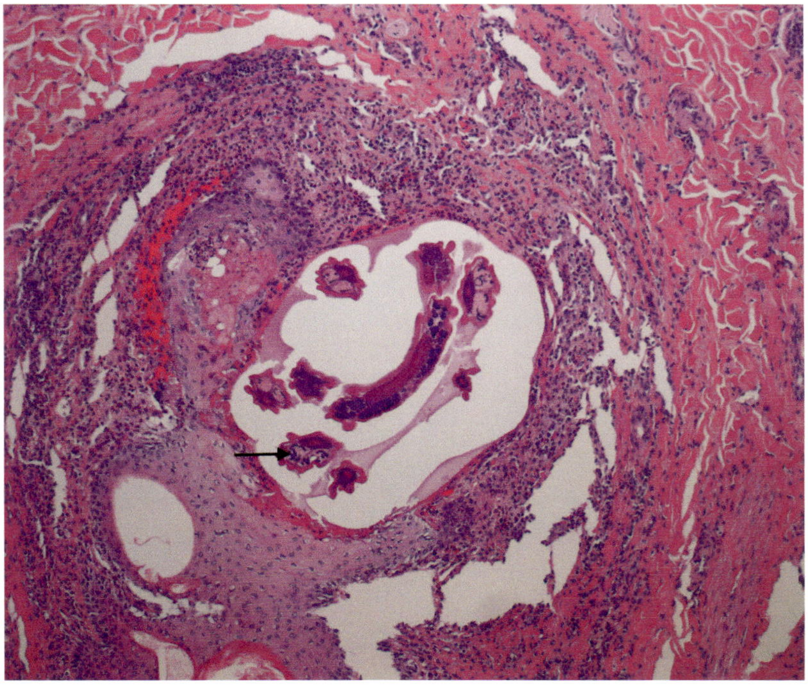

Fig. 12.96. Ox. Stephanofilariasis. Parasitic dermatitis. Histologic picture of follicle destruction, with cross and longitudinal sections of a typical nematode. The dark, crescent-shaped bodies within the nematodes are microfilaria (arrow) (H&E).

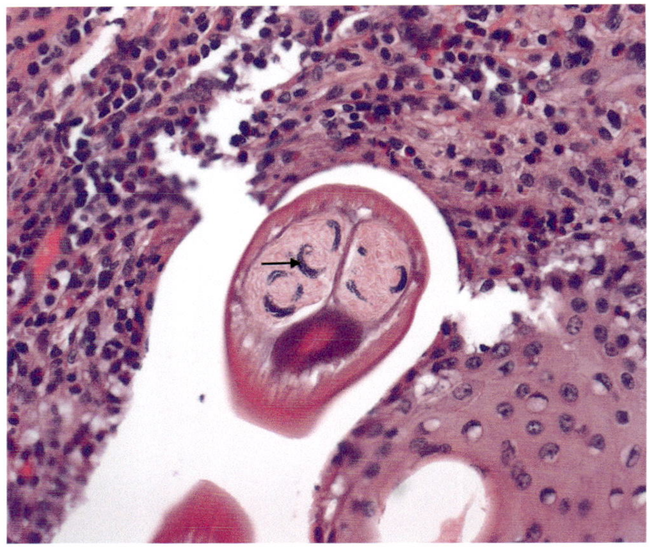

Fig. 12.97. Ox. Skin. Stephanofilariasis. Parasitic dermatitis. Close-up of one nematode, showing microfilaria within the uteri (arrow). Mixed inflammatory cells surrounding the nematodes are mononuclear cells and some eosinophils (H&E).

12.7.4 Pelodera dermatitis (rhabditic dermatitis)

Introduction. This nematode (*Rhabditis bovis*) is a free-living parasite that resides in wet bedding and soil. It only causes skin lesions when the skin is damaged, such as by constantly lying on excessively wet, soiled surfaces. The adults invade the hair follicles, causing eosinophilic folliculitis, furunculosis, and subsequent alopecia. Pruritis is variable.

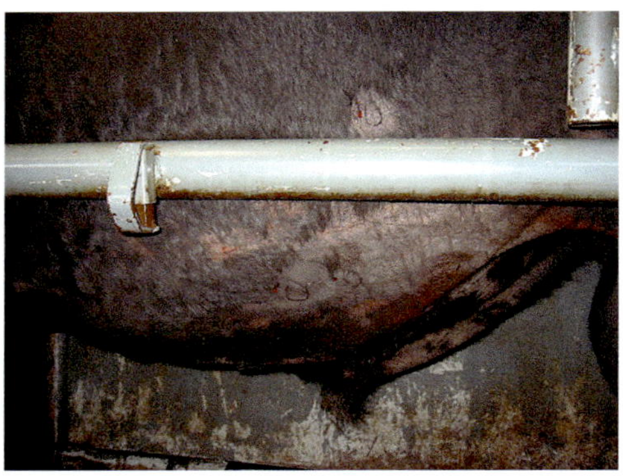

Fig. 12.98. Ox. Skin. Rhabditic dermatitis. Ventral abdomen of an adult Angus bull with typical alopecia, little crusting, and hyperkeratosis. Focal hemorrhages represent biopsy sites.

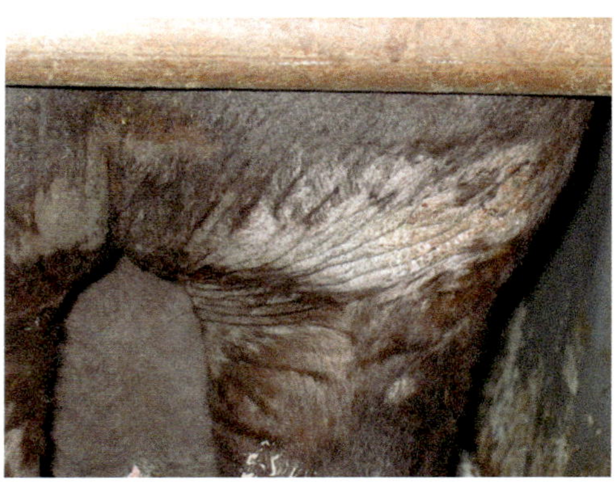

Fig. 12.99. Ox. Skin. Pelodera dermatitis. Proximal limb region of the same bull showing more crusting along with the alopecia.

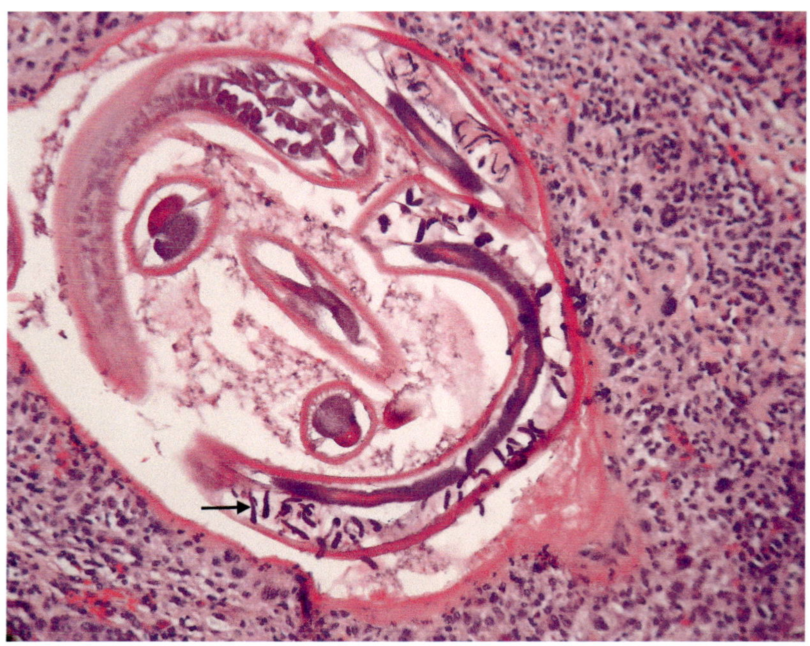

Fig. 12.100. Ox. Skin. Pelodera dermatitis. Longitudinal and cut sections of several nematodes residing in a follicle that has been destroyed. The comma-shaped, dark bodies represent microfilaria (arrow) (H&E).

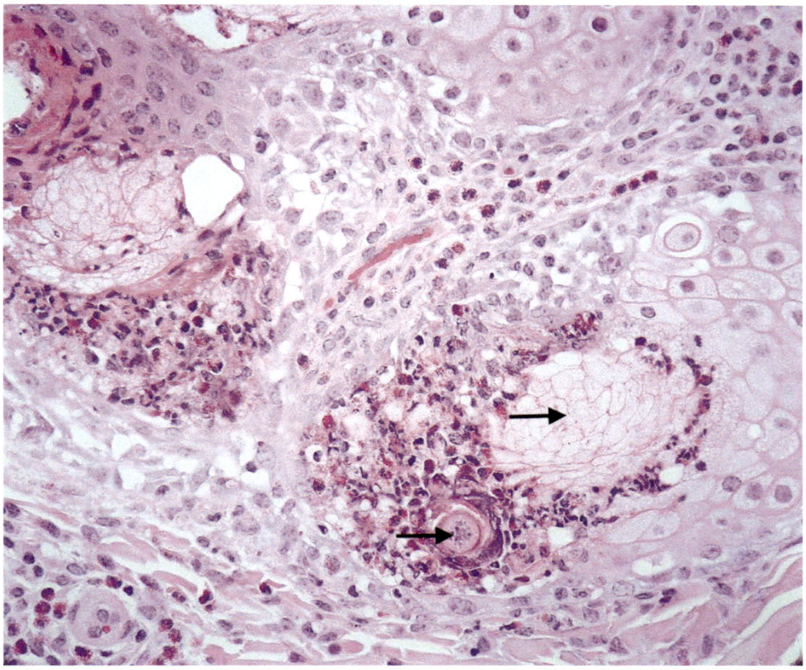

Fig. 12.101. Ox. Skin. Pelodera. Another site of folliculitis, necrosis with cell debris, eosinophils, and necrosis of a sebaceous gland, the latter probably a result of eosinophil degranulation (top arrow). Cut section of one nematode is present (bottom arrow) (H&E).

Other genera of skin helminths affecting cattle are *Onchocerca* spp. and *Parafilaria* spp. (Asia, Africa, and Europe).

12.7.5 Hypodermosis (warbles, cattle grubs)

Introduction. In the northern American hemisphere, *Hypoderma bovis* and *Hypoderma lineatum* are the cause, whereas in central South America, *Dermatobia hominis* is most prevalent. Other species occur in other parts of the world. The adult Hypoderma are known as heel flies that lay eggs on the hair of the heels and lower limbs. The larvae penetrate the skin and migrate through fascial planes to partially develop in the submucosal tissue of the esophagus (*H. lineatum*) or subdural fat along the spinal cord (*H. bovis*). The use of pour-on insecticides has made both of these infections very uncommon now. Swellings along the dorsum of the body, with breathing holes for the grubs, are classic findings.

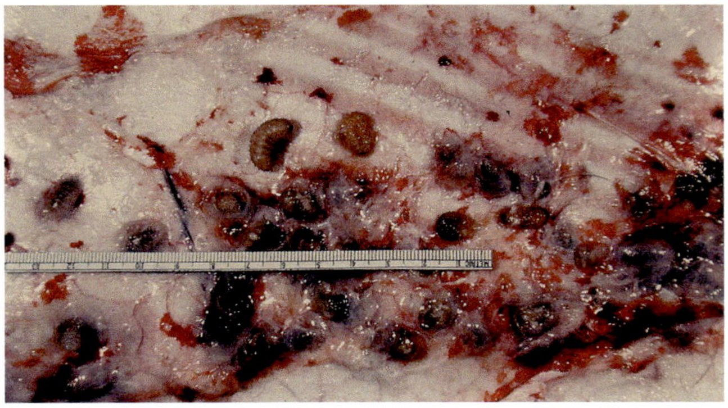

Fig. 12.102. Ox. Skin. Hypodermosis. A case of warble grubs under the skin, detected at slaughter.

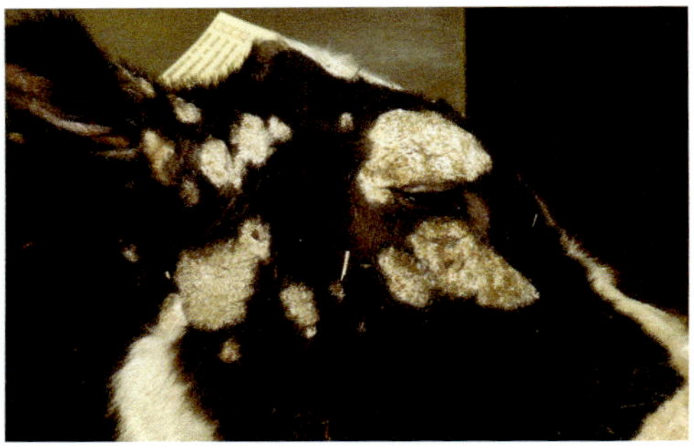

Fig. 12.103. Ox. Skin. Dermatophytosis. Exfoliative dermatitis and alopecia. Extensive white, crusted lesions periocular and on the ears and temporal regions.

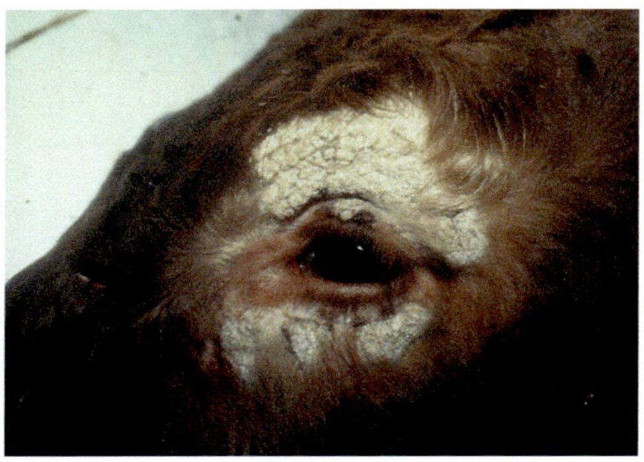

Fig. 12.104. Ox. Skin. Dermatophytosis. Exfoliative dermatitis. Close-up of periocular lesions. Focal alopecia and encrustations.

12.8 MYCOSES (FUNGAL INFECTIONS)

Introduction. The most common fungal infections in the bovine skin occur in fetuses aborted by various fungal agents causing placentitis, and these are covered in Chapter 10: Diseases of the Reproductive System.

12.8.1 Dermatophytosis ('ringworm')

Introduction. A common disease that occurs in cattle, especially under 1 year of age and in winter months in housed conditions. It can have a high incidence in a herd and is a zoonosis. *Trichophyton verrucosum* is most often involved, but *Trichophyton mentagrophytes* and several *Microsporum* spp. are less commonly identified. Lesions are most common around the head and face, but neck and rump can also have lesions. Typically, there is marked hair loss and heavy, white, thick crusts in localized areas.

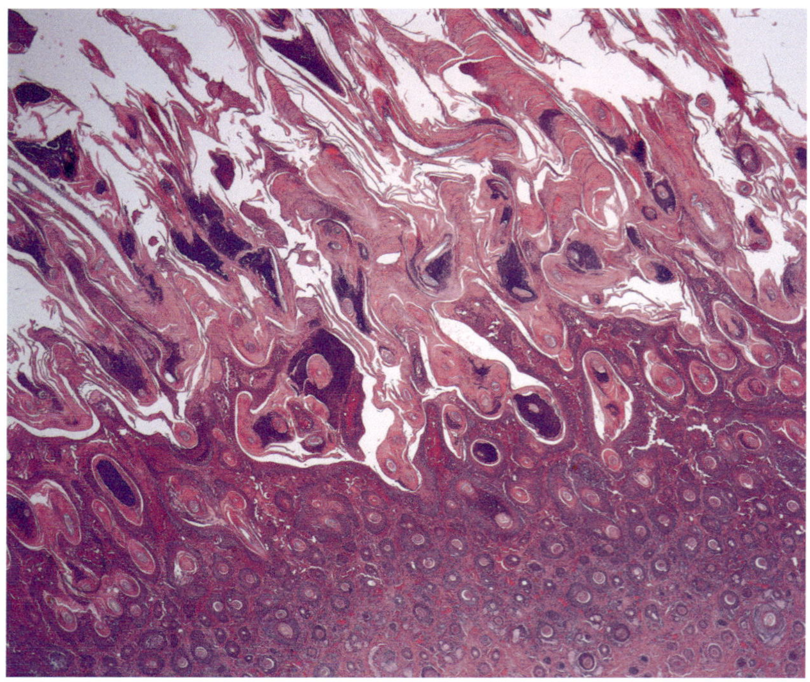

Fig. 12.105. Ox. Skin. Dermatophytosis. Purulent folliculitis. The diagnosis is usually easy to make without histopathology, but dermatophilosis is a differential diagnosis. This low-power photograph shows extensive hyperkeratosis in which hair shafts containing fungal elements are surrounded by neutrophils. In very chronic cases that may resolve without treatment, it is important to examine the surface crust material, with the best chance of seeing the organisms in hair shafts in the crust material using GMS (silver) and/or PAS stains (H&E).

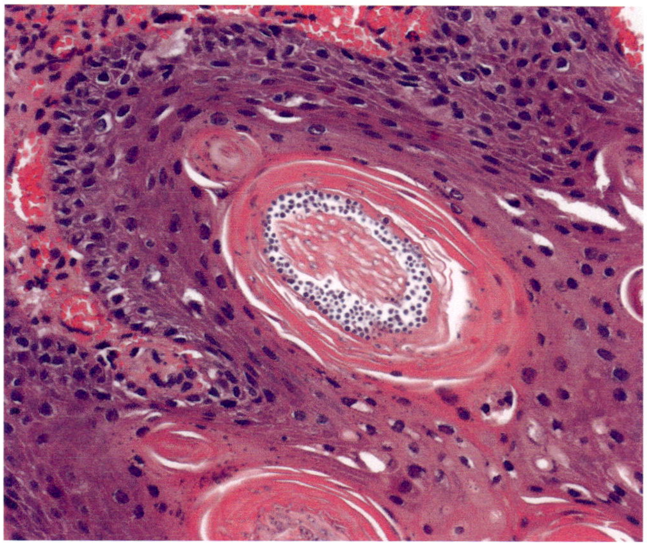

Fig. 12.106. Ox. Hair follicle. Dermatophytosis. Close-up of a hair follicle with arthrospores surrounding the hair shaft (ectothrix) and mycelia present within the hair shaft (H&E).

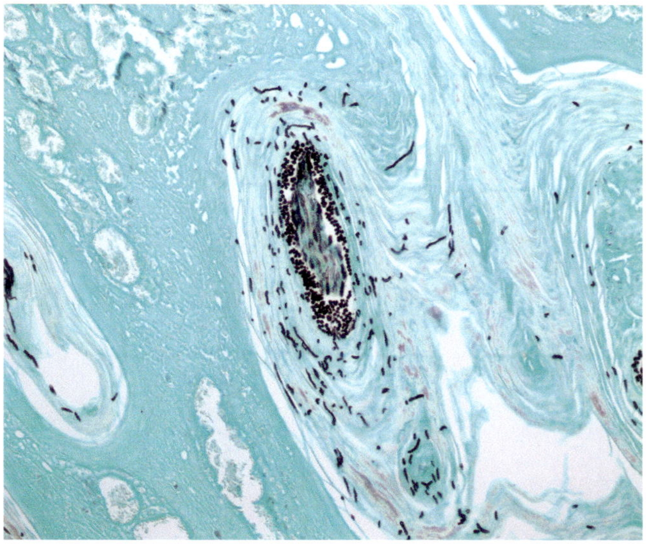

Fig. 12.107. Ox. Hair follicle. Dermatophytosis. A special stain of one or more follicles showing both mycelia and arthrospores (Grocott's silver).

12.8.2 Fungal granulomas

Introduction. Various saprophytic fungi can occasionally cause cutaneous fungal granulomas in cattle, as in other domestic species. These include *Aspergillus* spp., *Pythium* spp., *Alternaria* spp., and hyalohyphomycoses. Other genera can be isolated as well in cattle. In the case of phaeohyphomycosis, the fungal elements are pigmented, but other non-pigmented species can be seen.

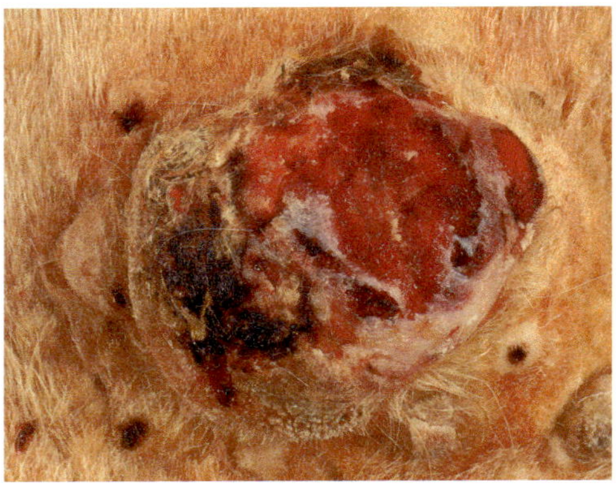

Fig. 12.108. Ox. Skin. Cutaneous lymphoma. A localized cutaneous growth with extensive ulceration.

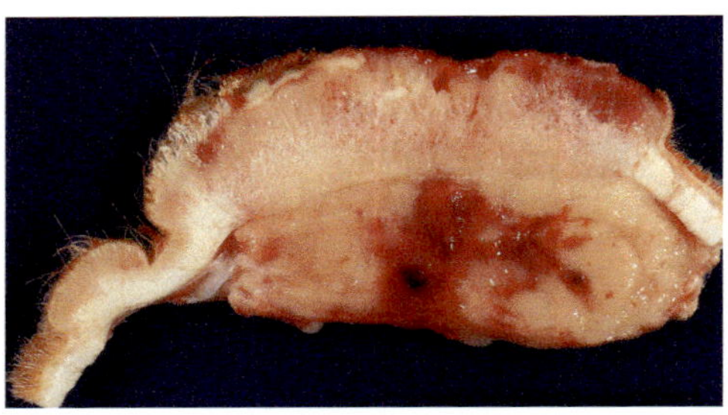

Fig. 12.109. Ox. Skin. Cutaneous lymphoma. The same growth on cut surface to show a large, gray dermal and subcutaneous lesion, as well as the epidermal ulceration.

12.9 NEOPLASTIC CONDITIONS

12.9.1 Cutaneous lymphoma (lymphosarcoma)

Introduction. For a more detailed discussion, see Chapter 11: Diseases of the Hematopoietic and Hemolymphatic System.

12.9.2 Squamous cell carcinoma (SCC)

Introduction. This malignant tumor involves the optic globe and eyelids of cattle very frequently and will be covered in Chapter 15: Diseases of Eye and Ear. Other sites include lower limbs, vulva, ears, and the muzzle. White-haired cattle in tropical and subtropical parts of the world and at higher altitude have the highest incidence. Sites of chronic skin damage, such as dehorning sites and branding are also predisposed to neoplasia.

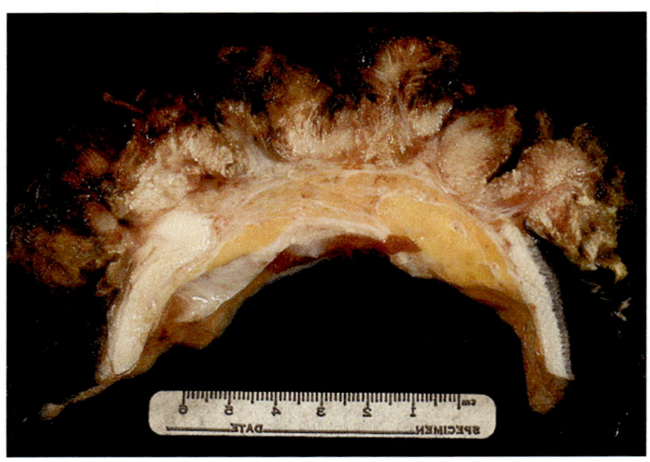

Fig. 12.110. Ox. Skin. Squamous cell carcinoma (SCC). Branding site squamous cell carcinoma showing papillary-like projections, epidermal ulceration, and surface crusting. The lesions are often called keratomas initially, but if left alone will often progress to SCCs.

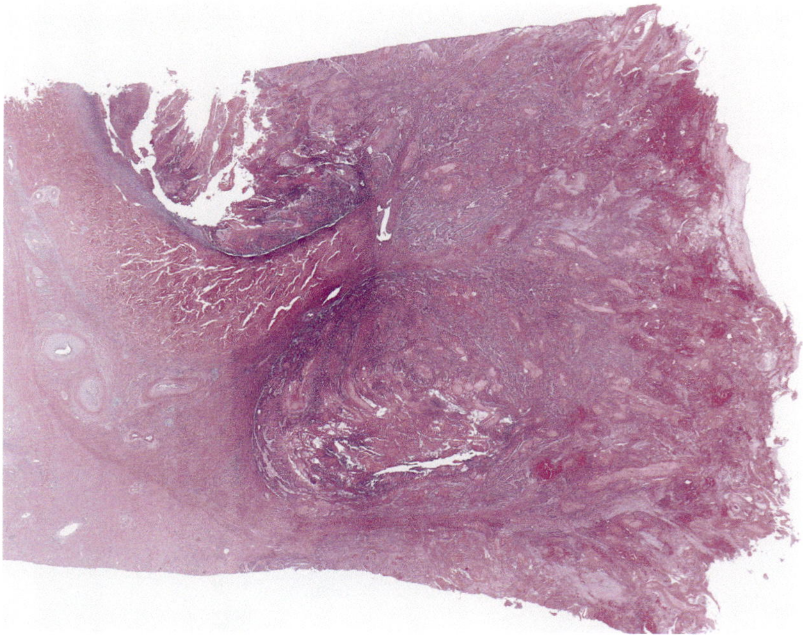

Fig. 12.111. Ox. Skin. Squamous cell carcinoma (SCC). Subgross histologic image of the same brand SCC showing loss of the epidermis and adnexal glands, with invasion of the deep dermis and subcutis by neoplastic keratinocytes (H&E).

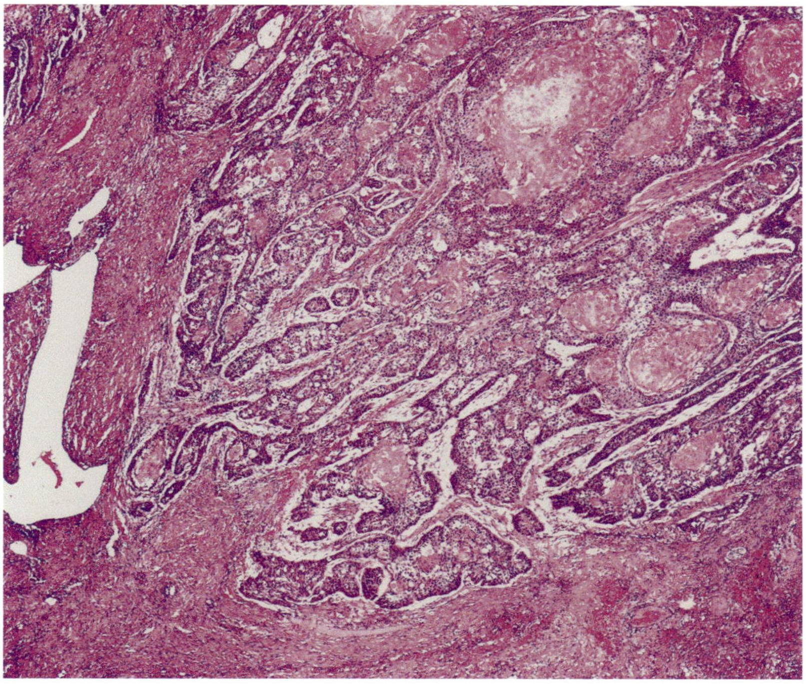

Fig. 12.112. Ox. Skin. Squamous cell carcinoma. Columns and irregular clusters of basiloid keratinocytes, with islands of more mature keratinocytes invading the deep subcutaneous connective tissues (H&E).

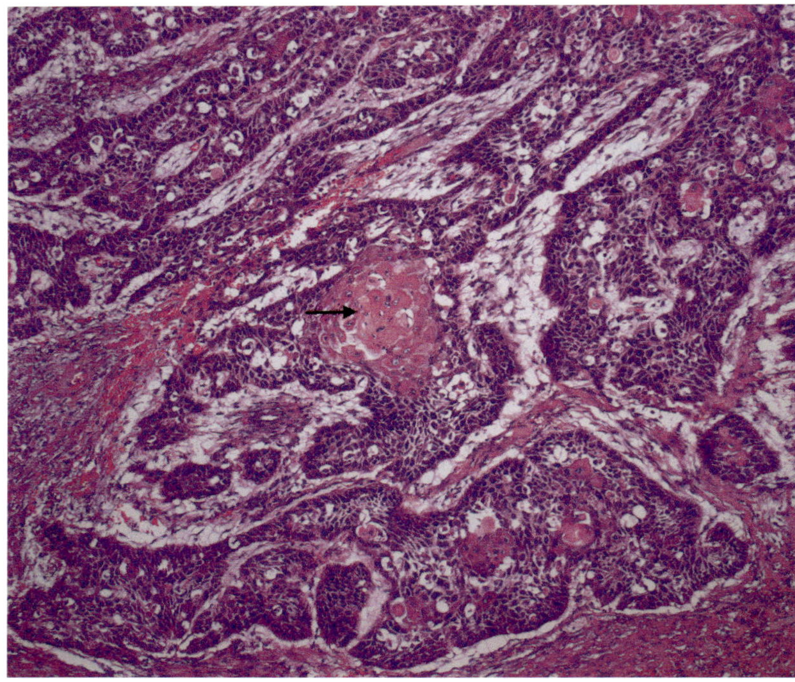

Fig. 12.113. Ox. Skin. Squamous cell carcinoma. Individual and clusters of more mature keratinocytes (arrow) among the predominant, more basophilic basiloid cells (H&E).

12.9.3 Mast cell tumor

Introduction. Not uncommon skin tumors, they can occur at any age, even congenitally on occasion. May develop anywhere on the body and may metastasize. They often ulcerate superficially.

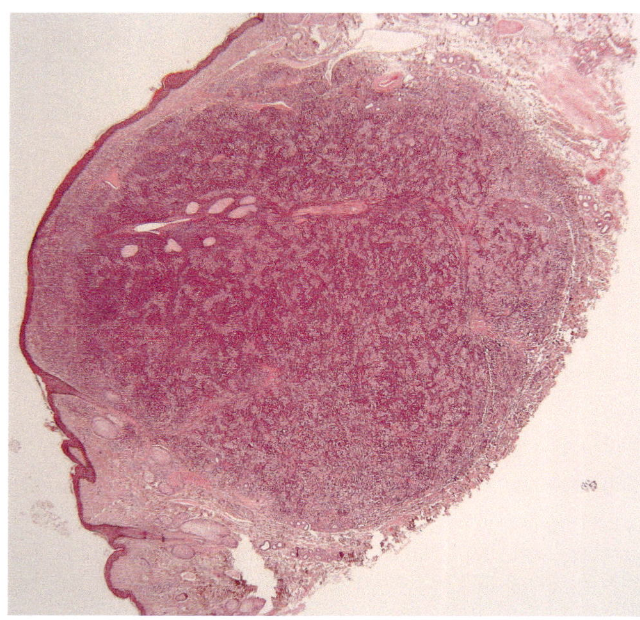

Fig. 12.114. Ox. Skin. Mast cell tumor. Subgross histologic picture of a well-delineated mast cell tumor extending from the epidermis deep into the subcutis. A hair follicle and adnexal glands are embedded. Eosinophils outnumber the tumor cells in this particular case, but may vary from case to case (H&E).

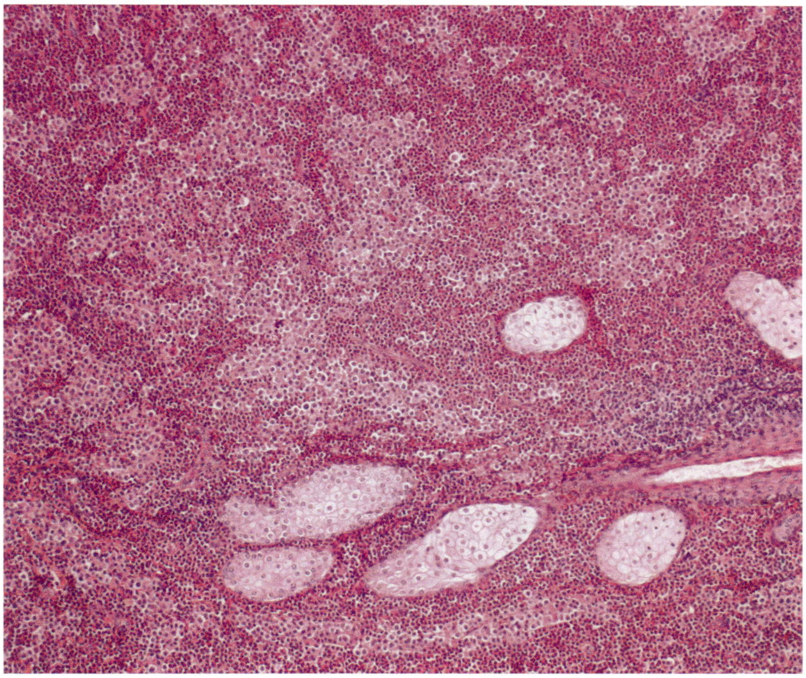

Fig. 12.115. Ox. Skin. Mast cell tumor. Higher-power view of the same tumor showing high numbers of eosinophils. The mast cells appear well differentiated, with no cytoplasmic granules present (H&E).

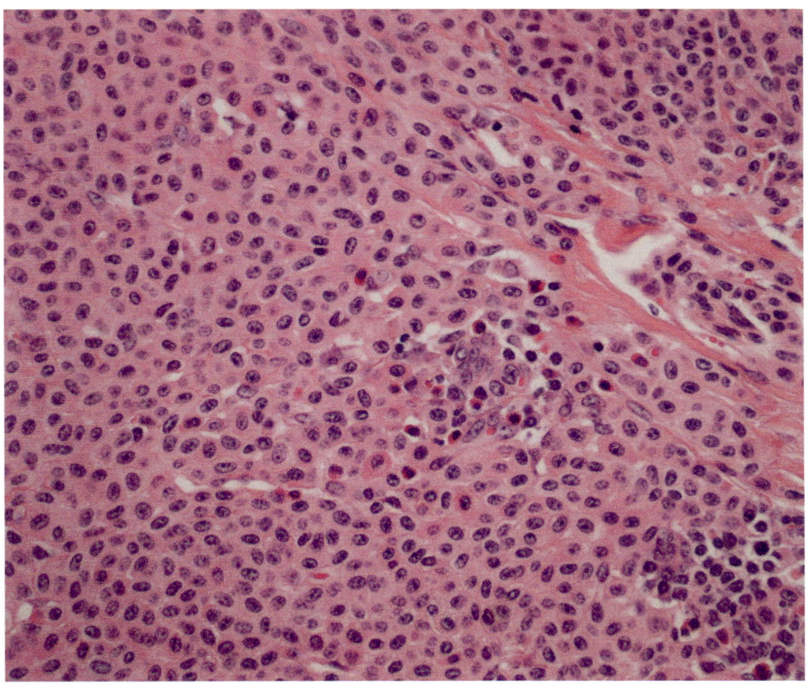

Fig. 12.116. Ox. Skin. Mast cell tumor. High-power view of another tumor with few eosinophils and very few cytoplasmic mast cell granules. No mitotic figures observed (H&E).

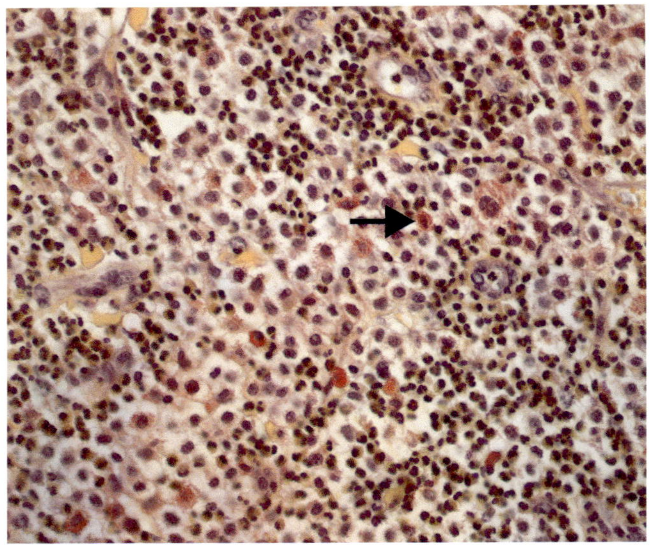

Fig. 12.117. Ox. Skin. Mast cell tumor. Another case using a neutral red stain to show the cytoplasmic granules (arrow). Giemsa, toluidine blue, and Duffy's stains also can be applied (neutral red).

12.9.4 Melanocytomas/melanomas

Introduction. Not uncommon, predominantly in adult cattle. A high percentage of these heavily pigmented tumors are benign. Their size, shape, and location on the body vary widely, with the majority being on the limbs.

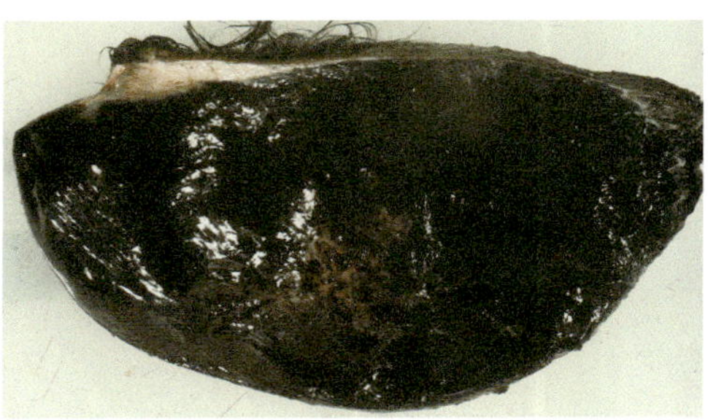

Fig. 12.119. Ox. Skin. Melanoma. Cut surface of a large melanoma with intense pigmentation.

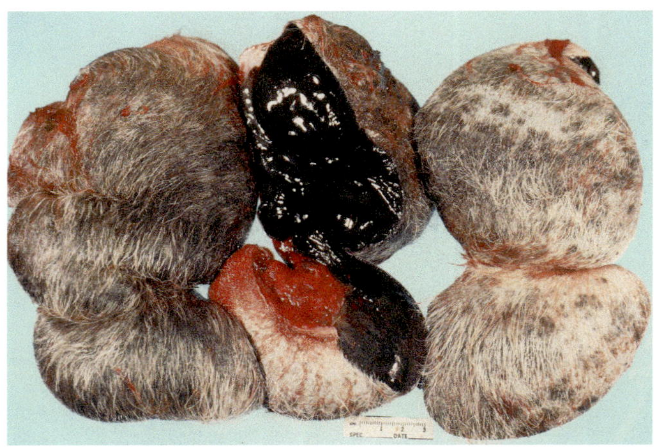

Fig. 12.118. Ox. Skin. Melanoma. Multiple sections of a large cutaneous melanoma. If large and pedunculated, they are frequently ulcerated.

12.9.5 Juvenile bovine angiomatosis

Introduction. These vasoproliferative growths may be hamartomas, and can be congenital or arise later in life. They can be multiple, and even develop in internal organs. Typical microscopic lesion in bovines is a non-encapsulated mixture of thin-walled channels lined by endothelial cells of varying differentiation, within a connective tissue stroma, that attempts to form blood or lymph vessels. Lesions can be accompanied by polymorphonuclear and mononuclear inflammatory infiltrations or fibroplasia with collagen deposition. Tending to be very dark red to black, they are by far most common in dairy cattle.

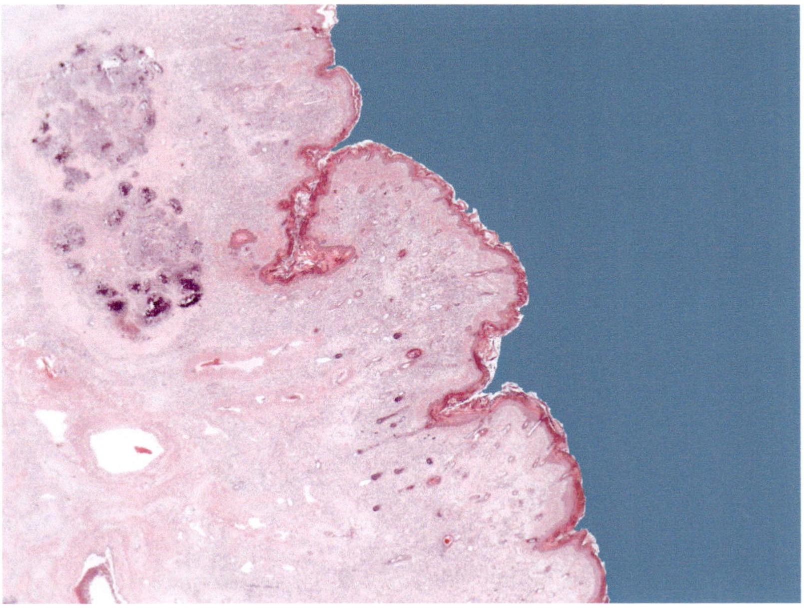

Fig. 12.120. Ox. Skin. Angiomatosis. Low-power histologic section of an angiomatosis mass that measured 10 cm × 6 cm diameter and was located on the dorsal neck region of a 14-day-old Charolais calf. It was described grossly as soft, with multifocal areas of dark brown coloration and multiple cavitations of variable size within the dermis and subcutis. Multiple raised areas of skin show hypercellularity of the dermis, with a large area of apparent mineralization (H&E).

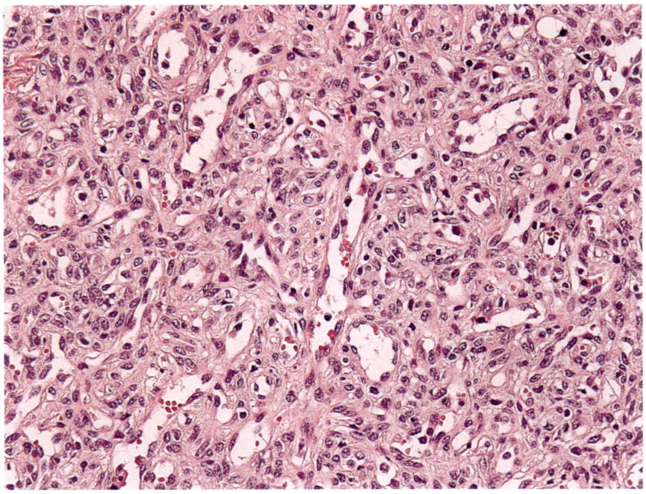

Fig. 12.121. Ox. Skin. Angiomatosis. Numerous endothelial cell-lined channels separated by thin collagen strands. A factor VIII-related IHC stain would confirm the endothelial cell population (H&E).

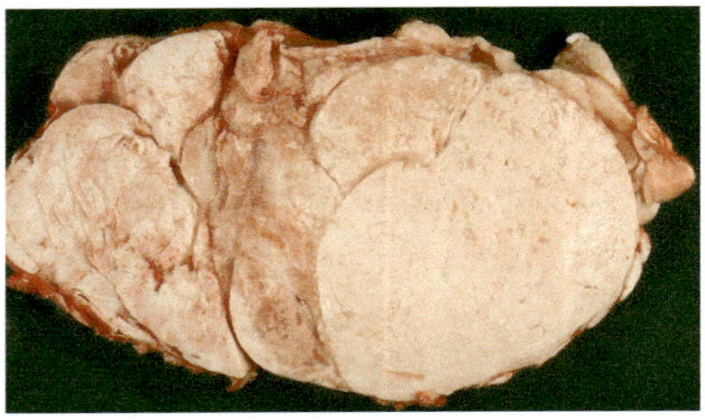

Fig. 12.122. Ox. Skin. Lipoma. Cut surface of a large cutaneous lipoma.

12.9.6 Cutaneous lipomas

Introduction. Seen on rare occasions, and most common in adult cattle. Often very large, with up to 50 cm diameter.

12.9.7 Fibromas, fibrosarcomas, and other spindle cell tumors

Introduction. Fibromas are more frequent in the bovine skin as compared to hemangiopericytomas or schwannomas/neurofibromas.

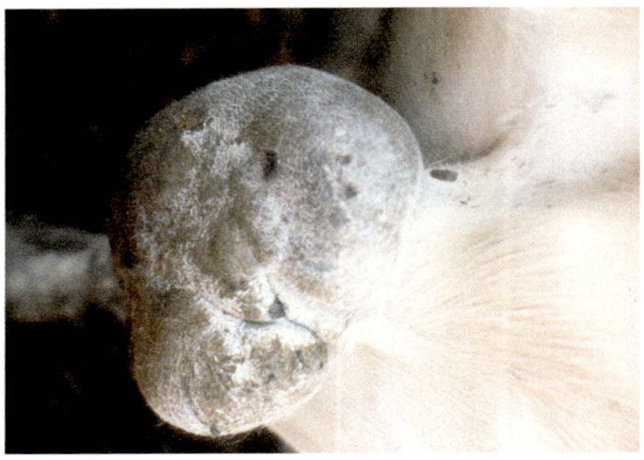

Fig. 12.123. Ox. Skin. Neoplasia. Large cutaneous tumor in an adult cow discovered as incidental findings prior to slaughter, and neither identified by histopathology. Spindle cell tumors, melanomas, or lipomas would all be possible diagnoses.

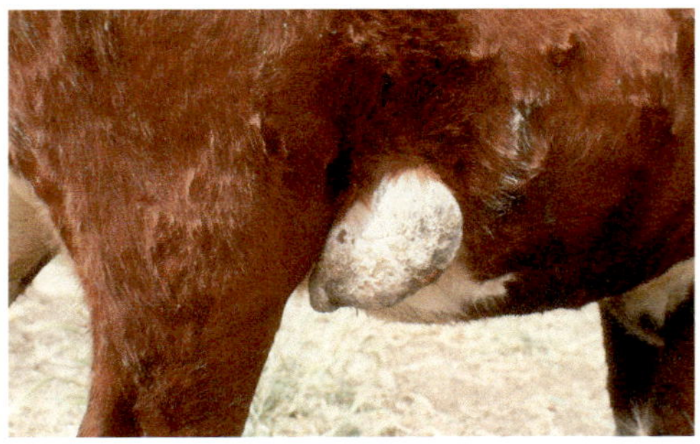

Fig. 12.124. Ox. Skin. Neoplasia. Large cutaneous tumor in an adult cow discovered as incidental findings prior to slaughter, and neither identified by histopathology. Spindle cell tumors, melanomas, or lipomas would all be possible diagnoses.

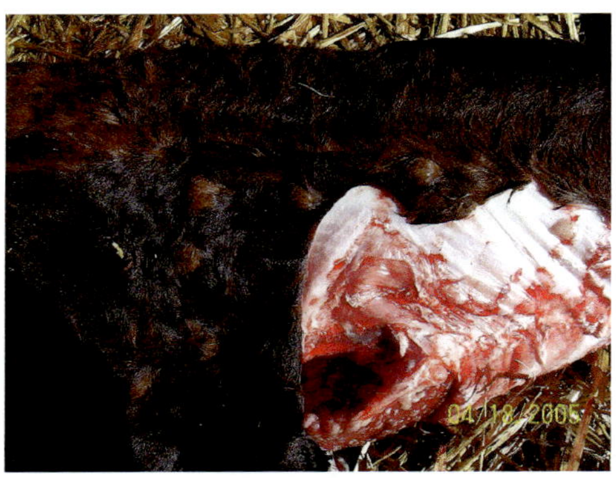

Fig. 12.125. Ox. Skin. Undifferentiated round cell tumor. Newborn Hereford calf showing numerous, multisystemic, smooth, white, round cell nodules.

12.9.8 Congenital, disseminated, undifferentiated round cell tumor

Introduction. Most congenital round cell tumors are lymphosarcomas, especially involving the thymus. On rare occasions, undifferentiated round cell tumors can be multisystemic. Also see Chapter 1: Diseases of Neonates and Calves, and Chapter 2: Diseases of the Nervous System.

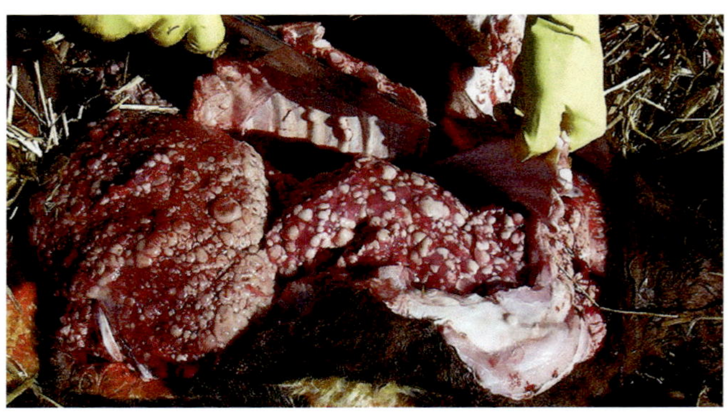

Fig. 12.126. Ox. Skin. Undifferentiated round cell tumor. Newborn Hereford calf showing numerous, multisystemic, smooth, white, round cell nodules.

12.10 MISCELLANEOUS CONDITIONS

12.10.1 Subcutaneous soft or fluctuant swellings

Introduction. The two main pathologic considerations are edema and hemorrhage. Trauma such as fractures or blunt trauma has to be considered, as well as pockets of purulent material (abscesses).

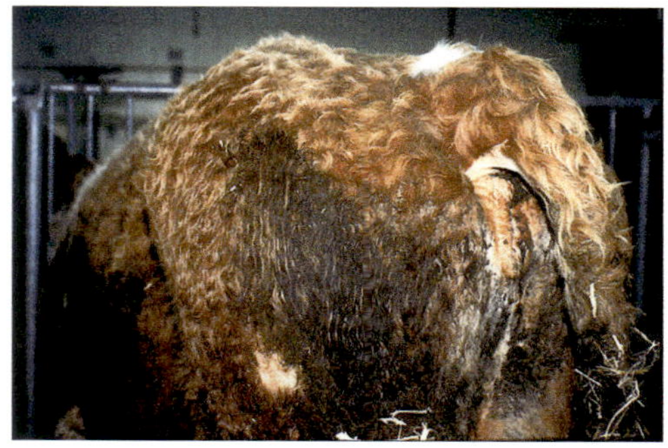

Fig. 12.127. Ox. Subcutis. Bleeding disorder. Swelling in the hindquarter of this Simmental bull is the result of a large area of hemorrhage from a congenital and inherited bleeding disorder in Simmental cattle due to a platelet malfunction. Their platelets have abnormal skeletal assembly and aggregation.

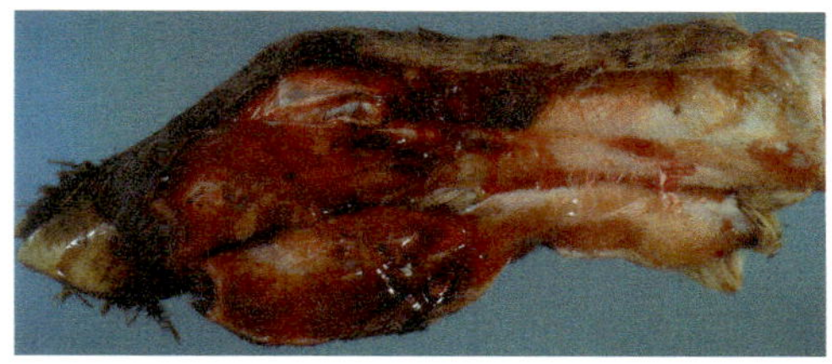

Fig. 12.128. Ox. Subcutis. Extravasation. Distal limb of a calf with severe hemorrhage and edema due to frostbite injury.

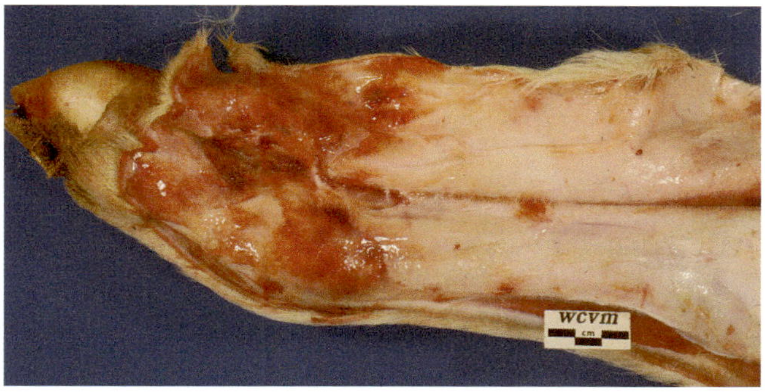

Fig. 12.129. Ox. Subcutaneous edema of the distal limb of a calf with mild frostbite injury.

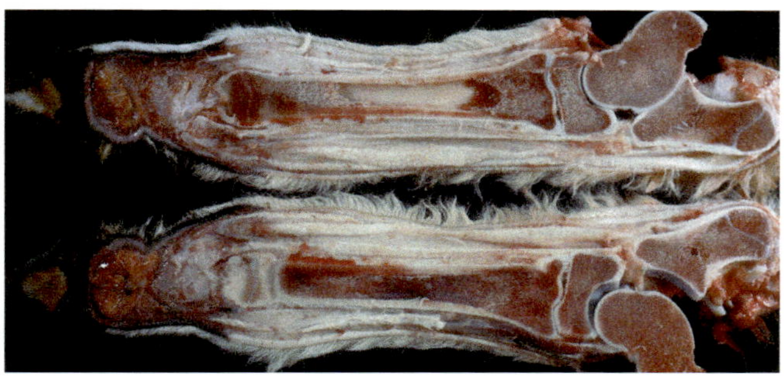

Fig. 12.130. Ox. Subcutis. Extravasation. Extensive hemorrhage in a newborn calf due to dicoumarol toxicity (sweet clover poisoning).

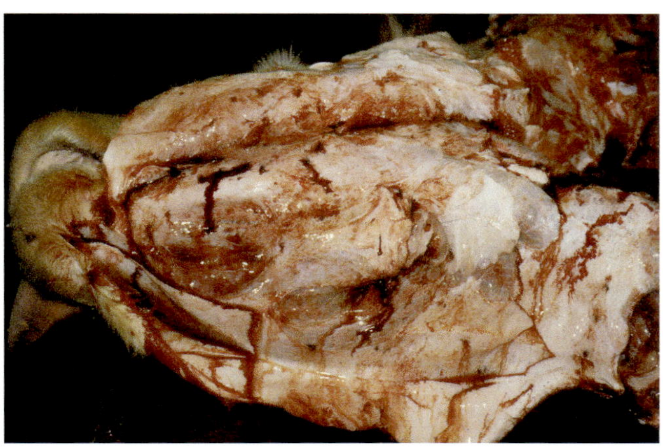

Fig. 12.131. Ox. Subcutis. Edema. Extensive submandibular edema due to congestive heart failure.

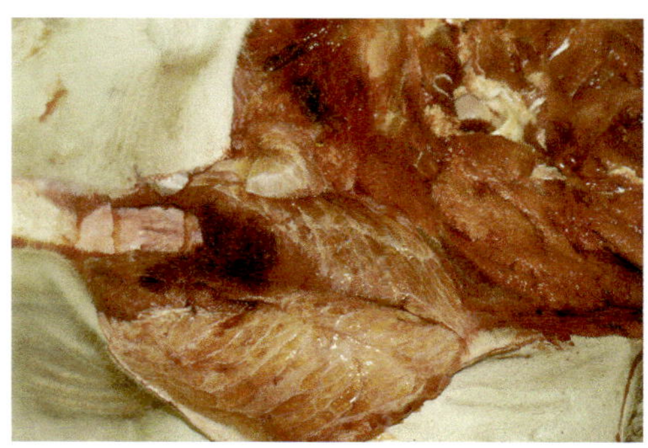

Fig. 12.132. Ox. Subcutis. Edema. Flank fold edema in a case of acute frothy bloat.

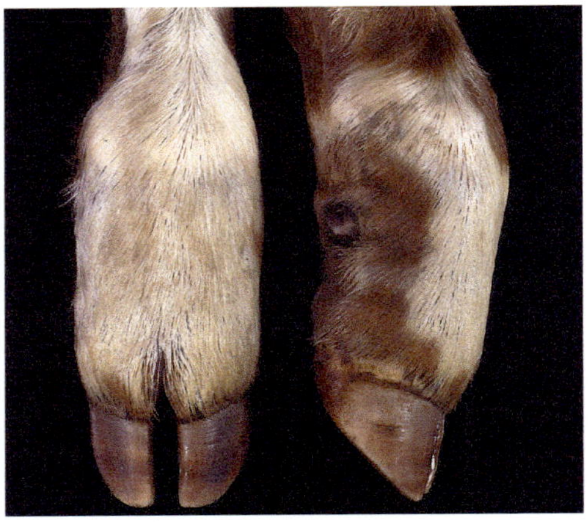

Fig. 12.133. Ox. Skin. Necrosis. Limb of a young calf with foot necrosis due to severe frostbite injury. This occurs most often in cold weather, when calves are in wet conditions or sick from dehydration.

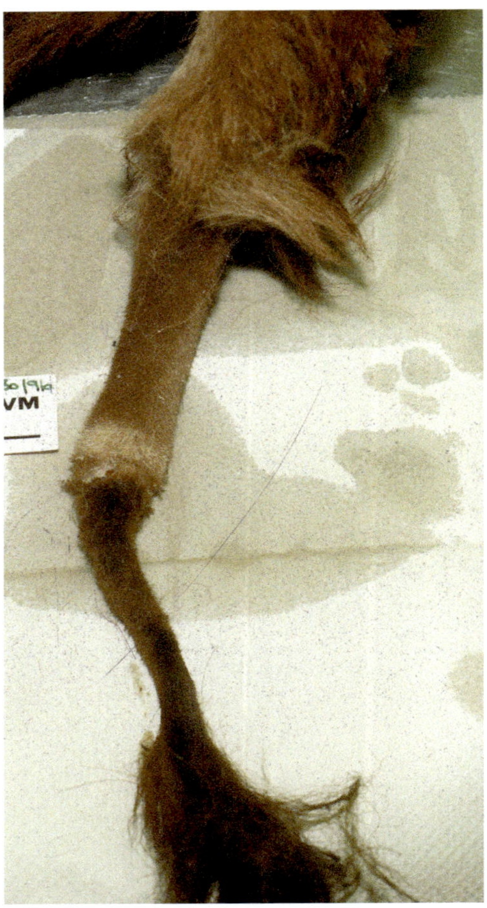

Fig. 12.134. Ox. Skin. Gangrene. Calf with gangrene of the distal tail. There is usually a sharp line of demarcation between necrotic and viable soft tissue and bone.

12.10.2 Distal extremity necrosis – dry gangrene

Introduction. In western Canada, the three most common causes for this condition are ergot and tall fescue grass toxicity, frostbite injury, and more rarely, BVDV as a transient infection causing vasculitis. The distal pelvic limbs, tips of the ears, and the tail tip are most commonly affected sites, but occasionally the teats may also be involved.

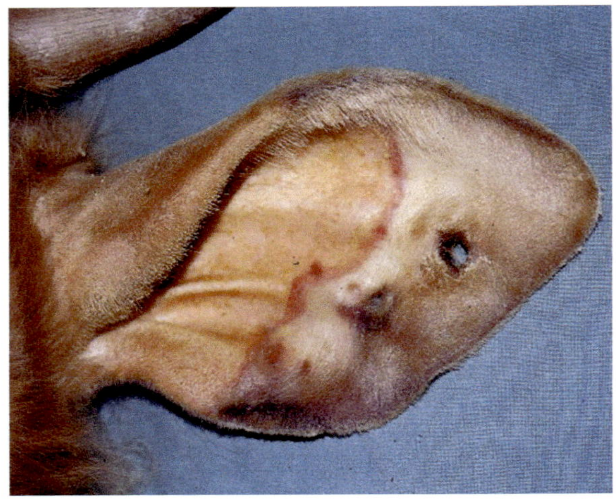

Fig. 12.135. Ox. Skin. Necrosis. Ear tip from a 5-month-old calf. Both ears, tip of the tail, and feet of both pelvic limbs were involved. Bovine viral diarrhea virus (BVDV) transient vasculitis was present in the soft tissues, and especially heart and ileum. The vessels were positive on IHC for BVDV. The exact mechanism of tissue necrosis has not been determined since vascular thrombosis was not seen.

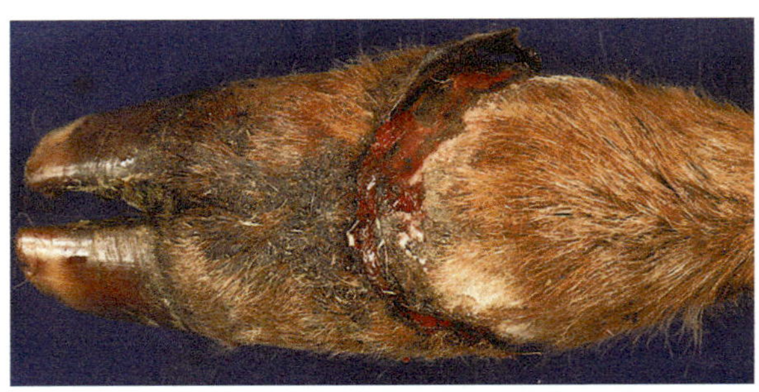

Fig. 12.136. Ox. Skin. Necrosis. Foot of a yearling animal with necrosis and skin separation due to ergot toxicity.

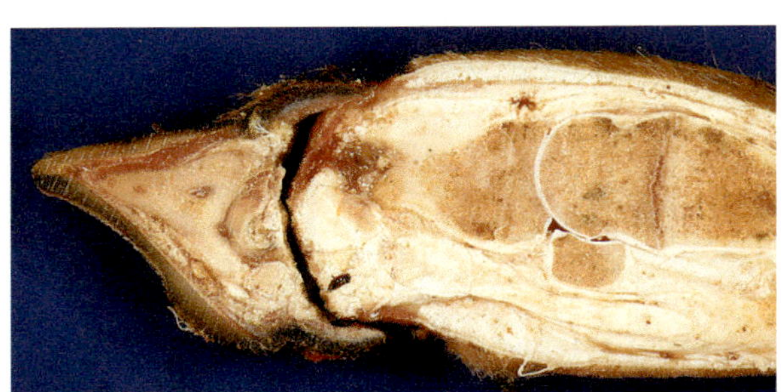

Fig. 12.137. Ox. Foot. Midsagittal section showing bone and soft tissue separation, with sloughing about to occur. Ergot toxicity.

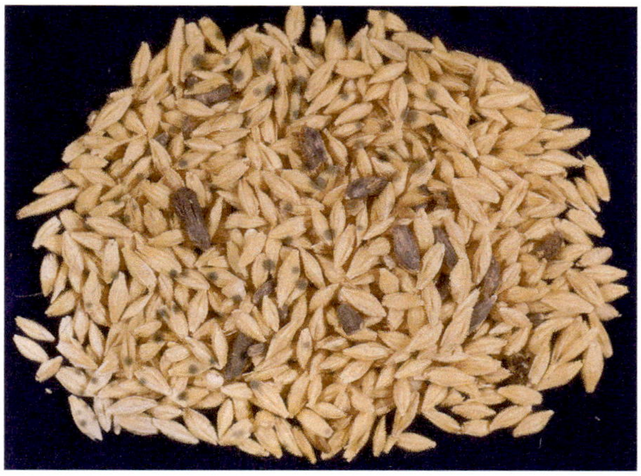

Fig. 12.138. Ox. Barley. A handful of barley kernels showing the black kernels due to fungal growth (*Claviceps purpurea* – producing the toxin ergotamine).

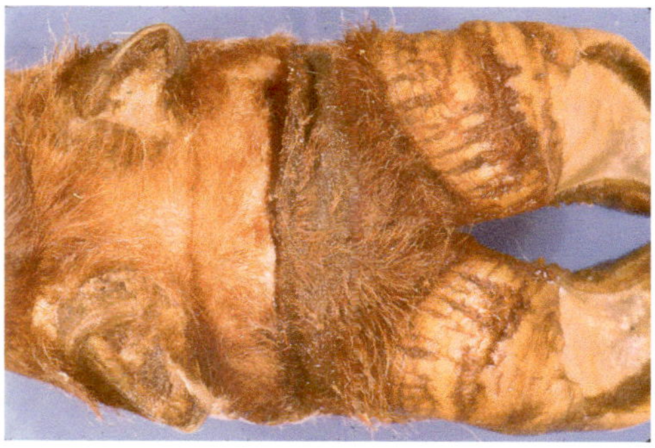

Fig. 12.139. Ox. Skin. Necrosis. Foot necrosis and early skin separation due to tall fescue grass infected with *Neotyphodium coenophialum* fungus producing a similar toxin. (Also see Chapter 13: Diseases of the Claw and Foot Skin.)

12.10.3 Allergic (type I hypersensitivity) dermatitis

Introduction. Milk allergy in high-producing dairy cattle (especially Jersey and Guernsey breeds) is the most common allergic skin disease in cattle, but hypersensitivity to various flies and insects is also encountered occasionally. The reactions are eosinophilic histologically. Confirmation of the etiologic agent is often necessary.

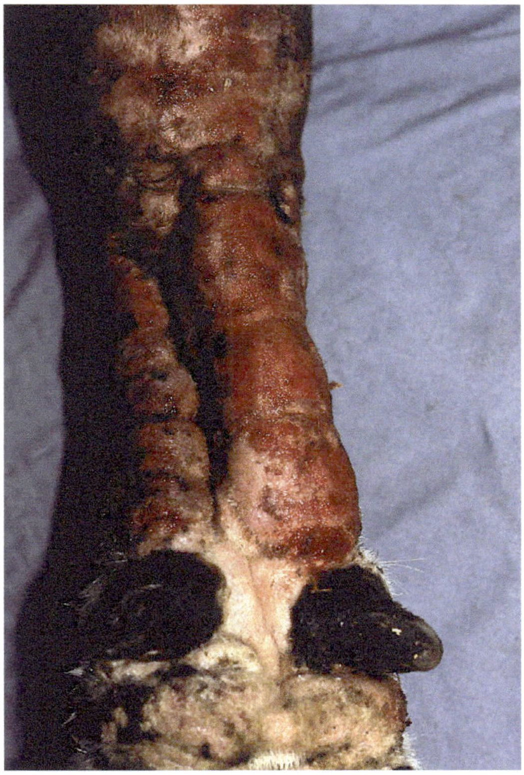

Fig. 12.140. Ox. Skin. Erythema. Severe eosinophilic pruritic dermatitis around the head and face of a young calf. Culicoides hypersensitivity was strongly suspected as the cause.

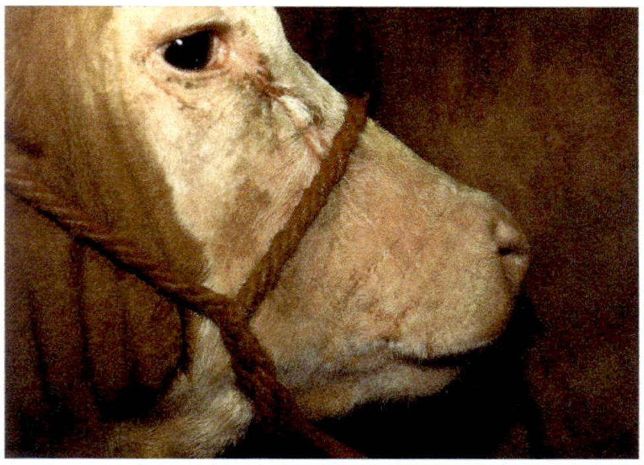

Fig. 12.141. Ox. Skin. Ulcerative dermatitis. Linear, swollen lesions on the distal forelimbs of a mature beef cow. Histologically, this was a severe eosinophilic dermatitis, with numerous eosinophils and mast cells in the biopsy specimens. A severe adverse reaction to food was highly suspected as the cause, as the condition was steroid responsive.

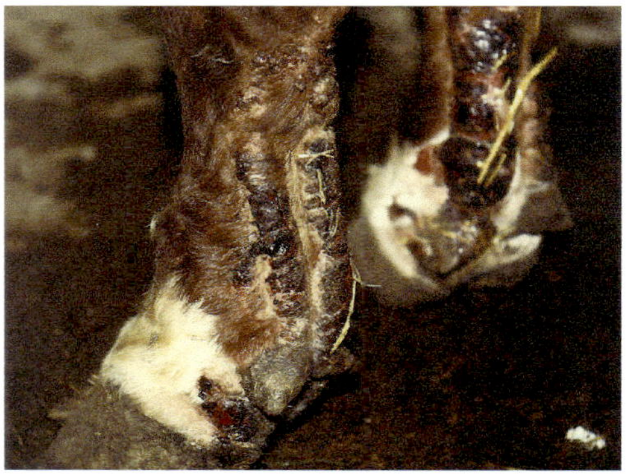

Fig. 12.142. Ox. Skin. Erosive dermatitis. Close-up of a thick, elongated linear lesion on the rear of the distal limb. Superficial skin erosions are present. Same case as Fig.12.141.

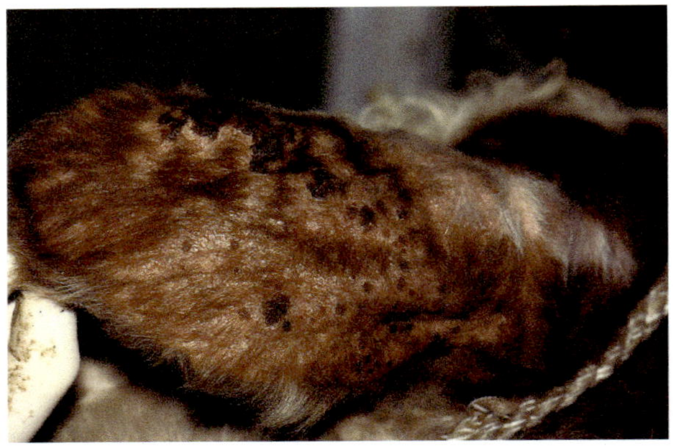

Fig. 12.143. Ox. Skin. Chronic dermatitis. Ears of the cow in Fig. 12.142, with raised crusted lesions. There were also linear skin lesions on the lateral thorax. Same case as Fig.12.141.

12.10.4 Photosensitivity dermatitis

Introduction. Skin necrosis, especially in white areas due to absorption and damage by ultraviolet light, occurs in three different situations: type I, or primary, is caused by certain plants or drugs; type II is an inherent inability to metabolize heme pigments, resulting in a build-up of hematoporphyrins that are photoreactive; and type III, or hepatogenous, is due to an accumulation of phylloerythrin, a breakdown product of chlorophyll from an immature or damaged liver. (Also see Chapter 6: Diseases of the Hepatobiliary System and Pancreas, and Chapter 16: The Pathology of Select Poisonous Plant-induced Diseases in Cattle.)

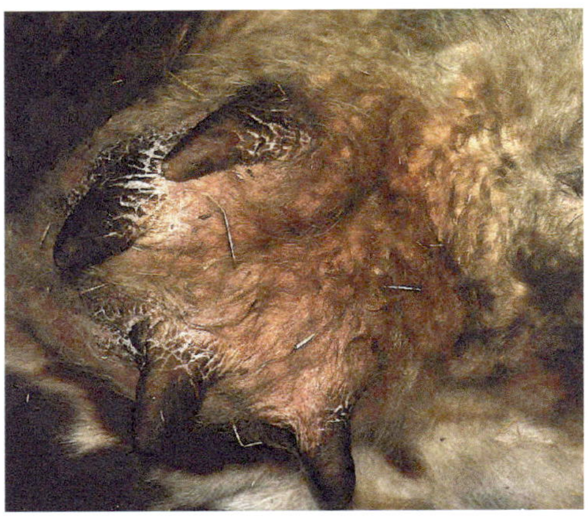

Fig. 12.144. Ox. Skin. Photosensitivity dermatitis. Teats of a mature cow with skin necrosis of type III, due to a pancreatic adenocarcinoma with extensive liver metastases.

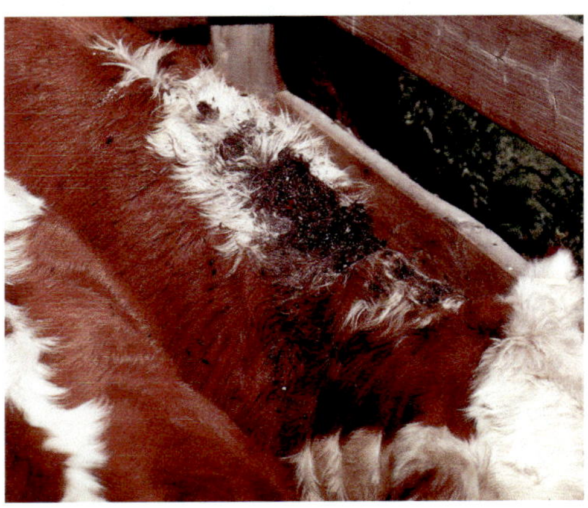

Fig. 12.145. Ox. Skin. Photosensitivity dermatitis. White skin area of a feedlot calf with focal necrosis. The cause of this particular case was not elucidated.

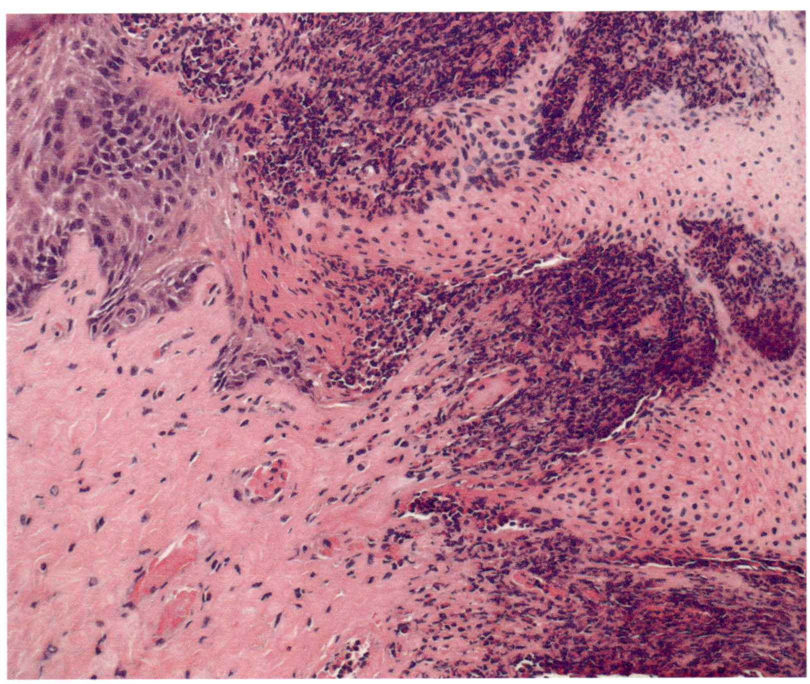

Fig. 12.146. Ox. Skin. Photosensitivity dermatitis. Typical microscopic lesion of a photosensitivity dermatitis case with extensive epidermal coagulation necrosis and underlying sheets of degenerate neutrophils. An adjacent intact epidermis area on the left for comparison (H&E).

12.10.5 Thermal burns

Introduction. The most common causes of skin necrosis due to burns in dairy cattle is lightning strike and barn fires. As most lightning strike cases show no skin or hair lesions, these cannot be relied upon to make a specific diagnosis. (Also see Chapter 17: Bovine Diseases without Lesions.)

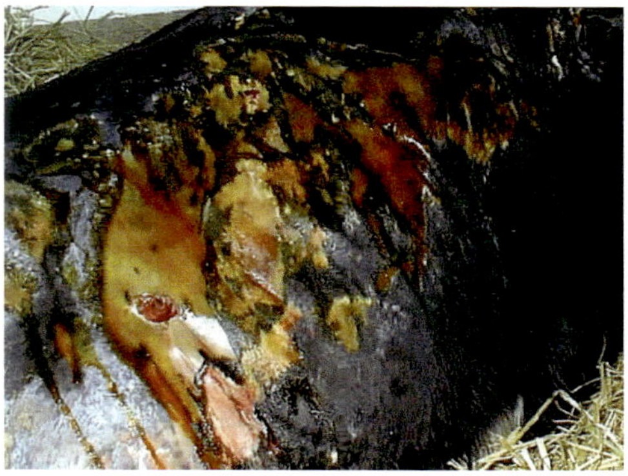

Fig. 12.147. Ox. Skin. Necrosis. Extensive acute multifocal skin necrosis due to a non-fatal barn fire.

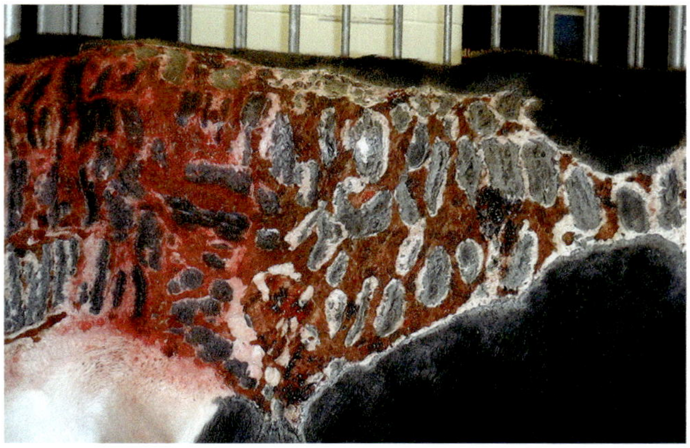

Fig. 12.148. Ox. Skin. Necrosis. Extensive chronic skin necrosis case due to a barn fire, with multiple successful skin grafts applied.

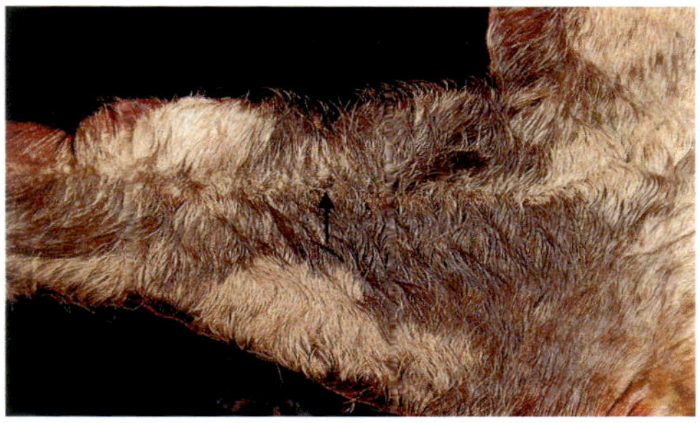

Fig. 12.149. Ox. Skin. Linear necrosis. A section of bovine skin showing a linear line of singed hair (arrow) due to lightning strike.

12.10.6 Generalized idiopathic dermatitis

Introduction. Occasionally observed as severe, acute onset, generalized dermatitis of unknown cause despite application of extensive PCR, IHC, and histologic examinations.

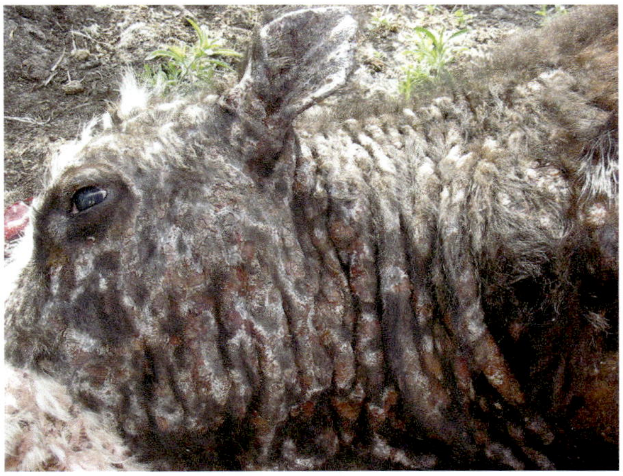

Fig. 12.150. Ox. Skin. Head and neck. Ulcerative dermatitis. A 10-month-old steer with severe generalized ulcerative dermatitis of unknown cause.

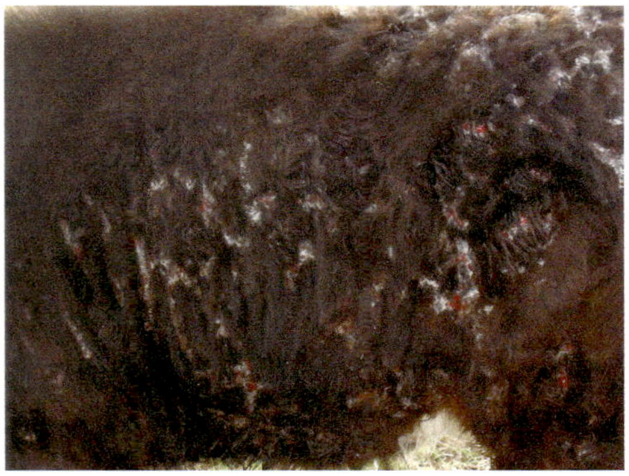

Fig. 12.151. Ox. Skin. Ulcerative dermatitis. The same animal as in Fig. 12.150 with involvement of the lateral trunk.

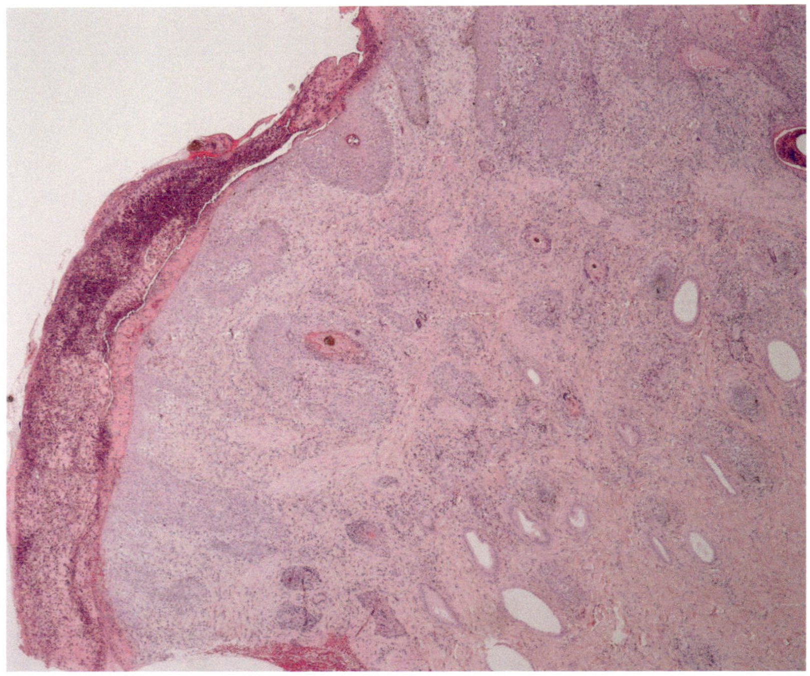

Fig. 12.152. Ox. Skin. Idiopathic ulcerative dermatitis. Histologic picture of the same case (see Fig. 12.150) showing irregular epidermal hyperplasia, areas of erosion, extensive surface serocellular crusting, and most hair follicles invaded by mixed mononuclear cells (H&E).

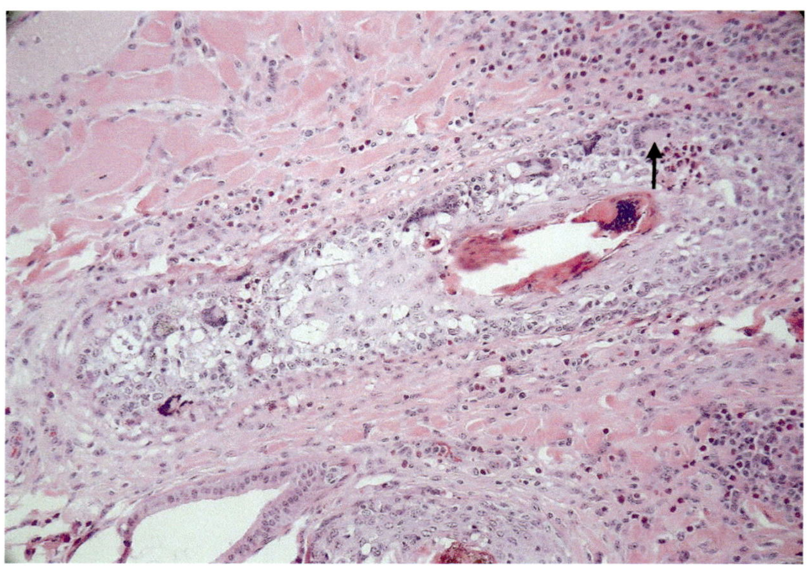

Fig. 12.153. Ox. Skin. Idiopathic ulcerative dermatitis. Close-up of a hair follicle showing vacuolation and mixed inflammatory cell infiltrations of a hair follicle, including multinucleated giant cells (arrow) (H&E).

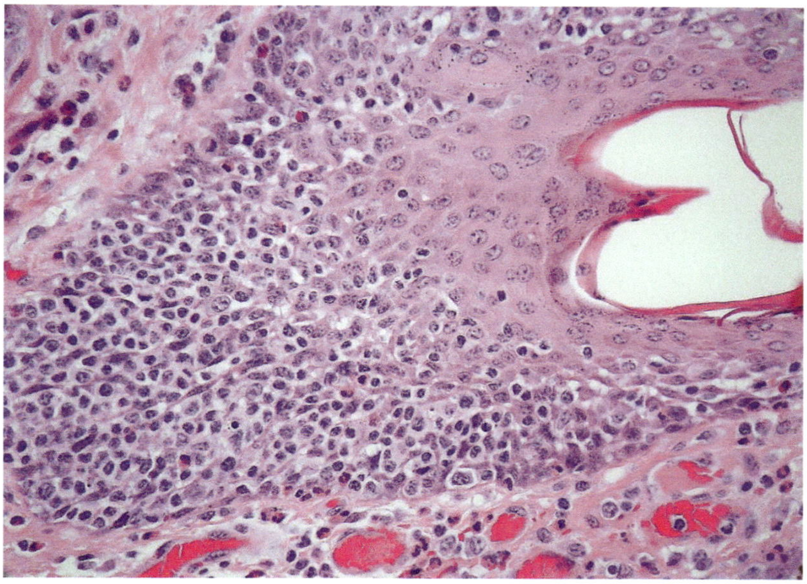

Fig. 12.154. Ox. Skin. Idiopathic ulcerative dermatitis. Another hair follicle with numerous lymphocyte and histiocytic cell infiltrations (H&E).

12.10.7 Cutaneous infarcts

Introduction. On rare occasions, if the hair is clipped, one can see or palpate patchy areas of skin necrosis that are infarcts due to thrombosis, or more rarely, vasculitis.

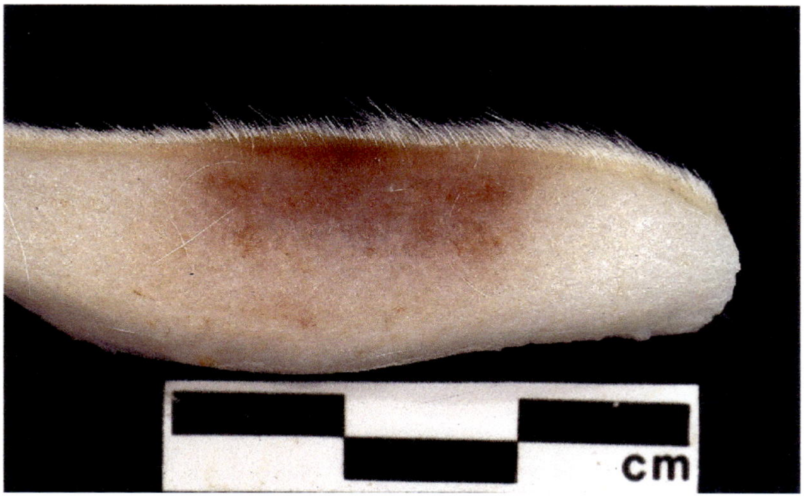

Fig. 12.157. Ox. Skin. Infarct. Cut surface of a small area with hyperemia due to acute infarction (H&E).

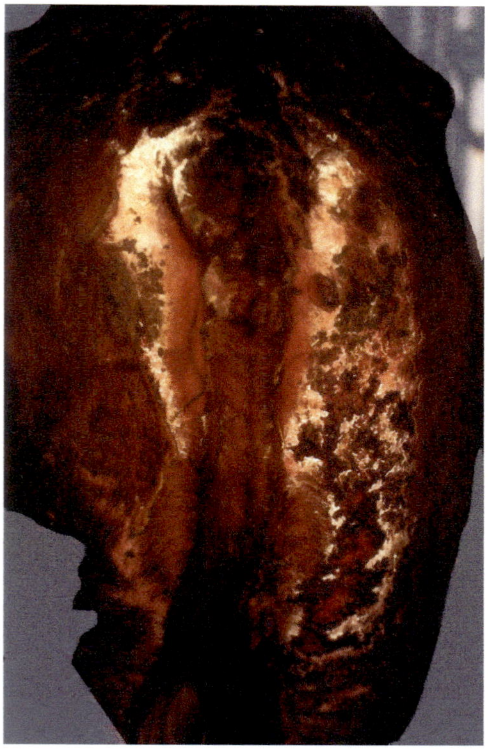

Fig. 12.155. Ox. Skin. Ulcerative dermatitis. Several new arrivals to a feedlot developed extensive pelvic limb and rump region areas of alopecia similar to that shown in the image. The cause was not determined but hairy vetch toxicity was considered, although not proven. The histologic changes were similar to Fig. 12.153, but with far more eosinophils scattered throughout the dermis.

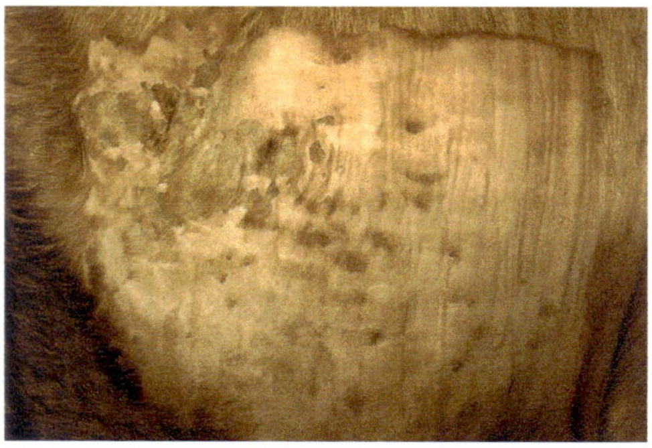

Fig. 12.156. Ox. Skin. Infarcts. Multiple, various sized areas of infarcted skin. This case was due to Salmonella septicemia.

SUGGESTED READING

Grant Maxie, M. (2016) *Pathology of Domestic Animals*, 6th edn. Elsevier, St Louis, Missouri, Vol 1, Chapter 6, Integumentary System, pp. 509–736.

Kahn, C.M. and Line, S. (2010) *The Merck Veterinary Manual*, 10th edn. Merck and Co., Inc., Whitehouse Station, New Jersey, pp. 757–895.

Scott, D.W. (2007) *Color Atlas of Farm Animal Dermatology*. Wiley-Blackwell, Ames, Iowa.

Zachary, J.F. and McGavin, M.D. (2012) *Pathologic Basis of Veterinary Disease*, 6th edn. Elsevier, St Louis, Missouri, Chapter 16, The Integument, pp. 972–1084.

CHAPTER 13

Diseases of the Claw and Foot Skin

Contributed by Jan K. Shearer
College of Veterinary Medicine, Iowa State University, Ames, Iowa, USA

13.1 Lesions of the Claw Horn Capsule
- 13.1.1 Laminitis (pododermatitis aseptica diffusa, coriosis)
- 13.1.2 Sole ulcer (pododermatitis circumscripta, Rusterholz ulcer)
- 13.1.3 White line disease (white line separation, white line fissure)
- 13.1.4 Thin soles and thin sole toe ulcers
- 13.1.5 Traumatic lesions of the sole (punctures of the sole)
- 13.1.6 Foreign body penetration of the sole
- 13.1.7 Vertical wall crack (sand crack)
- 13.1.8 Sepsis of the distal interphalangeal joint
- 13.1.9 Non-healing claw lesions
- 13.1.10 Degloving injuries, diseases, and lesions allegedly due to feeding with beta-antagonists

13.2 Infectious Disorders of the Foot and Foot Skin
- 13.2.1 Digital dermatitis (papillomatous digital dermatitis, foot warts, Mortellaro's disease)
- 13.2.2 Foot rot (interdigital phlegmon, foul in the foot)
- 13.2.3 Foreign body in the interdigital skin
- 13.2.4 Interdigital dermatitis (scald, slurry heel, stable foot rot)

13.3 Neoplasia
- 13.3.1 Interdigital fibroma (corn), interdigital hyperplasia
- 13.3.2 Warts

13.4 Miscellaneous
- 13.4.1 Heel horn erosion
- 13.4.2 Mud fever
- 13.4.3 Formalin burn
- 13.4.4 Screw claw (corkscrew claw)

INTRODUCTION

There are multiple disorders of the distal and proximal limb that result in lameness. For the purposes of organizing these into a logical order, these conditions have been broken down into the following categories: (i) disorders affecting the hoof (or claw) and the horn capsule; and (ii) infectious disorders of the foot and foot skin. With the exception of lesions caused by traumatic injury, congenital, inherited, or developmental conditions and metabolic disease, lameness disorders that involve the claw or claw horn capsule normally occur with greatest frequency on the lateral claw of the rear foot. Greater weight-bearing and claw horn overgrowth on the lateral claw of the rear foot creates mechanical overloading that, when combined with metabolic and physiologic factors, increases the potential for lameness to occur on the lateral claw.

The most common infectious disorders of the foot and foot skin are digital and interdigital dermatitis, foot rot, heel horn erosion, and mud fever. Unlike conditions that affect the hoof or claw, infectious lesions of the foot and foot skin are likely to respond to antimicrobial treatment when early treatment is instituted.

Major diseases of the chapter are depicted in the diagram.

Major Diseases of Brovine Claw

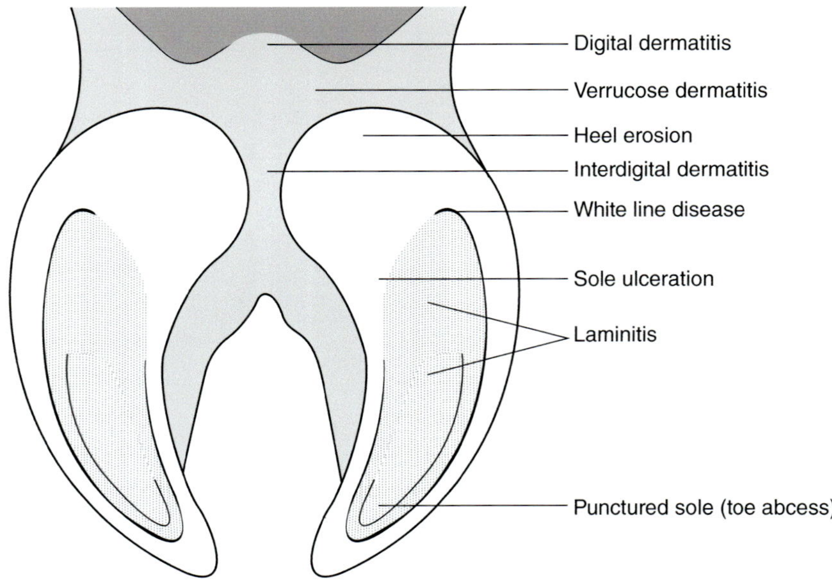

13.1 LESIONS OF THE CLAW HORN CAPSULE

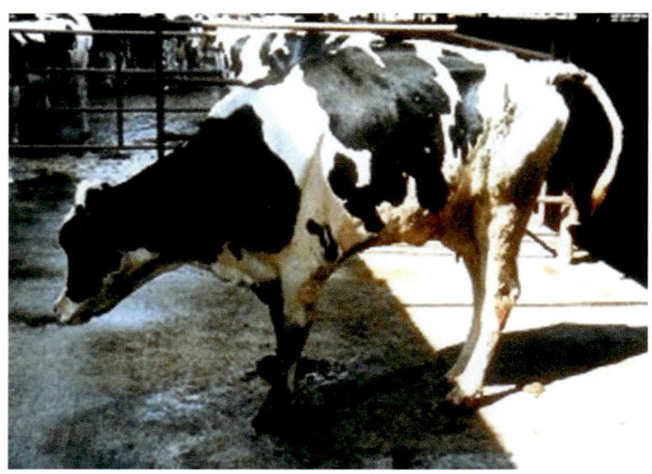

Fig. 13.1. Ox. Whole body. Acute laminitis. Typical 'camped under posture'.

13.1.1 Laminitis (pododermatitis aseptica diffusa, coriosis)

Introduction. Also known as founder, laminitis is an important underlying cause of claw disorders (i.e. sole ulcers and white line disease) in cattle. It is characterized by a disruption in blood flow to the corium, which results in inflammation and damage to tissues that suspend the third phalanx (P3) within the claw horn capsule. In cattle, laminitis is thought to be primarily a degenerative process affecting the dermal–epidermal junction and basal cell layer of the epidermis. Unlike the condition of laminitis in equines, the significance of inflammation in the pathogenesis of laminitis in cattle is unclear. Some believe that inflammation may be largely a secondary event occurring subsequent to an increase in interstitial tissue pressure resulting from vascular changes associated with vasodilatation, congestion, transudation, and diapedesis within the corium. Some have proposed the term 'coriosis' as a better term for this disease since it describes the condition more accurately as an inflammatory insult affecting all regions (i.e. laminar, coronary, solar, and perioplic) of the corium. Disrupted blood flow to tissues of the coronary corium reduces the keratinization of horn cells, resulting in concave dorsal walls and wall horn that flattens axially and abaxially as the coronary horn reaches the weight-bearing surface. The concurrent release of metalloproteinase enzymes during bouts of laminitis weakens the collagen fiber bundles within the laminar corium. This precipitates sinking and rotation of the P3 within the claw horn capsule, resulting in contusion of the solar and perioplic corium, which predisposes to the development of sole and heel ulcers. The potential for white line disease increases as a response to the production of dyskeratotic horn by a weakened and inflamed laminar corium.

A key factor in the pathogenesis of laminitis is vascular compromise that interferes with the metabolic exchange occurring between corium tissues and developing keratinocytes within the basal cell layer. Disrupted blood flow results in a decrease in the transfer of nutrients from capillaries within the corium to living cells within the stratum basale and stratum spinosum of the epidermis. The consequence of this is poorer, weaker horn, deformed hooves, and increased susceptibility to claw disease.

In contrast to the horse, where a physical separation of this connection is normally observed, in cattle the suspensory tissues of the corium are more likely to elongate or stretch in response to breakdown of the collagen fiber bundles within these structures. As a result, extreme compression of the corium beneath the apex of P3 in the toe is less likely; instead, the downward displacement of P3 and compression of the digital cushion and corium at the heel–sole junction are more likely to be the outcome. This is presumably why sole ulcers are a common claw disorder in cattle.

Clinical signs. Acute laminitis – extreme reluctance to walk and a 'camped under posture' when standing; chronic laminitis – concave dorsal walls, widened or flattened walls; subclinical laminitis – yellowish, discolored claw horn.

Differential diagnosis. Thin soles (from excessive wear).

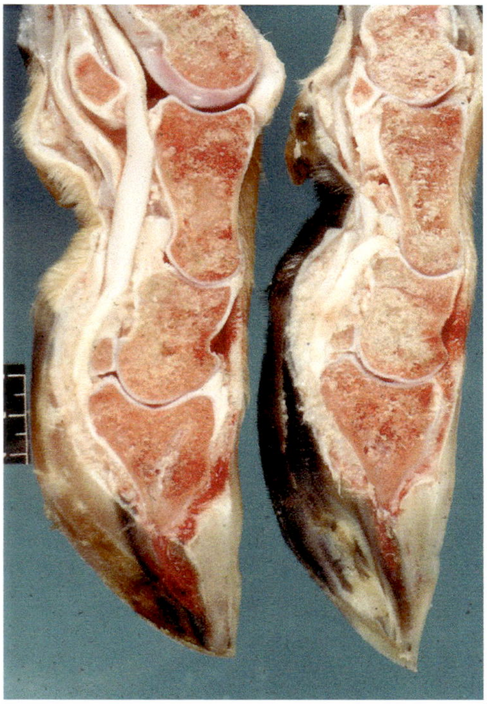

Fig. 13.2. Calf. P3. Severe laminitis. Note the extreme rotation of the apex of the third phalanx.

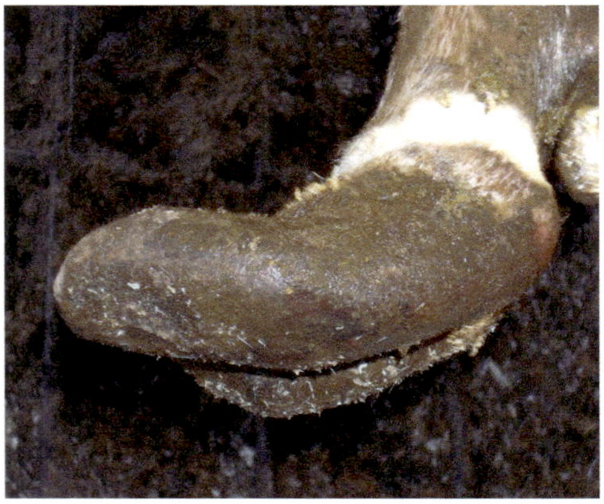

Fig. 13.3. Ox. Claw. Chronic laminitis. Foot exhibiting altered shape.

13.1.2 Sole ulcer (pododermatitis circumscripta, Rusterholz ulcer)

Introduction. An ulcer may be defined as a full thickness defect in the epithelium that exposes the underlying corium. In cattle, sole ulcers are largely a consequence of metabolic disorders and mechanical loading that contributes to injury of the solar, perioplic (corium of the heel), and

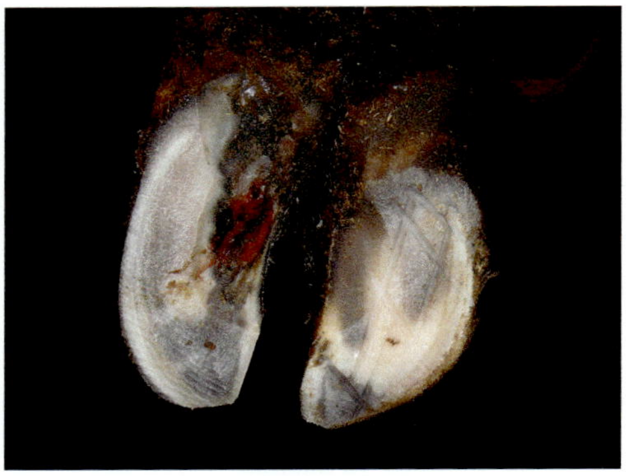

Fig. 13.4. Ox. Claw. Sole ulcer. A sole ulcer in the typical site.

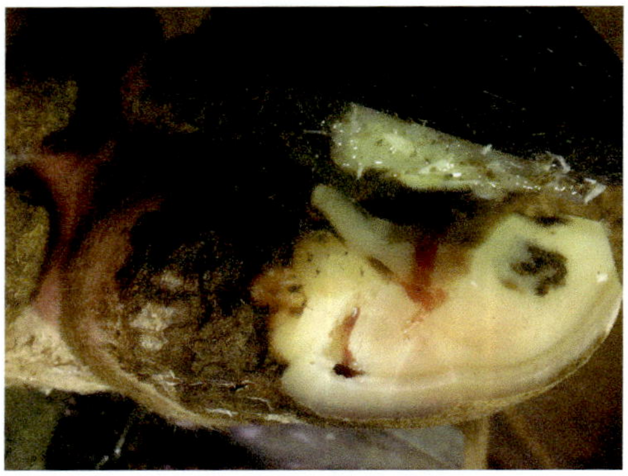

Fig. 13.5. Ox. Claw. White line disease. Location is in the abaxial heel of the lateral claw. Corrective trimming has exposed a tract and the drainage of purulent material from the abscess which had formed beneath.

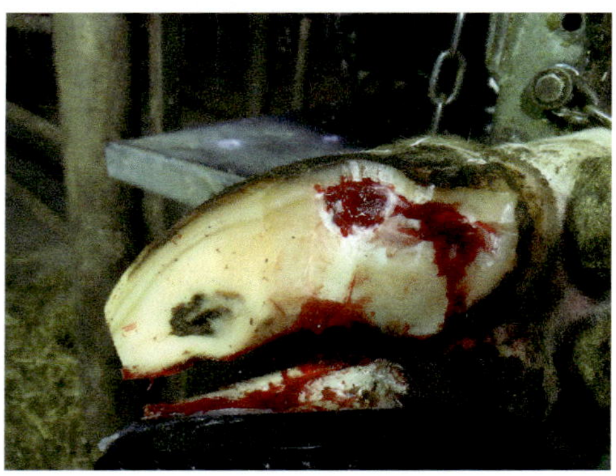

Fig. 13.6. Ox. Claw. White line disease. Lesion in Fig. 13.5 following corrective trimming. The exposed corium and extent of the abscess at the heel–sole junction and caudally in the heel are visible.

laminar corium. The most common metabolic conditions predisposing to claw lesions include rumen acidosis, coriosis/laminitis, activation of metalloproteinases, and hormonal changes, specifically relaxin (or relaxin-like hormone) and estrogen in the peripartum period.

Sole ulcers typically occur at the heel–sole junction (described by Toussanit Raven as the 'typical site'), whereby the corium becomes compressed between the flexor tuberosity of the third phalanx (P3) from above and the sole in contact with the floor beneath. Disturbances in the microvasculature of the contused compressed area of involved tissue lead to ischemia, hypoxia, and the development of an ulcer. Sole ulcers are one of the most common claw lesions in dairy cattle, particularly for animals housed on hard surfaces.

Clinical signs. Variable degrees of lameness, exposed corium at the heel–sole junction.

Differential diagnosis. Traumatic lesions of the sole that expose the underlying corium.

13.1.3 White line disease (white line separation, white line fissure)

Introduction. The white line is a three-part structure produced by the laminar corium and consists of an outer, intermediate, and inner zone. It is the softest and least resistant part of the claw horn capsule, and is subject to damage by mechanical shearing forces and the penetration of bacteria and foreign bodies such as coarse dirt and gravel. The area of the white line most commonly affected is the abaxial heel–sole–wall junction of the lateral claw. The white line in this region is naturally predisposed to a higher degree of mechanical force and wear during locomotion, since this area bears the impact of heel strike during the foot placement phase of the animal's stride.

Lesions within the white line normally begin as small cracks that become infiltrated with stones, dirt, or other types of organic matter. These cracks or fissures may be visualized as one or more dark lines within the white line running in an oblique direction. In other cases where separation is advanced and complicated by infection, the lesion may appear as a large area of loose necrotic horn within the white line. Anaerobic bacteria colonize in the necrotic horn of the white line and gradually ascend toward the corium. Abscess formation and pain leading to lameness occurs as the bacteria make contact with the corium. Purulent material accumulates in the subsolar region of the sole and heel, or in some cases it will migrate caudally toward the heel bulb. Some may migrate beneath the wall and eventually rupture, forming a sinus tract at the skin–horn junction.

Clinical signs. Severe lameness, draining tract at the skin–horn junction.

Differential diagnosis. Draining tracts associated with distal interphalangeal joint sepsis.

13.1.4 Thin soles and thin sole toe ulcers

Introduction. 'Thin soles' is a growing problem in confinement dairy operations throughout the USA. It is particularly prevalent in large freestall barns where cows may have limited relief from concrete flooring conditions. New concrete flooring surfaces tend to be more abrasive compared with older flooring systems and, when wet, these surfaces may be up to 80% more abrasive compared with dry concrete. Hoof wear is also complicated by the spatial layout of facilities that requires cows to walk long distances to and from the milking parlor. Sand, despite its benefits as a comfortable bedding material for cows, increases claw horn wear, and particularly when recycled multiple times, which makes the grain size larger or coarse and more abrasive. The use of water in sprinklers, misters, or foggers is essential for heat-stress abatement, but the increased moisture necessary for cow cooling also softens claw horn and increases horn wear rates.

The most common lesion observed secondary to thin soles is a thin sole toe ulcer (TSTU). This lesion normally occurs in the abaxial region near the toe. As the sole in this area thins, it becomes weaker and separates away from the white line, exposing the underlying corium. This change may be distinguished from white line disease by careful examination of the lesion, noting that soles are normally thin and flexible and that it is actually a separation in the sole.

Clinical signs. Sole flexible to finger pressure, ulcer in the abaxial region of the toe.

Differential diagnoses. White line disease, toe ulcer.

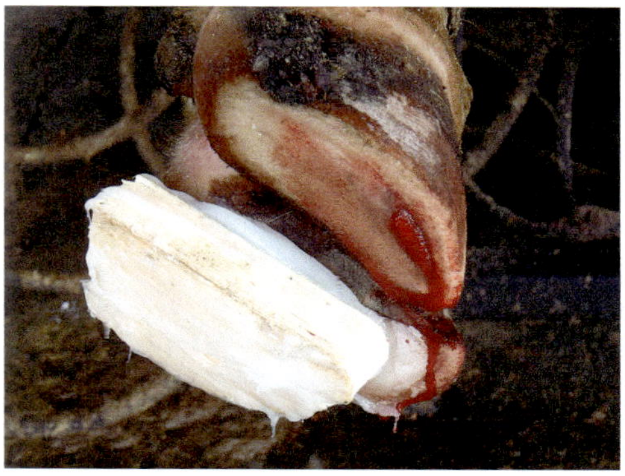

Fig. 13.7. Ox. Claw. Thin sole toe ulcer. Solar corium is protruding through a separation between the white line and the sole.

13.1.5 Traumatic lesions of the sole (punctures of the sole)

Introduction. Traumatic lesions of the sole occur when cows encounter sharp objects, such as a nail protruding through the concrete, a stone or other sharp object on the flooring surface that penetrates the sole. Large dairies attempting to control or reduce hoof wear often apply rubber to the floors. The rubber is oftentimes nailed down to secure it in place; however, when the rubber is dislodged inadvertently or lifted from the floor (as might occur when cleaning with a skid-steer loader type of machine), the nail or nail head remains and protrudes above the flooring surface. Cows stepping on to these protruding nails and nail heads are subject to traumatic sole lesions. Depending on the depth of penetration (i.e. into the bone), these kinds of lesions can have complicated outcomes.

Clinical signs. Severe lameness, subsolar abscess, and evidence of a puncture wound.

Differential diagnoses. White line disease, sole ulcer.

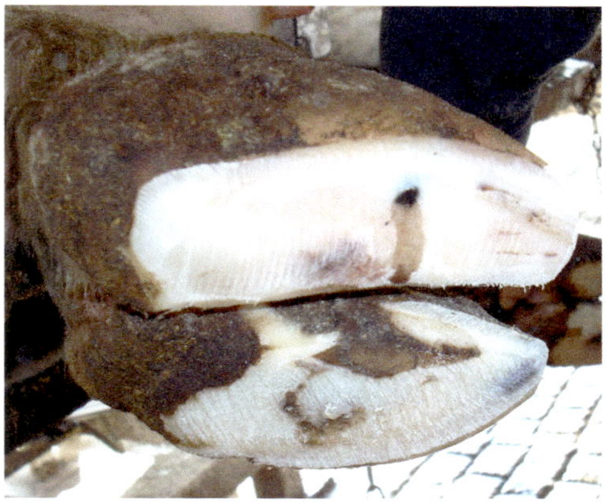

Fig. 13.8. Ox. Claw. Puncture. Traumatic sole lesion resulting from a protruding nail in the concrete, which was exposed when rubber flooring was dislocated inadvertently during manure removal and cleaning.

13.1.6 Foreign body penetration of the sole

Introduction. Claw lesions may occur as a consequence of foreign bodies that become lodged within the sole. Nails, hypodermic needles, and many other types of sharp objects may be found embedded in the sole. Some of these may penetrate sufficiently deep to make contact with the solar or perioplic corium, digital cushion, and bone. Severe lameness and abscess formation of the sole are commonly observed. Foreign bodies that penetrate sufficiently deep to make contact with the bone are likely to induce an osteitis that may have serious consequences.

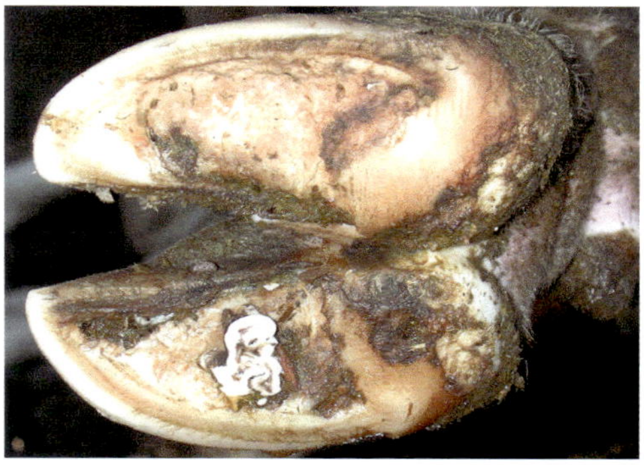

Fig. 13.9. Ox. Claw. Foreign bodies. Common causes of lameness. In the photograph, a tooth has become lodged in the sole, resulting in severe lameness.

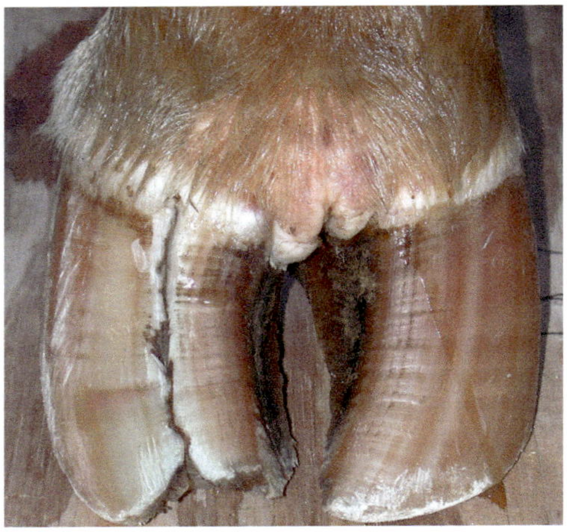

Fig. 13.10. Ox. Claw. Vertical wall crack. Location is on the lateral claw of a front foot.

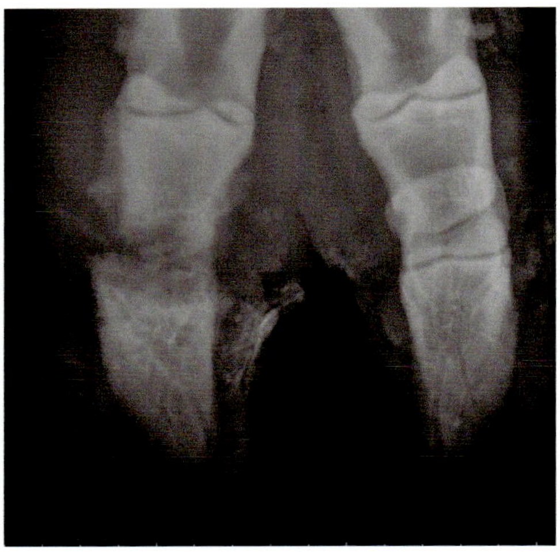

Fig. 13.11. Ox. Radiograph. Sepsis. Distal interphalangeal joint. Note the soft tissue swelling and lysis within the distal interphalangeal joint. (Courtesy of Dr J. Schleining, Iowa State University, USA.)

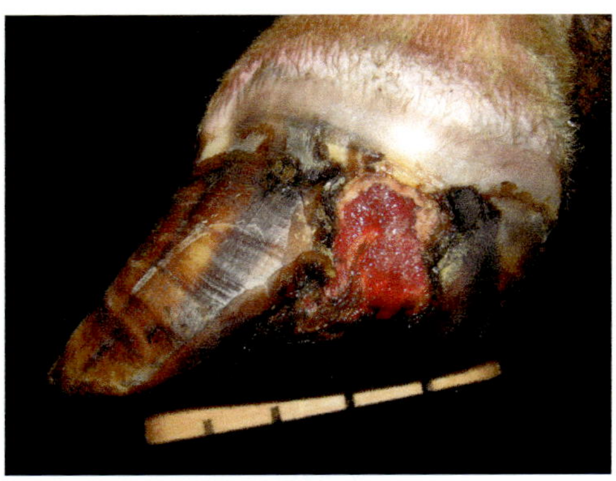

Fig. 13.12. Ox. Non-healing claw lesion. Corium exposed by corrective trimming several weeks earlier. Lesion has made little or no progress toward healing. The glistening surface of the lesion is typical of corium infected with digital dermatitis.

Clinical signs. Severe lameness, presence of a foreign body lodged in the sole.

Differential diagnoses. Subsolar abscess, sole ulcer, white line disease.

13.1.7 Vertical wall crack (sand crack)

Introduction. Cracks or fissures in the hoof wall are common in cattle. Those that run in a vertical direction (from the coronet to the weight-bearing surface) are referred to as vertical wall cracks, or sand cracks. Incidence rates as high as 64% have been reported in beef cattle, compared with less than 1% in dairy cattle. For reasons that are not completely understood, vertical wall cracks occur with greatest frequency (80% of the time) on the lateral claw of the front feet. The percentage of cows that may become lame with vertical wall cracks is generally low, but when lameness does occur, it may be difficult to treat or manage.

Clinical sign. Vertical wall cracks are visible on the surface of the hoof wall.

Differential diagnoses. White line disease, traumatic lesions of the hoof wall.

13.1.8 Sepsis of the distal interphalangeal joint

Introduction. Sepsis of the distal interphalangeal joint typically occurs secondary to complications that may occur with a white line disease abscess, sole ulcer, or foot rot. Lameness with this condition is severe, often resulting in extreme reluctance to bear weight on the affected digit. It is distinguished by swelling at the coronet, and in some cases a draining tract on the anterior-lateral aspect of the coronet, which some consider pathognomonic for this disorder in cattle. Long-standing infections are sometimes accompanied by osteitis and the proliferation of new bone. Options for treatment of septic interphalangeal joints include amputation, joint ankyloses and/or resection.

Clinical signs. Severe lameness and unilateral swelling and redness of the coronet of the affected claw. Radiographically, most exhibit separation and lysis in the distal interphalangeal site.

Differential diagnoses. Foot rot, retroarticular space abscess.

13.1.9 Non-healing claw lesions

Introduction. Post-treatment contamination of claw lesions with exposed corium is unavoidable in the environment of confined dairy cows. They are continually exposed to bacteria-laden manure and moisture. In recent years, anecdotal observation suggests that these 'non-healing claw lesions' seem to be particularly widespread in herds suffering a high prevalence of digital dermatitis. Careful examination of the lesion reveals a granular-appearing surface that is extremely sensitive if touched or otherwise disturbed. Typical lesions are often observed on the corium under loose, undermined horn associated with white line disease and sole ulcers.

In some cases, these lesions occur as a secondary complication on claw lesions where the corium had previously been exposed in the process of corrective trimming. One of the most common of non-healing lesions observed in dairy cattle is chronic toe lesions. These lesions are almost invariably infected with spirochetes associated with digital dermatitis.

Researchers report finding spirochetes on the surface, as well as deep within these lesions.

Effective treatments reported include tetracycline as a topical spray under a bandage and a paste of dexamethasone and oxytetracycline in combination applied under a loose wrap. Alternatives to topical treatment are amputation of either the affected claw or the apex of the affected digit. A study of 122 cattle over a 4-year period found that claw lesions occurring in the apex of P3 had the potential to spread rapidly to the distal phalanx.

Clinical signs. Chronic toe lesions: affected animals walk in such a way as to put most of the limb's weight toward the heel. This allows the toe of the claw to overgrow, becoming long and also very thick as a consequence of less wear of the sole at the toe.

Differential diagnosis. Claw lesion with exposed corium.

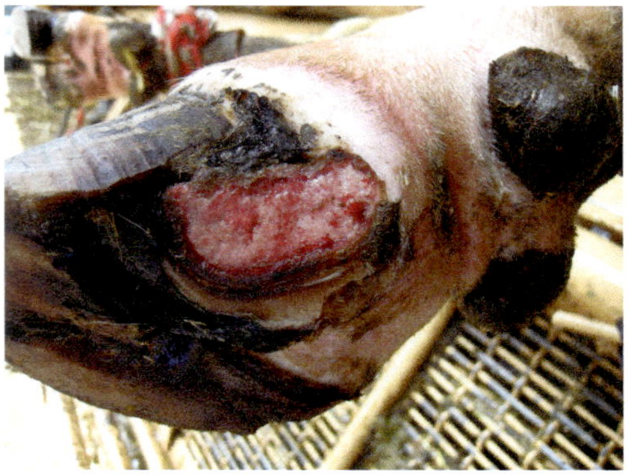

Fig. 13.13. Ox. Non-healing claw lesion. Lesion after 2 weeks of topical treatment with a combination of tetracycline solution and dexamethasone.

13.1.10 Degloving injuries, diseases, and lesions allegedly due to feeding with beta-antagonists

Introduction. Degloving injuries can result in severe and permanent damage. They are most often the result of a traumatic injury that occurs when a cow or calf gets one of its digits (or claws) caught or wedged between two stationary items, such as a fencepost and a gate. If the animal panics and forcefully jerks the foot away from the entrapment, it may remove part of, or the entire, hoof wall. This is a very painful lesion, requiring treatment in the form of the application of a foot block to the opposite uninjured claw to remove weight-bearing from the degloved claw and a protective bandage over the exposed corium. The outcome will be determined by the degree of damage to the corium. In worst-case scenarios, euthanasia may be the best option.

Disease-related causes of degloving-type lesions may also occur in cattle within a matter of weeks following the grazing of endophyte-infested tall fescue, particularly during the autumn and early winter months. The earliest lesions observed are lameness of one or both back feet, and swelling and redness at the coronet. If grazing continues on toxin-rich fescue, gangrene, necrosis, and eventually sloughing of the hooves or distal limb are potential outcomes. Affected cattle will also lose other body parts, such as the ear tips and tail ends. The toxins produced by the fungal endophytes are ergot alkaloids, the most prevalent of which is ergovaline. The toxic effects of ergovaline are related to vasoconstriction and severely restricted blood flow to peripheral body tissues. Extreme heat or bitterly cold temperatures may worsen tissue damage because of altered blood flow. In worst-case scenarios, affected animals may develop a line of demarcation resembling that of a wire being wrapped around the leg. Closer inspection will often reveal a gangrenous lesion that may ultimately result in sloughing of the lower limb. (Also see Chapter 12: Diseases of the Integument.)

Beta-agonists are growth promoters fed to cattle and swine for the purpose of partitioning nutrients to the synthesis of muscle rather than fat. They are normally only fed to cattle or swine during the last few weeks (normally 20–40 days) prior to slaughter. These additives have been very popular with the feeding industry because of the marked response in muscle mass observed in cattle supplemented with these compounds. They are often referred to as repartitioning agents, since they are able to increase muscle accretion and reduce body fat without affecting organ or bone mass. Beta-agonists act by binding with muscle cell receptors that are able to initiate the synthesis of protein.

A novel fatigue syndrome (FCS) of finished feedlot cattle has been reported recently. Factors such as stressful handling, transport, seasonal, and beta-receptor agonist application are thought to be responsible for the development of the condition. It has been hypothesized that the syndrome is not likely to be laminitis resulting from dietary feeding practices. The extreme end point of this syndrome is the sloughing of one or more hooves.

Clinical sign. Loss of the claw horn capsule.

Differential diagnoses. Trauma, fescue foot, laminitis, or fatigued cattle syndrome.

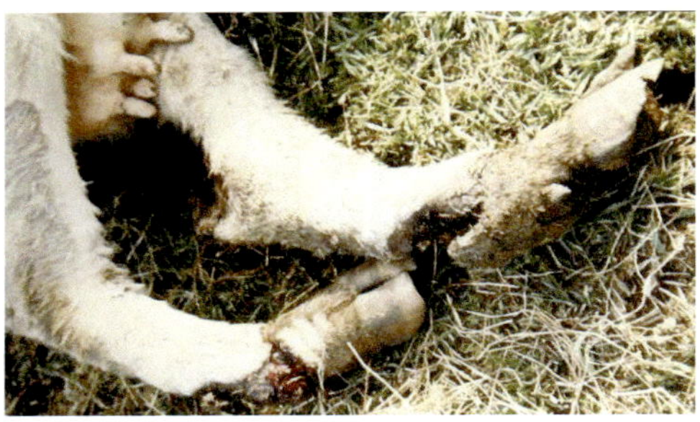

Fig. 13.15. Ox. Feet. Fescue poisoning. Distal gangrene. Affected limbs reveal sloughing of hoofs in lower limb and ulcerative dermatitis.

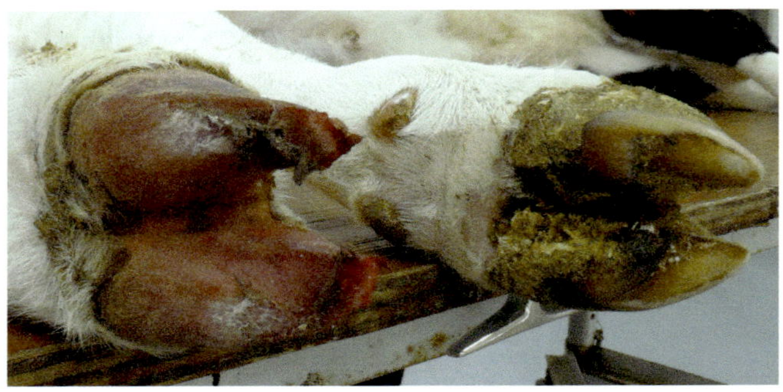

Fig. 13.14. Ox. Degloving injury. Degloving type of injury believed to be traumatic in origin. Maintenance of animals with these types of injuries on soft bedding is often sufficient for redevelopment of a hoof capsule.

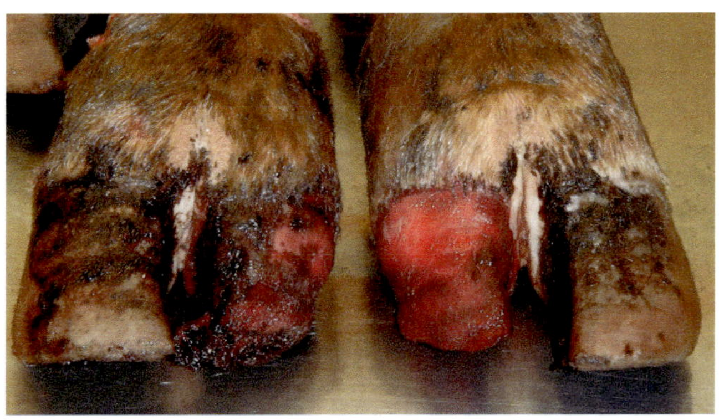

Fig. 13.16. Ox. Horn. Sloughing of capsule. Foot from an animal in which the medial claw hoof capsule has sloughed off, allegedly due to supplementation with the beta-agonist, Zilpaterol.

13.2 INFECTIOUS DISORDERS OF THE FOOT AND FOOT SKIN

13.2.1 Digital dermatitis (papillomatous digital dermatitis, foot warts, Mortellaro's disease)

Introduction. Digital dermatitis (DD) is considered to be the most common infectious disease affecting housed dairy cattle worldwide. It is estimated to affect nearly 100% of dairy herds and up to 20% of all dairy cattle. Lesions of DD are typically observed in one of three locations of the foot: (i) on the skin of the plantar aspect of the rear foot adjacent to the interdigital cleft; (ii) on the interdigital skin; and (iii) at the skin–horn junction of the heel bulbs. Less frequently, lesions may be observed near or above the dewclaws. Early lesions are generally a red, circular, or oval lesion, with a raw ulcerated surface located adjacent to the interdigital cleft. As the lesions mature, they develop a granular-appearing surface similar to that of a wart (thus the term, foot warts). The borders of mature lesions are clearly demarcated by the presence of hypertrophied hairs. More chronic lesions are characterized by a thick bed of granulation tissue, and in some cases epithelial outgrowths that appear as long hairs extending from the surface of the granulation tissue bed. Digital dermatitis lesions are extremely sensitive and very painful when touched or disturbed.

Mature and particularly chronic lesions are accompanied by significant erosion of the heel horn. The heel erosion may be diffuse, in the form of fissures, or in the shape of a 'V'. In some cases, the erosion may result in significant undermining of heel horn. Veterinarians and hoof trimmers know to examine a foot with an abnormally long heel or toe carefully, because the shape of a hoof is an important indicator of foot problems. For example, when lesions occur on the plantar surface of the foot, animals will favor the forward toe. This causes greater wear at the toe and less at the heel, permitting the heel to become abnormally long. Lesions occurring on the front of the foot will cause the animal to shift its weight to the heel, resulting in a longer toe and shorter heel. Therefore, claw conformation can be a very useful diagnostic indicator of DD lesions in cattle.

It is postulated that multiple pathogenic *Treponema* phylotypes, in addition to host genetics, immunity, and environmental risk factors, are involved in the etiopathogenesis of digital dermatitis. Some of the spirochetes may reside in ruminal fluid. Another hypothesis is that digital dermatitis is a polybacterial disease, with temporal changes in bacterial populations throughout the course of the disease.

Clinical signs. Pain, weight shifting.

Differential diagnoses. Interdigital dermatitis, foot and mouth disease, traumatic lesions of the foot.

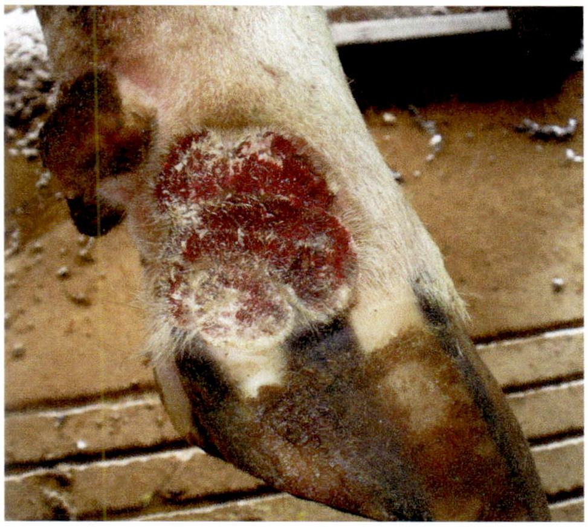

Fig. 13.17. Ox. Digital dermatitis. Location on the lateral aspect of the foot in a dairy cow. Erect hairs on the lesion periphery with granular surface of the lesion.

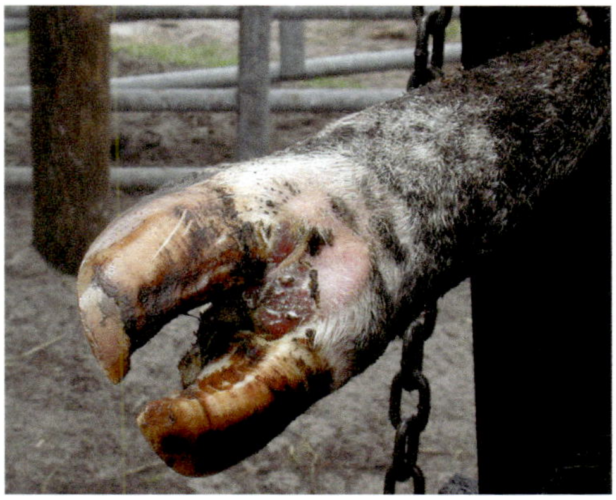

Fig. 13.18. Ox. Digital dermatitis. Anterior aspect of the foot. Lesion in the interdigital cleft extending into the interdigital space.

13.2.2 Foot rot (interdigital phlegmon, foul in the foot)

Introduction. Foot rot is a subacute or acute infection involving the soft tissues of the foot. It usually occurs as a unilateral condition causing severe lameness and generalized swelling of the foot. On closer examination, one will notice a foul-smelling, necrotic lesion in the interdigital skin. Most believe that the lesion is predisposed by softening

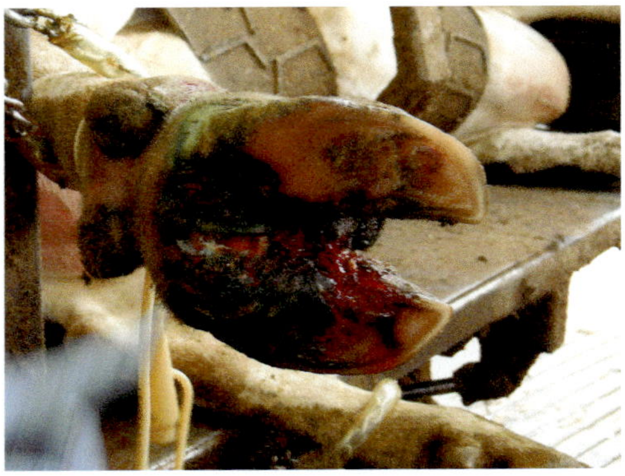

Fig. 13.19. Ox. Foot rot. Necrosis and swelling of the foot.

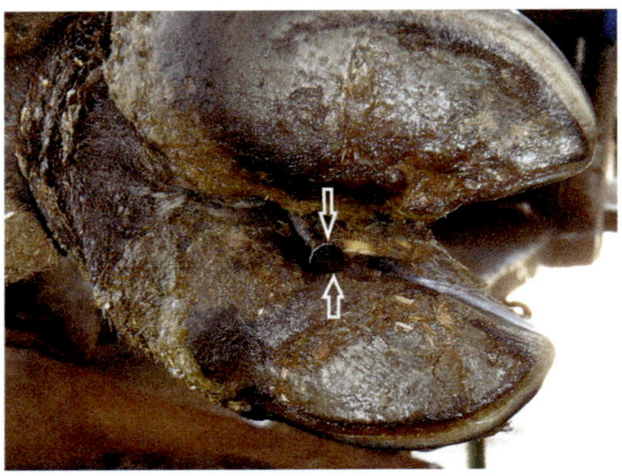

Fig. 13.20. Ox. Foreign body. Photograph shows the presence of a large nail in the interdigital space (arrows).

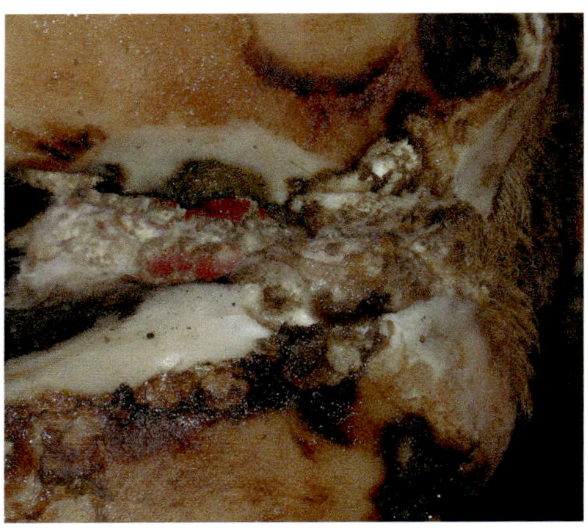

Fig. 13.21. Ox. Claws. Interdigital dermatitis (ID). Superficial inflammation.

of the interdigital skin followed by some type of mechanical injury that permits entry of the bacterial agents of this disease. In pasture conditions, the mere grazing of stubble on recently mowed pasture is sufficient to cause injury generating disease. In winter conditions, walking on hardened mud, stony ground or irregular ice-covered surfaces may cause injury to the interdigital skin and increase susceptibility to the disease. Organisms identified as likely agents in causing foot rot are *Fusobacterium necrophorum*, *Porphyromonas levii*, *Trueperella pyogenes*, and many others. The key to a successful outcome from therapy requires prompt diagnosis and treatment. A delayed or poor response to therapy increases the potential for secondary complications, leading to deep digital sepsis conditions. Confirmation of the disease may be achieved by examination of the interdigital skin for evidence of a necrotic interdigital lesion.

Clinical signs. Severe lameness and generalized swelling of the foot. Fever in the acute stages.

Differential diagnoses. Foreign body in the interdigital skin, deep digital claw sepsis.

13.2.3 Foreign body in the interdigital skin

Introduction. Foreign bodies that become lodged between claws, and particularly those that penetrate the interdigital skin and migrate deeply into the interdigital region, may have grave consequences for the animals affected. Whenever animals are presented for examination due to lameness, a careful inspection of the interdigital area is required. Secondary infections may ensue.

Clinical signs. Severe lameness and generalized swelling of the foot.

Differential diagnoses. Foot rot, deep digital sepsis.

13.2.4 Interdigital dermatitis (scald, slurry heel, stable foot rot)

Introduction. Despite significant differences in the clinical presentation of the two conditions, interdigital dermatitis (ID) is sometimes confused with foot rot. A major difference is the lack of swelling with ID as compared with foot rot. Complicating things still further is the opinion of some that ID and digital dermatitis (DD) are one and the same condition. Indeed, ID and DD share many similarities: both conditions cause erosion of the interdigital skin, have a distinctive foul odor, and are painful to the touch. The oozing of fluid from lesions leads to the formation of crusts and skin debris that are most likely the cause of the characteristic odor associated with animals affected with this disease. In most cases, ID is a benign condition that rarely causes lameness. Chronic or long-standing lesions are believed to predispose to interdigital fibromas, and most are accompanied by varying degrees of heel horn erosion. Interdigital dermatitis is an extremely common condition in confinement housed cattle. The only practical therapy is use of a footbath.

Clinical sign. Superficial dermatitis of the interdigital skin.

Differential diagnoses. Digital dermatitis, foot and mouth disease.

13.3 NEOPLASIA

13.3.1 Interdigital fibroma (corn), interdigital hyperplasia

Introduction. Chronic inflammation associated with interdigital dermatitis (ID) is believed to predispose to interdigital fibromas, or corns. In some cases, fibromas occur as a consequence of conformational features of the foot that subject the interdigital skin to physical stretching or physical trauma associated with splaying of the claws that permits contact between the interdigital skin and weight-bearing surface when the foot is placed on the ground.

Regardless of cause, interdigital fibromas rarely cause lameness. When they do, it is often a consequence of secondary infection, as with digital dermatitis or in association with foot rot. In these situations, it is important to treat and control these conditions. If lameness persists in the absence of these diseases, and it can be determined that the fibroma is the cause, then surgical removal is indicated.

Clinical sign. Interdigital fibromas are observed easily as callous-like structures within the interdigital space.

Differential diagnosis. Foreign bodies within the interdigital space

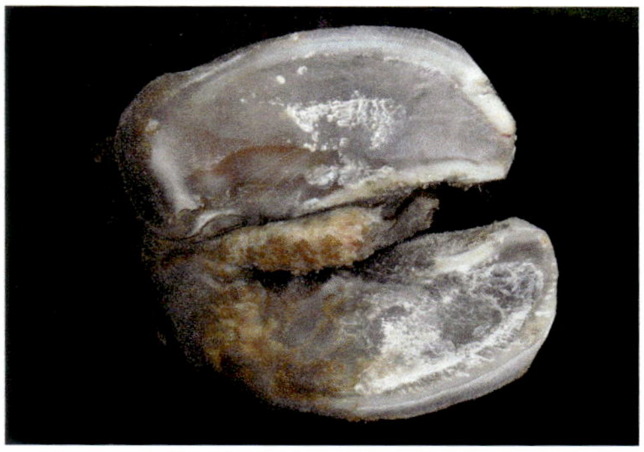

Fig. 13.22. Ox. Claws. Interdigital fibroma ('corn') callous that forms in the interdigital skin secondary to chronic inflammation.

13.3.2 Warts

Introduction. Virus-induced, finger-like proliferation on digital dermis leads to growths covering the claw. These lesions are self-healing.

Clinical sign. Locomotor discomfort.

Differential diagnosis. 'Hairy warts'.

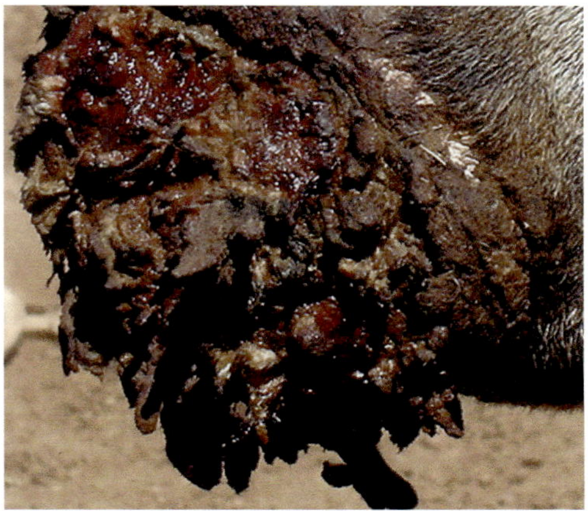

Fig. 13.23. Ox. Digit. Warts. Fibropapillomatous dermal proliferation.

13.4 MISCELLANEOUS

13.4.1 Heel horn erosion

Introduction. Heel horn erosion occurs as a diffuse pitting or fissuring of the horn of the heel bulb. It does not cause lameness, but when severe or chronic, it results in significant loss of heel horn. The incidence of heel horn erosion is near 100% in many confinement operations where exposure to manure, slurry, and moisture are unavoidable. The precise cause or etiology is unknown, but its consistent observation in cows affected with digital dermatitis and interdigital dermatitis suggests that heel erosion may share a common etiology with these diseases.

Clinical sign. A rough, pitted or fissure-like appearance to the horn of heel bulbs is characteristic of heel horn erosion.

Differential diagnosis. Heel cracks.

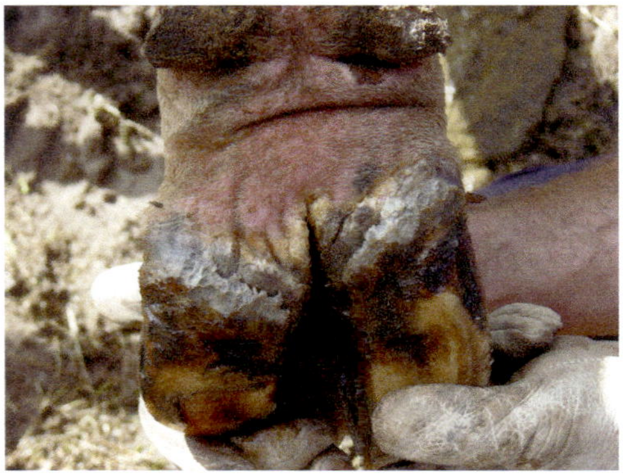

Fig. 13.24. Ox. Heel horn erosion. Loss of heel horn.

13.4.2 Mud fever

Introduction. Mud fever is a generalized dermatitis of the lower leg, often associated with cold, wet and muddy conditions. Occurrence is associated with the accumulation of muddy debris on the skin of the

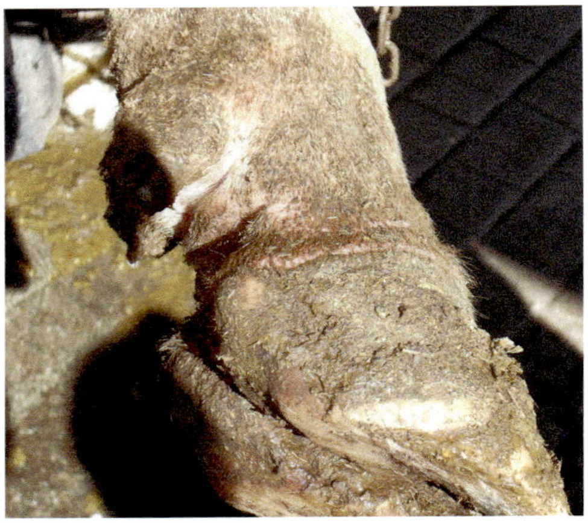

Fig. 13.25. Ox. Lower leg. Exfoliative dermatitis. The lower legs of this animal are reddened in response to muddy conditions that have resulted in mud fever.

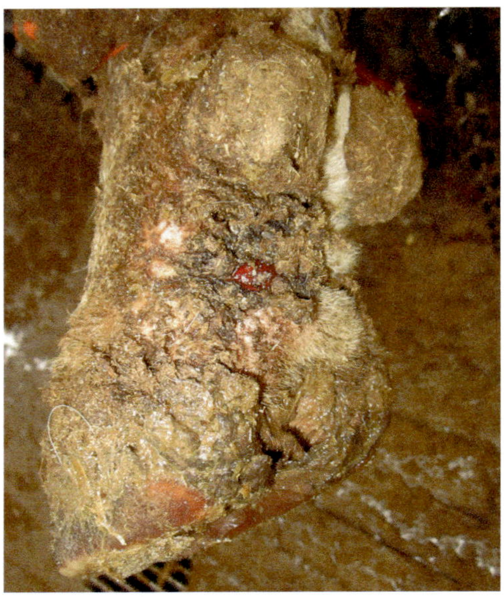

Fig. 13.26. Ox. Claws. Formalin burn. Exfoliative dermatitis. Skin lesion below the dewclaws. The darkened area of the lesion surrounds an ulcer adjacent to skin folds on the plantar pastern aspect of the foot.

lower leg. Rear legs seem to be affected more than front legs. In some cases, the dermatitis may extend as high as the hock joint. There is usually significant hair loss, and the skin appears reddened and thickened in response to inflammation. Although mud fever does not cause lameness, it does cause significant skin irritation. The precise cause or etiological agent(s) is unknown, but *Dermatophilus* spp. may be involved. Teat dip solutions containing emollients as a topical spray are recommended as a topical treatment. However, dry weather and reduced exposure to muddy conditions is the best option for control of the problem.

Clinical signs. Red and thickened skin of the lower legs, generalized dermatitis, small pustules in the skin.

Differential diagnosis. Generalized non-specific dermatitis.

13.4.3 Formalin burn

Introduction. Formaldehyde is frequently added to footbaths to create a disinfectant solution for treatment of infectious skin disorders of the foot. Most recommendations call for the addition of 1 gallon of 37% formaldehyde to be added to 19 gallons of water to create a 5% formalin solution. Some prefer a weaker solution of 2–3% formalin, which is generally less irritating to skin. Mixing errors are not uncommon, and often result in concentrations in excess of 5% formalin. Experience has shown that foot bathing over a period of 3–5 consecutive days with formalin above a concentration of 5% is likely to cause chemically induced lesions in the foot skin. These errors can have devastating consequences in large herd situations, when a large percentage of the herd may be affected with skin lesions. Organic matter frequently combines with skin exudates, forming encrusted material that collects on the periphery of ulcerated skin lesions. Healing of lesions is often prolonged, with culling of the most severely affected animals the best option. There is no specific treatment; however, many apply mild disinfectant solutions such as teat dip solutions with skin conditioners.

Clinical signs. Erythema, edema, and vesiculation of the skin, ulcers on the plantar aspect of the foot, plantar skin creases (or skin folds) on the caudal side of the pastern.

Differential diagnoses. Generalized dermatitis, traumatic skin lesions.

13.4.4 Screw claw (corkscrew claw)

Introduction. Corkscrew claw is most commonly observed in the lateral claw of the rear foot or the medial claw of the front foot. It is reported to be a heritable condition; however, other factors such as age, previous claw disease, and housing conditions are thought to influence its occurrence. It is characterized by rotation of the toe that displaces the sole, axial wall, and white line in an axial direction.

There are a couple of important abnormalities present in the heritable form of this condition: (i) a misalignment of the second and third phalanges on the lateral aspect; and (ii) a long and narrow third phalanx that has an abaxial to axial curve. This curving of the claw and its internal structures results in weight-bearing on the mid to caudal portion of the abaxial wall. The corkscrew claw is also normally larger and bears the majority of weight in the foot. This results in atrophy of the medial claw, because of reduced weight-bearing. These abnormalities contribute to a greater potential for the occurrence of sole ulcers, and also white line lesions in the abaxial region of the toe. White line lesions in the abaxial toe region are more likely since the corium is in abnormally close proximity to the weight-bearing surface in this region. In addition, white line horn in this region is frequently weaker and more easily compromised by external factors. Trimming generally requires great care, as it is quite easy to expose the corium in this region during the trimming process.

An acquired form of this condition is commonly seen in both dairy and beef cattle that feed from a manger. The acquired form of corkscrew claw affects the medial claw of the front foot, and is believed to be associated with the abnormal displacement of weight that occurs in the front claws of cows feeding at a feedbunk. When cows are feeding at a manger, they are required to stand with their front feet in a side-by-side posture. As the cow reaches for feed, an abnormal stress and load-bearing on front claws occurs that causes the toe of the medial claw to become thicker and rotate laterally. By comparison, cows at pasture normally graze with their front feet in a front-to-rear straddled posture. This posture balances weight-bearing more normally between claws, thus preventing abnormal weight distribution and screw claw development.
Clinical sign. Abnormal shape of affected claws.

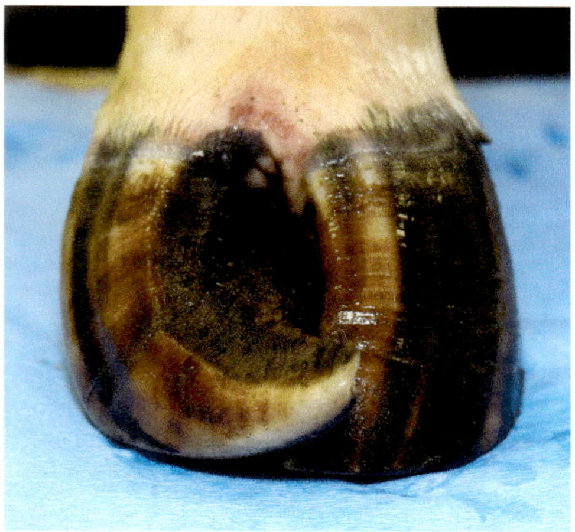

Fig. 13.27. Ox. Claw. Screw claw. Anterior view of a screw claw; note the rotation and upward deviation of the toe.

SUGGESTED READING

Atkinson, O. (2011) Non-healing hoof lesions in dairy cows. *Veterinary Record* 169, 561–562.

Blowey, R. and Weaver, D. (2011) *Color Atlas of Diseases and Disorders of Cattle*, 3rd edn. Mosby Elsevier Ltd, London.

Evans, N.J., Blowey, R.W., Timofte, D., Isherwood, D.R., Brown, J.M., *et al.* (2011) Association between bovine digital dermatitis treponemes and a range of 'non-healing' bovine hoof disorders. *Veterinary Record* 168, 214.

Greenough, P.R. (2001) Sand cracks, horizontal fissures, and other conditions affecting the wall of the bovine claw. *The Veterinary Clinics of North America: Food Animal Practice* 17, 93–110.

Leipold, H.W., Hiraga, T. and Dennis, S.M. (1993) Congenital defects of the bovine musculoskeletal system and joints. *Veterinary Clinics of North America: Food Animal Practice* 9, 93–104.

Lischer, Ch.J. and Ossent, P. (2000) The significance of the suspensory mechanism of the third phalanx and its fat bodies in the pathogenesis of sole ulcers in cattle. Part I: Macroscopic findings. In: *III International Conference on Bovine Lameness*, Parma, Italy.

Mulling, C. (2002) Theories on the pathogenesis of white line disease – an anatomical perspective. In: *12th International Symposium on Lameness in Ruminants*, Orlando, Florida.

Ossent, P. (1999) Subclinical bovine laminitis. *Cattle Practice* 7, 193–195.

Ossent, P. and Lischer, Ch.J. (1998) Bovine lamninitis: the lesions and their pathogenesis. *In Practice* 20, 415–427.

Ossent, P. and Lischer, Ch.J. (2000) The significance of the suspensory mechanism of the third phalanx and its fat bodies in the pathogenesis of sole ulcers in cattle. Part II: Microscopic findings. In: *III International Conference on Bovine Lameness*, Parma, Italy.

Raven, T. (1989) *Cattle Footcare and Claw Trimming*. Farming Press Ltd, Ipswich, UK.

Sanders, A.H., Shearer, J.K., DeVries, A. and Shearer, L.C. (2009) Seasonal incidence of lameness and risk factors associated with thin soles, white line disease, ulcers, and sole punctures in dairy cattle. *Journal of Dairy Science* 92, 3165–3174.

Shearer, J.K. (2009) Infectious disorders of the foot skin. In: Anderson, D.E. and Rings, D.M. (eds) *Current Veterinary Therapy, Food Animal Practice*. Saunders Elsevier, St Louis, Missouri, pp. 234–242.

Shearer, J.K. and van Amstel, S.R. (2011) Lameness in dairy cattle. In: Risco, C. and Melendez, P. (eds) *Dairy Production Medicine*. Wiley-Blackwell, Ames, Iowa, pp. 233–254.

Shearer, J.K., van Amstel, S.R. and Brodersen, B.W. (2012) Diagnostic pathology, clinical diagnosis of foot and leg lameness in cattle. *Veterinary Clinics of North America: Food Animal Practice* 28, 535–556.

Thomson, D.U., Loneragan, G.H., Henningson, J.N., Ensley, S.T. and Bawa, B. (2015) Description of a novel fatigue syndrome of finished feedlot cattle following transportation. *Journal of the American Veterinary Medical Association* 247, 66–72.

Van Amstel, S.R. and. Shearer, J.K. (2001) Abnormalities of hoof growth and development. *The Veterinary Clinics of North America: Food Animal Practice – Bovine Lameness* 17(1), 73–91.

Van Amstel, S.R. and Shearer, J.K. (2006) Review of pododermatitis circumscripta (ulceration of the sole) in dairy cows. *Journal of Veterinary Internal Medicine* 20, 805–811.

Van Amstel, S.R. and Shearer, J.K. (2008) Clinical report – characterization of toe ulcers associated with thin soles in dairy cows. *The Bovine Practitioner* 42, 189–196.

Whitlock, B.K. (2010) Heritable birth defects in cattle. In: *Applied Reproductive Strategies Conference Proceedings*, Nashville, Tennessee, pp. 146–151.

CHAPTER 14

Diseases of the Udder and Teats

14.1 Udder Diseases
- 14.1.1 Inflammation
  - 14.1.1.1 Udder dermatitis
  - 14.1.1.2 Udder cleft syndrome
  - 14.1.1.3 Staphylococcal dermatitis/impetigo
  - 14.1.1.4 Udder abscess
  - 14.1.1.5 Thrombophlebitis of milk vein
  - 14.1.1.6 Mastitis
- 14.1.2 Neoplasia

14.2 Teat Diseases
- 14.2.1 Inflammation
  - 14.2.1.1 Viral
  - 14.2.1.2 Bacterial
  - 14.2.1.3 Traumatic

INTRODUCTION

The lactating udder is the most overlooked organ in terms of its pathology and consequences to the cow's well-being. It is also one of the most economically exploited organs. Bovine mastitis is of worldwide importance. Little progress has been made in the prevention, treatment and control of udder inflammation. Decades of genetic selection for higher production has resulted in more susceptibility to mastitis.

The lactating udder plays an important physiological role in providing nutrition and protection to the newborn calf. The colostrum contains valuable antibodies, but also elements of cell-mediated response, protective enzymes, and cytokines. The mammary gland has an intrinsic mechanism of protection against pathogenic invaders. Resident neutrophils and macrophages are involved as effector cells in eliminating bacteria. In the teat, anatomic barriers including a sphincter are effective in protecting from environmental invaders.

For the pathologist, the udder should be removed from the body and each quarter investigated for lesions during the early phase of the necropsy in order to avoid overlooking changes that might have contributed to the animal's demise.

14.1 UDDER DISEASES

14.1.1 Inflammation

14.1.1.1 Udder dermatitis

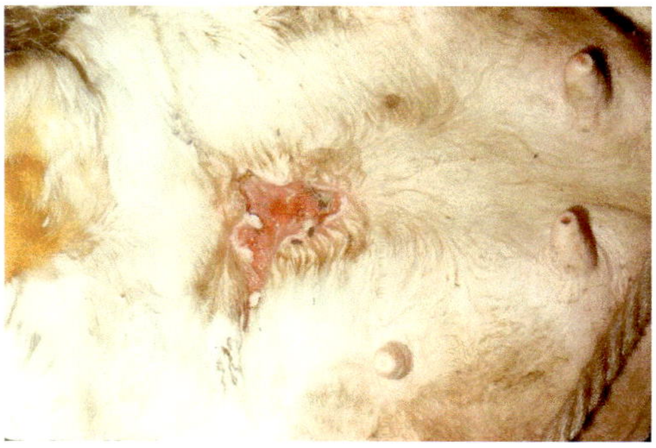

Fig. 14.1. Ox. Skin. Udder. Focal ulcerative dermatitis. A superficial, moist, ulcerative dermatitis with matting of the hair is located in front of the forequarters. Aspiration of pustule material and a stained smear should reveal *Staphylococcus* organisms to differentiate from viral material. (Courtesy of Dr R. Whitlock, University of Pennsylvania, USA.)

Introduction. Occurs soon after calving as superficial, moist inflammation between the inside of the thigh and medial attachment of the udder or between the forequarters and the ventral abdominal wall. It is a common

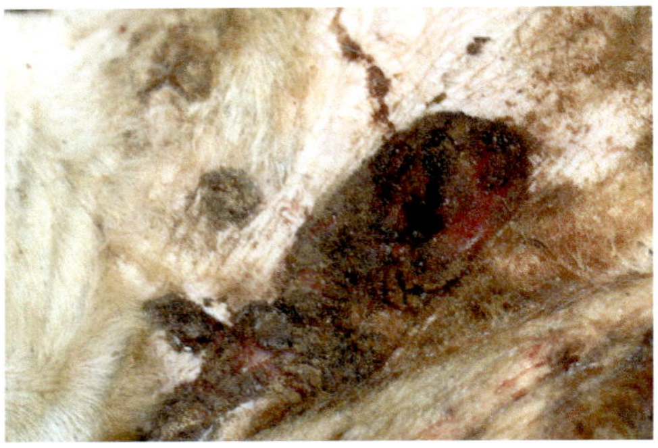

Fig. 14.2. Ox. Udder. Udder cleft syndrome. Gangrenous dermatitis. A deep, moist, exudative, odoriferous dermatitis is present in the skin fold between the udder quarters, with skin patches peeling off. The site is heavily infected by anaerobes, which may on occasion spread hematogenously to other organs such as the lung.

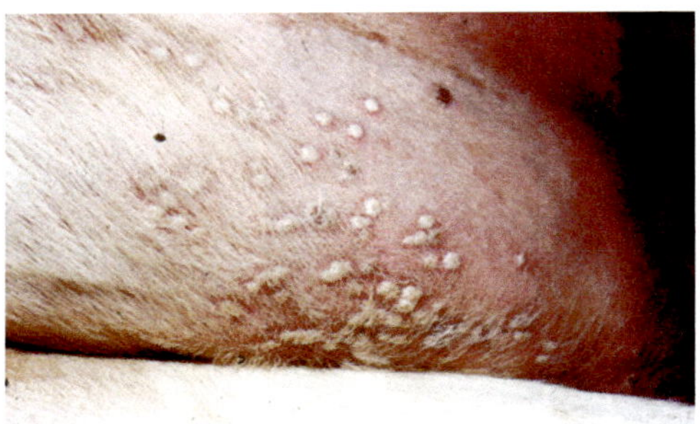

Fig. 14.3. Ox. Udder. Skin. Impetigo. Slightly raised white pustules are located in the epidermis over the udder, with a preference in the caudal aspect of the udder. Aspiration of the pustule material and a stained smear should reveal the organisms to differentiate from viral infection. (Courtesy of Dr R. Whitlock, University of Pennsylvania, USA.)

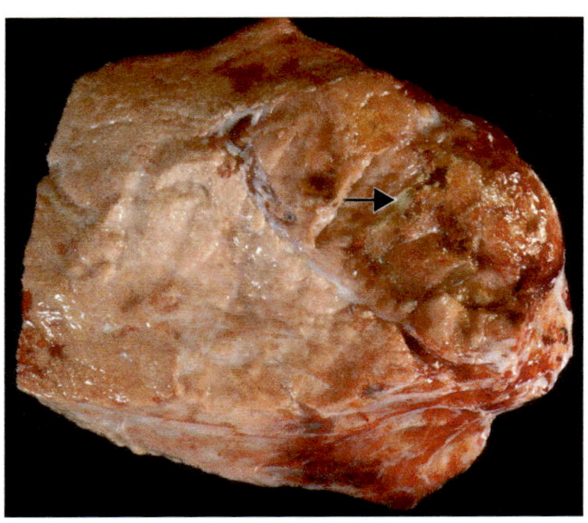

Fig. 14.4. Ox. Udder. Abscess. A circumscribed, red-tan elevated necrotic zone appears distinctly separated from the remaining normal udder parenchyma. The center of the abscess (arrow) is reflected by green discoloration. *Trueperella pyogenes* was isolated. (Courtesy of the Government of Alberta, Canada.)

skin condition that is predisposed by udder edema. Causes may be chemical, physical (photosensitization), bacterial (*Dermatophilus congolensis*), or fungal (*Trichophyton verrucosum*).

Clinical sign. Local pain.

Differential diagnosis. Impetigo (staphylococcal dermatitis).

14.1.1.2 Udder cleft syndrome

Introduction. Defined as a necrotic, gangrenous skin condition between udder halves or cranial to the front quarters at ventral midline, associated with foul odor and sloughing of skin. It is the result of friction to the skin, with secondary invasion of *Fusobacterium necrophorum* or *Trueperella pyogenes*. Transmission by mites has been incriminated. The condition is also known as 'udder rot'. Hemorrhage from erosion of adjacent blood vessels and thromboembolism to the lung can occur.

Clinical sign. Lameness.

Differential diagnosis. Inner thigh dermatitis.

14.1.1.3 Staphylococcal dermatitis/impetigo

Caused by *Staphylococcus aureus*, the condition occurs with staphylococcal mastitis in the herd. It may spread to the teats. Has zoonotic potential.

14.1.1.4 Udder abscess

Localized abscesses without evidence of associated mastitis occur after skin puncture and are contaminated with pyogenic anaerobes such as *T. pyogenes*. Milk from the affected quarter will be normal.

14.1.1.5 Thrombophlebitis of milk vein

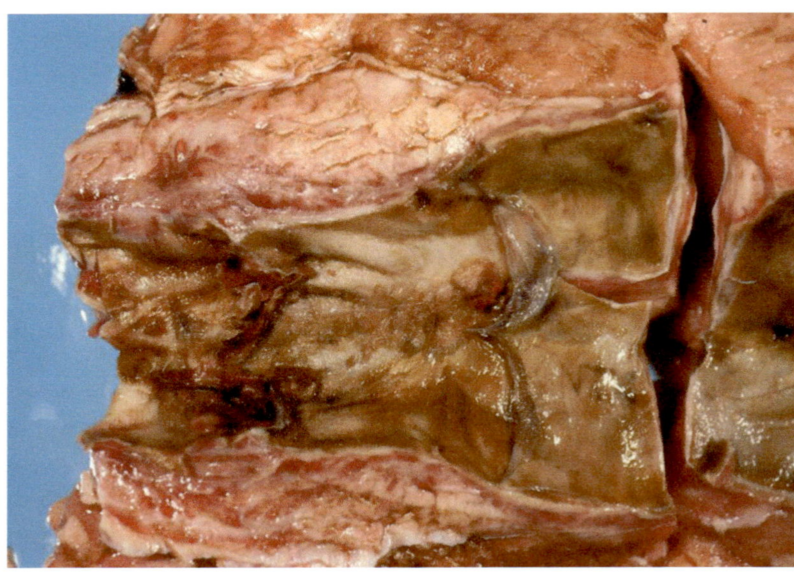

Fig. 14.5. Ox. Udder. Milk vein. Vegetative endophlebitis. Usually induced as a complication from venipuncture. Infected emboli may spread to the lung, or cause a vegetative valvulitis. Alternatively, the event is rarely the result of an extending infected deep dermatitis or udder cleft dermatitis with the potential of infectious emboli seeding the lung. (Courtesy of the Government of Alberta, Canada.)

14.1.1.6 Mastitis

Inflammation of the udder can be classified according to duration as acute or chronic, or according to the nature of the response as necrotizing (gangrenous), purulent, and (pyo)granulomatous. One or more quarters are involved. Infections may be sporadic or endemic within a herd. Galactophoritis is defined as inflammation of the lactiferous ducts.

NECROTIZING MASTITIS

Coliform mastitis

Introduction. An example of environmental and sanitation inefficiencies, coliform mastitis is life-threatening due to developing systemic disease from endotoxins released by the gram-negative bacteria. Causative organisms are *Escherichia coli*, *Enterobacter aerogenes*, *Pseudomonas aeruginosa*, and *Klebsiella pneumoniae*. Cows are most susceptible immediately post-partum.
Clinical signs. Depression, fever, inappetence, recumbency, shock.
Differential diagnoses. Post-parturient hypocalcemia, internal diseases.

Clostridial mastitis

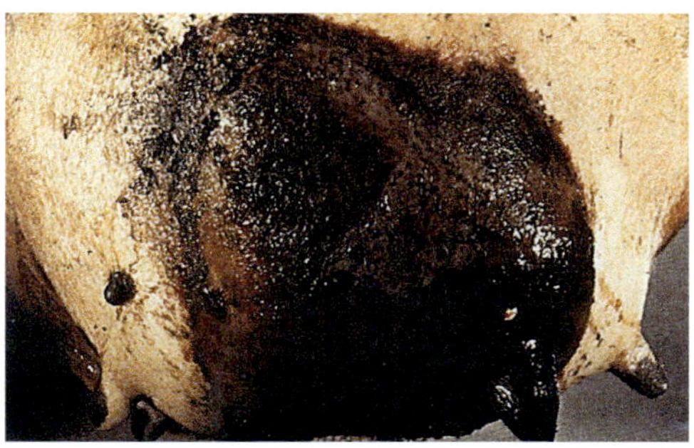

Fig. 14.8. Ox. Udder. Necrohemorrhagic mastitis. The quarter is dark red and swollen. *Clostridium perfringens* type A was isolated. Severe clinical signs similar to coliform mastitis can be expected.

Fusobacterium necrophorum mastitis

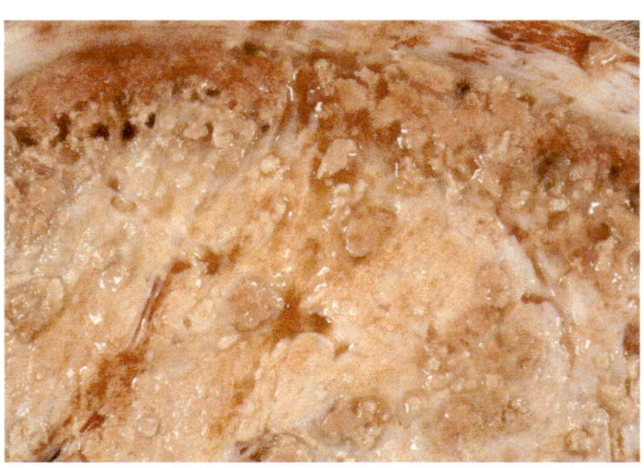

Fig. 14.10. Ox. Udder. Necrotizing mastitis. The parenchyma is moist, friable, granular on cut section. The organism releases endotoxins. Milk secretion is serous. (Courtesy of the Government of Alberta, Canada.)

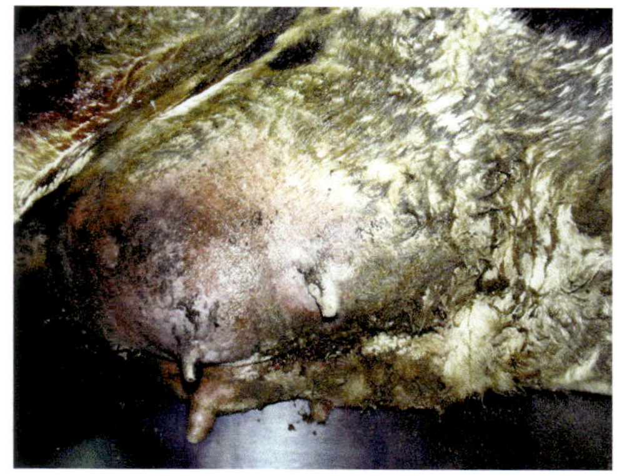

Fig. 14.6. Ox. Udder. Coliform mastitis. The affected quarters have a deep red gangrenous inflammation of the skin. Notice that the animal was kept in an unsanitary environment.

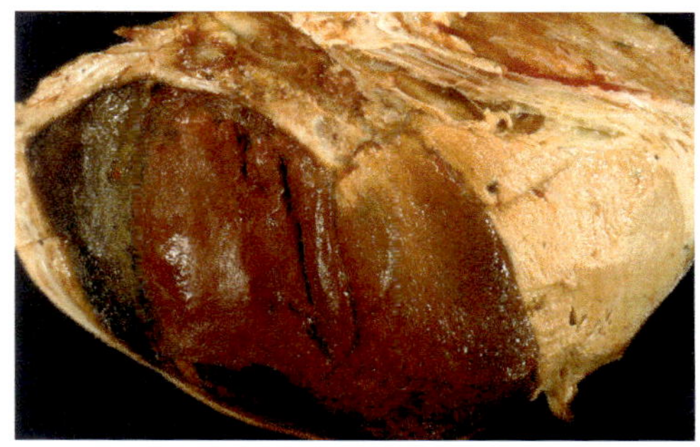

Fig. 14.7. Ox. Udder. Coliform mastitis. Necrotizing, gangrenous mastitis. The transverse section of the quarter is diffusely green, red discoloured, and moist.

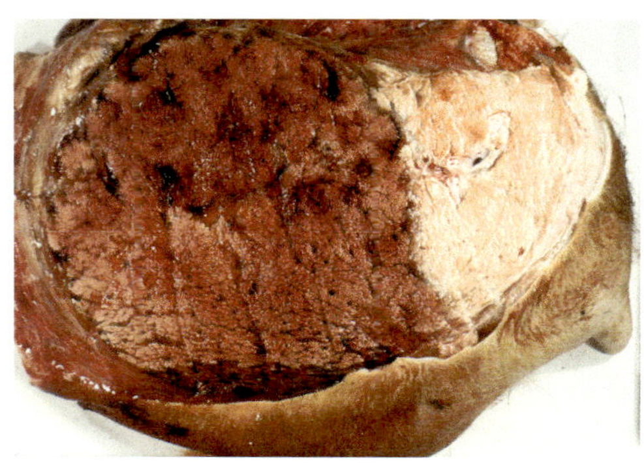

Fig. 14.9. Ox. Udder. Necrohemorrhagic mastitis. On transverse section, the quarter is dry, red and contains gas bubbles. There is subcutaneous edema. The junction to the adjacent normal quarter is well demarcated.

Pseudomonas aeruginosa mastitis

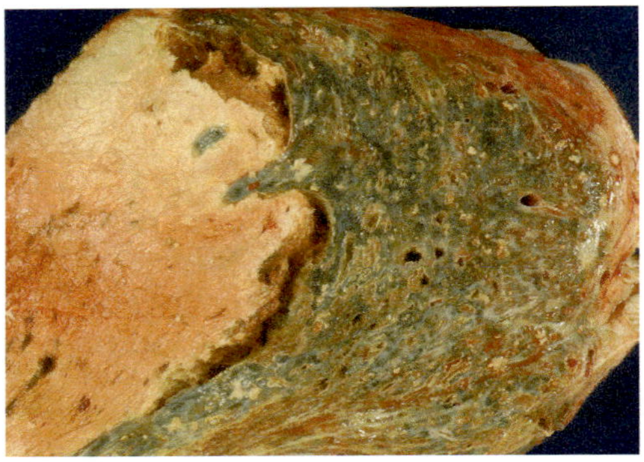

Fig. 14.11. Ox. Udder. Gangrenous mastitis. On cut section, green, necrotic material has collected around the mammary parenchyma and lactiferous ducts (perigalactophoritis). (Courtesy of the Government of Alberta, Canada.)

SUPPURATIVE MASTITIS

Streptococcus agalactiae, *Streptococcus dysgalactiae*, *Streptococcus uberis*, *Staphylococcus aureus*, *Mycoplasma bovis*, *Trueperella pyogenes* are typical isolates from this type of inflammation.

Staphylococcus aureus mastitis

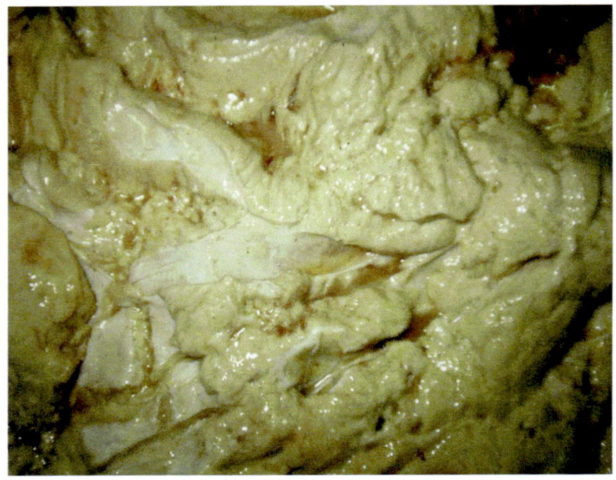

Fig. 14.12. Ox. Udder. Suppurative mastitis. The udder parenchyma is replaced diffusely by pus. The bacterium produces toxins that are dermonecrotic and vasoconstrictive, aiding in the development of gangrenous changes.

Streptococcus mastitis

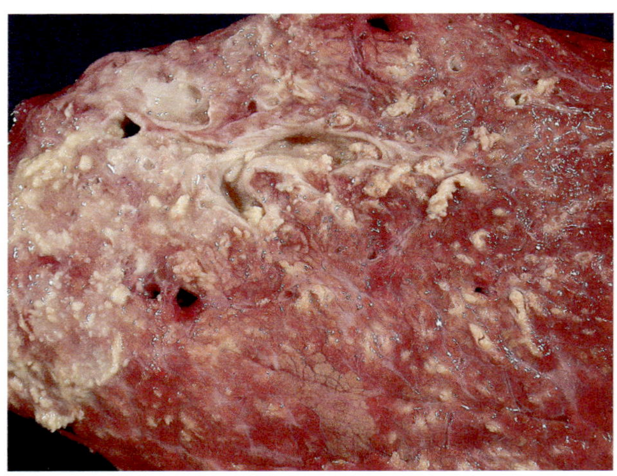

Fig. 14.13. Ox. Udder. Suppurative mastitis. Gray, purulent nodules have occupied the lactiferous sinus, ducts, and adjacent parenchyma. *Streptococcus agalactiae* has a higher prevalence in a herd than *Streptococcus dysgalactiae*.

Trueperella pyogenes mastitis

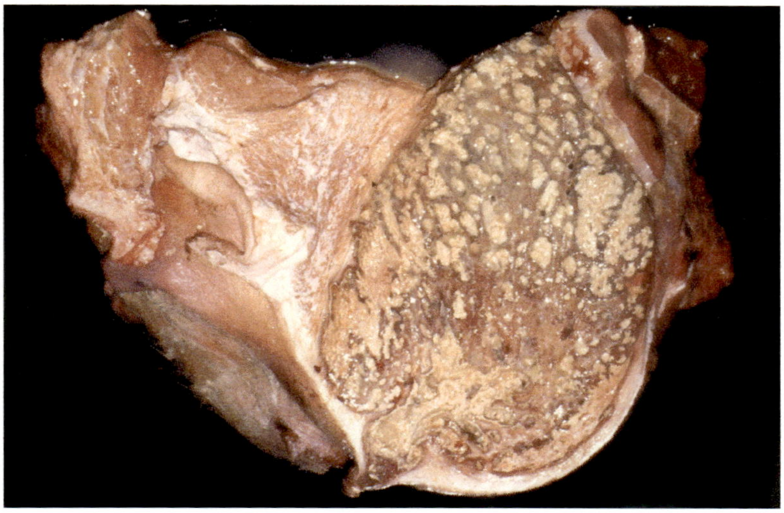

Fig. 14.14. Udder. Suppurative mastitis and galactophoritis. Multiple yellow foci seed the mammary parenchyma, lactiferous ducts, and sinus extending into the teat canal. Environmental organism.

CHRONIC MASTITIS

Mycoplasma mastitis

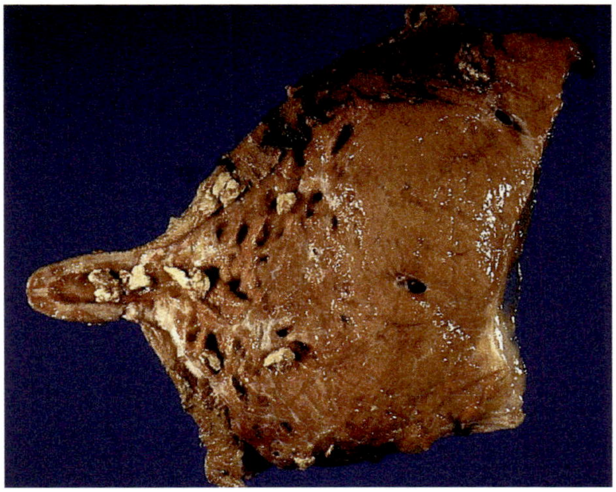

Fig. 14.15. Ox. Udder. Mycoplasmosis. Caseous galactophoritis and mastitis. *Mycoplasma bovis* is the most common isolate, but other mycoplasma species can participate. Infection may involve multiple quarters. Spread to the udder may occur from internal organs or from the environment. *Mycoplasma bovis* can be very devastating when introduced into a dairy herd.

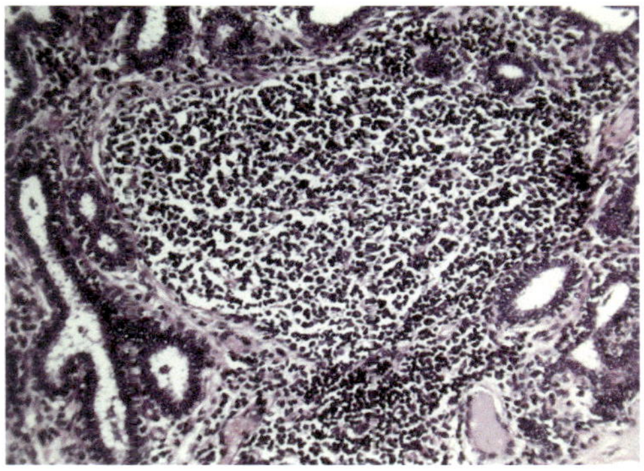

Fig. 14.16. Ox. Udder. Lymphocytic mastitis. The interstitium of the alveoli is markedly invaded and distended by lymphocytic aggregates, with destruction of alveoli. Histiocytes and plasma cells, as well as fibroblasts, may be interspersed. Surrounding alveoli are atrophic (H&E).

GRANULOMATOUS MASTITIS

Other than mycobacteria (pathogenic and atypical) and *Nocardia asteroides* or *farcinica*, fungi such as *Candida* spp., *Aspergillus* spp., *Cryptococcus* spp., and algae of *Prototheca* spp. have to be considered as causative agents gaining access from the environment or being installed from contaminated needles or milking equipment. Infected udders are enlarged and firm. System signs of illness are usually absent. Public health concern exists when unpasteurized milk is consumed.

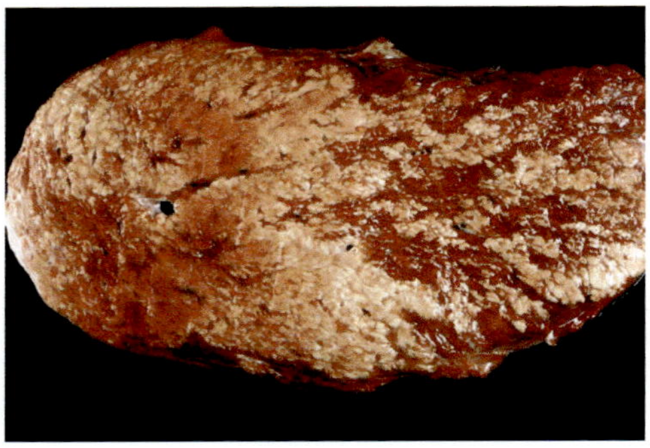

Fig. 14.17. Ox. Udder. Nocardiosis. Granulomatous mastitis. Affected lobules contain multiple and confluent, slightly raised, pale nodules, replacing most of the normal parenchyma. *Nocardia asteroides* was isolated.

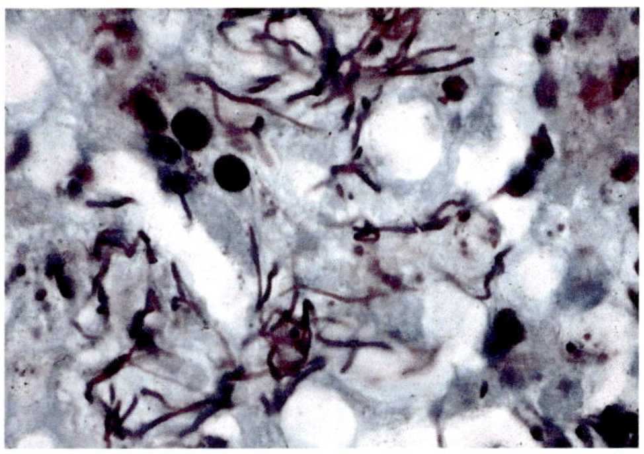

Fig. 14.19. Ox. Udder. Nocardiosis. An acid-fast stain demonstrates long-chained positive organism arranged in clusters (Ziehl–Neelsen).

Nocardia mastitis

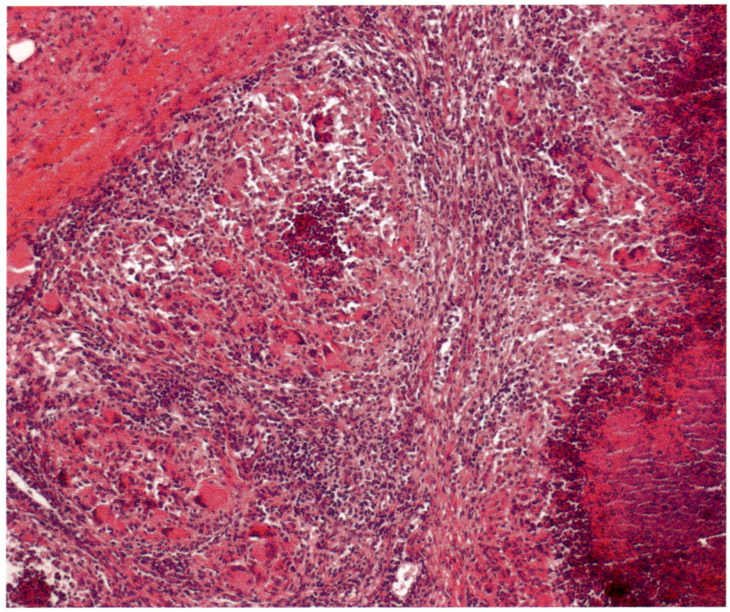

Fig. 14.18. Ox. Udder. Nocardiosis. Pyogranulomatous mastitis. The mammary tissue has been replaced by an inflammatory infiltrate composed of central necrosis and degenerate neutrophils with numerous histiocytes and multinucleate giant cells, as well as interspersed clusters of lymphocytes (H&E).

Prototheca mastitis

Wet, muddy, tropical or subtropical environmental conditions and insanitary milking procedures or needle infusion contribute to the spread of the algal organism *Prototheca zopfii* to the mammary gland.

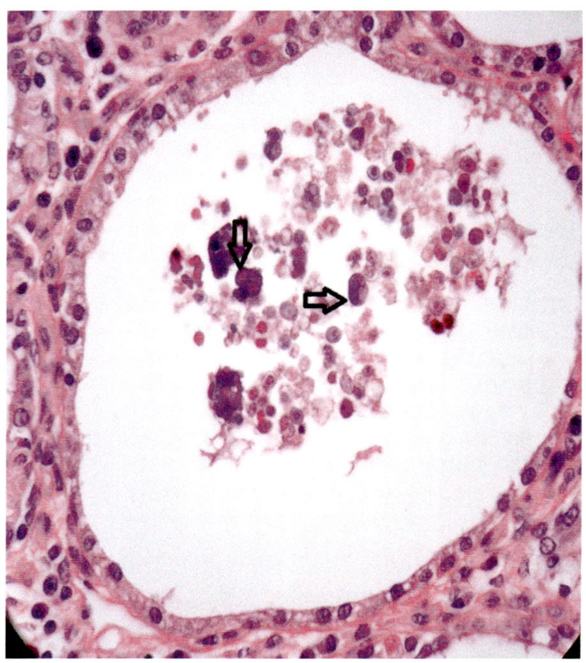

Fig. 14.20. Ox. Udder. Protothecosis. Unicellular sporangia and endospores (arrows) of algae are demonstrated within alveolus as round to ovoid, basophilic structures admixed with cellular debris. There is very little inflammation (H&E).

14.1.2 Neoplasia

The incidence of mammary tumors in cattle, except for fibropapillomas (skin of udder or teat), is extremely low. Occasional lymphosarcoma is encountered, as are sporadic squamous cell carcinomas or adenocarcinomas in older cows.

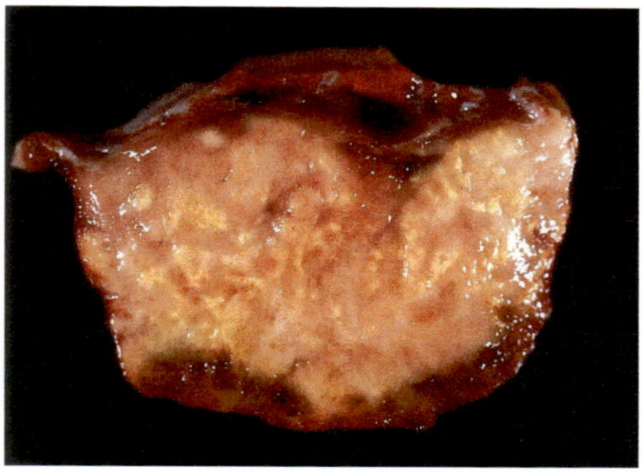

Fig. 14.21. Ox. Udder. Sarcoma. Multiple yellow, round or linear foci are scattered throughout section of the mammary gland. (Courtesy of the Government of Alberta, Canada.)

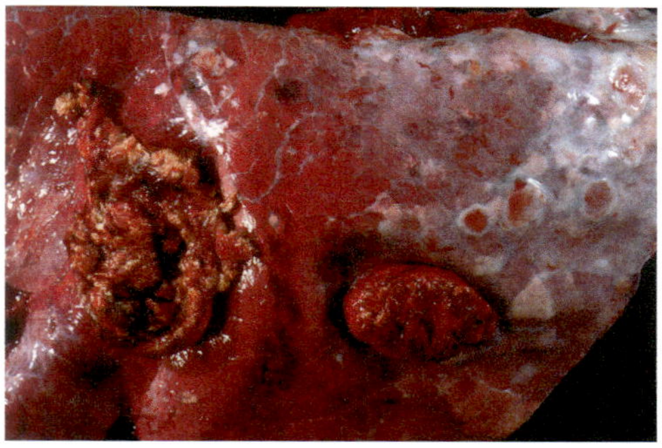

Fig. 14.22. Ox. Lung. Mammary gland sarcoma metastasis. Discrete nodules of varying size have spread within the lung. The larger nodules have a necrotic center. (Courtesy of the Government of Alberta, Canada.)

14.2 TEAT DISEASES

The teat is composed of skin, stroma, and mucosa. The streak canal is the most distal portion, and the exit for milk. It is encircled by a sphincter muscle and distally lined by keratinized mucosa, which functions as an external barrier and defense against mastitis development. The teats of the udder are extremely susceptible to injury and infection from environmental contamination. (Also see Chapter 12: Diseases of the Integument.)

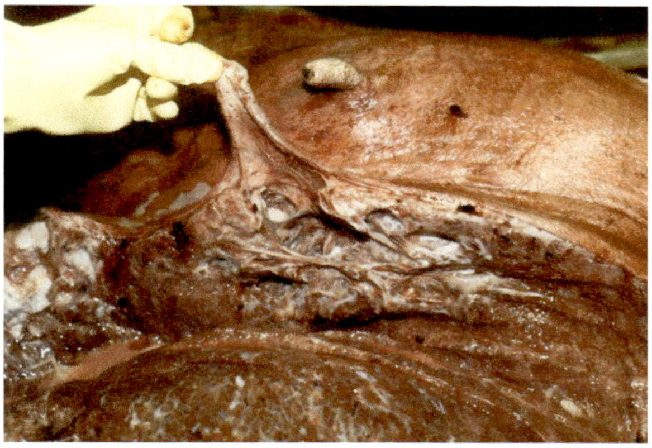

Fig. 14.23. Ox. Teat. Internal teat exposure. The mucosal surface and lumen of the teat canal are exposed, with the incision extending into the lactiferous sinus, lactiferous ductal system, and alveolar parenchyma. A pair of scissors should be used for the procedure and before the mammary gland and lactiferous sinuses are sectioned.

14.2.1 Inflammation

Inflammation of the teat is defined as thelitis.

14.2.1.1 Viral

Bovine herpes mammillitis (BHM)

Introduction. Bovine herpesvirus-2 (BHV-2) is the etiologic agent. The virus infects the skin of the teat and is the localized form of this virus infection. The virus induces vesicles that rupture to produce erosions, hemorrhage, and scabs. The infection may spread within a herd and to suckling calves (oral lesions).

Clinical signs. Pain, resentment to milking.

Differential diagnoses. Trauma, pseudocowpox, bluetongue, vesicular stomatitis.

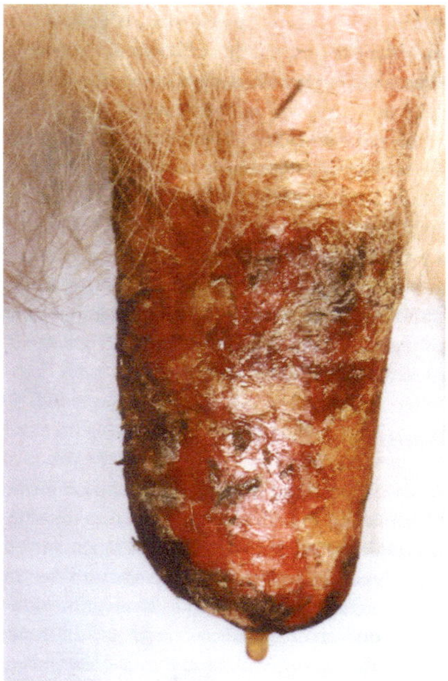

Fig. 14.24. Ox. Teat. Bovine herpes mammillitis (BHM). Hemorrhagic, erosive thelitis. The entire teat presents erythema, erosions, necrosis, and crusts. Mastitis is a severe complication.

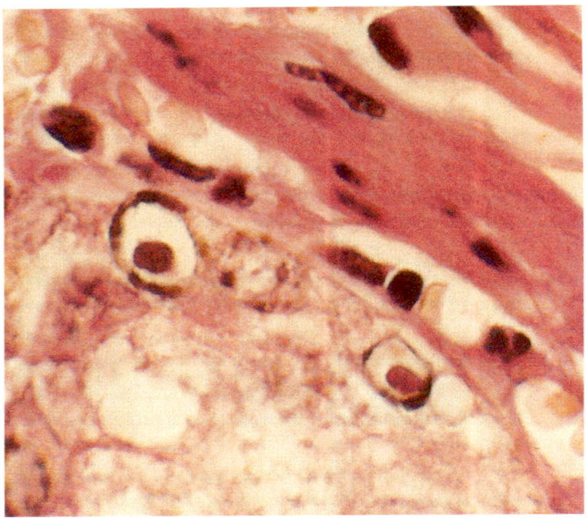

Fig. 14.25. Ox. Teat. Bovine herpes mammillitis (BHM). Intranuclear herpesvirus inclusions are visible in the vacuolated epithelial cells (H&E).

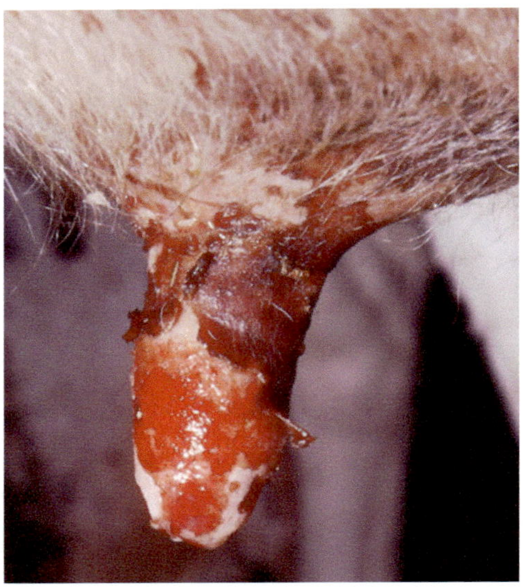

Fig. 14.26. Ox. Teat. Bovine herpes mammillitis (BHM). Ulcerative, necrotic, erosive, congested thelitis. Superficially, the entire skin sloughs off in the most severe cases. (Courtesy of Dr R. Whitlock, University of Pennsylvania, USA.)

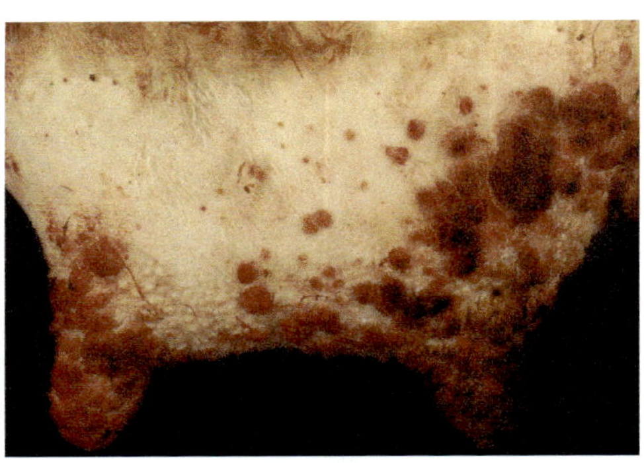

Fig. 14.29. Ox. Teat. Udder. Pseudocowpox. Papular thelitis. Circular, red-brown, raised, various-sized nodules are present in the skin. These may erupt to cause crusts and scabs. Mastitis is a complication. The condition is not associated with systemic disease. Of public health significance ('milker's nodules').

Bluetongue (BT)

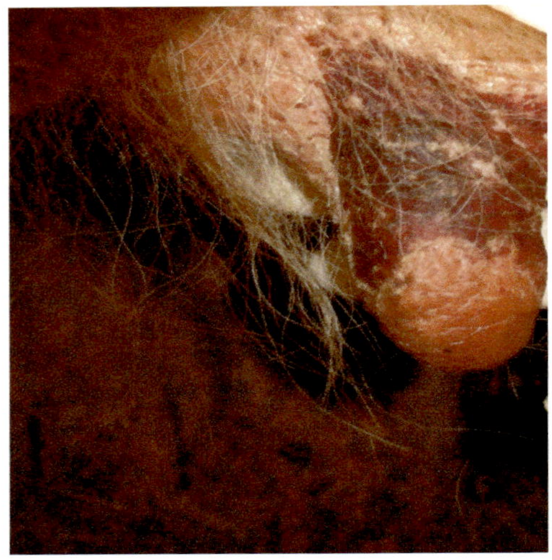

Fig. 14.27. Ox. Teat. Bluetongue (BT). Erosive, congested thelitis. Superficial blisters and breaks are present in the skin. Differential diagnosis should include photosensitization and vesicular stomatitis. (Courtesy of Dr Ch. Griot, EDI BLV, Vetsuisse, Bern, Switzerland.)

Vesicular stomatitis (VS)

In addition to stomatitis, vesicular lesions can be encountered in other parts of the body, such as the teat, coronary band, and interdigital space with this Rhabdovirus infection. Teat lesions may develop sporadically.

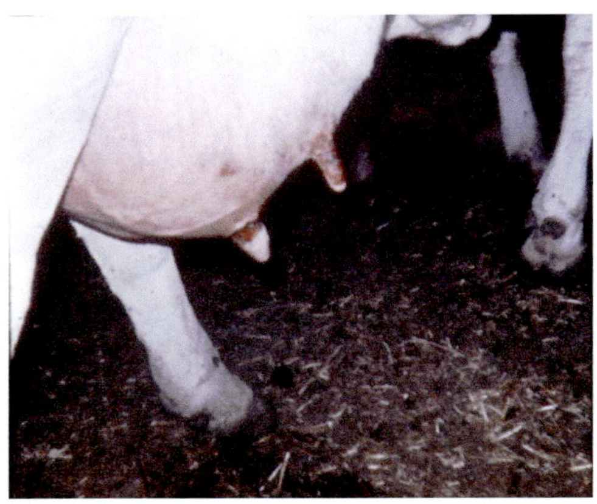

Fig. 14.28. Ox. Teat. Vesicular stomatitis (VS). Small vesicles are present in the skin of the teat of the right forequarter and right hindquarter. (Courtesy of Dr R. Whitlock, University of Pennsylvania, USA.)

Other viruses causing erosive changes on the teat are bovine viral diarrhea virus (BVDV), foot and mouth disease virus (FMDV) and rinderpest (officially eradicated).

Pseudocowpox

Infection is caused by a member of the genus *Parapoxvirus*, family Poxviridae.

Papilloma (bovine papilloma virus, BPV)

Viral-induced warts commonly develop in the skin at the lower end of the teat, sometimes obstructing the teat orifice. Flies are transmitting vectors.

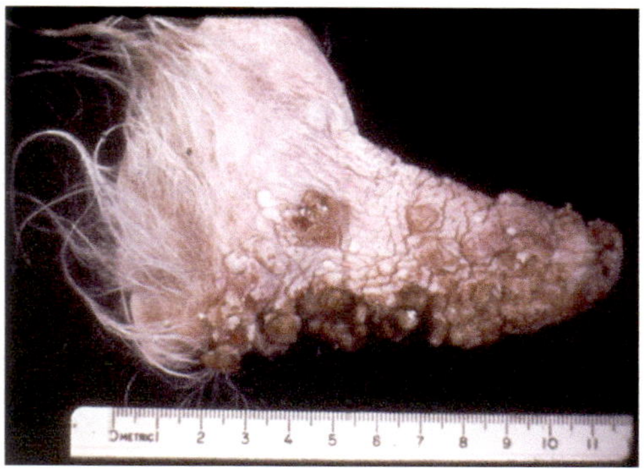

Fig. 14.30. Ox. Teat. Bovine papilloma virus (BPV). Multiple grain-like, raised nodules are scattered throughout the teat skin. (Courtesy of Dr R. Whitlock, University of Pennsylvania, USA.)

14.2.1.2 Bacterial

Impetigo

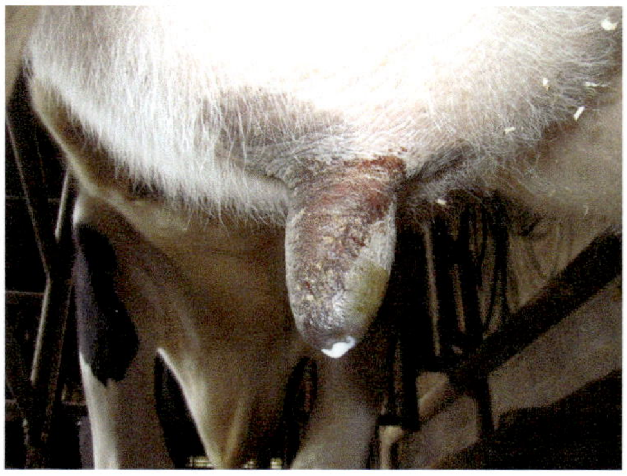

Fig. 14.31. Ox. Teat. Impetigo. Pustular thelitis. Small, fluctuating nodules arise from an erythematous skin. Etiology: *Staphylococcus aureus*. Of zoonotic potential.

14.2.1.3 Traumatic

Introduction. The teats are very susceptible to physical and chemical injuries. Physical causes include frostbite, sunburn, photosensitization, insect bites, self-inflicted trauma, milking machine. Chemical causes include dips and washes.

Clinical signs. Pain, non-cooperation with milking procedure.

Differential diagnoses. Infectious etiologies.

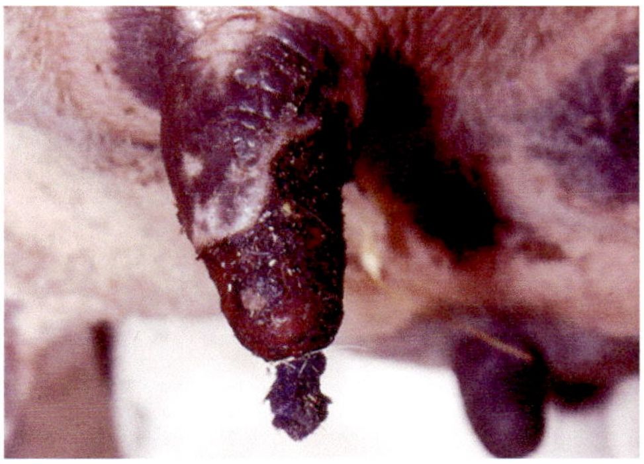

Fig. 14.32. Ox. Teat. Trauma. Necrotizing, ulcerative dermatitis. The skin over the distal portion of the teat sloughed, exposing the denuded teat to environmental contaminants. The skin in the upper portion is raised, leathery, and hemorrhagic. (Courtesy of Dr R. Whitlock, University of Pennsylvania, USA.)

SUGGESTED READING

Aalbaek, B., Stenderup, J., Jensen, H.E., Valbak, J., Nylan, B. and Huda, A. (1994) Mycotic and algal bovine mastitis in Denmark. *Acta Pathologica Microbiologica et Immunologica Scandinavia* 102, 451–456.

Corbellini, L.G., Driemeier, D. and Cruz, C.E. (2001a) Immunohistochemistry combined with periodic acid-Schiff for bovine mammary gland with protothecal mastitis. *Biotech Histochemistry* 76, 85–88.

Corbellini, L.G., Driemeier, D., Cruz, C., Dias, M.M. and Ferreiro, L. (2001b) Bovine mastitis due to *Prototheca zopfii*: clinical, epidemiological and pathological aspects in a Brazilian dairy herd. *Tropical Animal Health Production* 33, 463–470.

Costa, E.O., Ribeiro, A.R., Watanabe, E.T. and Melville, P.A. (1998) Infectious bovine mastitis caused by environmental organisms. *Zentralblatt Veterinaermedizin* B 45, 65–71.

Francoz, D., Bergeron, L., Nadeau, M. and Beauchamp, G. (2012) Prevalence of contagious mastitis pathogens in bulk tank milk in Quebec. *Canadian Veterinary Journal* 53, 1071–1078.

Gonzalez, R.N. and Wilson, D.J. (2003) Mycoplasmal mastitis in dairy herds. *Veterinary Clinics Northern American Food Animal Practice* 19, 199–221.

Jasper, D.E., Boothby, J.T. and Thomas, C.B (1987) Pathogenesis of bovine mycoplasma mastitis. *Israelic Journal of Medical Science* 23, 625–627.

Manninen, K., Smith, R.A. and Kim, L.O. (1993) Highly presumptive identification of bacterial isolates associated with the recent Canada-wide mastitis epizootic of *Nocardia farcinica*. *Canadian Journal of Microbiology* 39, 635–641.

Osman, K.M., El-Embawy, M.I., Ezzeldeen, N.A. and Hussein, H.M. (2009) Mastitis in dairy buffalo and cattle in Egypt due to *Clostridium perfringens*: prevalence, incidence, risk factors and costs. *Review Science Technology* 28, 975–986.

CHAPTER 15

Diseases of Eye and Ear

Contributed by Ingeborg Maria Langohr
Department of Pathobiological Sciences, School of Veterinary Medicine, Louisiana State University, USA

15.1 Congenital Ocular Diseases
15.1.1 Microphthalmia
15.1.2 Hypovitaminosis A
15.1.3 Lysosomal storage diseases
15.1.4 Dermoid
15.1.5 Entropion and ectropion
15.1.6 Colobomas
15.1.7 Albinism
15.1.8 Remnant hyaloid artery

15.2 Degenerative Ocular Diseases
15.2.1 Cataracts
15.2.2 Hemorrhage
15.2.3 Papilledema

15.3 Inflammatory Ocular Diseases
15.3.1 Blepharitis
15.3.2 Conjunctivitis, keratoconjunctivitis, and uveitis

15.4 Neoplastic Ocular Diseases
15.4.1 Papilloma
15.4.2 Squamous cell carcinoma
15.4.3 Lymphoma

15.5 Inflammatory Otic Diseases

15.6 Neoplastic Otic Diseases

EYES

INTRODUCTION

Cattle have laterally positioned eyes, providing them with a wide visual field, as is usual in herbivores. When the head is either raised or down to graze, and the body does not obscure the view, their combined field of vision covers nearly 360 degrees. This allows them rapid recognition of approaching predators, as well as assessment of ground conditions for both eating and escape. Ocular health is therefore critical to the well-being of the animal. This chapter summarizes both congenital and acquired degenerative, inflammatory, and neoplastic ocular diseases that affect cattle.

15.1 CONGENITAL OCULAR DISEASES

Congenital ocular anomalies are, like other developmental anomalies in cattle, of special concern in the management of breeding herds because they may be of genetic, nutritional, or *in utero* infectious origin. None the less, the cause of some abnormalities remains unknown.

15.1.1 Microphthalmia

Multiple congenital defects of the eye have been known in cattle for years, characterized by microphthalmia, microphakia, cataract, persistent hyaloid

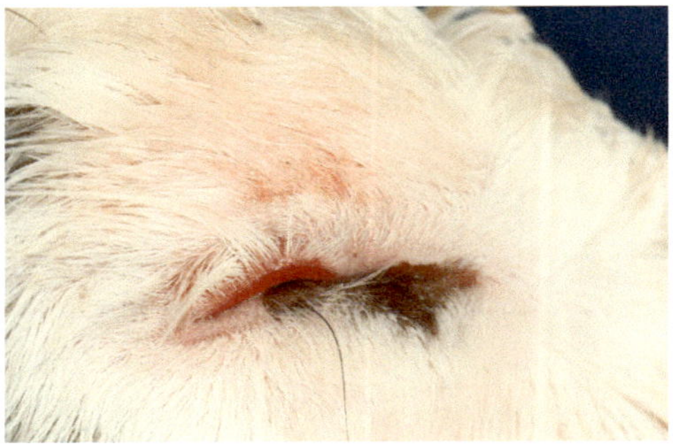

Fig. 15.1. Ox. Eye. Microphthalmia. The small palpebral fissure denotes very early interference with the formation of the optic vesicle and its contact with the fetal surface ectoderm. If the microphthalmia is as severe as in this case, it may mimic anophthalmia (complete absence of the eye). None the less, vestigial remnant of ocular tissue can almost always be found in the orbit, which is generally abnormally small in these cases. (Courtesy of Department of Veterinary Pathology, WCVM, University of Saskatchewan, Saskatoon, Canada.)

vessels, and retinal dysplasia and detachment. Such multiple ocular defects have been associated with a frameshift mutation in the *WFDC1* gene on chromosome 18 in Japanese Black cattle with the recessively inherited form of this disease. Multiple inherited ocular anomalies, including retinal dysplasia and internal hydrocephalus, have also been reported in Jersey, Hereford, and Shorthorn cattle.

Fetal malformations, including of the eyes, can also be the result of *in utero* exposure to bovine viral diarrhea virus (BVDV), either by natural infection or by vaccination of the dam with modified live virus vaccines at 100–150 days of gestation. Ocular malformations in these cases range from cortical cataract through retinal dysplasia/atrophy and gliosis of the optic nerve to microphthalmia. The variability of the degenerative ocular lesions may be due to differing stages of development at the time of viral infection, as well as the degree of virulence of the viral strain. Affected calves generally also have cerebellar hypoplasia. (See Chapter 2: Diseases of the Nervous System.)

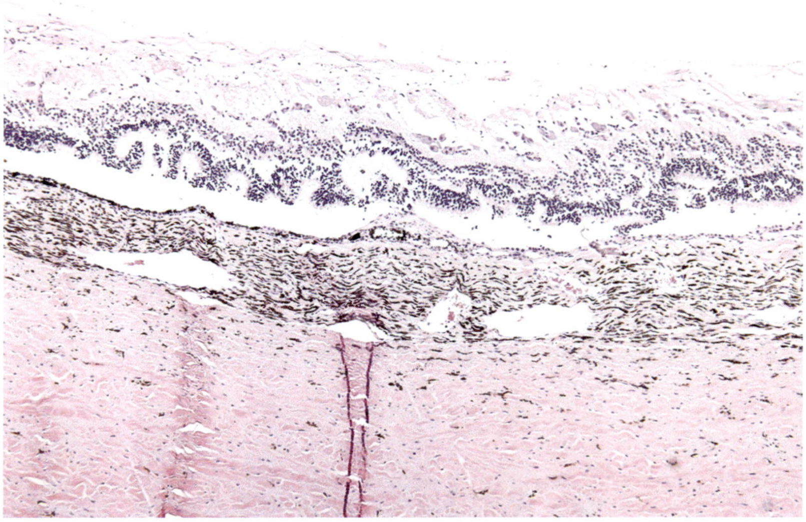

Fig. 15.2. Calf. Retina. Bovine viral diarrhea virus (BVDV) retinopathy. The outer retinal layers are somewhat disorganized and folded, and the retinal pigment epithelium has undergone multifocal mild spindle cell metaplasia. No sign of inflammation usually exists in these cases, although foci of retinitis have been observed in fetuses in experimental conditions during the 3rd and 4th week after viral inoculation of their dams (H&E). (Courtesy of Dr R. Dubielzig, Comparative Ocular Pathology Laboratory of Wisconsin, USA.)

15.1.2 Hypovitaminosis A

Maternal hypovitaminosis A is another cause of ocular malformations and blindness in cattle. Alterations include cataract, lens luxation, microphthalmia, and retinal folds and atrophy. Affected calves may also have doming of the forehead, associated with thickened occipital and sphenoid bones that constrict the optic nerves, leading to initial papilledema and eventual optic nerve atrophy. Because green forage is high in vitamin A precursors (carotene), maternal vitamin A deficiency is rare; however, it may occur with the feeding of lower-quality hay or silage during the winter. Adult vitamin A-deficient cattle have increased cerebrospinal fluid (CSF) pressure, resulting from failure of proper resorption of CSF through abnormal arachnoid villi, leading to papilledema. This by itself does not lead to blindness, however, unless it is accompanied by vascular compression and secondary ischemic damage to the optic nerve. (Also see Chapter 2: Diseases of the Nervous System.)

Differential diagnosis. Defective bone remodeling leading to hypoplastic foraminae and blindness associated with defects in the optic nerve is also seen in Black Angus cattle with osteopetrosis expressed as an autosomal recessive trait.

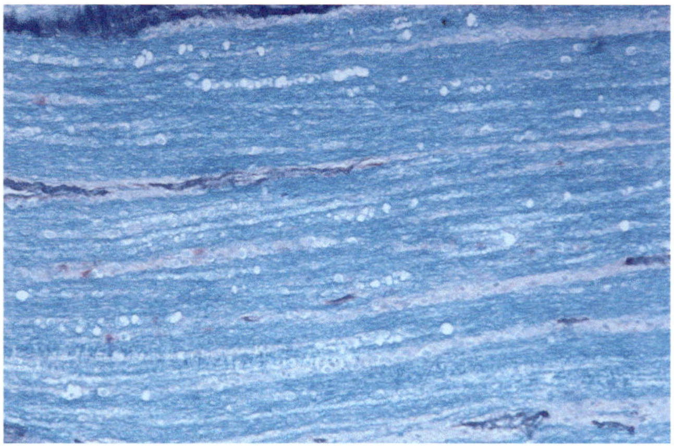

Fig. 15.3. Ox. Eye. Optic nerve degeneration. This calf had hypovitaminosis A, which in growing cattle leads to papilledema and optic nerve degeneration characterized by the depicted dilated myelin sheaths, many of which contain cross sections of swollen axons (spheroids). Optic nerve atrophy and retinal degenerative alterations can lead to eventual vision loss of affected calves. If the diet is adjusted soon enough, however, the alterations are reversible (Luxol fast blue). (Courtesy of Department of Veterinary Pathology, WCVM, University of Saskatchewan, Saskatoon, Canada.)

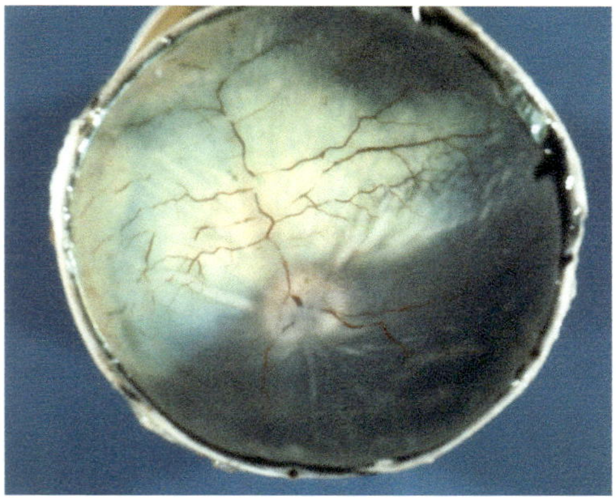

Fig. 15.4. Ox. Eye. Papilledema. While papilledema can be seen with hypovitaminosis A, the swollen optic disk with blurred margins, characteristic of this condition, is most often indicative of increase in cerebrospinal fluid pressure within the optic nerve. In this particular animal, it developed in association with polioencephalomalacia. (Courtesy of Department of Veterinary Pathology, WCVM, University of Saskatchewan, Saskatoon, Canada.)

15.1.3 Lysosomal storage diseases

Several inherited lysosomal storage diseases with ocular alterations have been reported in cattle, including gangliosidosis and mannosidosis.

GM_1-gangliosidosis is seen in Holstein calves related to a generalized metabolic deficiency in beta-galactosidase and beta-glucuronidase. The most striking ocular finding is ganglion cell vacuolar degeneration.

Salers calves with beta-mannosidase deficiency have narrow palpebral fissures and slightly domed head with mild prognathism. The characteristic microscopic cytoplasmic vacuolation seen in many cells throughout the body is also present in corneal stromal and endothelial cells, outer and inner epithelial cells of the ciliary body, cells along the anterior border of the iris, retinal bipolar cells, photoreceptor cells, retinal pigment epithelial cells, glial cells of the optic nerve, and vascular endothelial cells and fibroblasts throughout the globe.

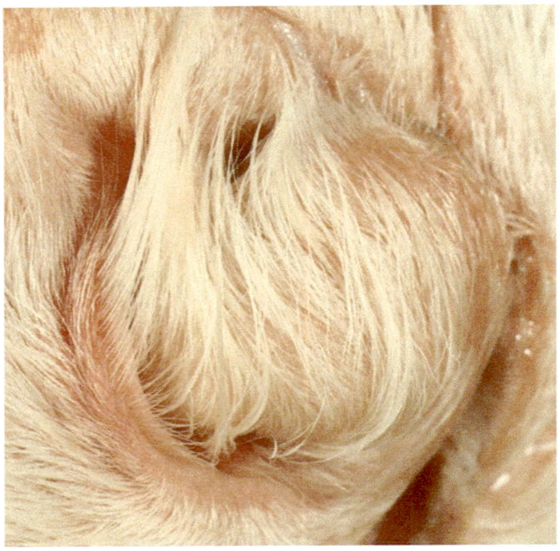

Fig. 15.5. Ox. Eye. Corneal dermoid. Primarily in a case like this, in which the abnormal plaque of haired skin obscures the entire cornea, is this congenital anomaly regarded as of clinical significance. Surgical removal is recommended. (Courtesy of Department of Veterinary Pathology, WCVM, University of Saskatchewan, Saskatoon, Canada.)

15.1.4 Dermoid

Ocular dermoid is the result of abnormal differentiation of the conjunctival and/or corneal surface ectoderm resulting in ectopic haired skin formation. Herefords have a higher predisposition for this lesion, which is of autosomal recessive and polygenic inheritance. The lesion, which can be uni- or bilateral, may cause various degrees of visual impairment related to irritation by the dermoid, leading to keratoconjunctivitis and corneal ulceration.

15.1.5 Entropion and ectropion

The conditions are defined as inversion and eversion, respectively, of the eyelid margins, and can occur in cattle as well. Congenital entropion has been reported in the Simmental breed, but acquired, cicatricial entropion is more common. Ectropion has been similarly associated with developmental and cicatricial causes.

15.1.6 Colobomas

Colobomas of the choroid, at the level of the optic disc, are relatively common in cattle, particularly in Hereford and Charolais cattle. Colobomas are bilateral and often small, but not necessarily symmetrical. Their effect on vision will depend on their size and depth, with many animals seemingly not much affected.

15.1.7 Albinism

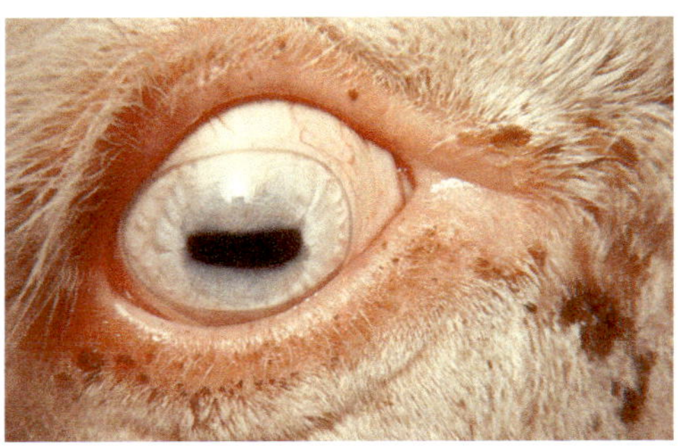

Fig. 15.6. Ox. Eye. Albinism. This newborn Hereford calf had incomplete albinism, characterized by a mainly white hair coat and a white iris with a fainter center. Albinism has a genetic background in this breed of cattle. (Courtesy of Department of Veterinary Pathology, WCVM, University of Saskatchewan, Saskatoon, Canada.)

Hereford cattle may have colobomas of the optic disc associated with the dominant form of incomplete albinism. Complete albinism, characterized by pink skin and complete lack of pigment in the choroid, iris, eyelids, and muzzle has been rarely documented in cattle. Affected animals have clinically normal vision, but may have variable photophobia, and possibly nystagmus. Incomplete albinism is more common, with colored muzzle, ears, eyes, and lower limbs. Recessive alleles associated with genetic pigment dilution exist in low frequencies in Braunvieh, Brown Swiss, and other breeds. Affected Hereford herds may include normal colored animals with heterochromia irides, associated with iridal hypoplasia and reduced uveal pigmentation. Heterochromia irides has also been reported in various other cattle breeds, including Ayrshire, Holstein, Angus, Brown Swiss, and Guernsey.

15.1.8 Remnant hyaloid artery

In calves, a non-patent remnant of the hyaloid artery, known as the Bergmeister's papilla, is often present at the center of the optic disc. Some remnant of this vessel will still be present in 80% of older cattle.

15.2 DEGENERATIVE OCULAR DISEASES

15.2.1 Cataracts

Congenital bilateral cataracts, which are usually mature when calves are 4–11 months of age, are autosomal recessively inherited in several breeds of cattle, including Jersey, Hereford, and Holstein. Non-progressive, nuclear congenital cataracts have also been reported. As mentioned previously, congenital cataracts have been documented in association with other ocular abnormalities as well, attributed either to a genetic defect or to BVDV exposure *in utero*.

Acquired cataracts develop secondary to trauma and inflammation.

Lens opacity can also be induced transiently by reducing temperature, causing the so-called 'cold cataract'. Such lens opacity first appears in the nuclear region when the temperature drops below 12°C, and is densest and most extensive at a temperature of 1°C. Warming causes the lens opacity to disappear completely at 16.5°C. (Also see Chapter 1: Diseases of Neonates and Calves.)

15.2.2 Hemorrhage

Intraocular hemorrhage may occur from trauma, thrombocytopenia (e.g. BVDV infection, bracken fern toxicity), or another clotting abnormality.

15.2.3 Papilledema

As mentioned previously, papilledema, i.e. non-inflammatory swelling of the optic disc, generally indicates increased intracranial pressure, such as seen with hydrocephalus, polioencephalomalacia, space-occupying brain lesions, meningoencephalitis, and hexachlorophene toxicity. Optic neuropathy with papilledema and peripapillary hemorrhage has also been observed with male fern poisoning (*Dryopteris filix-mas*).

15.3 INFLAMMATORY OCULAR DISEASES

15.3.1 Blepharitis

Blepharitis, or inflammation of the eyelids, is most often due to infection or photosensitization. The periocular region is frequently involved with dermatophytosis (ringworm). Photosensitization due to ingestion of a photodynamic agent (primary photosensitization) or accumulation of phylloerythrin due to liver damage or biliary duct occlusion (secondary photosensitization) affects the periocular region most frequently in cattle with little periocular pigmentation.

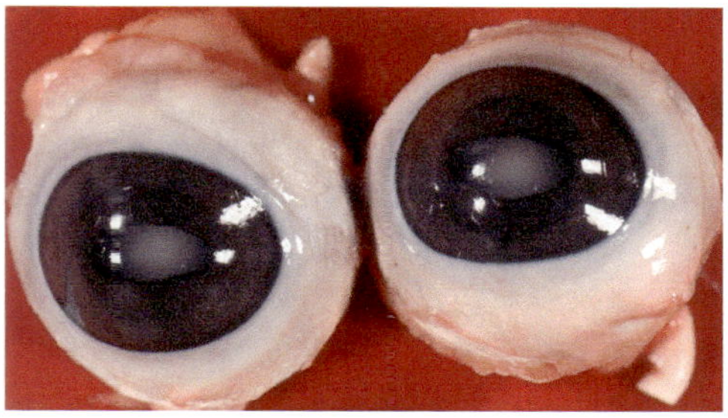

Fig. 15.7. Ox. Eye. Cataracts. Lens opacity is an overall rare condition in cattle. It may occur as a congenital or acquired alteration, which can lead to blindness if severe. (Courtesy of Department of Veterinary Pathology, WCVM, University of Saskatchewan, Saskatoon, Canada.)

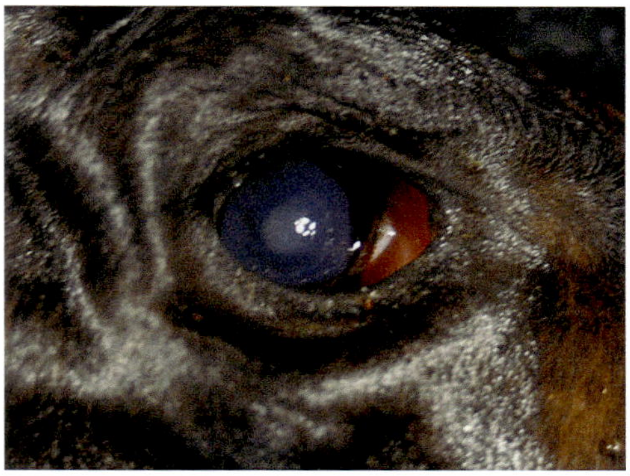

Fig. 15.8. Ox. Eye. Cataract. Mild transient lens opacity as seen in this calf, which died of diarrhea and was maintained at low temperature prior to necropsy, can be induced by reducing the temperature, causing the so-called 'cold cataract'. The eye is also deeply sunken in the orbit, denoting marked dehydration.

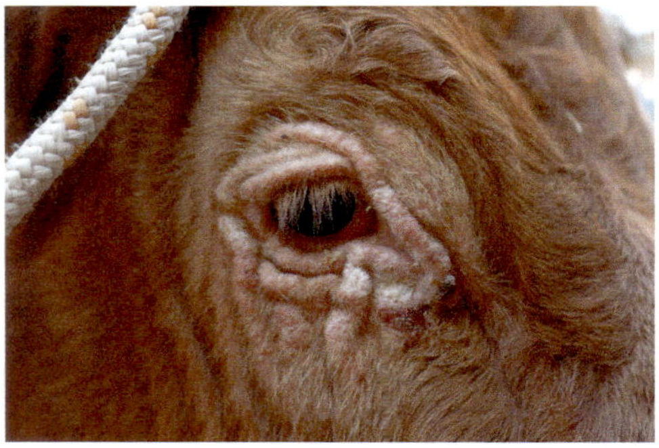

Fig. 15.9. Ox. Eyelid. Besnoitiosis. The eyelids are one of the best sites to observe the alopecia and intradermal indurations seen in the chronic stage of *Besnoitia besnoiti* infection, considered an emerging protozoal disease in cattle in Europe. Severe acute disease is characterized by pyrexia, lethargy, subcutaneous edema, conjunctivitis, nasal discharge, salivation, and lameness. (Also see Chapter 12: Diseases of the Integument.) (Courtesy of Dr E. Lepri, University of Perugia, Italy.)

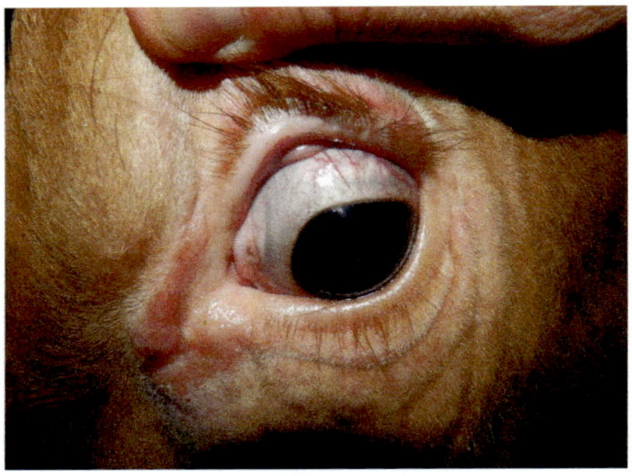

Fig. 15.10. Ox. Eye. Besnoitiosis. Many animals infected with *Besnoitia besnoiti* remain asymptomatic. In these animals, the only sign of the infection is the presence of protozoal cysts in the sclera (and in cows also in the vulvar region). (Courtesy of Dr E. Lepri, University of Perugia, Italy.)

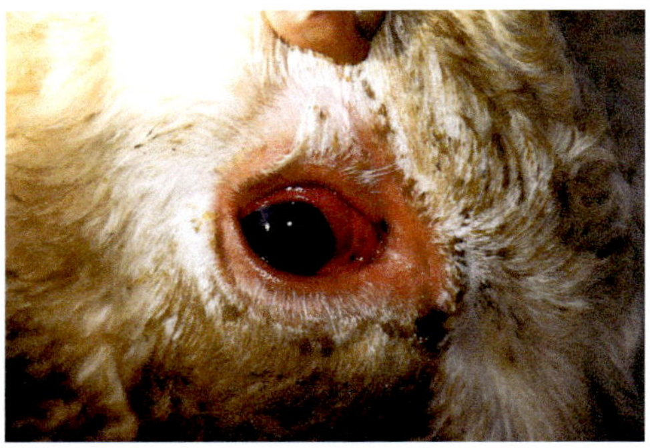

Fig. 15.11. Ox. Eye. Bovine herpesvirus 1-associated conjunctivitis. Cattle with the respiratory form of infectious bovine rhinotracheitis (IBR) will often also have conjunctivitis with profuse, initially serous, ocular discharge. The cornea is usually unaffected; however, in cases with secondary bacterial infection, keratitis and corneal ulceration can follow.

The main **differential diagnosis** in cases with excessive periocular crusting is dermatophilosis. Sarcoptic and demodectic mange have additionally been implicated as a cause of periocular dermatitis in cattle. (Also see Chapter 12: Diseases of the Integument.)

15.3.2 Conjunctivitis, keratoconjunctivitis, and uveitis

Conjunctivitis represents an important disease, not only from an economic standpoint but also for the well-being of the affected animals. Infectious agents, in particular *Moraxella bovis*, but also other agents such as chlamydophila, are the most common cause of conjunctivitis in cattle, often in conjunction with keratitis. None the less, one should also examine the conjunctival sac for the presence of foreign bodies or nematodes (*Thelazia* spp.), although there has been a marked decline of the latter in the past several decades, likely related to the use of macrocyclic lactone endectocides.

Animals fed silage, in particular when fed big-bale silage in ring feeders or directly from clamps, can develop listerial keratoconjunctivitis and uveitis, also known as 'silage eye', as a primary condition not associated with other signs of listeriosis. Most lesions are unilateral and clinically characterized by epiphora, photophobia, corneal opacity, and hypopyon.

Uveal changes distinguish ocular listeriosis from infectious bovine keratoconjunctivitis (IBK), also known as 'pinkeye', caused primarily by *M. bovis.* IBK is a highly contagious disease regarded as the most important ocular disease affecting cattle worldwide. Signs can vary from mild to severe, with profuse lacrimation, blepharospasm, photophobia, conjunctival swelling, corneal edema, and central corneal ulceration. Animals may recover spontaneously with varying degrees of corneal scarring, but occasionally perforation of the corneal ulcer occurs, followed by iris prolapse, leading to permanent blindness. Predisposing factors include breed and age of the animal (*Bos taurus* breeds, in particular Herefords, and calves are generally more susceptible), host immune system, bacterial strain, UV light exposure, concurrent pathogens (including *Moraxella bovoculi*), and dry climate and pasture conditions that may create mechanical injury to the eye (e.g. dust, tall grasses, and weeds). IBK occurs most commonly in the summer and autumn when flies, which act as a mechanical vector, are active. *M. bovis* can also be transmitted by animal handlers, direct animal-to-animal contact with nasal and ocular discharges of infected animals, and contact with fomites.

Malignant catarrhal fever (MCF) has an ocular component clinically characterized by purulent ocular discharge. Affected animals frequently also have uveitis, featured by the presence of keratic precipitates, aqueous flare, hypopyon, fibrin in anterior chamber, and miosis, the improvement of which appears to be prognostic for survival. The histologically lymphocytic keratitis with endotheliitis, uveitis and vasculitis is probably immune mediated. With the 'head and eye' form of the disease, nystagmus may also be seen. (Also see Chapter 2: Diseases of the Nervous System and Chapter 5: Diseases of the Gastrointestinal System.)

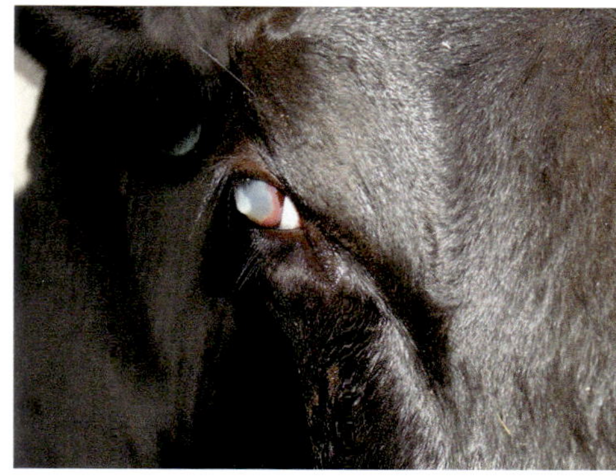

Fig. 15.12. Ox. Eye. Infectious bovine keratoconjunctivitis. Central corneal ulcer leading to abscess with stromal liquefaction is typical for this condition, likely because of lysis of the infiltrating neutrophils, triggered by *Moraxella bovis*-derived leukotoxins. Keratomalacia led to forward coning (keratoconus) of the weakened, inflamed central cornea in this cow. The remaining corneal stroma is edematous, with a prominent peripheral rim of vascularization extending from the limbus. (Courtesy of Dr F. Furlan, Universidade do Estado de Santa Catarina, Brazil.)

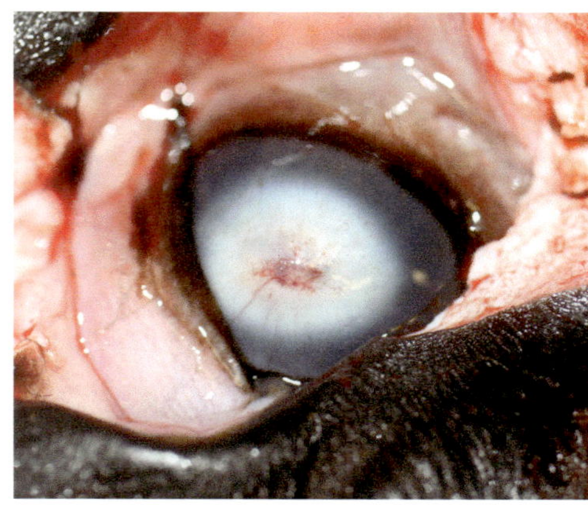

Fig. 15.13. Ox. Eye. Infectious bovine keratoconjunctivitis. A dense axial corneal scar (leukoma) developed after healing of the severe stromal defect in this 3-month-old Holstein calf. Infection by *Moraxella bovis* was suspected, but this bacterium was not recovered, even with the use of special cultures, probably due to the chronicity of the lesion. (Courtesy of Dr G. Rimoldi, CAHFS, University of California, USA)

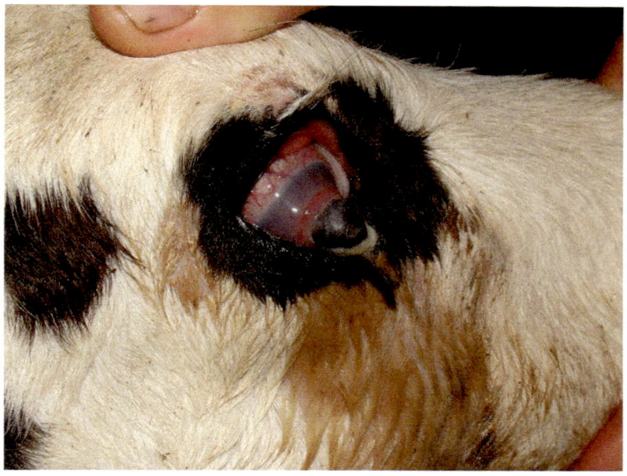

Fig. 15.14. Ox. Eye. Infectious bovine keratoconjunctivitis. Iris prolapse. Corneal rupture and prolapse of the iris are other possible, albeit overall uncommon, sequelae of the *Moraxella bovis*-induced corneal ulcer, leading to permanent blindness of the animal. (Courtesy of Dr F. Furlan, Universidade do Estado de Santa Catarina, Brazil.)

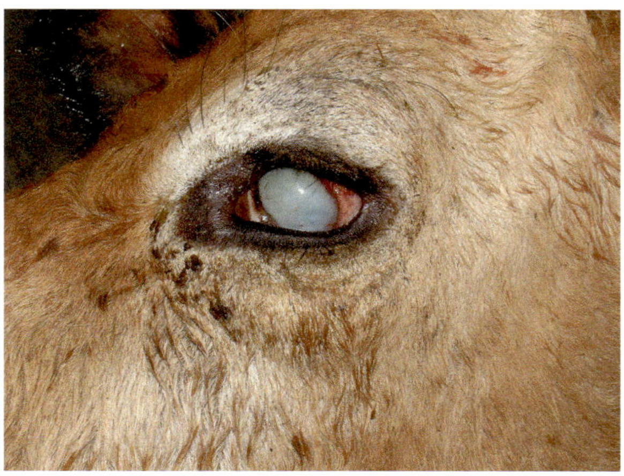

Fig. 15.15. Ox. Eye. Malignant catarrhal fever. Corneal edema, ocular discharge, and conjunctival hyperemia are among the most common clinical ocular findings with this disease. (Courtesy of Dr F. Furlan, Universidade do Estado de Santa Catarina, Brazil.)

Differential diagnoses. If nystagmus is noted in addition to neurologic disease in cattle, rabies virus infection and polioencephalomalacia should be considered in the differential diagnoses. Corneal disease characterized by bilateral edema can rarely be seen either at or soon after birth associated with an autosomal recessive endothelial disease. Corneal edema has also been seen in calves with bluetongue virus *in utero* infection and with phenothiazine toxicity.

Uveitis per se does not have a specific causative diagnosis. Instead, it is often associated with systemic disease (e.g. neonatal septicemia and septicemia associated with severe mastitis, metritis, traumatic reticuloperitonitis or reticulopericarditis, and thrombotic meningoencephalitis). Hypopyon, iris swelling, and miosis appear as predominant signs of acute uveitis, particularly in calves, where they are an important diagnostic indicator of septicemia, often of poor prognosis. When chronic, uveitis may be accompanied by posterior synechiae, predisposing to cataract formation.

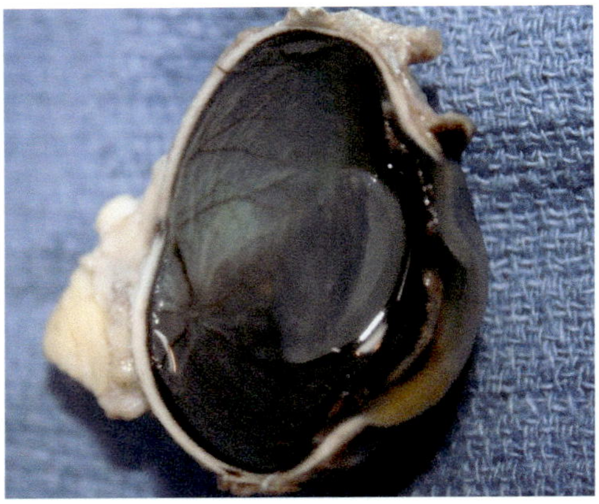

Fig. 15.16. Ox. Eye. Malignant catarrhal fever. Serofibrinous inflammatory exudate in the anterior chamber is indicative of uveitis and is another frequent finding with this disease. (Courtesy of Dr A. Berkowitz, University of Pennsylvania, USA.)

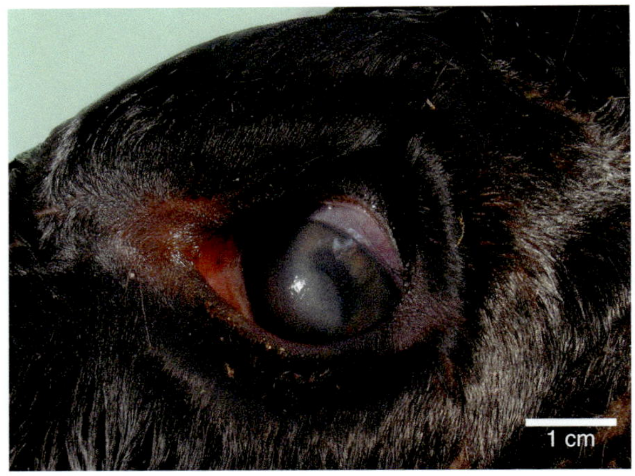

Fig. 15.17. Ox. Eye. Hypopyon. The purulent effusion in the anterior chamber in this calf should raise immediate suspicion of neonatal infection and sepsis (see Chapter 1: Diseases of Neonates and Calves). It occurs most frequently in calves with failure of passive transfer and, through multisystemic inflammation, can culminate in multiple organ dysfunction syndrome and death. If diagnosed in time and treated properly, however, the affected animal can recover. (Courtesy of Dr P. Mouser, Indiana Animal Diagnostic Laboratory, USA.)

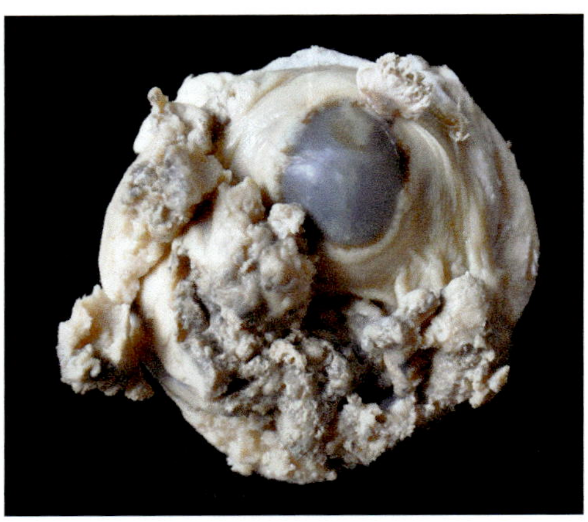

Fig. 15.18. Ox. Eye. Papilloma and squamous cell carcinoma. Ocular tumors of squamous epithelium often begin as a smooth, raised plaque that can progress to an exophytic squamous papilloma, as evident at the corneoscleral junction on the superior aspect of this globe. While some ocular papillomas will regress spontaneously, others develop into squamous cell carcinoma, as occurred at the inferior aspect of this globe. (Courtesy of Drs D. Driemeier and W. Panziera, Universidade Federal do Rio Grande do Sul, Brazil.)

15.4 NEOPLASTIC OCULAR DISEASES

Of the food animal species, cattle are the ones most affected by ocular and periocular neoplasms, with the great majority consisting of squamous cell carcinomas, followed by retrobulbar lymphomas. Papillomas can occur on the eyelids or corneoscleral junction, and predispose to ocular squamous cell carcinoma. Other ocular tumors are rarely reported in cattle and have included hemangiosarcoma, lymphangiosarcoma, Meibomian gland tumor, uveal melanoma, iridociliary adenoma, and optic meningioma.

15.4.1 Papilloma

Papillomas, or fibropapillomas if accompanied by stromal proliferation, may be sessile or pedunculated and, when large, may interfere with vision.

15.4.2 Squamous cell carcinoma

Squamous cell carcinoma (SCC) is the most common malignancy affecting the ocular region in cattle. The most common affected sites within the eye are the lower lid, the third eyelid, and the corneoscleral junction (limbus). The carcinoma arises typically within an epithelial plaque or papilloma. European breeds, in particular those with light corneoscleral pigmentation, such as Herefords, are predisposed to this neoplasm, with prevalence increasing with age. The prevalence of the neoplasm is also higher in geographical regions with higher levels of sunlight and, consequently, higher exposure to solar ultraviolet radiation. A viral cause has been suspected for many years. In particular, bovine papillomavirus has been thought to contribute to the induction, although not the maintenance, of this neoplastic lesion. Bovine herpesviruses, in particular BHV-5, have also been implicated in the development of ocular SCC, but further studies are required to verify this hypothesis. SCC tends to be locally aggressive. Thus, the best outcome is seen when lesions are treated early through surgical excision. The likelihood of metastases depends on the location of the SCC, with neoplasms in the eyelids showing a higher frequency of metastases to the regional lymph nodes, or even lungs, than neoplasms of the cornea and the limbus.

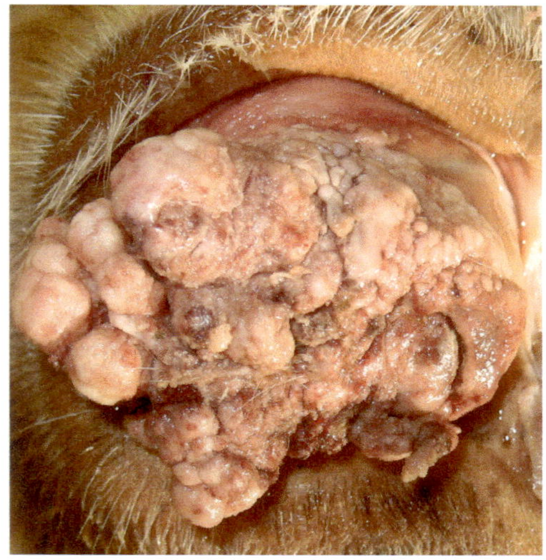

Fig. 15.19. Ox. Eye. Squamous cell carcinoma. Approximately 9 months earlier, this old Hereford cross cow had a squamous cell carcinoma removed from the third eyelid using cryosurgery. The neoplasm returned more aggressively, extending over the entire cornea.

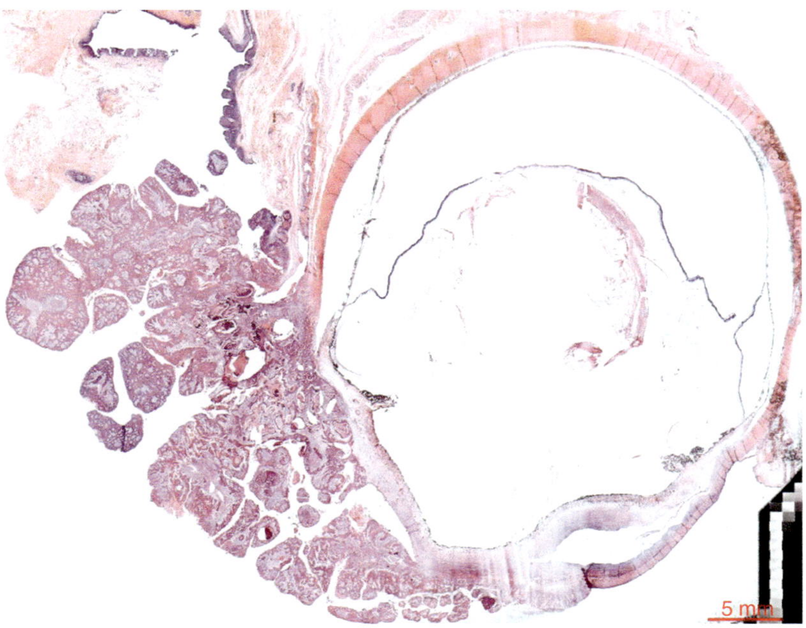

Fig. 15.20. Ox. Eye. Squamous cell carcinoma . Microscopically, the neoplasm consisted of a large, exophytic, papillomatous epithelial proliferation that spread extensively from the limbus region into the cornea. The corneal stroma was extensively fibrotic, with discontinuous Descemet's membrane (not evident in this section) and broad anterior synechiae (H&E).

15.4.3 Lymphoma

Lymphoma affecting the retrobulbar tissues is the most common cause of unilateral or bilateral exophthalmos in cattle, with or without strabismus. Accompanied by peripheral lymphadenomegaly, it is a common clinical presentation in cattle with multicentric bovine leukemia virus (BLV)-induced B-cell lymphoma. When protrusion of the affected globe becomes severe, exposure keratitis may occur.

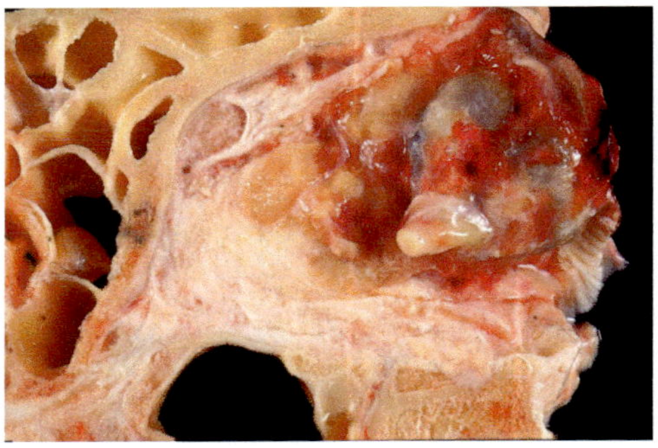

Fig. 15.22. Ox. Eye. Retrobulbar neoplasm. The retrobulbar neoplasm leading to unilateral proptosis in this cow was initially suspected to be due to lymphoma, the most common cause of orbital tumors in cattle. In aged cattle, nasal adenocarcinoma with spread into the retrobulbar space is another, rare cause of exophthalmos. In this case, the proptosis was determined to be due to a rare case of nasal adenosquamous tumor. (Courtesy of Dr M. Rebelatto, Indiana Animal Disease Diagnostic Laboratory, USA.)

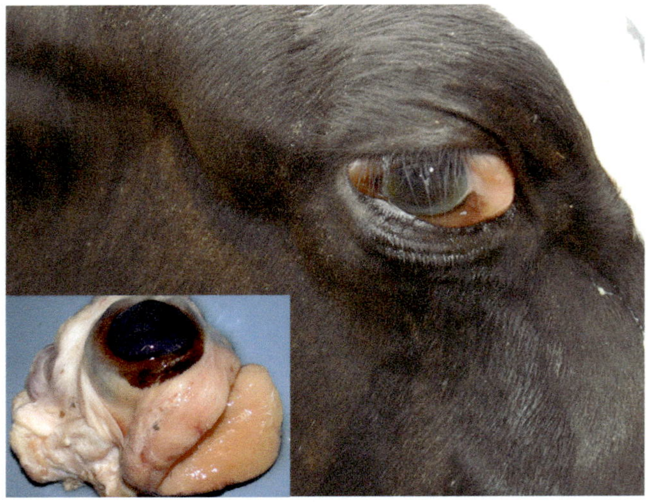

Fig. 15.21. Ox. Eye. Lymphoma. This cow with bovine leukosis had bilateral exophthalmos and conjunctival swelling as the result of enlarged retrobulbar lymph nodes that, on the exposed cut surface, had the characteristic tissue effacement by yellow-tan, homogeneous, diffuse cell infiltrate seen with lymphoma (inset). (Courtesy of Dr D. Driemeier, Universidade Federal do Rio Grande do Sul, Brazil.)

Differential diagnoses. Marked bilateral exophthalmos in calves can develop with daily dexamethasone treatment, leading to increased retrobulbar fat deposition. Exophthalmos can also be seen with inflammatory orbital disease secondary to trauma, puncture wounds of the eyelids or conjunctiva, foreign-body migration from the mouth, and actinobacillosis.

EARS

INTRODUCTION

Hearing is an important sense in livestock, although used less for localization of the source of the sound than vision. Of the livestock species, cattle have the most acute hearing, with Holstein cattle more sensitive to sound than beef cattle.

15.5 INFLAMMATORY OTIC DISEASES

Otitis externa in cattle is primarily associated with infestation by free-living rhabditiform nematodes and by *Raillietia auris* mites. Both parasites are found in the external auditory meatus of cattle. Otitis caused by nematodes of the genus *Rhabditis* mainly affects mature Zebu cattle with long, pendant, and gutter-shaped ears, in particular breeds with downward-growing horns, such as of the Gyr breed. Accumulation of secretion, in particular cerumen, likely promotes the growth and multiplication of the parasites, with larger horns probably contributing to increased parasitism by compressing the ear canal. The occurrence of parasitic otitis by *Rhabditis* seems to correlate with humid and hot climate, possibly due to a concurrent increase in fly populations, which have been recognized as vectors of the nematode. Raillietiosis affects a number of ruminant species, including cattle. Infestation is most frequently asymptomatic, but heavy parasitic infestations, often accompanied by secondary bacterial infections, can lead to weight loss, tympanic membrane rupture, otitis media, and even meningitis, microabscesses in the brain stem, and cranial nerve paralysis. Associated clinical signs include head tilt, head shaking, hearing loss, and ataxia. Though considered overall rare, otic parasitism in cattle may be overlooked. Secondary fungal and bacterial infections, such as caused by *Malassezia*, *Candida, Aspergillus, Pseudomonas, Proteus*, and *Trueperella pyogenes*, may complicate cases of parasitic otitis.

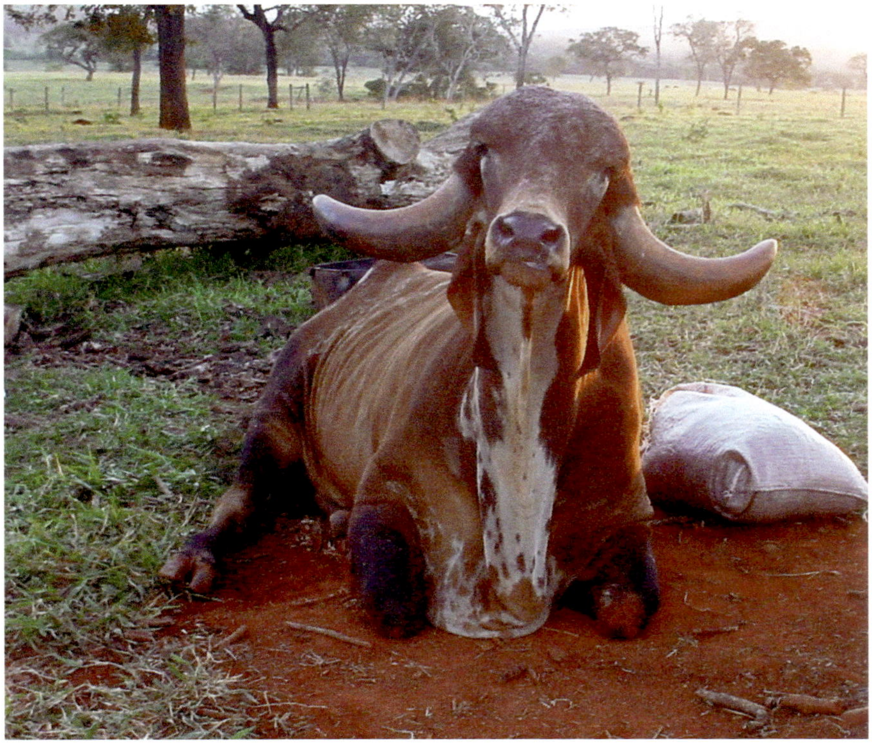

Fig. 15.23. Ox. Ear. *Rhabditis* otitis. Horned 8-year-old Gyr steer in recumbency due to ataxia, left head tilt, and drooping of the ipsilateral lip and eyelid (indicative of vestibulocochlear and facial nerve paralysis). In tropical regions, horned Gyr cattle are much more likely to be infested with *Rhabditis* compared to polled Gyr cattle (90% versus 40% prevalence), with older cattle more severely affected than younger animals. (Courtesy of Dr E. Facury Filho, Universidade Federal de Minas Gerais, Brazil.)

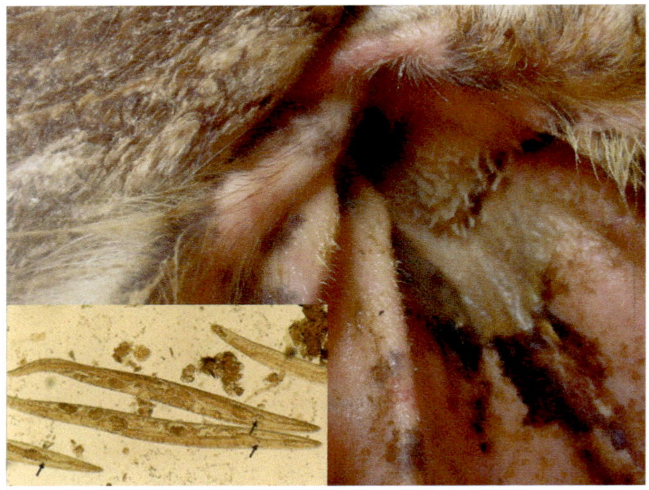

Fig. 15.24. Ox. Ear. *Rhabditis* otitis. External auditory meatus with secretion in a 5-year-old Gyr cow with rhabditiform nematode infestation. Inset: the minute nematodes have a characteristic rhabditiform esophagus, with a corpus, isthmus and the readily apparent bulb (arrows). (Courtesy of Dr E. Facury Filho, Universidade Federal de Minas Gerais, Brazil.)

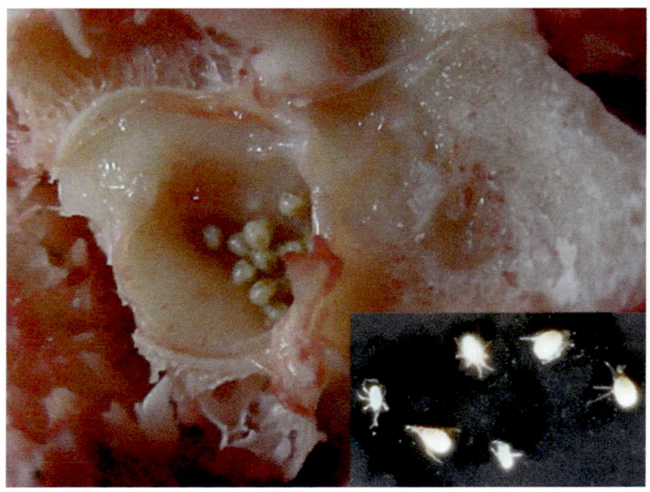

Fig. 15.25. Ox. Ear. Raillietiosis. Mites in the middle ear of a Nelore cow. While the cattle ear mite, *Raillietia auris*, is generally found in the external auditory meatus, it can also perforate the tympanic membrane and result in otitis media. Inset: detail of the mites. (Courtesy of Dr E. Facury Filho, Universidade Federal de Minas Gerais, Brazil.)

Primary otitis media and interna is most frequently seen in 1- to 2-month-old dairy calves. *Mycoplasma bovis* is the most common isolated agent from these animals. Feeding of infected milk is thought to be the most probable mode of transmission, with the infection likely extending from the pharynx via the auditory tube into the middle ear. (Also see Chapter 1: Diseases of Neonates and Calves.) Two other *Mycoplasma* species, *Mycoplasma bovirhinis* and *Mycoplasma alkalescens*, have been isolated from cows with mastitis, and from calves with otitis as well. Other bacterial agents occasionally associated with otitis in calves, in particular in pasture-raised beef calves, include *Histophilus somni*, *Mannheimia haemolytica*, *Pasteurella multocida*, *Streptococcus* spp., and *Trueperella pyogenes*, all agents involved in the bovine enzootic pneumonia complex.

Clinical signs include droopy ears, otorrhea, head tilt, facial nerve paralysis, and other neurologic signs. Some animals may also have evidence of pneumonia and polyarthritis.

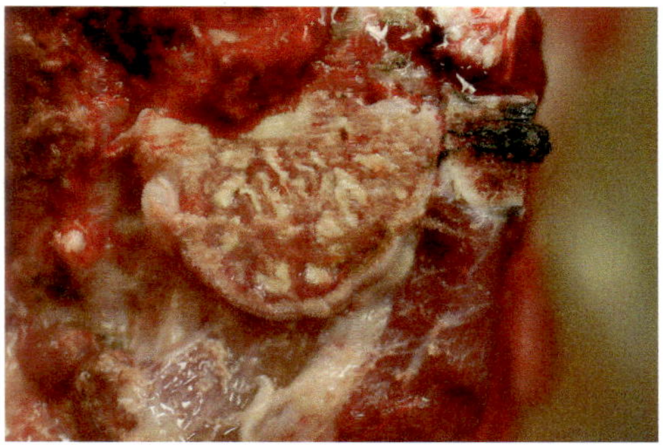

Fig. 15.26. Ox. Middle ear. Suppurative otitis media. Otitis media in calves is frequently associated with pneumonia. Also, this 5-week-old Jersey calf had bilateral cranioventral suppurative pneumonia in addition to the otitis media. From both the lung and the middle ear, *Mannheimia haemolytica* was isolated and *Mycoplasma* spp. was detected by PCR. *Mycoplasma bovis* appears to be the organism lasting the most in infections of this type. (Courtesy of Dr G. Rimoldi, CAHFS, University of California, USA.)

15.6 NEOPLASTIC OTIC DISEASES

Cutaneous neoplasms can also affect the external ear, although they are generally rare in this location. Cases of auricular papilloma, mast cell tumor, and melanoma have been reported in cattle.

SUGGESTED READING

Alexander, D. (2010) Infectious bovine keratoconjunctivitis: a review of cases in clinical practice. *Veterinary Clinics of North America: Food Animal Practice* 26, 487–503.

Duarte, E.R. and Hamdan, J.S. (2004) Otitis in cattle, an aetiological review. *Journal of Veterinary Medicine B Infectious Diseases and Veterinary Public Health* 51, 1–7.

Gollnick, N.S., Scharr, J.C., Schares, G. and Langenmayer, M.C. (2015) Natural *Besnoitia besnoiti* infections in cattle: chronology of disease progression. *BMC Veterinary Research* 11, 35.

Tsujita, H. and Plummer, C.E. (2010) Bovine ocular squamous cell carcinoma. *Veterinary Clinics of North America: Food Animal Practice* 26, 511–529.

Zemljič, T., Pot, S.A., Haessig, M. and Spiess, B.M. (2012) Clinical ocular findings in cows with malignant catarrhal fever: ocular disease progression and outcome in 25 cases (2007–2010). *Veterinary Ophthalmology* 15, 46–52.

CHAPTER 16

The Pathology of Select Poisonous Plant-induced Diseases in Cattle

Contributed by Bryan L. Stegelmeier
USDA/ARS Poisonous Plant Research Laboratory, Logan, Utah, USA

16.1 Neurotoxic Plants
16.1.1 Swainsonine/calystegine
16.1.1.1 Swainsonine or locoweed intoxication
16.1.1.2 Calystegine toxicity
16.1.1.3 Castanospermine
16.1.1.4 Ryegrass toxicity
16.1.1.5 *Delphinium* spp.
16.1.1.6 Nitrotoxins
16.1.1.7 Hemlocks
16.1.1.8 Lupines
16.1.1.9 Death camas

16.2 Hepatotoxic Plants
16.2.1 Dehydropyrrolizidine alkaloids
16.2.2 Saponin-containing plants
16.2.3 Cocklebur (*Xanthium strumarium*) and other potent hepatotoxic plants
16.2.4 Plants containing fungal hepatotoxins
16.2.4.1 Fumonisins
16.2.4.2 Lupinosis
16.2.4.3 Sporidesmin
16.2.4.4 Lantana

16.3 Myotoxic Plants
16.3.1 Cardioactive glycoside-containing plants
16.3.2 Rayless goldenrod and white snakeroot
16.3.3 Thermopsis and other myotoxic plants
16.3.4 *Cassia* or *Senna* spp.
16.3.5 Seleniferous plants
16.3.6 Yew (*Taxus cuspidata* – Japanese yew; *Taxus baccata* – common yew; and *Taxus media* – hybrid common and Japanese yew)

16.4 Teratogenic Plants
16.4.1 Lupine

16.5 Nephrotoxic Plants
16.5.1 Oak
16.5.2 Oxalate-containing plants
16.5.3 *Amaranthus* spp. (pigweeds)
16.5.4 Calcinogenic glycoside-containing plants

16.6 Other Toxic Plants
16.6.1 Pine needles
16.6.2 Cyanogenic plants
16.6.3 Nitrate-accumulating plants
16.6.4 Photosensitizing plants
16.6.4.1 Hypericism
16.6.4.2 Fagopyrism
16.6.4.3 Furocoumarins
16.6.5 Bracken fern
16.6.6 Hairy vetch (*Vicia villosa* Roth)

INTRODUCTION

Under most pasture or range conditions, toxic plants only occasionally poison cattle; however, when toxic plants contaminate prepared feeds, alternative safe forages are not available, or some change such as grazing pressure, soil disruption, cultivation, or herbicide treatment increases plant availability, palatability, or toxicity, poisoning can be epidemic and devastating. Toxic plants rarely produce characteristic gross and histologic lesions; consequently, diagnostics are challenging and require multidisciplinary cooperation to identify definitively. The objectives of this chapter are to review the pathologic changes characteristic of disease in cattle produced by toxic plants.

16.1 NEUROTOXIC PLANTS

16.1.1 Swainsonine/calystegine

16.1.1.1 Swainsonine or locoweed intoxication

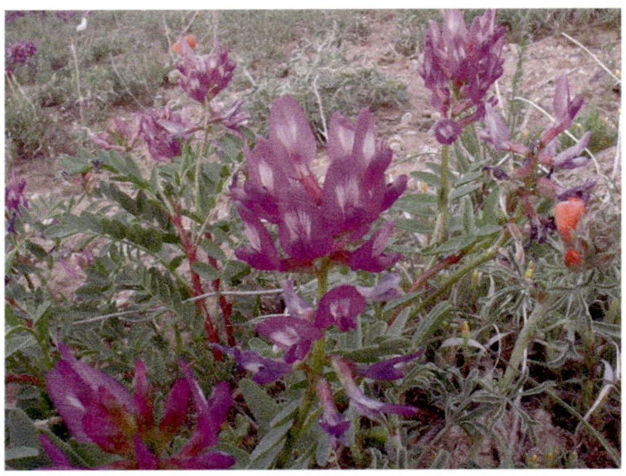

Fig. 16.1. *Oxytopis lambertii*, or Lamberts locoweed, is a North American perennial that occasionally poisons cattle. All locoweed poisoning is caused by endophyte-produced swainsonine. Endophyte infection is spread vertically in the seed coat, and infections vary between and within plant populations. Swainsonine and endophyte infection has been identified in over 30 *Astragalus* and *Oxytropis* species in the Americas and Asia. Other swainsonine-containing plants include *Swainsona* spp. of Australia, and *Ipomoea* and *Physalis* species in South America.

Locoweeds are *Astragalus* and *Oxytropis* species that contain swainsonine. Swainsonine inhibits cellular mannosidases, producing an induced storage disease similar to genetic mannosidosis. Poisoning requires continuous enzyme inhibition, and when cattle ingest locoweed for 2 weeks, they develop subtle neurologic disease.

Clinical signs. With continued exposure, animals become weak and develop obvious proprioceptive deficits and intention tremors. Chronically poisoned cattle have dull and rough-appearing coats that may not shed in season, and their eyes appear dull or less transparent. Months of extended exposure produce severe neurologic signs, including depression, disorientation, and obvious loss of proprioception, excitability, irregular gait with hypermetria, and incoordination. Chronically poisoned animals have severe anorexia and they become emaciated and recumbent. Poisoning is generally not fatal and emaciated cattle are often euthanized.

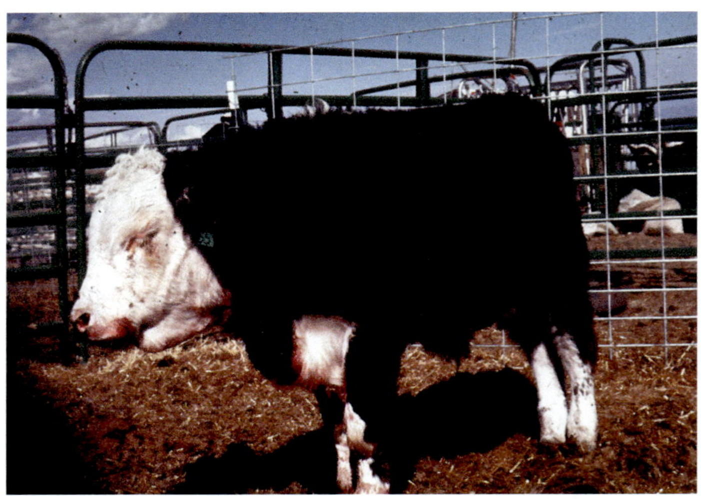

Fig. 16.2. Ox. Whole body. Steer poisoned with *Oxytropis sericea* at about 3000 m altitude. Notice the marked subcutaneous edema in the sternum, neck, and jaw secondary to altitude-related congestive heart failure (high-mountain disease). In this study, all locoweed-poisoned steers developed congestive heart failure compared to none of the controls.

Gross changes. Locoweed-induced reproductive lesions include disrupted estrus cycles, as many cattle have enlarged and cystic ovaries. Others develop anestrus or dysfunction reproductively due to massive neurologic deficits. Though early gestational poisoning does not alter embryogenesis, implantation, or placentation, it is fetotoxic and results in fetal resorption or abortion. Late-gestation poisoning often results in hydrops amnii. Transplacental and transmammary poisoning results in fetal and neonatal visceral and neurologic lesions similar to adults. Poisoning in bulls alters both spermatogenesis and spermatozoal maturation. Both male and female locoweed-induced lesions are reversible and functionally restored within several estrus cycles if neurologic damage is not so severe it alters behavior and libido. Locoweed-poisoned cattle also develop pulmonary hypertension and, when at high altitudes, many will develop congestive heart failure (high-mountain disease).

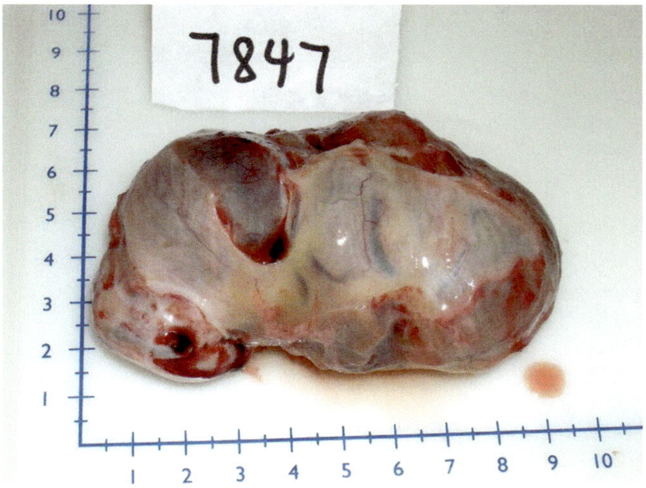

Fig. 16.3. Ox. Ovary. Cysts. Left ovary from an animal poisoned with *Astragalus lentiginosus.* Notice the large cysts that were identified as both follicular and large luteal cysts. The cysts were functional, resulting in abnormal estrus behavior. When locoweed ingestion was discontinued, the right ovary, which was left *in situ*, returned to normal, and regular estrus behavior resumed with 42 days.

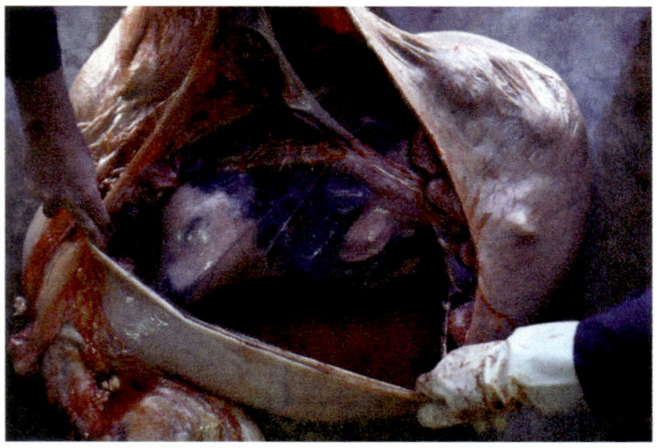

Fig. 16.4. Ox. Hydrops amnii. Fluid-filled uterus in a cow that was poisoned with *Oxytropis sericea.* Notice the excessive fluid in the amniotic sac. The fetus had neurologic and visceral vacuolation similar to the cow.

Microscopic changes of locoweed poisoning are characterized by widespread visceral and neurologic cytoplasmic vacuolation. These lesions are most severe and prominent in GABAergic neurons of the cerebellum and basal ganglia. Other neurons and even oligodendroglia develop fine vacuolation with extended exposures. Additional changes that are less obvious via light microscopy include loss of dendritic connections, axonal dystrophy, and abnormal neuritic processes that involve meganeurite formation at the axonal hillock, and aberrant synapses and dendritic outgrowths. Severely poisoned animals have fewer cerebellar Purkinje cells (seen as empty axonal baskets), with subsequent axonal degeneration and spheroid formation. Cattle also develop vacuolation of the exocrine pancreas, thyroid follicular epithelium, renal tubular epithelium, macrophages and histiocytic cells, and various other tissues. The visceral lesions resolve within a couple of weeks of discontinuing exposure. If neurologic damage is not extensive, poisoned animals will recover. However, severely poisoned animals may develop irreversible neurological deficits, and these animals should be considered dangerous and unfit for work.

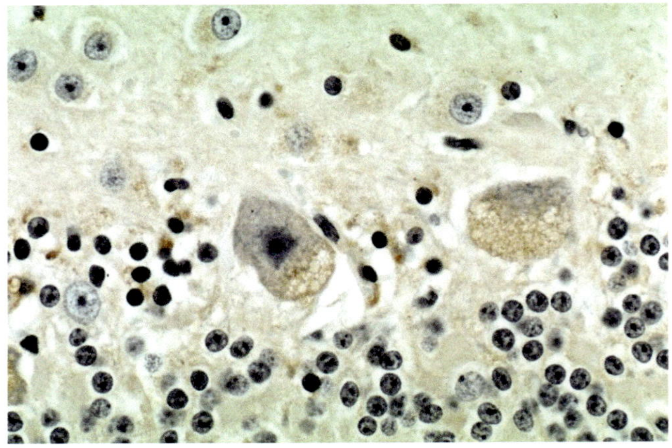

Fig. 16.5. Ox. Cerebellum. Cow was poisoned with *Astragalus lentiginosus* at a rate of 1.8 mg swainsonine/kg/day for 45 days. Notice the swelling and fine vacuolation in the cytoplasm of the Purkinje cells. These vacuoles are stained with lectin concanavalin A, marking the remaining mannose-rich oligosaccharides within the neuron cell body (lectin stain).

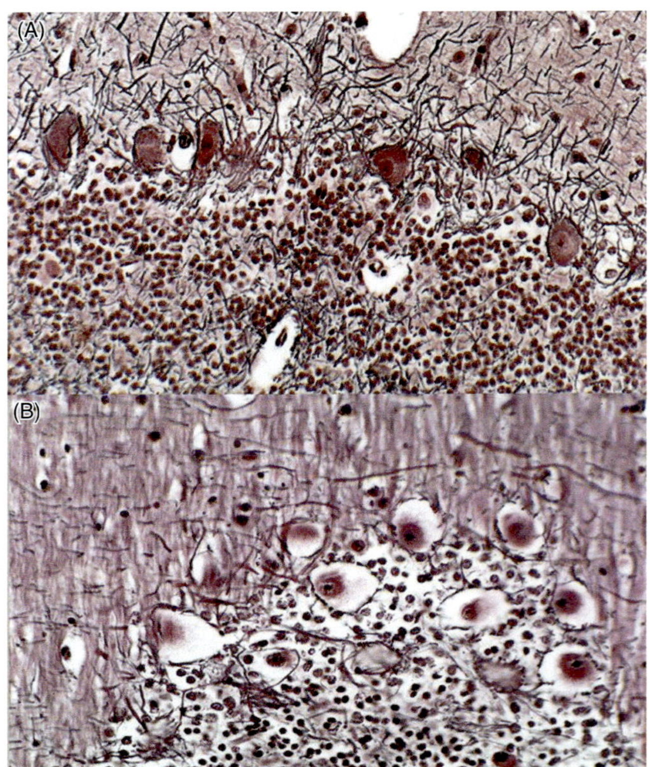

Fig. 16.6. Ox. Cerebellum. Cerebellum from a control (A) and an animal poisoned with *Astragalus lentiginosus* at a rate of 1.5 mg swainsonine/kg/day for 45 days (B). These sections are stained with modified Bodian silver stain (Yamamoto and Hirano) to visualize axon–Purkinje cell interactions. Note the Purkinje cell swelling, with marked decreases in axon interations in locoweed-poisoned animals (silver stain).

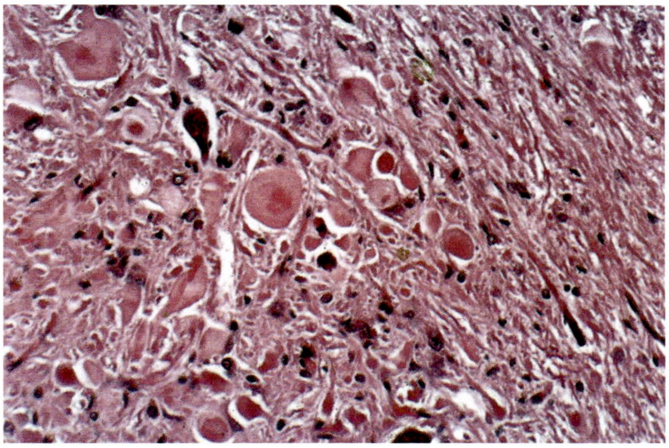

Fig. 16.7. Ox. Cerebrum. Nucleus gracilis near the obex in an animal poisoned with *Astragalus lentiginosus* at a rate of 1.5 mg swainsonine/kg/day for 45 days. Notice the focally severe axonal swelling and dystrophy with large eosinophilic spheroids (H&E).

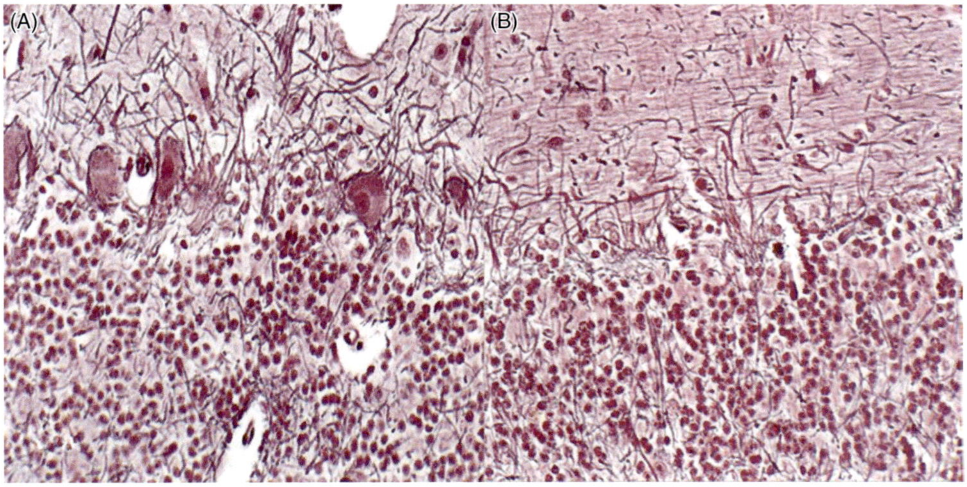

Fig. 16.8. Ox. Cerebellum. Cerebellum from a control (A) and an animal poisoned with *Astragalus lentiginosus* at a rate of 1.5 mg swainsonine/kg/day for 45 days (B). These sections are stained with a modified Bodian silver stain (Yamamoto and Hirano) to visualize axons and highlight empty baskets where Purkinje cells have died and disappeared. Notice the numerous empty baskets in the locoweed-poisoned animals (silver stain).

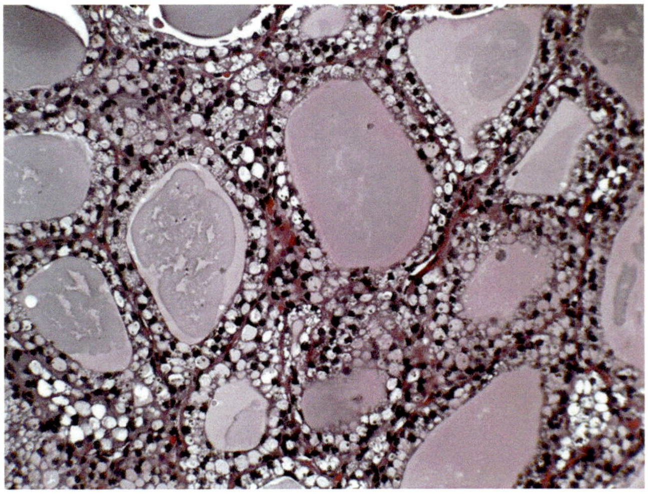

Fig. 16.9. Ox. Thyroid. Cow poisoned with *Astragalus lentiginosus* at a rate of 1.8 mg swainsonine/kg/day for 45 days. Notice the swelling and fine vacuolation in the thryroid epithelial cells (H&E).

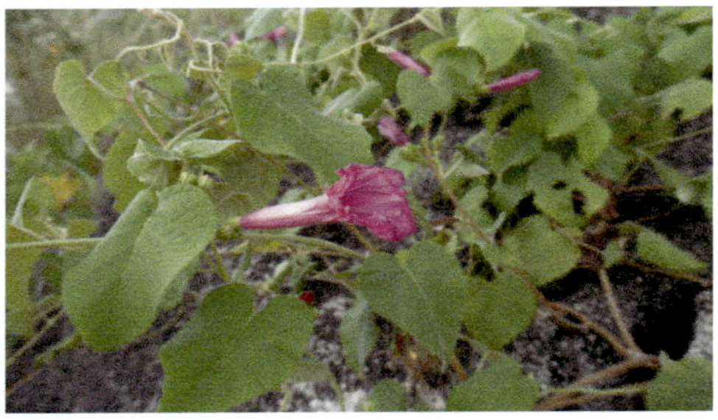

Fig. 16.10. *Ipomoea carnea* from near Campina Grande, Brazil. Although it is not highly palatable, animals become poisoned during times of drought when alternative forages are not available. This *I. carnea* contained 0.0029% swainsonine and 0.0045% of a mixture of calystegines B_1, B_2, B_3, and C_1. Poisoning is probably due to both calystegine and swainsonine, as the described clinical disease is more severe and lethal than disease produced by swainsonine alone.

16.1.1.2 Calystegine toxicity

Calystegines are glycosidase-inhibiting alkaloids that have been identified in *Calystegia sepium*, *Atropa belladonna*, *Convolvulus arvensis*, and various other *Solanum*, *Scopolia*, *Hyoscyamus*, *Morus*, *Datura*, *Physalis*, and *Ipomoea* species. The calystegines inhibit ß-glucosidase and α-galactosidase and ß-xylosidase, but most plants associated with animal poisoning have both swainsonine and calystegines. With some exceptions, clinical signs and lesions are similar to locoweed-induced disease. Calystegine-associated diseases include an ataxic syndrome in cattle grazing *Ipomoea muelleri* and *Ipomoea lonchophylla* in north-west Australia, 'crazy cow syndome' in Texas, associated with *Solanum dimidiatum*, and 'mad-drunk disease' in South Africa, associated with *Solanum kwebense*. Cerebral dysfunction with severe neuronal vacuolation has been described in these diseases; however, none have been reproduced experimentally with calystegines alone.

16.1.1.3 Castanospermine

Castanospermine is structurally similar to swainsonine and is a potent inhibitor of α-glucosidase. The castanospermine-containing Morton Bay chestnut tree (*Castanospermum australe*) in Australia has been shown to produce fatal gastroenteritis with myocardial degeneration and nephrosis in cattle and horses.

16.1.1.4 Ryegrass toxicity

Two different 'ryegrass toxicity' syndromes are caused by *Lolium* (Poaceae) spp.; however, the toxins, clinical disease, lesions, and the outcome are different.

Perennial ryegrass staggers. This is a reversible Australian disease that occurs when cattle graze *Lolium perenne* that contains endophyte-produced tremorgenic lolitrem B and ergovaline. Disease develops after livestock graze ryegrass for 7–14 days.
Clinical signs include incoordination, staggering, trembling, and collapse with muscular spasms. Disease resolution is within a couple of days if exposure is discontinued. Poisoning is usually not fatal, although chronically poisoned animals may become emaciated and have to be culled.
Histologic changes are generally related to wasting, but subtle vacuolation and degeneration of cerebellar granular and Purkinje cells have been described.

Annual ryegrass toxicity. This is a fatal neurologic disease of Australian and South African livestock grazing annual or Wimmera ryegrass (*Lolium rigidum* Gaud.) that is parasitized by the nematode *Anguina funesta*. The nematode is infected with *Rathayibacter toxicus* that produces corynetoxins. Corynetoxins inhibit *N*-acetylglucosamine-1-phosphate transferase (GPT), resulting in accumulation of *N*-linked glycoproteins in the endoplasmic reticulum.
Clinical signs. Poisoned animals lag behind, and when forced to move, they may collapse, become recumbent, and develop convulsion-like trembling and paddling. Other signs include muscle tremors, head nodding, opisthotonus, teeth grinding, nystagmus, and hypersalivation.

Gross lesions include an enlarged, friable, and yellowish liver, with gall-bladder distension and ocassional petechial serosal hemorrhages on the gall bladder and epicardium.

Microscopic changes. Affected hepatocytes are swollen with eosinophilic cytoplasmic expansion or inclusions (most likely distended endoplasmic reticulum). The neurologic lesions are minimal eosinophilic deposits of protein-like fluid in the subarachnoid space and along small vessels. There is also loss of Purkinje cells, and there is neuronal eosinophilia of both Purkinje cells and granular cells.

16.1.1.5 Delphinium *spp.*

Larkspurs (*Delphinium* spp.) are common in pastures and ranges of western North America. Cattle are uniquely susceptible, and poisoning is reported by *Delphinium barbeyi*, *Delphinium occidentale*, *Delphinium glaucescens*, and *Delphinium glaucum* (tall larkspurs); *Delphinium nuttallianum*, *Delphinium bicolor*, *Delphinium andersonii* (low larkspurs), and *Delphinium geyeri* (plains larkspur). Toxic *Delphinium* alkaloids are nicotinic acetylcholine (nACh) receptor antagonists that effectively block neuromuscular transmission. As binding appears to be competitive, cholinergic potentiating drugs neostigmine and physostigmine are useful for reversing many of the clinical signs.

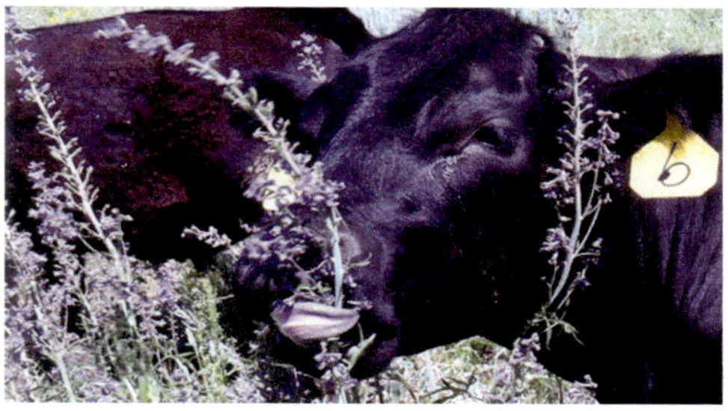

Fig. 16.11. *Delphinium barbeyi* (tall or Barbey's larkspur) is a perennial that grows to 1.5 m tall in subalpine and alpine zones, where it often dominates some plant communities of the western USA. In some ranges, it consistently encangers cattle, and stock losses have often been calculated as up to 10% per year.

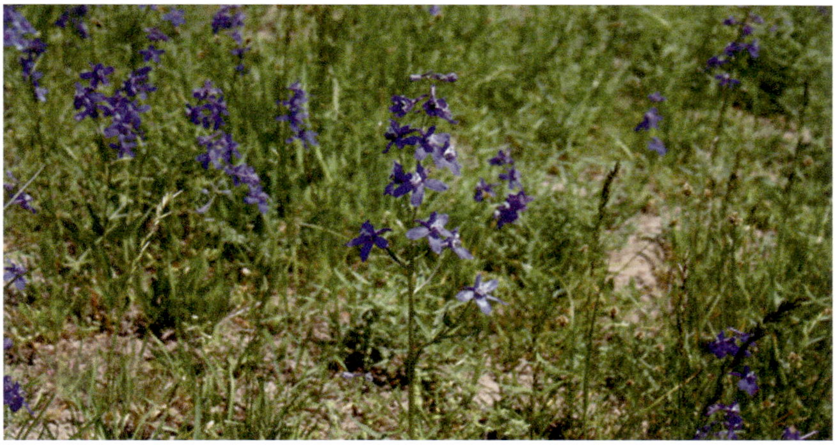

Fig. 16.12. *Delphinium andersonii* (low or Anderson's larkspur) is an annual larkspur common in meadows and fields of the western USA. Its populations cycle with available precipitation, resulting in seasonal population expansions that can produce epidemic poisoning. This larkspur grows in the early spring; quickly flowers and produces seed; and then quickly senesces. Cattle poisonings can be avoided by waiting until the senescence, when pods have shattered in early June before allowing cattle access.

Clinical signs. Initially, poisoning produces restlessness and agitation, followed by muscular tremors, frequent urination, incomplete defecation, and increased shallow respiration, tachycardia, and severe general muscular weakness. Severely poisoned animals collapse, and when limited in lateral recumbency, they develop dyspnea as a result of respiratory paralysis, rumen distension, and tympany.

Gross lesions include rumen tympany and pulmonary emphysema. As these are non-specific lesions, diagnosis is generally made by documenting exposure, clinical signs, the lack of pathologic leisons, and chemical identification of *Delphenium* alkdaloids in ingesta or tissues.

16.1.1.6 Nitrotoxins

In plants, the nitrotoxins (3-nitropropanol or 3-nitropropanoic acid) are generally glycosides called miserotoxins. They have been identified in 263 North American *Astragalus* species or varieties. The nitrotoxin glycosides and esters are hydrolyzed rapidly and oxidized to nitropropionic acid (NPA). NPA is a metabolic toxin that also oxidizes hemoglobin, producing methemoglobinemia, which has been used as an indicator of disease. GABAergic neurons appear to be highly sensitive to NPA-induced damage, and the basal ganglion leisons, though difficult to detect in clinical cases, have been described in various experimental models.

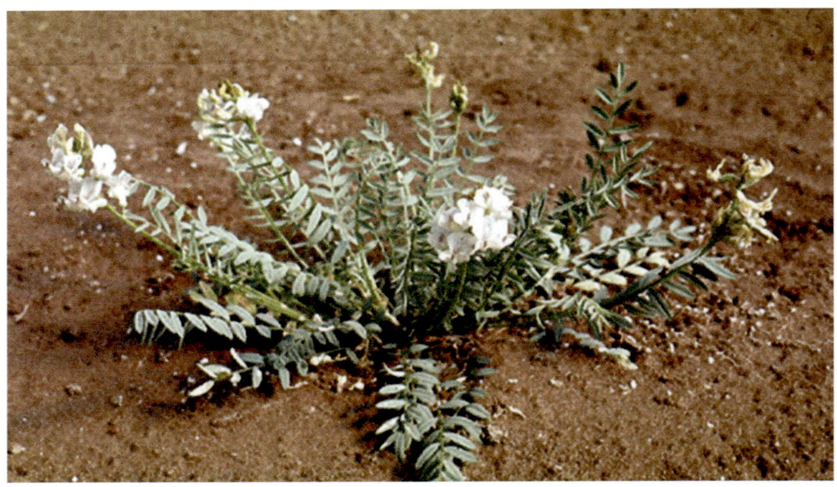

Fig. 16.13. *Astragalus miser* (timber milk vetch) is a perennial herb, with various varieties found through the western USA. These are a low-growing legume that frequently dominates plant communities in moist, shaded areas in alpine and subalpine zones.

Clinical signs. Poisoned cattle become dyspneic, with muscular incoordination and weakness, frequent urination, cyanotic mucous membranes, collapse, and recumbency. Severe poisoning is usually lethal within 25 h, and exercise exacerbates clinical disease.

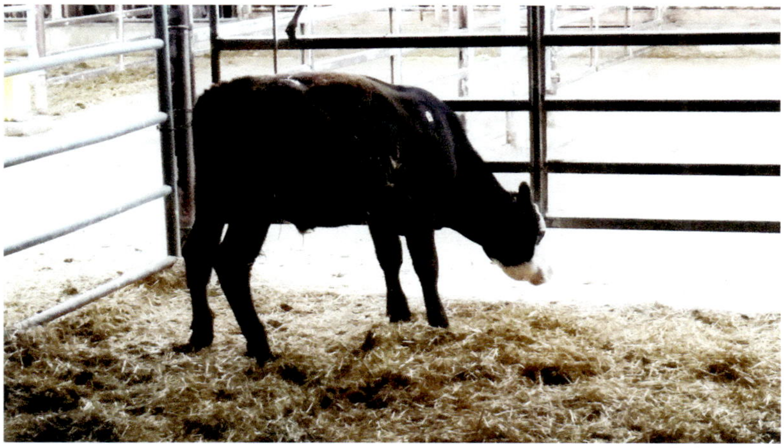

Fig. 16.14. Ox. Whole body. Steer poisoned with *Astragalus miser.* Notice the dyspnea in this animal, seen as extended neck and open-mouth breathing. He was also weak and reluctant to stand. Electrodes are visible that were used to monitor his electrocardiogram. This steer had a normal cardiac rhythm other than tachycardia, which was probably related to the increased physical exertion required to walk and stand.

Gross lesions include pulmonary edema, and the subsequent dyspnea results in extensive interlobular edema and emphysema.

Histologic lesions include degeneration and necrosis of neurons of the thalamus, patchy cerebellar Purkinje cell necrosis, spongiosis of the white tracts in the globus pallidus, distension of the lateral ventricles, and Wallerian degeneration of the ventral and lateral columns of the spinal cord and of the sciatic nerves.

16.1.1.7 Hemlocks

The toxic hemlocks include *Conium maculatum* (poison hemlock) and *Cicuta* spp. (water hemlock). Poison hemlock is a biennial that grows to about 2 m tall, with white flowers and distinguishing purple spots on the stem. Poison hemlock toxins include γ-coniceine and coniine, which are nicotinic acetylcholine receptor agonists.

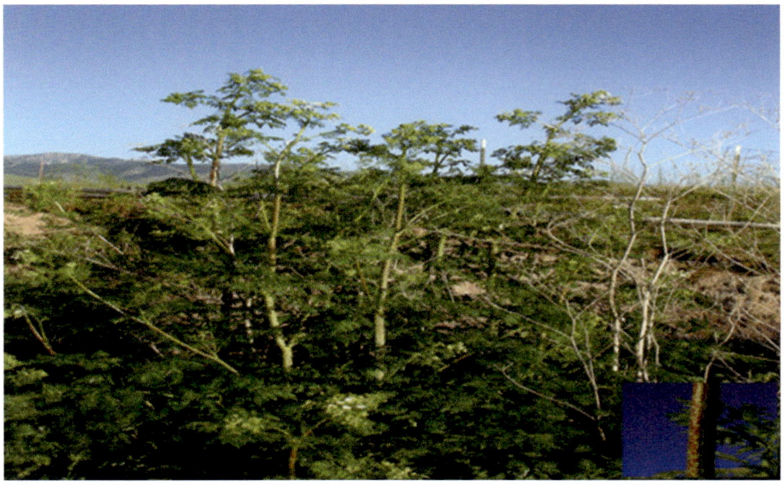

Fig. 16.15. *Conium maculatum* (poison hemlock) is a tall, 1–2 m plant, with a carrot-like leaf that sprouts early, often making it the first and often the only green plant in the spring. Identification is facilitated by the characteristic dark, almost purple spots on the stems (inset). Poisoning occurs in the early spring when there are few other forage options, or when it is chopped and fed to cattle fresh.

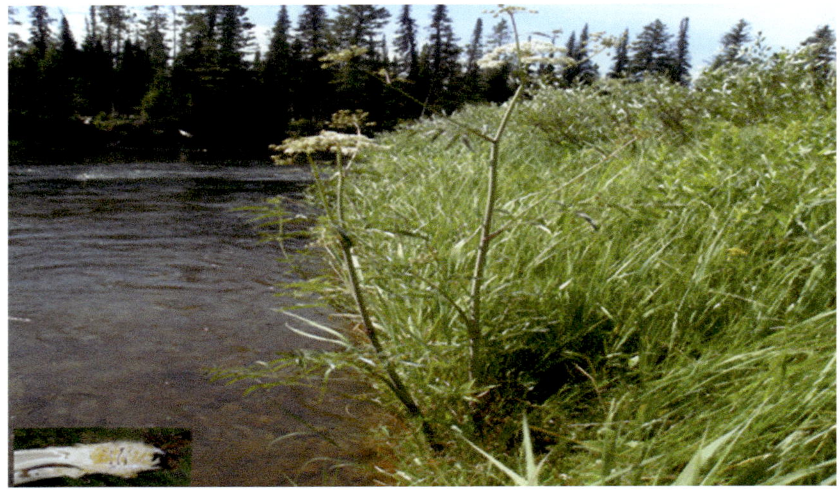

Fig. 16.16. *Cicuta maculata* (water hemlock) is a tall, carrot-like plant that commonly grows along streams and ditches. Identification is helped by examination of the root, which is chambered when sectioned (inset).

Clinical disease is characterized by initial stimulation, seen as nervousness, with frequent urination and defecation, rapid pulse, temporarily impaired vision (the nictitating membrane fails to retract), muscular weakness, muscle fasciculations, ataxia, incoordination, followed by depression, recumbency, collapse, and death from respiratory failure. Water hemlock is a similar tall biennial, but it has tuberous, chambered roots and grows in wet habitats along stream beds and ditch banks. The water hemlock toxin, cicutoxin, is a potent convulsant thought to interact with GABA receptors.

Clinical signs. Posonining is characterized by ataxia, dyspnea, muscular tremors, and weakness that progress to spastic head and neck movements, and then to intermittent grand mal seizures. If the seizures are not controlled, they lead to prolonged asphyxia and death.

The post-mortem and histologic lesions with both types of hemlock poisoning are lacking, with minimal, non-specific changes relating to the animal's agonal condition. Some are subtle, including seizure-related subcutaneous bruising and dermal abrasions.

16.1.1.8 Lupines

Lupines are legumes with worldwide distribution that may contain a variety of quinolizidine and piperidine lupine alkaloids, which generally act as agonists at nicotinic acetylcholine receptors. This produces several differing toxic syndromes ranging from congenital abnormalities, hepatotoxicity, and acute neurologic disease. The neurologic disease is described historically as livestock that eat toxic lupine seed pods.

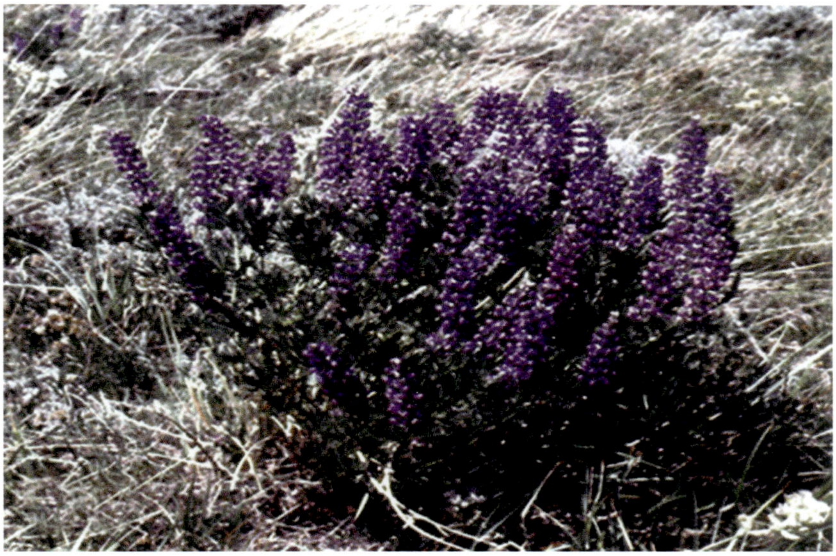

Fig. 16.17. *Lupinus caudatus* (tailcup lupine) is an example of the many lupine species. They are flowering legumes that have many different phenotypes and chemotypes, suggesting that different populations may have very different toxin types and concentrations. As taxonomy is difficult, sampling for accurate identification and chemical analysis is indicated to best predict risk.

Clinical signs. Poisoned animals become nervous, with increased urination and defecation, depression, frothing at the mouth, ataxia, muscular fasciculations, weakness, lethargy, collapse, recumbency, respiratory failure, and death.

Post-mortem and histologic examinations of poisoned animals are generally unremarkable. The teratogenic effects of lupine will be discussed later.

16.1.1.9 Death camas

Toxicoscordion or *Zigadenus* spp. (death camases) are found in North and Central America, where they grow in the early spring and quickly senesce in the early summer. Recent poisonings in cattle indicate that in wet spring weather and when combined with low larkspur (*Delphenium* spp.), cattle can be fatally poisoned, with high morbidity and mortality. Death camas contains several toxins but zygadenine predominates in most plants, and it has been used to monitor exposure and identify poisoned animals.

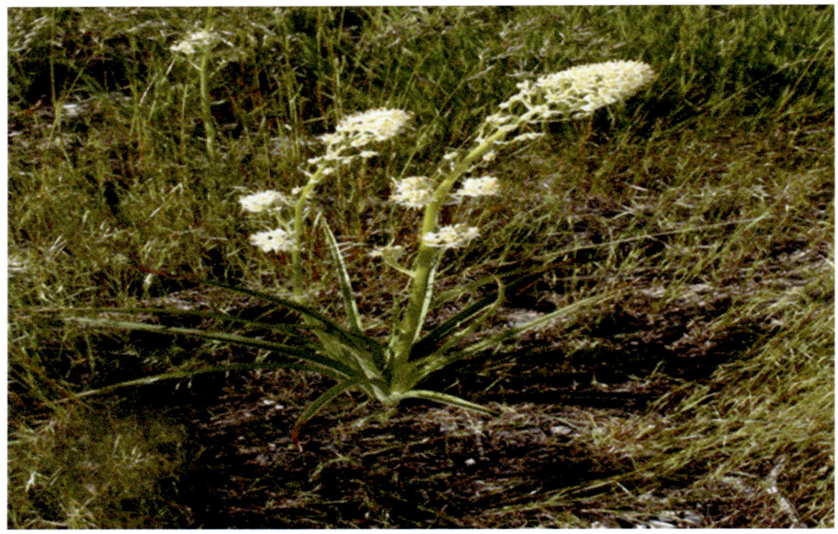

Fig. 16.18. *Toxicoscordion venenosum* (previously *Zigadenus venenosum*) is a grass-like plant that sprouts from a bulb, grows, flowers, produces seeds, and senesces in the spring and early summer. Identification can be difficult, and submission of the entire plant in flower is recommended.

Clinical signs. Poisoning is characterized by frothy hypersalivation, hypothermia, depression, nausea, vomiting, retching, colic, and grinding of the teeth. With more severe poisoning, animals develop trembling, incoordination, severe depression, and weakness. With fatally poisoned animals, the syndrome progresses to severe tachycardia and dyspnea, recumbent coma, and death. The diagnosis is made using exposure, clinical signs, the lack of gross and microscopic lesions, and chemical identification of zydadenine in ingesta and tissues.

16.2 HEPATOTOXIC PLANTS

16.2.1 Dehydropyrrolizidine alkaloids

Hepatotoxic dehydropyrrolizidine alkaloids (PAs) are found in plants throughout the world. Plants associated with poisoning livestock include species of *Senecio*, *Heliotropium*, *Echium*, *Symphytum*, *Crotalaria*, *Cyanoglossum*, and *Trichodesma* genera. Cattle are highly sensitive to PA poisoning.

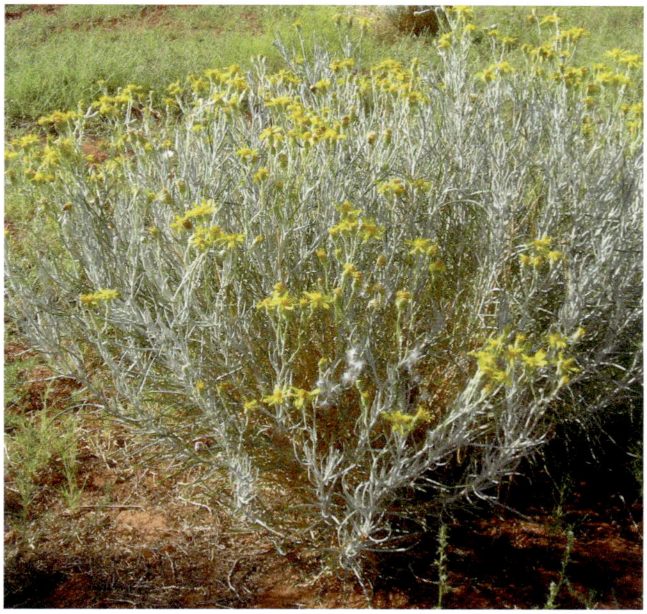

Fig. 16.19. *Senecio longilobus* (threadleaf or wooly groundsel) is found in desert zones of the south-west USA. As with other dehydropyrrolizidine alkaloid (DHPA)-containing plants, it is not very palatable and is generally avoided by livestock. Cattle are poisoned when there are no other forages available. Many other DHPA-containing plants are invasive and contaminate feeds and food.

Clinical signs. Acutely intoxicated animals develop acute liver failure, with signs of anorexia, depression, icterus, visceral edema, and ascites. Poisoned animals will have massive elevations in serum enzyme activity (AST, SDH, ALK, and GGT), and increased serum bilirubin, and bile acids. Many animals also develop hepatogeneous photosensitivity.

Gross lesions of acute poisoning are prominent panlobular hepatocellular necrosis accompanied by hemorrhage, with minimal inflammation. Chronic poisoning is less severe with minimal clinical signs, minimal change in serum enzyme activities, bilirubin or bile acids, and minimal hepatic fibrosis and hepatocyte damage.

Histologic lesions vary according to the exposure, but classically lesions include hepatic necrosis, fibrosis, biliary hyperplasia, and megalocyte production. Certain potent alkylating toxins such as aflatoxins should be considered as differential diagnoses. The variability of presentation and lesions often makes a definitive diagnosis difficult.

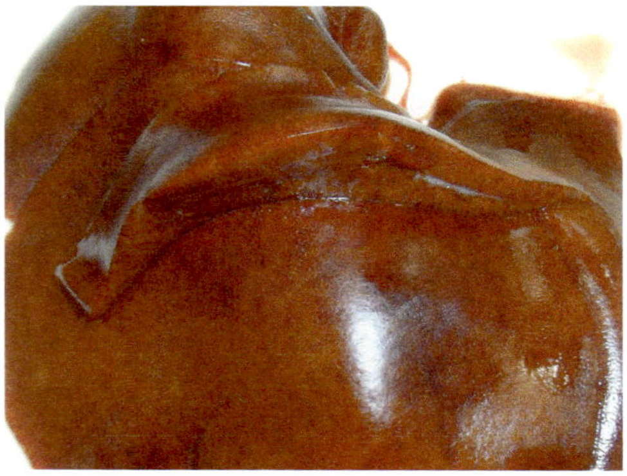

Fig. 16.20. Ox. Liver. Necrosis. Notice the lobular hemorrhage, necrosis, and hepatic icterus.

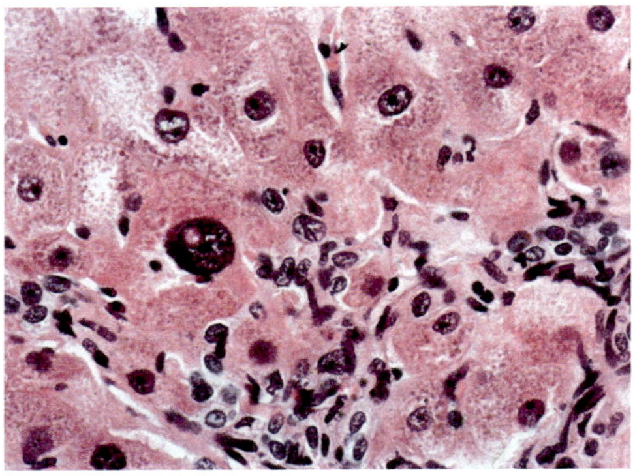

Fig. 16.22. Ox. Liver. Megalocytosis. Animal chronically poisoned with *Cynoglossum officinale*. Notice the minimal piecemeal necrosis and single large hepatic megalocyte. Megalocytosis development is dependent on PA characteristics as well as the dose and the duration, as it is not seen in all presentations (H&E).

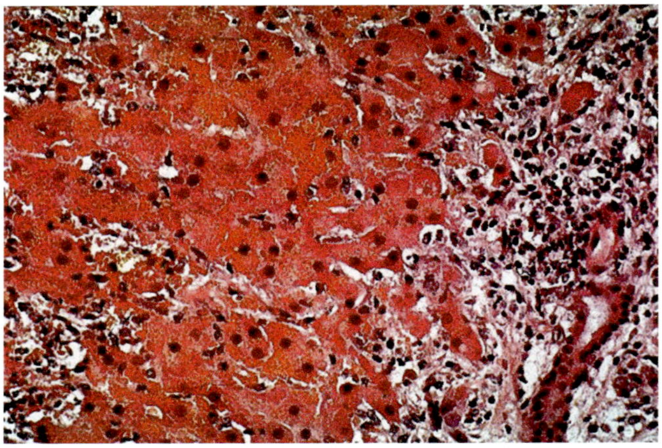

Fig. 16.21. Ox. Liver. Necrosis. Cow acutely poisoned with *Senecio jacobea*. Notice the extensive hemorrhagic necrosis, collapse of hepatic sinusoids, and early proliferation of biliary epithelium (H&E).

16.2.2 Saponin-containing plants

Plant saponins are glycosides with distinctive foaming characteristics. Toxic saponin-containing plants include *Tribulus terrestris*, *Narthecium ossifragum*, *Agave lechuguilla*, and various species of *Brachiaria*, *Panicum*, and *Sesbania* genera.

Clinical signs. Secondary or hepatogenous photosenstivity. This photoirradiation-induced dermatitis (photosensitivity) affects lightly haired, unpigmented, or unprotected skin. Conjunctivitis and subsequent photophobia are common presentations. In lactating cows, the udder may be burned severely, resulting in premature weaning of calves and marked loss of production.

Histologic lesions. Other than the radiation-associated necrotizing dermatitis, the primary reported histologic lesion is crystalline hepatopathy, which is characterized by the inclusion of eosinophilic crystalline material in bile canuliculi and hepatocytes. These crystals are calcium salts of sapogenic glucuronides that inhibit or block biliary function. The diagnosis is made by ruling out other causes of hepatogenous photosensitivity and identifying saponin-containing plants. If hepatic damage is not extensive, most animals recover hepatic function and the photosensitivity resolves.

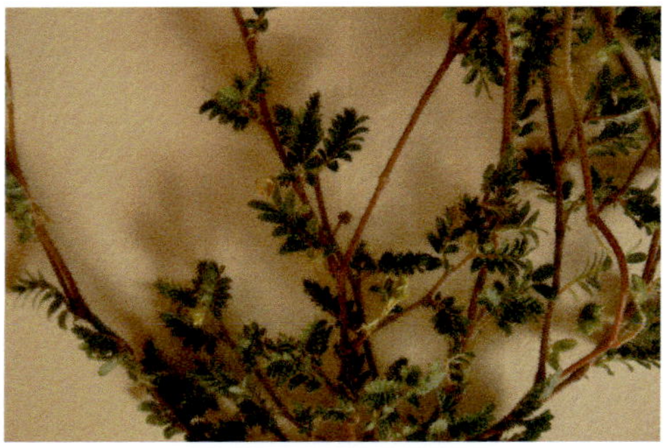

Fig. 16.23. *Tribulus terrestris* (goats head or puncture vine) is an invasive annual found throughout the world. Poisoning occurs when cattle have no alternative forages.

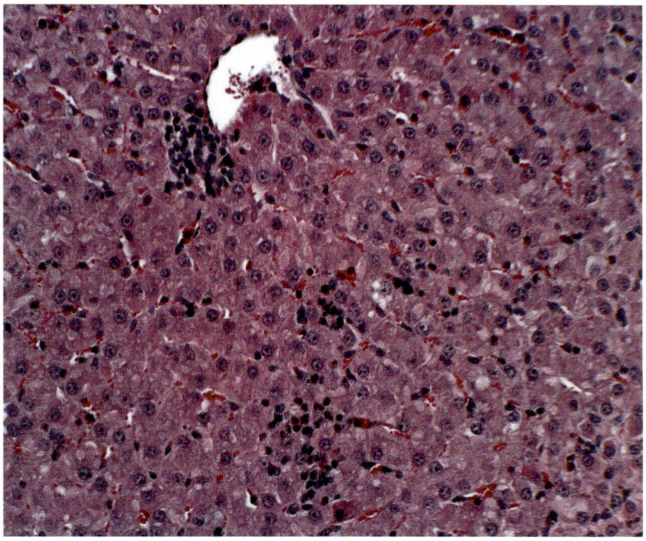

Fig. 16.24. Ox. Liver. Clefts. Animal poisoned with switchgrass (*Panicum virgatum*). The calcium salts have been removed when the tissues were processed. Notice the eosinophilic material and clefts or empty areas in hepatocytes and the small adjacent canuliculi (H&E).

16.2.3 Cocklebur (*Xanthium strumarium*) and other potent hepatotoxic plants

Cocklebur poisoning is most often associated with livestock eating seedlings or young plants in the cotyledon stage. But mature plants including the spiney seeds contain carboxyatractyloside and have poisoned cattle.

Clinical disease is related to acute liver failure and includes neurologic signs (hyperexcitability, blindness, spastic gait, falling, and convulsions) that are probably precipitated by hepatic encephalopathy. Serum biochemistry is dependent on disease duration and can include massive elevations in enzymatic activity as well as increases in serum bilirubin and bile acids.

Gross lesions may include ascites, a pale swollen liver with a prominent, often red, mottled, or nutmeg-like pattern.

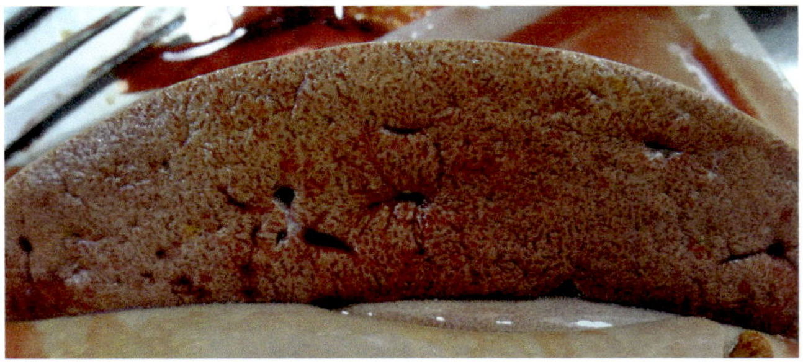

Fig. 16.26. Ox. Liver. Hepatomegaly. Cow poisoned with *Xanthium strumarium* (cocklebur). Notice the swollen liver with rounded edges and lobular necrosis, seen as a prominent red lobular pattern on the cut edge.

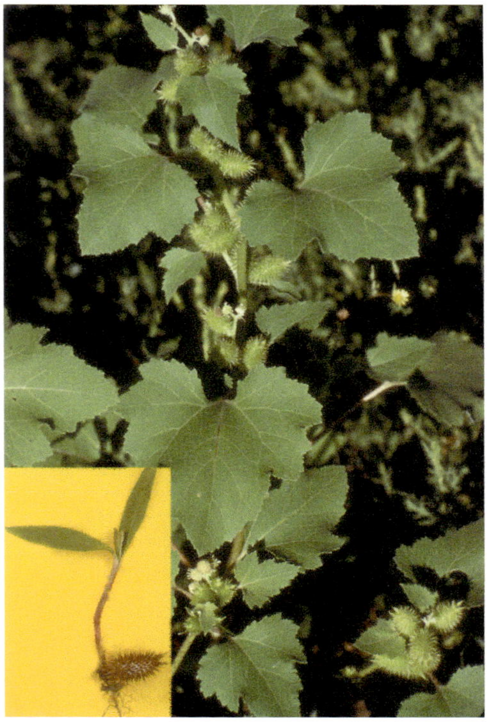

Fig. 16.25. *Xanthium strumarium* (rough or common cocklebur) is a North American annual that expands and dominates disturbed or marginal areas. Seeds and seedling plants are most toxic, but all parts are toxic and can poison livestock. Inset: seedling. (Courtesy of A. Knight, Colorado State University, USA.)

Histologic changes include severe centrilobular hepatocellular degeneration and necrosis, with hemorrhage and sinusoidal collapse. Severe poisoning is usually quickly fatal. A small number of severely affected animals may develop fibrotic hepatic lesions that are thought to progress to cirrhosis and chronic liver failure. Diagnosis may be assisted by identifying carboxyatractyloside and intact burrs in the rumen. Non-fatally poisoned animals recover with little detectable hepatic change.

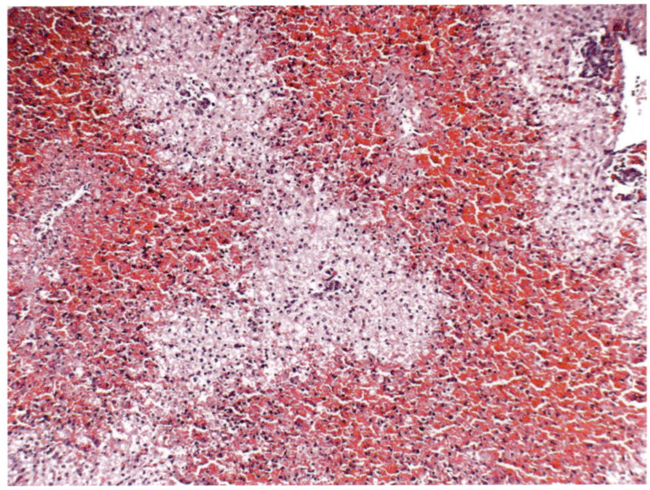

Fig. 16.27. Ox. Liver. Necrosis. Cow poisoned with *Xanthium strumarium* (cocklebur). Notice the massive centrilobular necrosis and hemorrhage with collapse and sinusoids (H&E).

Kochia scoparia (Kochia weed) is an invasive weed that is commonly associated with nitrate poisoning. It is also intermittently associated with a severe liver disease similar to cocklebur poisoning that is characterized by massive centrilobular hepatic necrosis and liver failure. Identifying the cause or toxin has been difficult as the disease has not been duplicated with feeding trails in cattle or various other animal models. Recent work suggests Kochia-related hepatic necrosis may be due to another plant or aflatoxin.

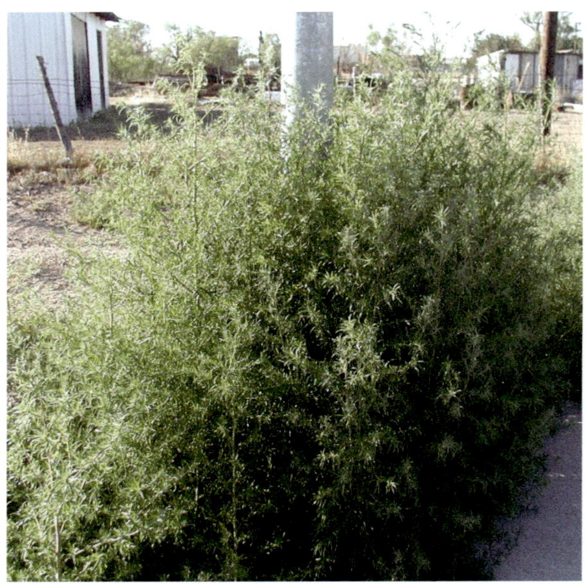

Fig. 16.28. *Kochia scoparia* (Kochia weed, ragweed, or fireweed) is a large annual invasive Eurasian plant that has invaded much of North America. It is commonly associated with nitrate poisoning and flourishes in disturbed soils like field edges and roadsides.

16.2.4 Plants containing fungal hepatotoxins

16.2.4.1 Fumonisins

There are numerous fungal toxins or aflatoxins that can be produced when fungi infect plants and grain. In cattle, *Fusarium verticillioides* (formerly *moniliforme*)-produced fumonisins cause hepatocellular necrosis, fibrosis, and biliary proliferation similar to DHPAs.

16.2.4.2 Lupinosis

Cultivated lupins have been selected so that they do not contain teratogenic quinolizidine alkaloids, and they are generally considered safe as forage. However, when infected with *Diaporthe toxica* (previously *Phomopsis leptostromiformis*), lupins can be contaminated with phomopsins. The phomopsins are potent hepatoxins that result in severe liver disease, with subsequent photosensitization in sheep and less frequently in cattle. Clinical signs of poisoning are seen as loss of appetite, jaundice, and pronounced secondary photosensitization.

Histologic changes are variable and are characterized by focally extensive hepatocellular degeneration with lipid accumulation and necrosis. Proliferative regenerative hepatocytes often have abnormal chromatin with bizarre, abnormal mitoses. The sinusoids are dilated and contain debris-filled Kupffer cells. Chronic lesions are fibrotic, with patchy small foci of hepatocyte necrosis and occasional megalocytosis. Phomopsins are antimitotic, as they arrest cells in metaphase of mitosis by inhibiting the polymerization of α and β tubulin dimers. Though lupinosis is not common in North America, it has been speculated that many of the local hepatic lipidosis syndromes (hard yellow liver disease, local hepatic encephalopathy, pronghorn antelope fatty liver) may be phomopsin-related.

16.2.4.3 Sporidesmin

Sporidesmin is produced by *Pithomyces chartarum*, which infects grasses, especially *Lolium perenne* (perennial rye). Poisoning is common in New Zealand, where it is called facial eczema, a photosensitization disease of sheep and cattle.

Clinical poisoning is characterized by diarrhea, anorexia, and agalactia, followed by liver failure, jaundice, and photosensitization. Most animals develop clinical disease with 7–24 days of exposure to the fungus-contaminated feed.

Gross lesions include hepatic swelling and edema, followed by icterus and hepatocellular degeneration and necrosis, seen grossly as a prominent lobular pattern. With continued poisoning, the liver shrinks with extensive periportal fibrosis. In severe chronic cases, the liver becomes cirrhotic, with continued hepatocellular necrosis, fibrosis, and pericholangitis.

16.2.4.4 Lantana

Lantana camara, *Lantana indica*, *Lantana involucrata*, *Lantana trifolia*, *Lantana lilacina*, and other species are toxic American shrubs that are often used as ornamentals, but in many places, they have escaped cultivation and become an invasive noxious weed. Its expansive nature and allelopathic ability to reduce competition have allowed *Lantana* to dominate many plant communities. Lantadene A and lantadene B are pentacyclic triterpenoids that are two of the primary hepatotoxic and allelopathic lantana toxins. They are present in the roots, leaves, stems, and unripe fruit, and small doses of <5 g of dried leaves can be fatal for cattle and sheep. It is thought that the lantadenes inhibit the sodium ATPase in biliary epithelium.

Clinical signs begin with anorexia, leading to icterus and photosensitization. Clinical signs and lesions are dose dependent.

Gross lesions include swollen, pale yellow and fragile liver, the gall bladder is distended, with dark black viscous fluid, and the gall bladder epithelium is thick and black.

Microscopically, the liver has marked intracellular cholestasis, with variable biliary epithelial proliferation, fibrosis, and hepatocellular degeneration and necrosis. The biliary epithelium and wall are edematous, with inflammatory infiltrates of lymphocytes and neutrophils. The proximal convoluted tubules of the kidney are multifocally degenerative and necrotic with cellular swelling, vacuolation, and occasional pyknosis and cellular disruption. Some tubules are dilated and filled with debris and fibrin. Some poisoned animals also have multifocal myocardial swelling and necrosis, and there are multifocal hemorrhages. These animals may also have pulmonary edema and emphysema (see Chapter 6: Diseases of the Hepatobiliary System and Pancreas).

16.3 MYOTOXIC PLANTS

16.3.1 Cardioactive glycoside-containing plants

Numerous plants, some of which have been used medicinally, contain toxic cardenolide and bufadienolide cardioglycosides (CGs). Cattle are very sensitive to poisoning, and small doses quickly produce severe cardiac arrhythmias and heart blocks, including ventricular tachycardia and first- and second-degree conduction blocks.

Clinical signs of poisoning include rapid breathing, cold extremities, and a rapid, weak, and often irregular pulse. These are potent toxins, and poisoning is generally fatal within 24 h of ingestion. The gross and microscopic lesions are related to the dose and duration, and high doses quickly produce fatal cardiac arrhythmias before heart lesions develop.

Gross changes. With lower doses, poisoning produces patchy myocardial degeneration that is seen as pale, soft streaking of the myocardium. These lesions are often most severe in the papillary and superficial ventricular myocardium. Other lesions vary as they occur secondary to heart failure and cardiovascular collapse. These include serosal hemorrhages, edema, and congestion of visceral organs.

Microscopically, ischemia-sensitive tissues such as the kidney may have ischemic-type glomerulopathy, tubular nephrosis, and lungs may have patchy atelectasis. The myocardial lesions include mild, non-suppurative myocardial degeneration with mononuclear inflammation.

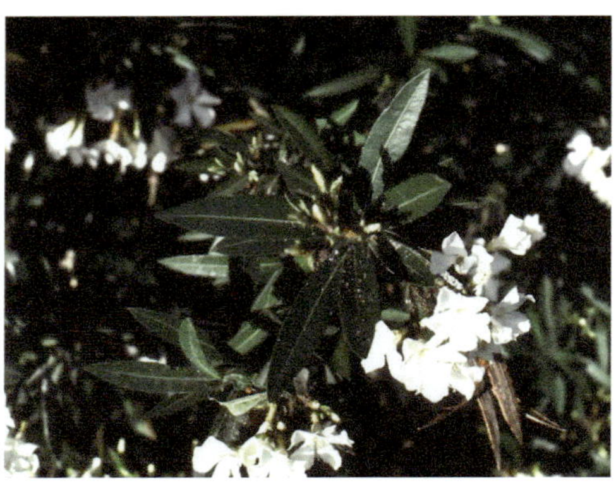

Fig. 16.29. *Nerium oleander* (oleander) is a Mediterranean plant that is commonly used as an ornamental. Livestock poisonings most often occur when clippings are inadvertently fed or included in feeds. Less commonly, cattle may be poisoned when they eat plants that have grown along fences and roadsides, or invaded fields and pastures. Other cardiac glycoside-containing plants, such as *Adonis microcarpa* (pheasant's eye), can be highly invasive, allowing them to invade fields, contaminate feeds, and poison livestock.

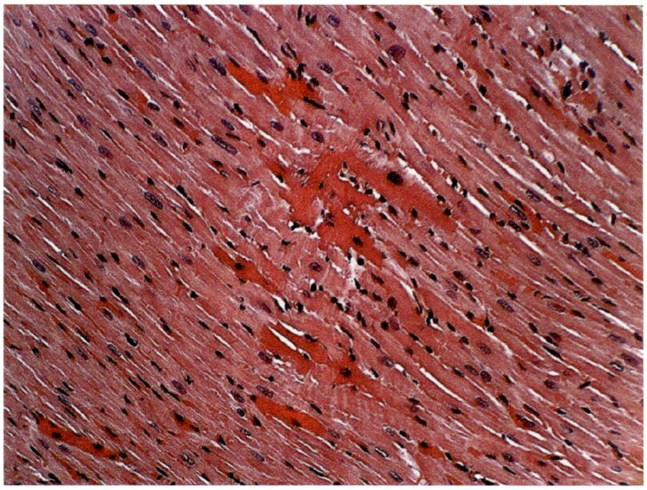

Fig. 16.30. Ox. Heart. Myodegeneration. Notice the focal myocyte swelling and hypereosinophilia. Pheasant eye cardiac glycosides are very toxic, and most animals die before developing myocardial lesions (H&E).

16.3.2 Rayless goldenrod and white snakeroot

White snakeroot (*Ageratina altissima*) and rayless goldenrod (*Isocoma pluriflora*) poison livestock in the Midwest and south-western USA, respectively. Though they are different species and they grow in different habitats, proposed toxins are similar in composition. Initial work suggested the toxin was trematol. This is misleading, as the toxins are mixtures of trematol, tremetone, dehydrotremetone, 3-oxyangeloyl-tremetone, and 3-hydroxytremetone (refered to as benzofuran ketones – BFKs).

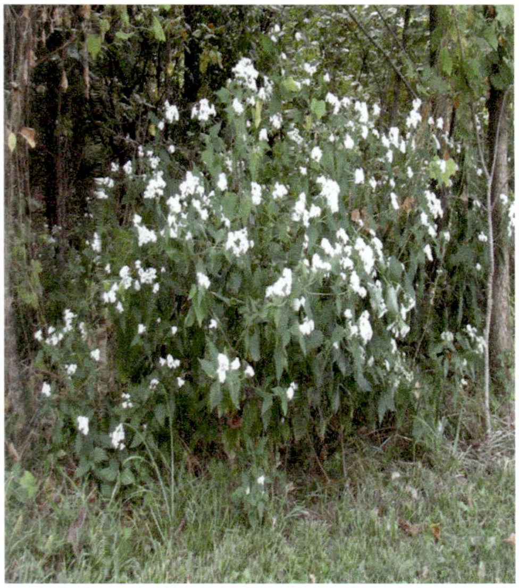

Fig. 16.31. *Ageratina altissima* (white snakeroot) is a perennial plant native to central and eastern North America. It grows to about 1.5 m tall, and commonly grows in the shade. Poisoning usually occurs in the autumn or early winter, when other forages are less available.

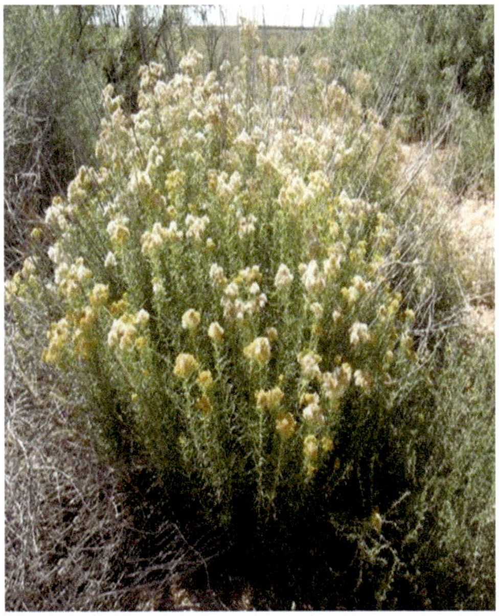

Fig. 16.32. *Isocoma pluriflora* (rayless goldenrod or jimmyweed) is a bush-like plant found in the desert south-west of the USA. Poisoning generally occurs in the winter, when alternative forages are not available or are covered with snow.

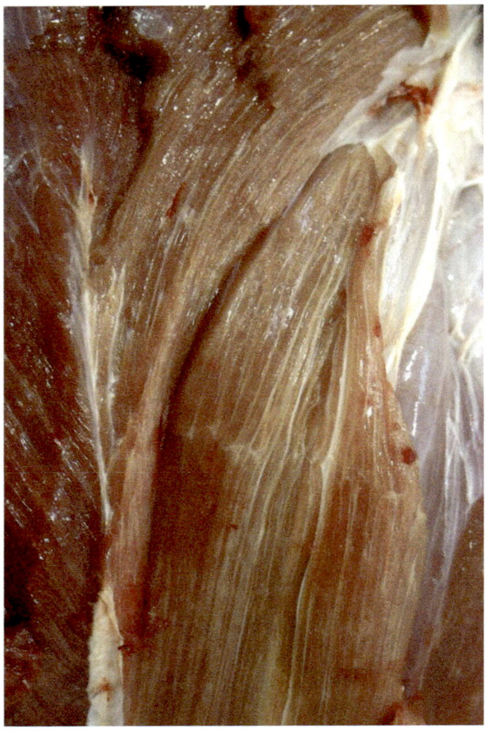

Fig. 16.33. Ox. Skeletal muscle. Myodegeneration. Cow poisoned with rayless goldenrod (*Isocoma pluriflora*). Notice streaks of soft, pale myofibers with edema.

Clinical disease usually develops after 5–7 days of BFK exposure. As the BFKs are lipid soluble, transmammary intoxication is common and has been referred to as 'milk sickness'. Initial signs of poisoning include depression, reluctance to move and eat, and inactivity. Extended intoxication includes fine muscle tremors of the face, flanks, and legs, especially following exercise or activity. Severely affected animals will often have tachypnea, tachycardia, a stiff gait, and altered posture with appendicular hyperextension (peg legs) and an arched back. Nursing young are predisposed to intoxication, while lactating mothers may be clinically normal.

At necropsy, poisoned animals will have swelling, edema, and pallor of many skeletal muscles: though lesions have been described in all skeletal muscles, the large appendicular muscles (semimembranosus, semitendinosus, biceps femoris, gluteus medius, supraspinatus, and triceps brachii) were the most frequently damaged. Other gross lesions include myoglobinuria, serosal petechial hemorrhages, and mild pericardial and thorasic effusions.

Histologic lesions are characterized by extensive monophasic degeneration and necrosis of skeletal muscle. The sequelae of poisoning are largely unknown, but such extensive lesions are likely to affect the athletic ability of previously poisoned animals permanently.

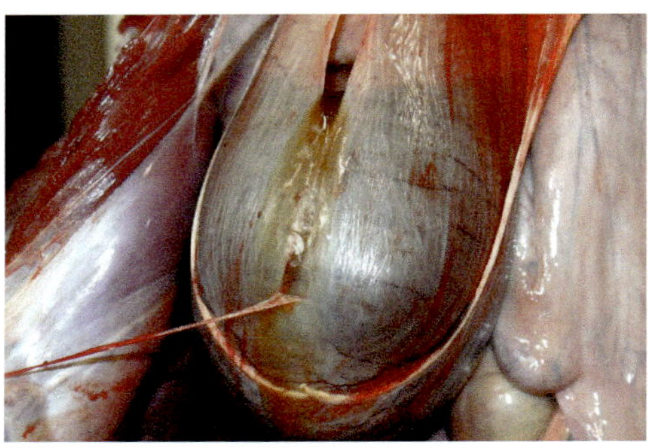

Fig. 16.34. Ox. Urinary bladder. Myoglobinuria. Cow poisoned with rayless goldenrod (*Isocoma pluriflora*). Notice brownish red discolored urine.

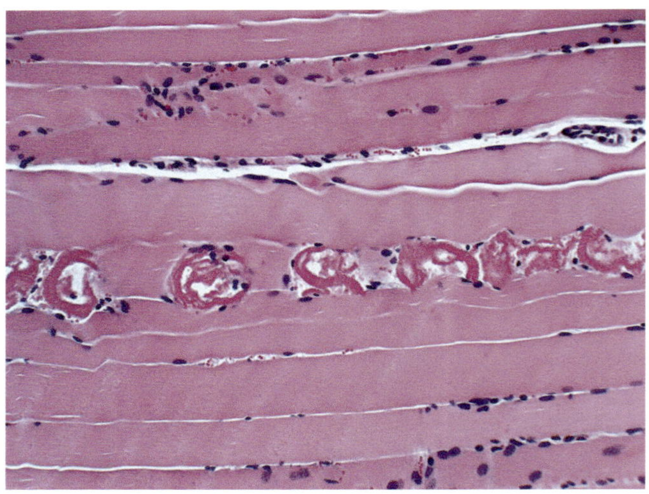

Fig. 16.35. Ox. Skeletal muscle. Myodegeneration. Cow poisoned with rayless goldenrod (*Isocoma pluriflora*). Notice the myocyte hypereosinophilia with focally extensive myocyte degeneration and necrosis (H&E).

16.3.3 Thermopsis and other myotoxic plants

Thermopsis rhombifolia var. *montana* has occasionally been associated with livestock poisoning in North America.

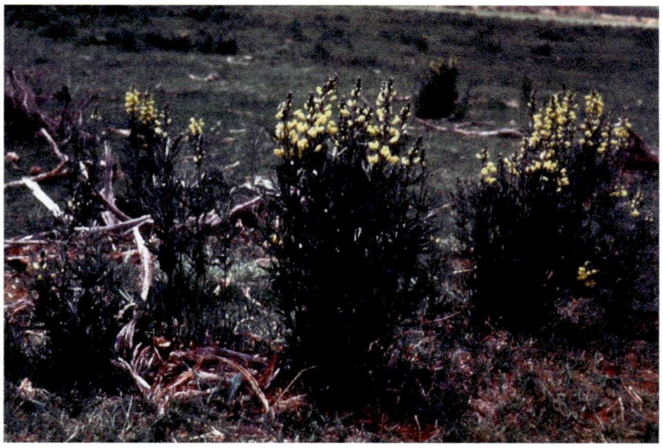

Fig. 16.36. *Thermopsis rhombifolia* var. *montana* (prairie thermopsis or buffalo flower) is a 30-cm legume found in the western plains of North America. Most poisoning has been associated with contaminated hay, when *Thermopsis* is harvested with other forages.

Clinical signs. Poisoned animals become weak, stiff, and reluctant to move, which can progress to recumbency, dehydration, malnutrition, and death. Biochemical changes include marked increases in CK, AST, and LDH activities.

Gross changes. These are usually only minimal and include pallor and softening of skeletal muscle, and loss of adipose tissue and body condition. Many poisoned animals may recover, but the permanent sequelae of poisoning have not been identified. Toxins isolated from *Thermopsis* include anagyrine, thermopsine, cytisine, and N-methylcytisine. Several of these are teratogens, and their contribution to myonecrosis is unknown.

Microscopically, there is prominent skeletal muscle degeneration and necrosis, with coagulation and clumping and myofibers. Some myocytes are swollen with hypereosinophilia (hyaline degeneration).

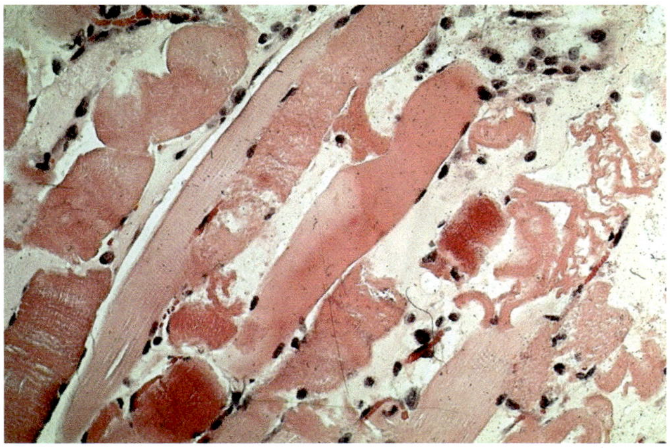

Fig. 16.37. Ox. Skeletal muscle. Coagulative necrosis. Calf poisoned with *Thermopsis rhombifolia*. Notice the coagulation and clumping of protein with monocyte and lymphocyte inflammation (H&E).

16.3.4 *Cassia* or *Senna* spp.

The *Cassia* species are generally not palatable to livestock; however, *Cassia occidentalis*, *Cassia obtusifolia*, *Cassia roemeriana*, *Cassia fasciculata*, *Cassia lindheimeriana*, and *Cassia nictitans* have been reported to poison animals. Most are weedy plants that expand along fences and roads, filling disturbed areas and invading fields and pastures. Multiple toxins have been proposed, including anthraquinones, emodin, chrysarobin, and N-methylmorpholine. More research is needed to identify the toxic agents and better determine their mechanism of toxicity.

Clinical signs. Poisoning is characterized by diarrhea, colic, tenesmus, weakness, recumbency, myoglobinuria, and wasting. As with other causes of myonecrosis, serum CK and AST activities are increased markedly. In severely poisoned animals, death has been attributed to cardiac fibrillation secondary to myonecrosis-induced hyperkalemia. In nearly all species, high doses are likely to produce hepatic necrosis, and in some cases severely affected animals develop hepatic encephalopathy.

Gross lesions include muscle pallor, softening, and secondary changes of nephrosis, or severe hepatic softening and congestion (see Chapter 8: Diseases of the Musculoskeletal System).

Histologically, there is skeletal muscle necrosis and degeneration that may not be monophasic. There is hepatic necrosis. This makes it challenging to differentiate from other nutritional myopathies. *Cassia*-induced liver disease is characterized by extensive centrilobular hepatocyte necrosis that, at times, can be massive with hemorrhage.

16.3.5 Seleniferous plants

Selenium (Se) is an essential nutrient that is a common nutritional supplement which has an extremely narrow safety margin. Poisoning is often due to errors in supplement and feed ration formulation. However, some soils have high Se that accumulates in plants that can poison livestock and wildlife. Se poisoning has been classified historically as chronic or acute poisoning to both dose and duration. Chronic Se toxicosis occurs when animals consume forages with 10–30 ppm over periods of weeks to months. Acute Se toxicosis is caused by ingestion of high Se doses (plants or feed with Se in thousands ppm range) over durations of hours. Plants that accumulate such high concentrations are often called 'accumulator' or 'indicator' plants, including *Astragalus bisulcatus*, *Astragalus praelongus*, or *Stanleya pinnata*. These plants have a characteristic smell, and generally they are not palatable to most livestock. Other plants such as *Aster* or *Grindelia* spp., or even common forages such as alfalfa (*Medicago sativa*), when grown in high Se soils, can passively accumulate slightly lower Se concentrations (hundreds to thousands ppm). Poisoning by these plants have become common in Se-contaminated areas such as around mine tailings and zones of evaporation from contaminated water. Different forms of Se have different toxicities, with methylselenocysteine the most toxic, followed by selenomethionine, selenate, and selenite.

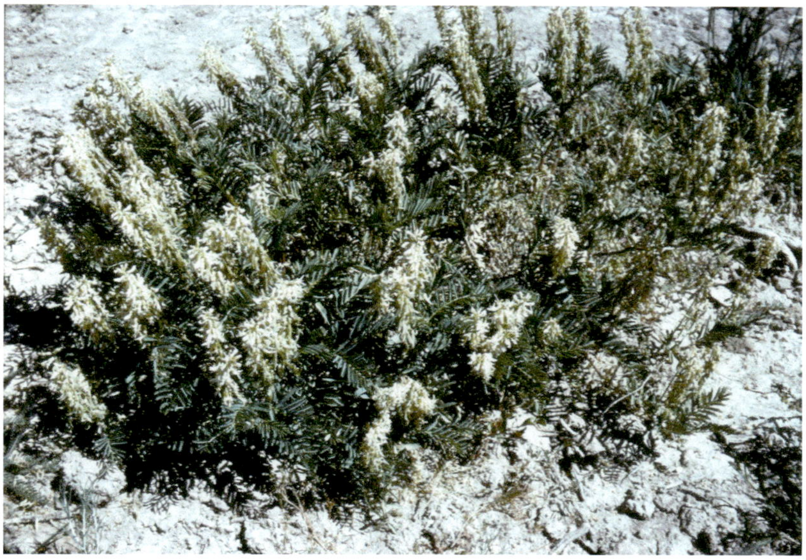

Fig. 16.38. *Astragalus bisulcatus* (two-grooved milkvetch or silver-leafed milkvetch) is a leafy perennial which grows on selenium-rich soils. Two-grooved milkvetch has been called an indicator plant, as it is found in seleniferous areas. It is not palatable and rarely poisons animals; however, it does make selenium available to adjacent facultative accumulating plants.

Clinical signs of acute poisoning include dyspnea, pulmonary edema, and sudden death. Lower doses over longer duration may produce chronic heart failure, with subsequent edema, thoracic and abdominal transfusions, hepatic congestion and degeneration, and vascular distension that is seen with a jugular pulse.

Grossly, affected animals develop extensive myocardial necrosis, fibrosis with adjacent edema. At lower, non-fatal doses, poisoned animals have minimal change, with altered hair and hoof growth that can progress to sloughing and loss of hooves, extreme lameness, and marked alopecia, especially of the tail.

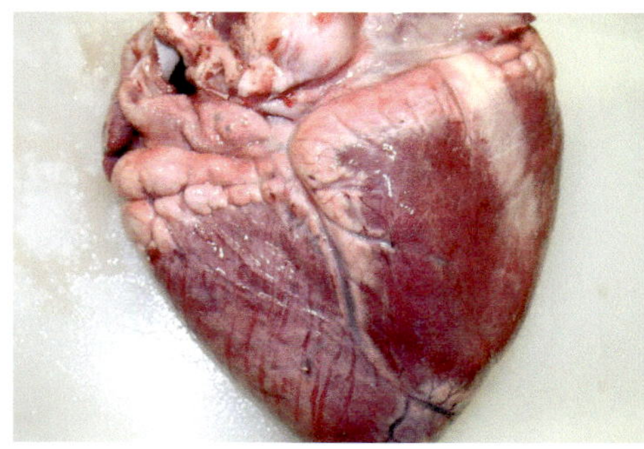

Fig. 16.39. Ox. Heart. Myocardial hemorrhage. Cow that survived nearly 2 weeks after ingesting highly seleniferous plants. Notice the extensive myocardial pallor with lymphatic dilation.

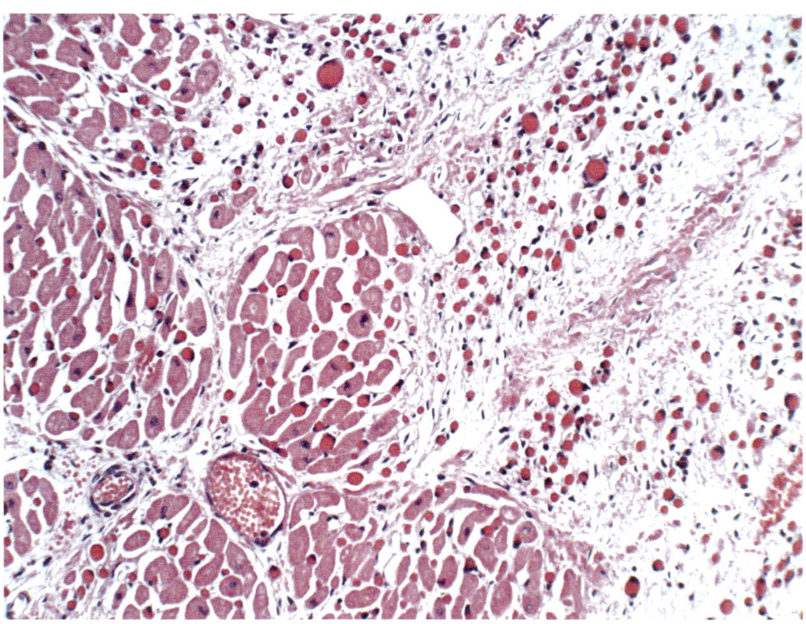

Fig. 16.40. Ox. Heart. Myocardial fibrosis. Cow with Se-induced chronic myocardial degeneration, necrosis, and fibrosis. Notice the myofiber swellings as they are entrapped by fibrous connective tissue. There is also extensive interstitial edema and minimal lymphocytic inflammation (trichrome stain).

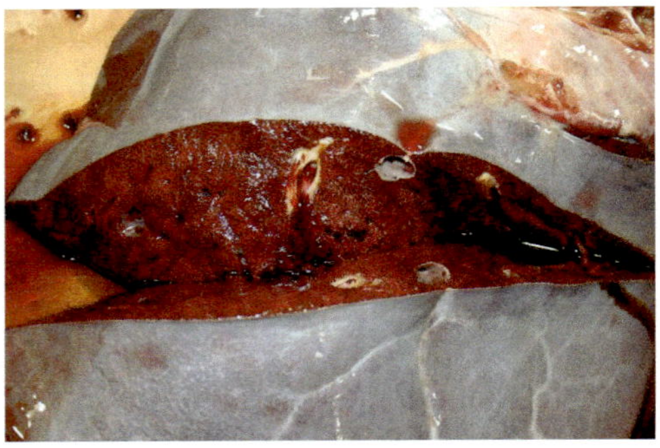

Fig. 16.41. Ox. Liver. Chronic passive congestion. Cow with heart disease caused by chronic selenosis. Notice the prominent lobular pattern (nutmeg-like appearance) characteristic of chronic heart failure.

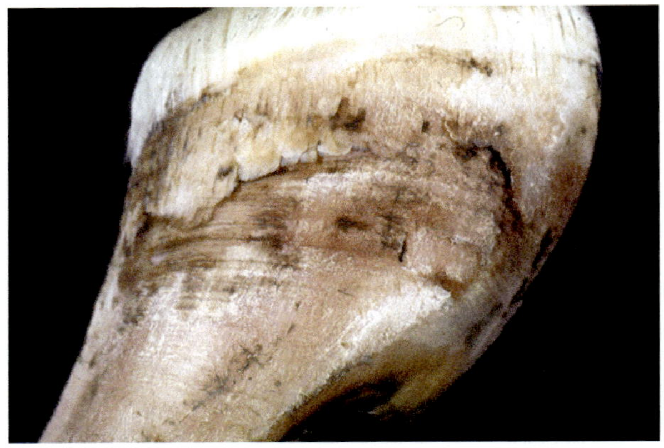

Fig. 16.42. Ox. Claw Coronary band. Cow with chronic selenosis. Notice the prominent growth ridges and abnormally rapid epithelial growth (chronic laminitis).

16.3.6 Yew (*Taxus cuspidata* – Japanese yew; *Taxus baccata* – common yew; and *Taxus media* – hybrid common and Japanese yew)

Yews are small to medium-sized evergreen trees that are commonly used as ornamental or decorative plants. All parts of the plant are toxic, but the leaves contain the most taxine (the yew toxin). Cattle are especially susceptible, and as little as 4.5 g wet plant material/kg body weight can be fatal.

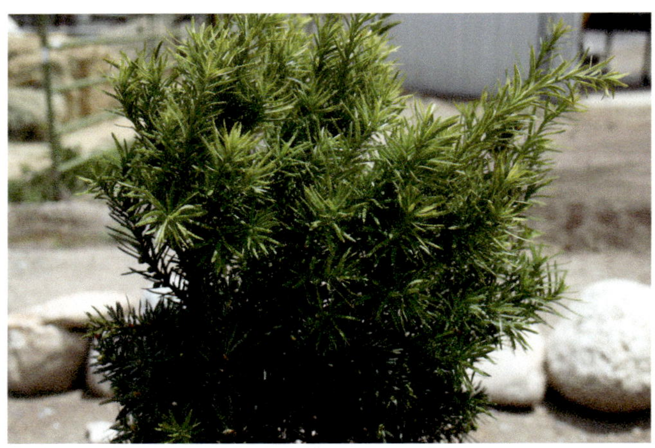

Fig. 16.43. *Taxus cuspidata* (Japanese yew) is an ornamental tree found throughout the world. It has flat needles that are highly toxic. Most poisoning occurs when yew clippings are fed to cattle. Fresh, wilted, and dry leaves are all toxic and have poisoned cattle.

Clinically, poisoning is characterized by ataxia, tachycardia, dyspnea, muscle tremors, convulsions, and cardiac arrest. Taxine inhibits Na/Ca channels blocking myocardial conduction, stopping the heart in diastole. As poisoning is nearly always short and fatal without toxin-specific lesions, diagnosis depends on documenting exposure, identifying yew plant in rumen contents, or by chemically identifying taxines in rumen or gastric contents (see Chapter 17: Bovine Diseases without Lesions).

16.4 TERATOGENIC PLANTS

16.4.1 Lupine

The lupines are usually considered nutritious legumes; however, they can contain several toxic and teratogenic alkaloids. As mentioned previously, some lupines are neurotoxic, but the most common condition in cattle relating to lupine ingestion is 'crooked calf disease'. In cattle gestation, days 40–100 are susceptible to lupine-induced birth defects. Similar inhibition of fetal movement and subsequent teratogenesis has been described with poison hemlock (*Conium*) and wild tree tobacco (*Nicotiana glauca*). The incidence of lupine-induced crooked calf disease varies with lupine populations, alternative forages, and breeding patterns. When lupine populations expand, alternative forages are lacking, and susceptible animals are exposed, incidence can be nearly 100%, producing epidemic outbreaks and economic devastation. Fetal lesions vary with dose and duration.

Clinical signs. Crooked calf disease is a congenital condition characterized by deformed calves born with skeletal contracture-type malformations and cleft palate after their mothers have grazed lupines during sensitive periods of pregnancy.

Gross features of the terata are characterized by arthrogryposis with scoliosis, torticollis, kyphosis, and cleft palate. Some articulations may be fused or functionally immobile due to malalignment of the articular surfaces, insertions, or prominences. In severe cases, there is axial rotation and ankylosis of the cervical and thoracic vertebrae.

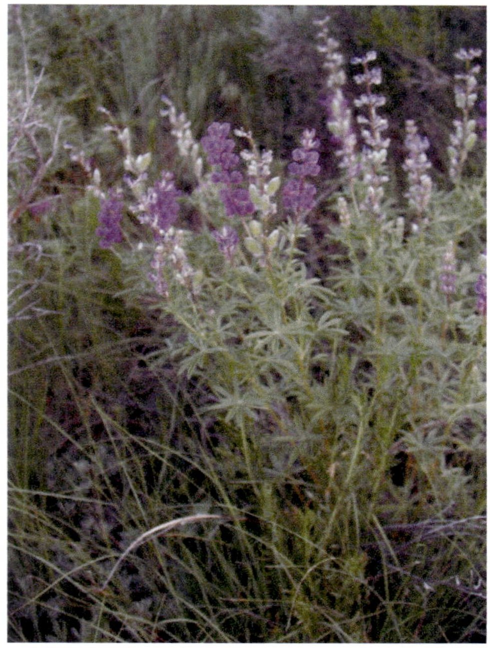

Fig. 16.44. *Lupinus wyethii* (Wyeth's lupine) is one of many lupine species that appear similar and are difficult to classify. Among the lupines, there are large population and chemotype differences. To assess risks accurately, testing lupine populations for known teratogens (anagyrine or ammodendrine) can be helpful.

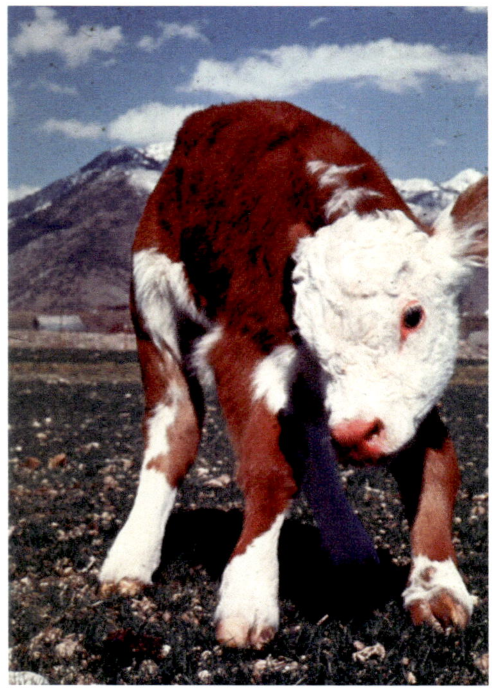

Fig. 16.45. Ox. Whole body. Calf with 'crooked calf disease'. Notice the angular limb deformities, with lateral rotation of the front legs. There is also prominent kyphosis and lordosis.

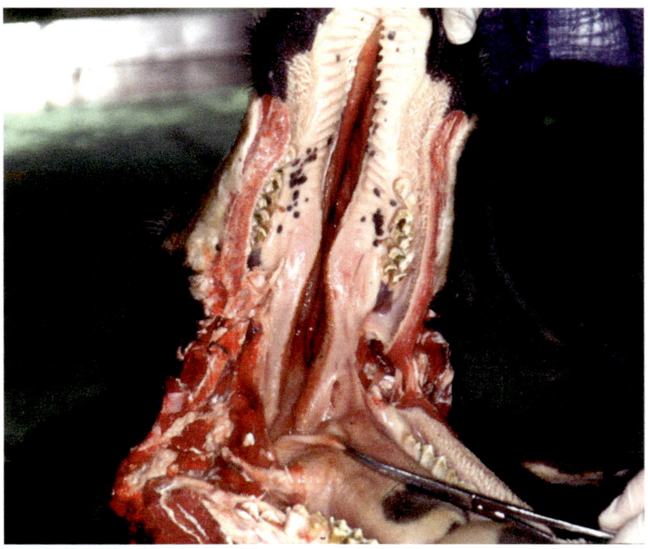

Fig. 16.46. Ox. Head. Palatoschisis. Calf with 'crooked calf disease'. Notice the full or complete cleft palate affecting both the hard and soft palate.

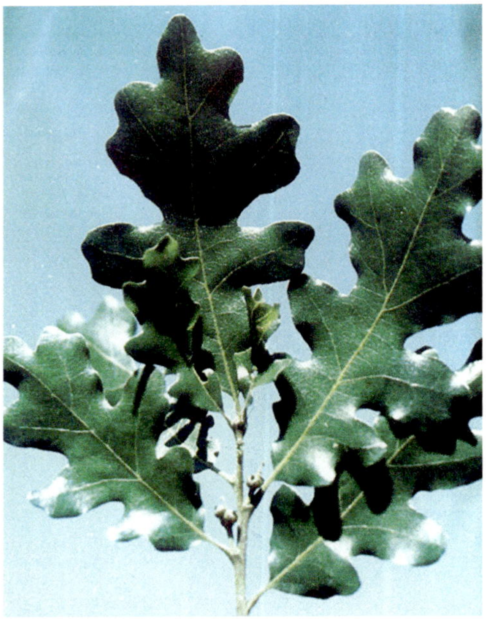

Fig. 16.47. Oak (*Quercus* spp.) are trees or shrubs found throughout the world. They vary from massive trees to small scrub and bushes. In North America, shinnery oak and Gambel or scrub oak are most commonly associated with livestock poisoning.

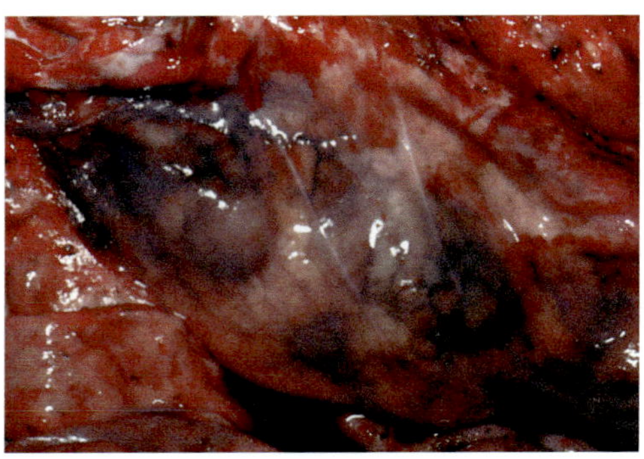

Fig. 16.48. Ox. Kidney. Perirenal edema. Calf poisoned with 'scrub oak'. Notice the extensive fluid surrounding kidney.

16.5 NEPHROTOXIC PLANTS

16.5.1 Oak

Oaks (*Quercus* spp.) are woody plants, ranging from smaller shrubs to large trees, that are all potentially toxic. Poisoning is commonly caused by seedlings, early bud growth, and acorns, usually because there are few alternative forages. Drought and overgrazing also potentiate poisoning, which frequently occurs in early spring or autumn. Oak toxins are primarily thought to be tannins that produce oxidative radicles that cross-link proteins and other macromolecules, denaturing proteins and altering protein interactions. Poisoning occurs when large doses are ingested over several days to weeks. Poisoning is most common in calves and usually includes gastroenteritis with nephrotoxicity. High doses may also be hepatotoxic.

Clinical signs of poisoning initially include lethargy, constipation, tenesmus, polydypsia and polyuria that progress into hemorrhagic diarrhea, abdominal pain, rumen atony, and anorexia. Severe poisoning is fatal. Oak-induced renal disease includes isosthenuria, glucosuria, proteinuria, and hematuria.

Gross lesions of acute poisoning include the presence of oak material/acorns in the digesta, subcutaneous edema, perirenal edema, edema of the mesenteric lymph nodes, ascites, hydrothorax, pale kidneys with petechial hemorrhage, and multifocal ulcerative and hemorrhagic rumenitis, gastritis, and enteritis.

Histologic findings include diffuse cortical renal tubular degeneration and necrosis, characterized by loss of tubular epithelium and formation of hyaline, granular, and cellular casts. In some tubules, the remaining tubular epithelial cells form a flattened epithelium with large nuclei (regeneration). The medullary tubules are generally spared, or only mildly affected. In cases with liver disease, the hepatocellular degeneration and necrosis is characterized by swelling, degeneration, and necrosis of hepatocytes with focally extensive hemorrhage.

Diagnosis of poisoning is generally made using exposure, clinical presentation, and pathologic findings. Chemical detection of pyrogallol has limited diagnostic use as it is metabolized quickly. Poisoning can be prevented by limiting the intake of oak materials to less than 50% of the diet.

16.5.2 Oxalate-containing plants

Oxalate-containing plants include species of the *Agave*, *Beta*, *Bassia*, *Chenopodium*, *Halogeton*, *Oxalis*, *Pennisetum*, *Rheum*, *Rumex*, *Sarcobatus*, and *Setaria* genera. Ruminants are usually poisoned when they ingest plants quickly that contain relatively high oxalate concentrations. Allowing cattle to adapt with low-dose exposure to soluble oxalates for 8–25 days will decrease the risk poisoning.

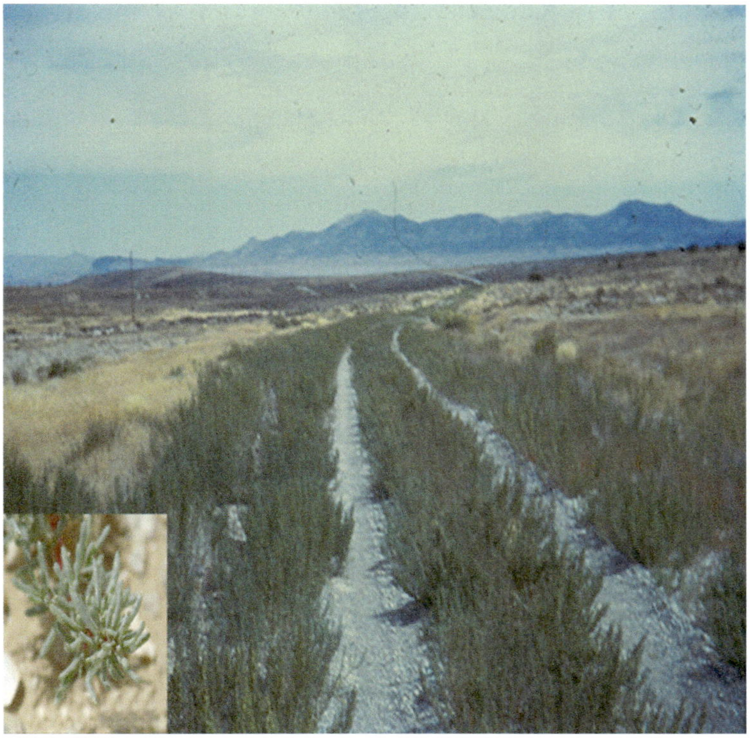

Fig. 16.49. *Halogeton glomeratus* (halogeton or saltlover) is a noxious weed and it has expanded and dominated many disturbed areas in the high mountain deserts. It commonly grows along roadsides or heavily used areas around feedlots, feed, or water. Poisoning often occurs when hungry animals are left in such areas, where they eat too much too quickly and are fatally poisoned. Inset: close-up view.

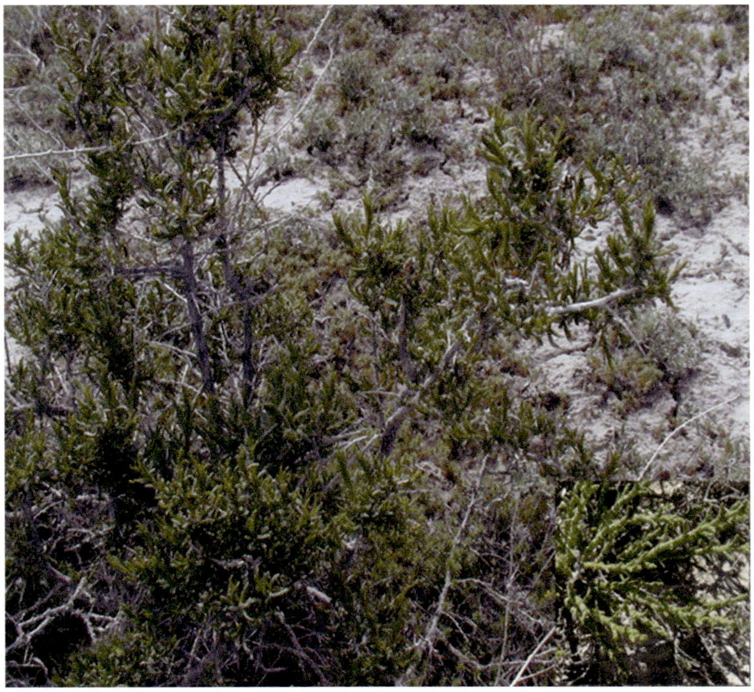

Fig. 16.50. *Sarcobatus vermiculatus* (greasewood) is a green-leafed shrub common in the dry desert zones of North America. As with halogeton, animals can become adapted to greasewood toxins. Poisoning generally occurs when there are few alternative forages and cattle ingest a toxic dose.

Gross changes. Acute poisoning, is characterized by crystalline-associated nephrosis.

Histologic lesions include vasculitis. Insoluble crystals form in areas of highest oxalate concentration, and they are often seen in rumen vasculature and renal tubules. Crystals may also be present in other vessels, including cerebral vessels, which may contribute to the neurologic changes seen in some animals. Deposition of birefringent crystals occurs in the renal tubules, abomasal mucosa, and gastric vasculature. Renal tubules are typically distended with crystalline material and have flattened and degenerative cortical tubular epithelium in acute cases (see Chapter 7: Diseases of the Urinary System).

16.5.3 *Amaranthus* spp. (pigweeds)

Amaranthus retroflexus and several additional species of this genus have poisoned ruminants, pigs, and, rarely, horses. The pigweeds contain nitrates, oxalates, and several unknown nephrotoxic and myocardiotoxic (pigs) factors. Both the myocardial or renal toxins require 5–10 days of ingestion before disease develops.

Clinically, renal disease is characterized by weakness, muscle tremors, ataxia, and knuckling of pasterns. These can progress to more severe recumbence, paralysis, hemorrhagic diarrhea, hemorrhages, coma, and death. Serum biochemistry changes include increases in potassium, phosphorus, blood urea nitrogen (BUN), and creatinine.

Grossly, ascites and hydrothorax develop, and the kidneys are swollen with prominent perirenal edema.

Microscopically, there is marked degeneration and necrosis of the convoluted renal tubular epithelium with interstitial edema.

16.5.4 Calcinogenic glycoside-containing plants

Solanum malacoxylon, *Solanum verbascifolium*, *Solanum torvum*, *Nierembergia veitchii*, *Trisetum flavescens*, and *Cestrum diurnum* are calcinogenic, as they contain glycosides of 1,25-dihydroxycholecalciferol (calcitriol) or physiologically similar compounds that act as active vitamin D (cholecalciferol). Poisoning causes hypercalcemia with metastatic calcification. Poisoning is reported in livestock throughout the world.

Clinical signs are characterized by a progressive depression, weakness, weight loss, infertility, anorexia, cardiac arrhythmias, and impaired stilted gait. With continued poisoning, animals become lame, recumbent, and death is often attributed to emaciation, heart and respiratory failure, and renal disease. There are elevations in BUN, creatinine, and phosphorus.

At necropsy and radiologically, mineralization of organs, vessels, and tissues is easily seen (see Chapter 4: Diseases of the Cardiovascular System).

Microscopically, there is mineralization of many tissues, bronchioles, alveoli, endocardium, vessel walls, and walls of the intestine and stomach (see Chapter 4: Diseases of the Cardiovascular System).

Poisoned animals rarely recover as they become emaciated, non-productive, and are culled.

Table 16.1. Calcinogenic plants. (Adapted from *Haschek and Rousseaux's Handbook of Toxicologic Pathology* (Stegelmeier *et al*., 2013).)

Country	Plant	Disease
Argentina	*Solanum malacoxylon*	Enteque seco
Brazil	*Solanum malacoxylon*	Espichamento
	Nierembergia veitchii	Calcinosis
Uruguay	*Solanum malacoxylon*	Calcinosis
USA	*Cestrum diurnum*	Enzootic calcinosis
	Solanum torvum	Naalehu disease
Jamaica	*Cestrum diurnum*	Manchester
	Solanum torvum	wasting disease
Cuba	*Cestrum diurnum*	Calcinosis
New Guinea	*Solanum torvum*	Calcinosis
Australia	*Solanum esuriale*	Humpy back
South Africa	*Solanum verbascifolium*	Calcinosis
Austria	*Trisetum flavescens*	Weidekrankheit Kalzinose
Germany	*Trisetum flavescens*	Enzootische Kalzinose
Switzerland	*Trisetum flavescens*	Enzootische Kalzinose

16.6 OTHER TOXIC PLANTS

16.6.1 Pine needles

Ponderosa pine (*Pinus ponderosa*), lodgepole pine (*Pinus contorta*), and Monterey cypress (*Cupressus macrocarpa*) cause abortion in late-term cattle. Both the fresh green needles and old dry needles are abortifacient, as is the dry material around the tree and dried slash (branches and needles) that might have fallen.

Clinical signs. The abortion is often complicated, with retained placenta, endometritis, and subsequent loss of reproductive capacity.

Cattle and bison are uniquely susceptible to abortion. Though the exact physiologic mechanism has not been identified, the abortifacient toxins (isocupressic acid, agathic acid, and dihydroagnathic acid) have been identified. It has been suggested that these toxins reduce blood to the fetus and subsequently initiate abortion. Factors including the gestation stage, dose, duration, animal condition, environmental stress, and nutritional status all influence abortion incidence. Abortion occurs within a couple of days to as long as several weeks after exposure. Cows in late gestation are most susceptible, and most abortions occur during the late winter or early spring, when storms force near-term pregnant cattle into the pine trees for shelter. Abortion is characterized by weak uterine contractions, incomplete cervical dilation, and vaginal mucus discharge. This results in dystocia, and though many are viable, the calves are weak and require nursing for survival. Cows that have aborted will not have milk, but they often have retained fetal membranes, endometritis, rumen stasis, and if untreated, some die. Diagnosis of pine needle abortion can, in some cases, be confirmed by analysis of sera samples for metabolites of isocupressic acid. (Also see Chapter 10: Diseases of the Reproductive System.)

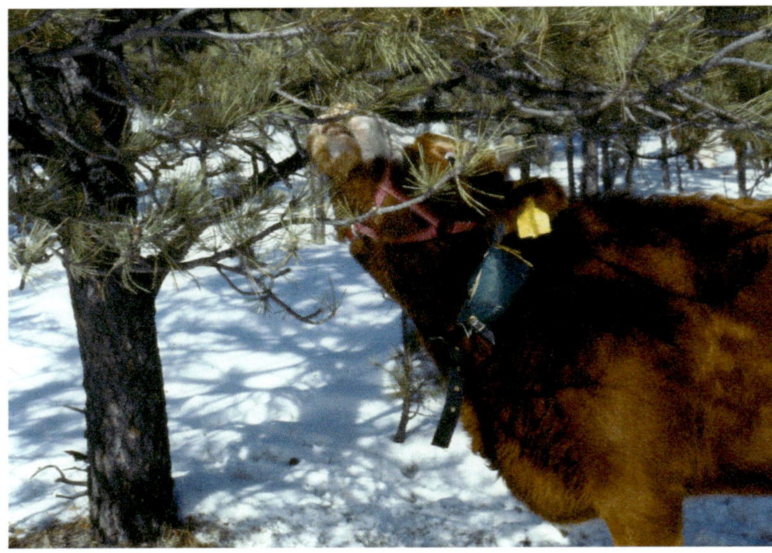

Fig. 16.51. Cow eating needles of ponderosa pine (*Pinus ponderosa*). Green needles, dry needles, bark, and pine needle duff from the ground are all abortifacient in cattle.

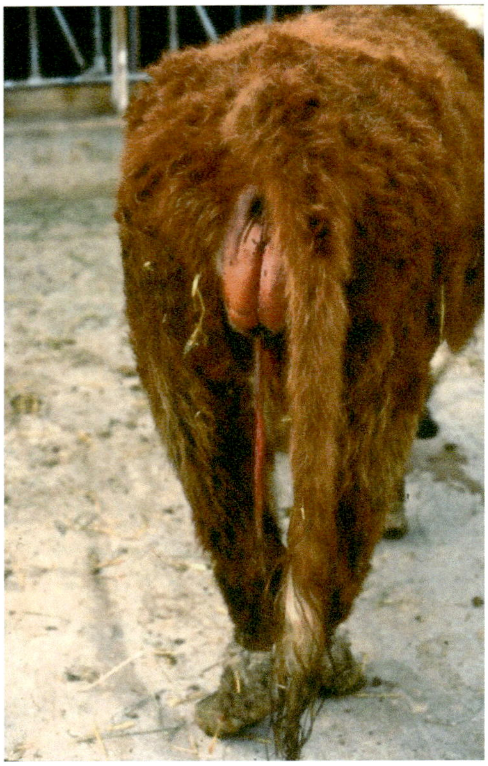

Fig. 16.52. Ox. Placenta. Retention. Cow aborting from pine needle ingestion. Notice the retained placental membranes that occur in nearly all pine needle-induced abortions.

16.6.2 Cyanogenic plants

Cherries (*Prunus* spp.), elderberry (*Sambucus* spp.), service berry (*Amelanchier alnifolia*), various sorghum, Johnson and Sudan grasses (*Sorghum* spp.), maize (*Zea* spp.), vetches (*Vicia sativa*), white clover (*Trifolium repens*), birdsfoot trefoil (*Lotus* spp.), and arrowgrass (*Triglochin* spp.) contain cyanogenic glycosides – amygdalin, prunasin, lucumin, and others. These glycosides become toxic when they are hydrolyzed by plant enzymes that are activated by crushing, chewing, freezing, or wilting. Plant toxicity varies, and it is highest in young, rapidly growing plants that are heavily fertilized and stressed with frost, drought, or herbicides. Drying or ensiling the plants decreases toxicity, as the cyanide is degraded slowly. Cyanide binds avidly with iron in cellular cytochrome oxidase, inhibiting cellular respiration. This produces oxyhemoglobin, which discolors blood and tissues 'cherry red'.

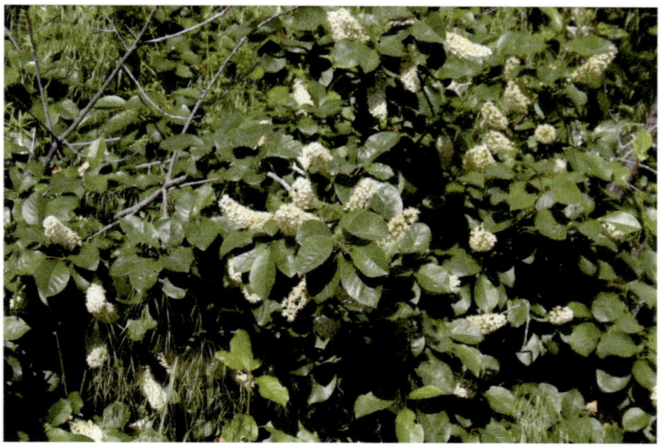

Fig. 16.53. *Prunus virginiana* (chokecherry) is a native North American bush. The leaves and pits are toxic, but as the plant is not palatable, poisoning occurs when there are no alternative forages for cattle.

Clinical signs of poisoning have been described as hyperventilation, dyspnea, hypotension, and staggering that progresses to convulsions, paralysis, and death. Post-mortem, these colored tissues deoxygenate quickly, losing the red discoloration. Most poisoned animals are found dead.

Gross findings are minimal and include petechial hemorrhages on the abomasum, endocardium, and epicardium.

A diagnosis is made linking exposure with clinical signs, sudden death, and lack of other gross and microscopic lesions. Recommendations to avoid poisoning include avoiding harvesting and feeding these plants when they are likely to be toxic. Plants that are toxic sporadically should be tested to determine their cyanogenic potential and potential risk.

16.6.3 Nitrate-accumulating plants

Many pasture and forage plants occasionally accumulate toxic nitrates. Toxicity requires that the nitrates be reduced in the gastrointestinal tract to nitrites, which oxidizes hemoglobin to methemoglobin. Cattle are highly sensitive to poisoning, and bovine fetal hemoglobin is especially sensitive to nitrite oxidation, and poisoning often results in abortion that may be seen in the absence of other clinical signs. All plant parts can contain nitrates, with concentrations highest in the stalks and leaves. Nitrates are usually lowest in the seeds, which are generally considered safe.

Clinical signs of poisoning include exercise intolerance, weakness, trembling, brown or cyanotic mucous membranes, dyspnea, brown discolored blood, abortion, and death. Chemical analysis of maternal and fetal blood, serum, and ocular fluids has been used to identify poisoned animals.

Gross lesions of nitrate poisoning include chocolate-colored or brown discoloration of the blood and tissues. As methemoglobin is reduced post-mortem, the brown discoloration diminishes. In most cases, the animals die quickly and treatment is usually not effective.

Nitrate poisoning is diagnosed by recognizing crops, weeds, and forages that are likely to accumulate nitrates, and testing forages to avoid using toxic feeds in susceptible species. Contaminated forages can still be used if they are diluted with good feed or fed to less susceptible species. (Also see Chapter 11: Diseases of the Hematopoietic and Hemolymphatic System.)

16.6.4 Photosensitizing plants

Photosensitization is radiation-induced dermatitis caused by increased light sensitivity due to photodynamic toxins in the skin. These chromophore toxins absorb light energy and transfer that energy to adjacent molecules, damaging proteins, nucleic acids, and lipid molecules.
Clinical signs of photosensitization include dermatitis of lightly pigmented areas with little hair protection, especially the muzzle, ears, eyelids, face, tail, vulva, udder, and coronary bands. Affected cattle develop conjunctivitis with photophobia.
Lesions include edema, serous exudation, scab formation, and skin necrosis. The resulting inflammation may be extensive, resulting in epidermal necrosis, sloughing of necrotic layers, and extensive suppurative exudate. These photodynamic chromophores are most often plant or fungal products, drugs, chlorophyll metabolites, or other chemicals. Photosensitization has been divided mechanistically into primary photosensitization, where the chromophores are exogenous and usually of plant origin, and secondary or hepatogenous photosensitization, where the chromophores are chlorophyll metabolites, such as phylloerythrin that accumulates because of defective liver excretion (see Chapter 6: Diseases of the Hepatobiliary System and Pancreas, and Chapter 12: Diseases of the Integument).

16.6.4.1 Hypericism

Hypericum perforatum, or St John's wort, goat weed, Tipton weed, amber, or Klamath weed, is an invasive weed in the western USA, Europe, Australia, New Zealand, and South America. Many plant parts, especially the leaves, are infected with an endophyte that produces hypericin, a potent chromatophore.

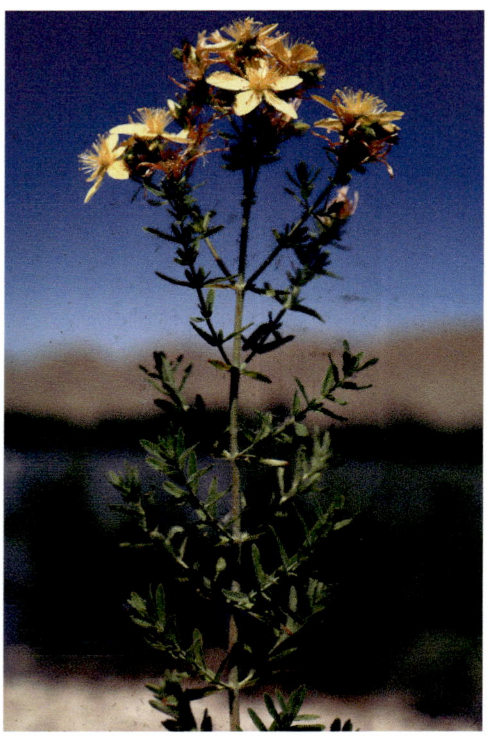

Fig. 16.54. *Hypericum perforatum* (St John's wort), a native of Eurasia that has spread and become an invasive weed in Africa, China, and North America. It spreads via rhizomes and seeds, and often dominates disturbed areas such as roadsides, gravel pits, and waste areas.

16.6.4.2 Fagopyrism

Buckwheat species, *Fagopyrum esculentum*, *Fagopyrum tataricum*, and other *Fagopyrum* spp. are Asian natives that have been used as a summer cover crop, and, in some areas, have escaped cultivation, growing in marginal areas and invading pastures and fields. The buckwheats produce fagopyrin, photofagopyrin, and pseudohypericin, which are structurally and functionally similar to hypericin.

16.6.4.3 Furocoumarins

Furocoumarins are both primary plant compounds and phytoalexins from spring parsley (*Cymopterus watsonii*), *Cymopterus* spp., bishop's weed (*Ammi majus*), Dutchman's breeches (*Thamnosma texana* and *Thamnosma montana*), and celery and parsnip. Various species of these fungal phytoalexins have been identified (xanthotoxin and tripsoralen). They should be monitored in infected plants.

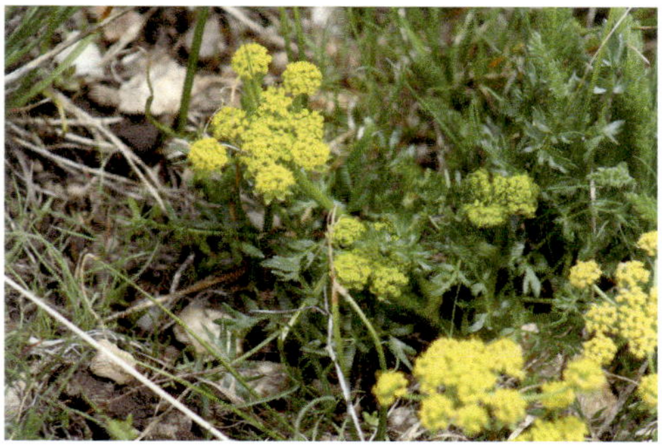

Fig. 16.55. *Cymopterus watsonii* (spring parsley) is a perennial that is native to North America. It grows early in the spring and often is the only green forage, as the grasses have not begun to grow. Ingestion results in plant-induced photosensitivity.

16.6.5 Bracken fern

Bracken ferns (*Pteridium aquilinum*) are found throughout the world, and they often expand and dominate local plant communities. Cattle are poisoned when alternative forages are not available, or when bracken fern contaminates stored and prepared feed. Cyanogenic glycosides, thiaminases, thiamine-inhibiting compounds, several steroid-like compounds, and ptaquiloside have been identified in bracken, and their dose, duration, and the species poisoned determine the type of poisoning. The best described toxin is ptaquiloside, a norsequiterpene glucoside that is mutagenic, clastogenic, and carcinogenic. It initially damages proliferating bone marrow and gastrointestinal cells, resulting in hemorrhage and alimentary and urinary tract neoplasms. Bracken-induced clinical syndromes include acute hemorrhagic disease, bovine enzootic hematuria, bright blindness, upper alimentary carcinomas, and thiamine deficiency.

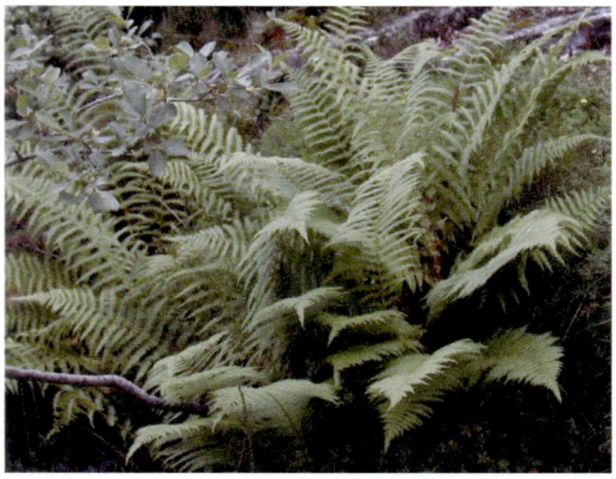

Fig. 16.56. *Pteridium aquilinum* (bracken fern) is found throughout the world. It grows in disturbed areas, often in shaded areas. Poisoning is often cumulative and chronic, as cattle may ingest bracken fern for months before developing disease.

Acute hemorrhagic disease and enzootic hematuria

Clinical signs. Being the most common presentation in cattle, it is characterized by chronic intermittent hematuria and anemia. Poisoned cattle are weak and lose weight rapidly. Later, cattle are anemic, which is seen clinically as dyspnea and pale mucosal membranes. Many develop hemorrhages ranging from petechiae and effusive serosal hemorrhages to massive gastrointestinal hemorrhages. Poisoning is almost always fatal.

Post-mortem examinations usually reveal multiple serosal and soft tissue hemorrhages and bruises. The urinary bladder and urethral mucosa nearly always have numerous vascular, fibrous, and epithelial neoplasms. Some cattle may present with extensive hematuria, often termed 'enzootic hematuria', which has hemorrhagic and neoplastic lesions that are most severe in the urinary tract. Both, the hemorrhage and neoplastic transformation are caused by ptaquiloside-induced neoplastic transformation, thrombocytopenia, and pancytopenia (see Chapter 5: Diseases of the Gastrointestinal Tract, Chapter 7: Diseases of the Urinary System, and Chapter 11: Diseases of the Hematopoietic and Hemolymphatic System).

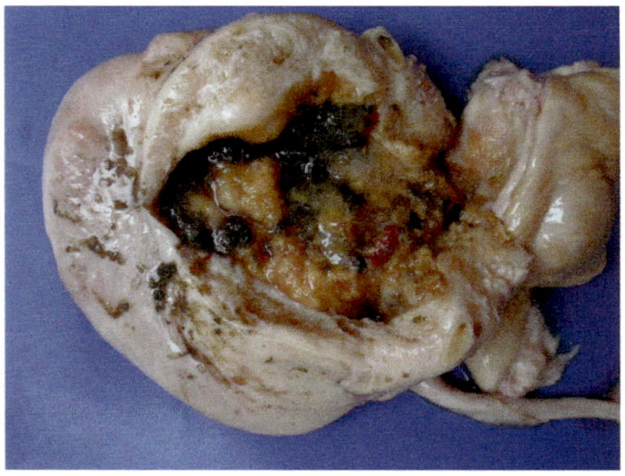

Fig. 16.57. Ox. Urinary bladder. Transitional cell carcinoma. Cow chronically poisoned with bracken fern. A sessile, fungiform growth is embedded in the mucosa. The bladder wall has been invaded by neoplastic cells. (Courtesy of Dr C. Barros, Universidade Federal de Santa Maria, Brazil.)

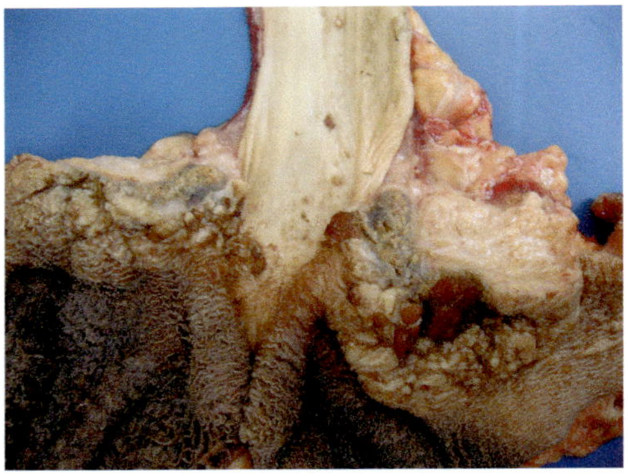

Fig. 16.58. Ox. Rumen. Squamous cell carcinoma. Gastrointestinal tract from a cow chronically poisoned with bracken fern (*Pteridium aquilinum*). Notice the carcinomas on the margin of the squamous epithelium and rumen mucosa. (Courtesy of Dr G. Kommers, Universidade Federal de Santa Maria, Brazil.)

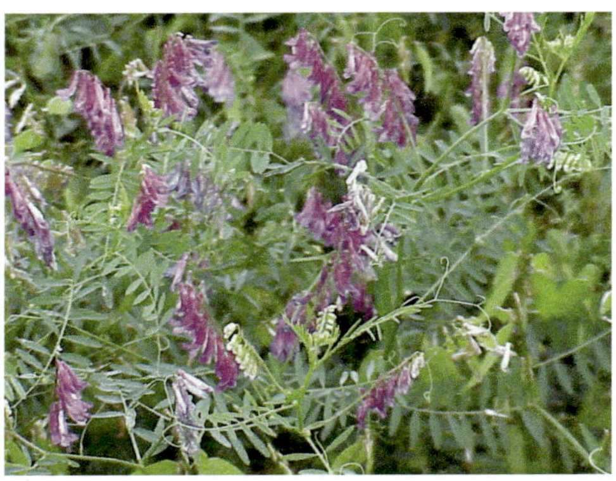

Fig. 16.59. *Vicia villosa* (hairy vetch) is a perennial legume that is commonly grown as a cover crop in many parts of the world. It has a hard, long-lived seed that shatters early in the season, leading to it persisting in fields and becoming weedy. It commonly invades fields and can contaminate hay and grain.

Upper alimentary carcinomas

Chronic, low-dose bracken fern exposures are more likely to be solely carcinogenic, resulting in neoplasms in the upper gastrointestinal tract. The effects appear to be cumulative, as many animals are exposed intermittently and exposures may occur over years before disease develops. Ptaquiloside-induced neoplasms have been described in many species, and cattle neoplastic transformation is exacerbated by bovine papilloma virus infection.

All of these bracken-related diseases are fatal and essentially untreatable.

16.6.6 Hairy vetch (*Vicia villosa* Roth)

Vicia plants produce disease in older cattle (>3 years) characterized by granulomatous inflammation of the skin and various other organs (see various organ systems). Hairy vetch and several related vetches are often used as cover crops, forages, and grow wild in many parts of the world. Presentation is dependent on exposure. Ingestion of seeds produces neurologic disease, probably related to seed cyanogenic glycosides, whereas ingestion of vegetative plants produces granulomatous dermatitis and inflammation of many organs. Morbidity is usually low, but it can be high. Black cattle (Angus and Holsteins) are most commonly affected after ingesting vetch for 10–14 days.

Clinical disease is characterized by dermatitis, puritis, diarrhea, and wasting.

Grossly, nodules and military foci are present in liver, spleen, kidney, adrenal glands, heart, pancreas.

Microscopically, the skin, liver, pancreas, kidneys, heart, adrenal glands, and various other tissues can be infiltrated with monocytes, lymphocytes, plasma cells, eosinophils, and multinucleated giant cells.

Affected animals may die weeks after exposure is discontinued. The several proposed pathogeneses include vetch-induced type IV hypersensitivity, or that vetch lectins directly activate T-lymphocytes, resulting in granulomatous inflammation. It should be mentioned that citrus pulp toxicosis, inducing comparable granulomatous lesions in multiple organs, has a similar pathogenesis and should be considered as a differential diagnosis.

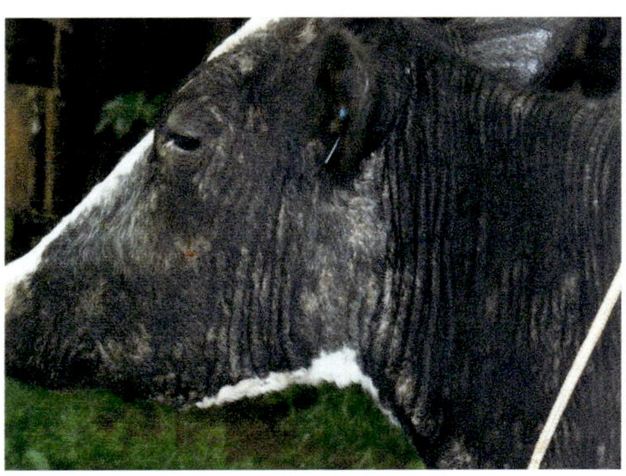

Fig. 16.60. Ox. Skin. Granulomatous dermatitis. Cow poisoned with *Vicia villosa*. Notice the thickened skin with raised, hard foci of nodular inflammation. (Courtesy of Dr C. Barros, Universidade Federal de Santa Maria, Brazil.)

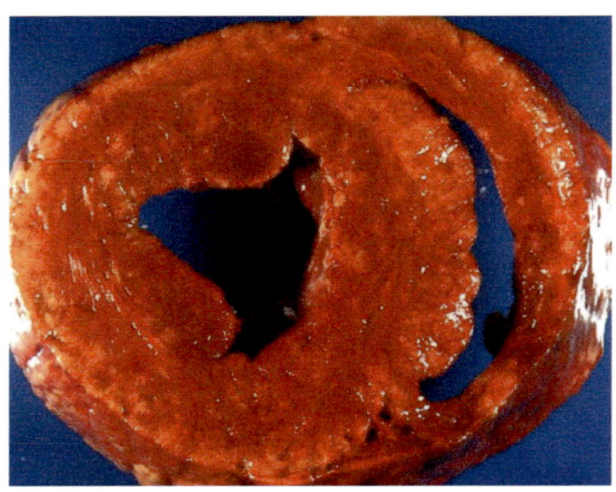

Fig. 16.61. Ox. Heart. Granulomatous myocarditis. Cow poisoned with *Vicia villosa*. Notice the pale to white foci that extend into the deep myocardium. (Courtesy of Dr C. Barros, Universidade Federal de Santa Maria, Brazil.)

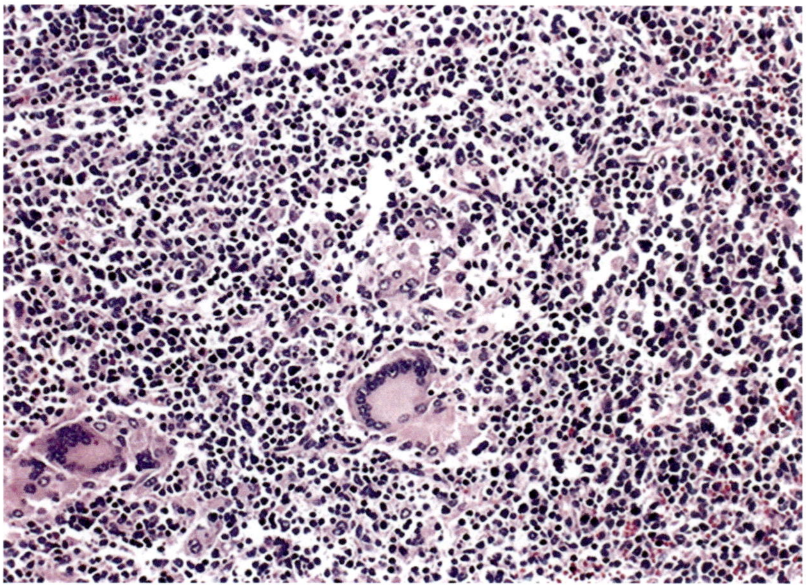

Fig. 16.62. Ox. Spleen. Granulomatous splenitis. Cow poisoned with *Vicia villosa*. Notice the white pulp is expanded with infiltrates of monocytes, macrophages, lymphocytes, and multinucleated giant cells (H&E). (Courtesy of Dr C. Barros, Universidade Federal de Santa Maria, Brazil.)

SUMMARY

Toxic plants poison cattle and often produce specific diseases with characteristic clinical, gross, and histologic lesions. This is a brief summary of the diseases and lesions produced by several select poisonous plants. Readers are referred to recent reviews for more complete descriptions, diagnostic techniques, and treatments (Kingsbury, 1964; Burrows and Tyrl, 2001; Knight and Walter, 2001; Stegelmeier *et al.*, 2013).

SUGGESTED READING

Bandara, V., Weinstein, S.A., White, J. and Eddleston, M. (2010) A review of the natural history, toxicology, diagnosis and clinical management of *Nerium oleander* (common oleander) and *Thevetia peruviana* (yellow oleander) poisoning. *Toxicon* 56, 273–281.

Burrows, G.E. and Tyrl, R.J. (2001) *Toxic Plants of North America*. University of Iowa Press, Iowa City, Iowa.

Gardner, D.R., James, L.F., Panter, K.E., Pfister, J.A., Ralphs, M.H. and Stegelmeier, B.L. (1999) Ponderosa pine and broom snakeweed: poisonous plants that affect livestock. *Journal of Natural Toxins* 8, 27–34.

Hanichen, T., Plank, P. and Dirksen, G. (1970) Enzootic calcinosis in cattle. II. Histomorphological studies of soft tissues. *Deutsche Tieraerztliche Wochenschrift* 77, 338–342.

Johnson, B., Moore, J., Woods, L.W. and Galey, F.D. (1992) Systemic granulomatous disease in cattle in California associated with grazing hairy vetch (*Vicia villosa*). *Journal of Veterinary Diagnostic Investigation* 4, 360–362.

Kingsbury, J.M. (1964) *Poisonous Plants of the United States and Canada*. Prentice-Hall, Inc, Englewood Cliffs, New York.

Knight, A.P. and Walter, R.G. (2001) *A Guide to Plant Poisoning*. Teton Newmedia, Jackson Wyoming.

Morton, J.F. (1994) Lantana or red sage (*Lantan camara* L. [Verbenaceae]), notorious weed and popular garden flower; some cases of poisoning in Florida. *Economic Botany* 48, 259–271.

Panter, K.E., Molyneux, R.J., Smart, R.A., Mitchell, L. and Hansen, S. (1993) English yew poisoning in 43 cattle. *Journal of the American Veterinary Medical Association* 202, 1476–1477.

Panter, K.E., James, L.F. and Gardner, D.R. (1999) Lupines, poison-hemlock and *Nicotiana* spp.: toxicity and teratogenicity in livestock. *Journal of Natural Toxins* 8, 117–134.

Panter, K.E., Gardner, D.R., Stegelmeier, B.L., Welch, K.D. and Holstege, D. (2011) Water hemlock poisoning in cattle: ingestion of immature *Cicuta maculata* seed as the probable cause. *Toxicon* 57, 157–161.

Pickrell, J.A. and Oehme, F. (2003) Cyanogenic glycosides. In: Plumlee, K.H. (ed.) *Clinical Veterinary Toxicology*. Mosby, St Louis, Missouri, pp. 391–392.

Sharma, O.P., Sharma, S., Pattabhi, V., Mahato, S.B. and Sharma, P.D. (2007) A review of the hepatotoxic plant *Lantana camara*. *Critical Reviews in Toxicology* 37, 313–352.

Shupe, J.L., Binns, W., James, L.F. and Keeler, R.F. (1967) Lupine, a cause of crooked calf disease. *Journal of the American Veterinary Medical Association* 151, 198–203.

Stegelmeier, B.L., James, L.F., Panter, K.E., Ralphs, M.H., Gardner, D.R., *et al.* (1999) The pathogenesis and toxicokinetics of locoweed (*Astragalus* and *Oxytropis* spp.) poisoning in livestock. *Journal of Natural Toxins* 8, 35–45.

Stegelmeier, B.L., Lee, S.T., James, L.F., Gardner, D.R., Panter, K.E., *et al.* (2007) The comparative pathology of locoweed poisoning in livestock, wildlife and rodents. In: Panter, K.E., Wierenga, T.L. and Pfister, J.A. (eds) *Poisonous Plants: Global Research and Solutions*. CAB International, Wallingford, UK, pp. 359–365.

Stegelmeier, B.L., Davis, T.Z., Green, B.T., Lee, S.T. and Hall, J.O. (2010) Experimental rayless goldenrod (*Isocoma pluriflora*) toxicosis in goats. *Journal of Veterinary Diagnostic Investigation* 22, 570–577.

Stegelmeier, B.L., Field, R.A., Panter, K.E., Hall, J.O., Welch, K.D., *et al.* (2013) Selected poisonous plants affecting animal and human health. In: Haschek, W.M., Rousseaux, C.G., Willig, M.A., Bolon, B., Ochoa, R. and Mahler, B.W. (eds) *Haschek and Rousseaux's Handbook of Toxicologic Pathology*, 3rd edn. Academic Press, San Diego, California, pp. 1259–1314.

Stegelmeier, B.L., Colegate, S.M. and Brown, A.W. (2016) Dehydropyrrolizidine alkaloid toxicity, cytotoxicity, and carcinogenicity. *Toxins* Nov 29 8(12), pii, E 356.

Stuart, B.P., Nicholson, S.S. and Smith, J.B. (1975) Perirenal edema and toxic nephrosis in cattle, associated with ingestion of pigweed. *Journal of the American Veterinary Medical Association* 167, 949–950.

Witte, S.T., Osweiler, G.D., Stahr, H.M. and Mobley, G. (1990) Cocklebur toxicosis in cattle associated with the consumption of mature *Xanthium strumarium*. *Journal of Veterinary Diagnostic Investigation* 2, 263–267.

Yadav, J.P., Arya, V., Yadav, S., Panghal, M., Kumar, S. and Dhankhar, S. (2010) *Cassia occidentalis*: a review on its ethnobotany, phytochemical and pharmacological profile. *Fitoterapia* 81, 223–230.

Yamamoto, T. and Hirano, A. (1986) A comparative study of modified Bielschowsky, Bodian and thioflavin S stains on Alzheimer's neurofibrillary tangles. *Neuropathology and Applied Neurobiology* 12, 3–9.

CHAPTER 17

Bovine Diseases Without Lesions

17.1 Botulism
17.2 Tetanus
17.3 Hypocalcemia
17.4 Hypomagnesemia
17.5 Nervous Ketosis
17.6 Urea Toxicity (Ammonia Toxicosis)
17.7 Acute Organophosphate Poisoning
17.8 Lightning
17.9 Japanese Yew (*Taxus cuspidata*)
17.10 Nervous Coccidiosis

INTRODUCTION

There are conditions in which individual or several animals die unexpectedly without manifesting pathologic changes after complete necropsy and thorough microscopic tissue examination. Broad categorization for etiologies to consider include toxins, toxic plants, metabolic disorders, and some infectious agents. In some of these instances, observed premonitory signs prior to death, detailed history, environmental conditions, and management changes may provide clues for a presumptive etiologic diagnosis. Additional ancillary testing is recommended for specific diagnosis depending on economic circumstances. Positive test results are helpful; negative results do not exclude the disorder. Since these disease entities lack morphologic lesions, key clinical signs of affected animals are added to some disorders in this chapter to create awareness of any of the specific diseases presented.

17.1 BOTULISM

Introduction. *Clostridium botulinum*, the causative agent, is a ubiquitous, spore-forming organism producing eight types of potent, lethal neurotoxins interfering with neurotransmitter release at the neuromuscular junction. The bacterium proliferates in decaying animal carcasses, improperly fermented silage, or contaminated feed or water sources. Toxins enter the bloodstream of the animal through the intestinal tract or infected skin wounds. Death results from respiratory failure. Diagnosis is made by culturing spores, analyzing for toxins via mouse inoculation of feed or fecal contents extracts, and polymerase chain reaction (PCR) for neurotoxin genes in feed, fecal, and gastrointestinal samples.

Clinical signs. Ataxia, paralysis (tongue), recumbency.

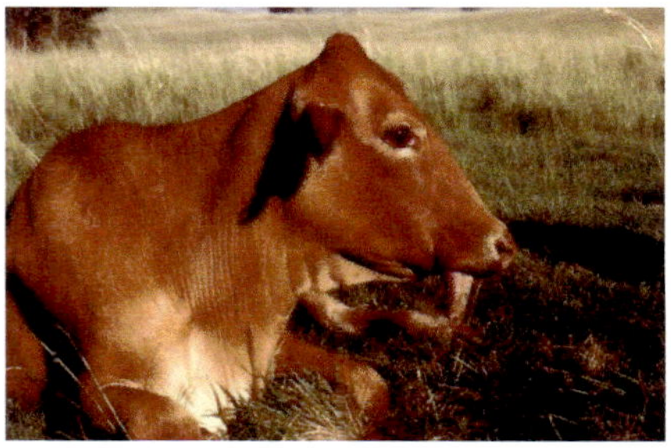

Fig. 17.1. Ox. Botulism. Motor paralysis of tongue. Protruding tongue in recumbent cow. (Courtesy of Dr D. Driemeier, Universidade Federal do Rio Grande do Sul, Brazil.)

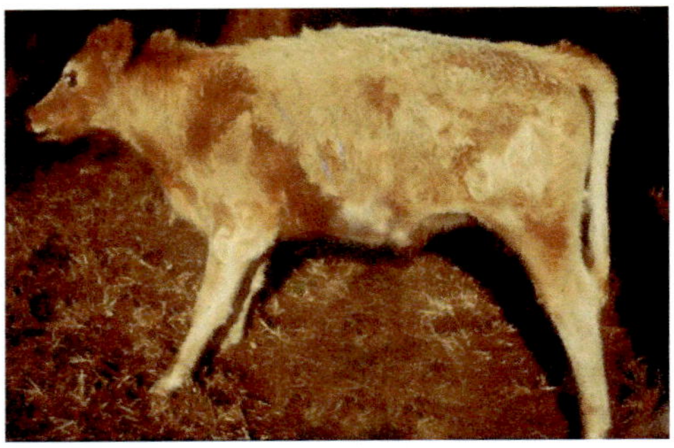

Fig. 17.2. Ox. Tetanus. Limb rigidity and expression of anxiety. (Courtesy of Dr D. Driemeier, Universidade Federal do Rio Grande do Sul, Brazil.)

Differential diagnoses. Rabies, bovine spongiform encephalopathy (BSE), other neurologic disorders, trauma.

17.2 TETANUS

Introduction. *Clostridium tetani* entering through puncture skin wounds produces a neurotoxin reaching the brain and spinal cord via the retrograde nerve pathway. Another common cause for tetanus to develop are elastrator bands used for castration. The spore-forming organism is commonly found in soil.

Clinical signs. Gait rigidity, bloat, third eyelid prolapse, elevated tail, 'locked jaw'.

Differential diagnoses. Hypomagnesemia, various central nervous system (CNS) diseases, musculoskeletal injuries.

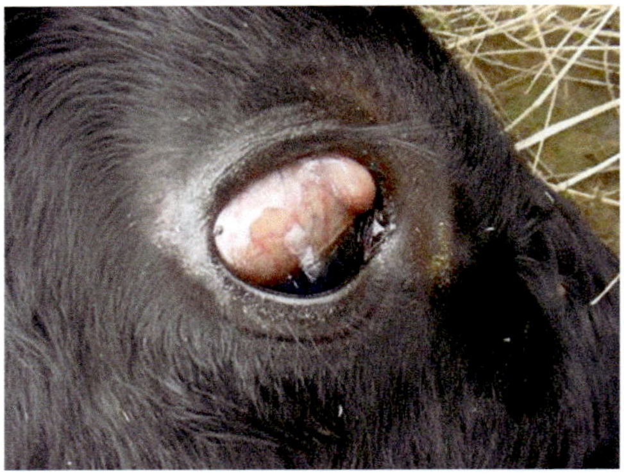

Fig. 17.3. Ox. Tetanus. Prolapse of nictitans membrane. (Courtesy of Dr D. Driemeier, Universidade Federal do Rio Grande do Sul, Brazil.)

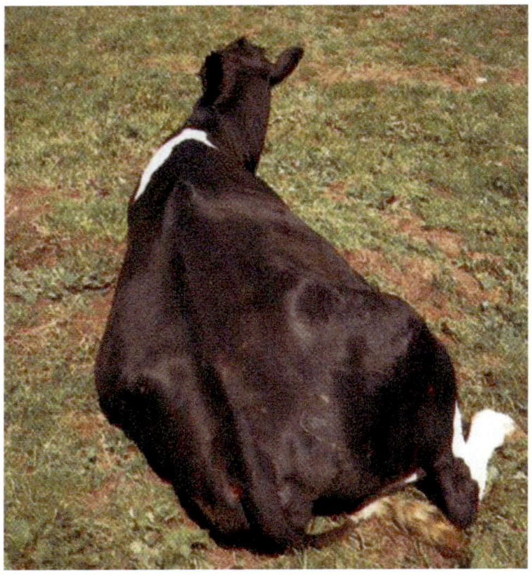

Fig. 17.4. Ox. Hypocalcemia. The neck is bent 'S' shaped. The head may rest on front legs. Affected animals are also seen in lateral recumbency, with gaseous distension since they cannot eructate normally. (Courtesy of Dr D. Driemeier, Universidade Federal do Rio Grande do Sul, Brazil.)

17.3 HYPOCALCEMIA

Introduction. (Post-) parturient hypocalcemia ('milk fever') immediately follows parturition, with blood calcium concentration dropping below 8.5 mg/dl.

Clinical signs. Affected animals become recumbent and unable to rise.

Differential diagnoses. Trauma, botulism, ketosis.

17.4 HYPOMAGNESEMIA

Introduction. Also known as grass tetany, the metabolic disorder occurs in spring pastured dairy and beef cows. Ocular, urine, and CNS fluid magnesium levels are 1.0 mg/dl or less.

Clinical signs. Stiffness, leg paddling, leg spasm, convulsions, muscle fasciculation, recumbency.

Differential diagnoses. Nervous ketosis, hypocalcemia, CNS diseases.

17.5 NERVOUS KETOSIS

Introduction. Nervous ketosis (azotemia) is associated with blood ketone bodies, ketonemia, and ketonuria. Occurs in high-producing cows.

Clinical signs. Licking, behavioral changes such as aggression, staggering, recumbency, blindness.

Differential diagnoses. Rabies, BSE, listeriosis, polioencephalomalacia, metabolic diseases.

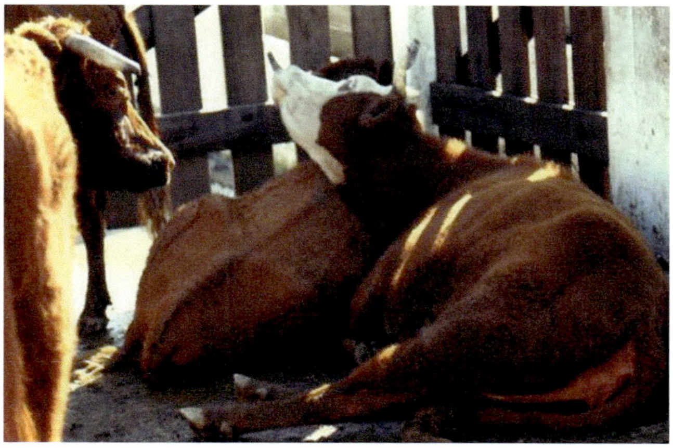

Fig. 17.5. Ox. Nervous ketosis. Opisthotonos. (Courtesy of Dr D. Driemeier, Universidade Federal do Rio Grande do Sul, Brazil.)

17.6 UREA TOXICITY (AMMONIA TOXICOSIS)

Introduction. The non-protein nitrogen (NPN) feed supplement when offered in too high concentrations (mixing error) in feed mixture (more than 3%) becomes toxic, causing the sudden death of multiple animals. There is a relative lack of gross and microscopic findings in cases of urea poisoning, with the exception of subjective ruminal tympany and a subjectively relative advanced stage of post-mortem autolysis. Feed analysis and determination of urea concentration (non-protein nitrogen) in feed and aqueous humor are recommended for the definitive diagnosis of urea poisoning. An additional recommendation is the determination of blood and vitreous ammonia (>1.0 mg/dl) levels. (Also see Chapter 5: Diseases of the Gastrointestinal Tract.)

Clinical signs. Colic, convulsions, paresis, recumbency, mucosanguinous nasal discharge.
Differential diagnoses. Lightning, chemical or plant toxicoses.

17.7 ACUTE ORGANOPHOSPHATE POISONING

Introduction. Used in herbicides and pesticides, the utilization of the compound is prohibited in many countries. The compound inhibits cholinesterase activity, with acetylcholine accumulation in synaptic junctions. Gross and microscopic lesions are absent in the CNS in acute cases of toxicosis. Analysis of adipose tissue and/or fresh brain for cholinesterase levels is recommended for diagnosis.
Clinical signs. Proprioceptive deficits (paresis, ataxia), muscle twitching, salivation.
Differential diagnoses. Urea poisoning.

17.8 LIGHTNING

Introduction. Lightning is a powerful electrical spark during a thunderstorm with a potential of up to millions of volts. Lightning, when striking an animal, will cause electrical injury to the skin and cardiovascular and nervous systems without leaving morphologic marks, making the specific diagnosis extremely difficult. The search for finding singe marks in the skin as a clue is almost always unsuccessful. Hemorrhages in the subcutis and on serosal surfaces are non-specific and may be just agonal. The environment of the demised animal is more supportive for the diagnosis of lightning. A loss of tree bark or several dead carcasses surrounding a tree, fence, or post are indicators to suspect lightning as cause of death, as is the procurement of the most recent local weather report. Local weather casts and reports may be helpful as well.
Clinical sign in survivors. Visual impairment.
Differential diagnoses. Anthrax, clostridial diseases, electrocution.

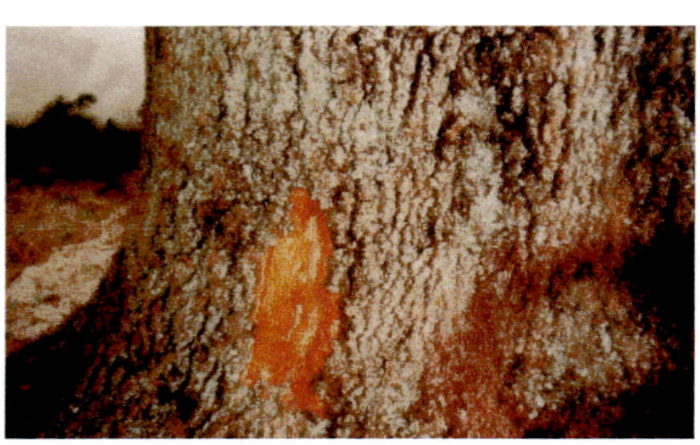

Fig. 17.7. Ox. Lightning. Loss of tree bark.

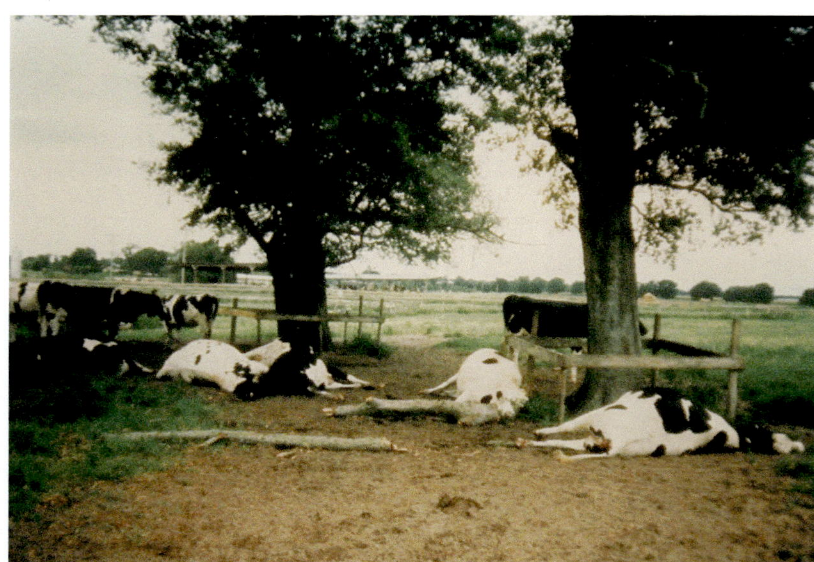

Fig. 17.6. Ox. Lightning. Multiple corpses around trees after a thunderstorm.

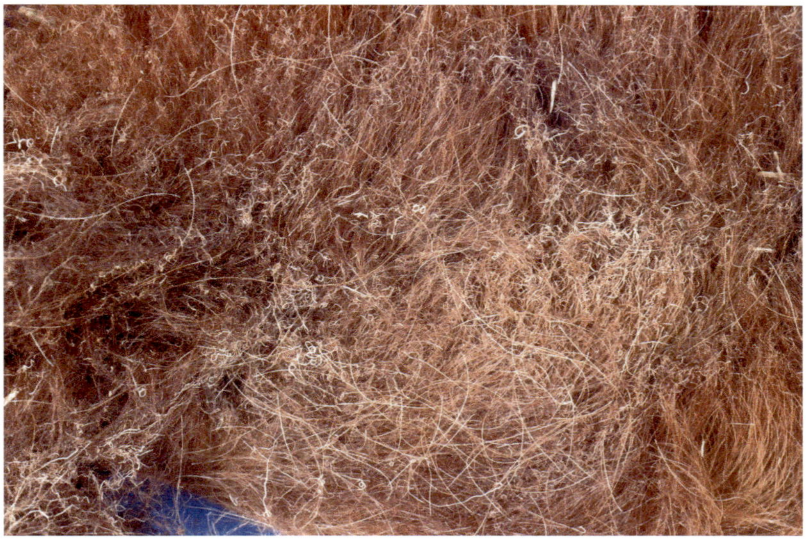

Fig. 17.9. Ox. Lightning. Hair singeing. Widespread scattering of detached, dry, burned hair as indirect evidence of lightning. (Courtesy of Department of Veterinary Pathology, WCVM, University of Saskatchewan, Saskatoon, Canada.)

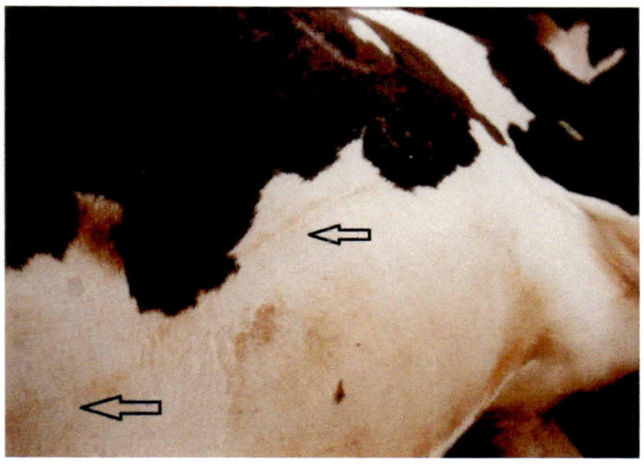

Fig. 17.8. Ox. Lightning Burn line. Continuous line of singed hair (arrows) expanding across lateral abdomen and thorax. This is a rare finding associated with lightning in livestock. (See Chapter 12: Diseases of the Integument.)

17.9 JAPANESE YEW (*TAXUS CUSPIDATA*)

Introduction. Leaves of *Taxus cuspidata*, an ornamental shrub, are highly toxic to livestock. Death occurs suddenly and fast due to cardiac dysrhythmia that is not usually associated with histologic lesions. Often, demised animals contain *Taxus* leaves in their mouth. The toxicity of yew leaves is due to the presence of alkaloids known as taxines, of which taxine B is suspected as being one of the most poisonous. Taxines act on cardiac myocytes. Chromatography or mass spectrometry of ruminal contents are recommended detection methods (see Chapter 16: The Pathology of Select Poisonous Plant-induced Diseases in Cattle).

17.10 NERVOUS COCCIDIOSIS

Introduction. Mainly seen in beef calves, it has been observed in dairy calves suffering from a heavy load of protozoa in conjunction with adverse weather conditions. Clinical signs mimic polioencephalomalacia. Mouse inoculation of serum from calves showing nervous signs resulted in neurologic signs in the mice similar to calves, suggesting that the calf serum might contain a neurotoxin. (Also see Chapter 5: Diseases of the Gastrointestinal Tract.)

SUGGESTED READING

Boeve, M.H., Huijben, R., Grinwis, G. and Djajadinningraf-Laanen, S.C. (2004) Visual impairment after suspected lightning strike in a herd of Holstein-Friesian cattle. *Veterinary Record* 154, 402–404.

Campagnolo, E.R., Kasten, S. and Banerjee, M. (2002) Accidental ammonia exposure to county fair show livestock due to contaminated drinking water. *Veterinary Human Toxicology* 44, 282–285.

Johnson, A.L., McAdams-Gallagher, S.C. and Sweeney, R.W. (2014) Quantitative real-time PC for detection of neurotoxin genes of *Clostridium botulinum* types A, B and C in equine samples. *The Veterinary Journal* 199, 157–161.

Khan, O. (2001) Organophosphate poisoning in a group of replacement heifers and dry cows. *Canadian Veterinary Journal* 42, 561–563.

Kopcha, M. (1987) Nutritional and metabolic diseases involving the nervous system. *Veterinary Clinics of North America: Food Animal Practice* 3, 119–135.

Sula, M.J., Morgan, S., Bailey, K.L., Schumpert, M. and Njaa, B.L. (2013) Characterization of cardiac lesions in calves after ingestion of Japanese yew (*Taxus cuspidata*). *Journal of Veterinary Diagnostic Investigation* 25, 522–526.

Vanneste, E., Weyens, P., Poelman, D.R., Chiers, K., Deprez, P. and Pardon, B. (2015) Lightning related fatalities in livestock: veterinary expertise and the added value of lightning location data. *Veterinary Journal* 203, 103–108.

Wilson, J.R., Sauer, J. and Hooser, S.B. (2001) Taxines: a review of the mechanism and toxicity of yew (*Taxus* spp.). *Toxicon* 39, 175–185.

INDEX

abdominal wall defects 5
abomasum
  displaced/rotated 135
  erosions/ulcers 21, 137
  hairballs 21
  hemorrhagic abomasitis 21–22, 138
  neoplasia 140, 285
  obstruction 136
  parasites 139–140
  salmonellosis 18, 138
abortion 240, 260
  bacterial infections 245, 257
    brucellosis 246–247
    campylobacteriosis 245, 251–252
    epizootic 252–253
    leptospirosis 247–249
    listeriosis 249–250
    ureaplasmosis 251
  diagnostic testing 259–260
  fungal infections 254
  plant toxins 259, 409–410
  protozoal infections
    neosporiasis 255–257
    trichomoniasis 254–255
  viral infections 245
    BHV-1 240–242
    bluetongue 244
    BVDV 210–211, 242–244
    IBR 242
    Schmallenberg 244
abscesses
  brain/spinal cord 47
  liver 170–171
  lung 87
  pituitary 218
  spleen 281
  udder 358
acantholysis, familial 298
actinobacillosis 119–120, 316–317
actinomycosis (lumpy jaw) 208, 209, 315–316
adenovirus 10
adrenal gland
  amyloidosis 221
  BHV-1 infection 242
  citrus pulp toxicosis 222
  hemorrhage 220
  neoplasia 221
aflatoxins 162–163
Ageratina altissima (white snakeroot) 398–399
albinism 370
allergic dermatitis 337–338
Allium spp. 282
alopecia 300–302, 304
Amaranthus spp. (pigweeds) 408
ammonia toxicosis 130, 419–420
amnion, epithelial plaques 238
amoebiasis, cerebral 49–50
amorphous globosus 238
amyloidosis 183, 221
anaplasmosis 175, 272
anemia, hemolytic 272–274, 282, 413
angiomatosis 333
anthrax 271, 280–281
aorta
  Marfan syndrome 106
  paratuberculosis 153
  vasculitis 105
aplasia
  cerebellum 3
  intestines 3
  uterine horns 231
aplasia cutis (epitheliogenesis imperfecta) 294
arthritis, septic 23, 24, 26, 79, 212–213
arthrogryposis 244, 258, 405
ascarid worms 20, 154
Aspergillus spp.
  aflatoxins 162–163
  infections 82, 131, 171, 254
aspiration pneumonia 84
Astragalus spp.
  nitrotoxins 388–389
  selenium toxicity 402, 403
  swainsonine 382–385
astrovirus, neurotropic 42–43
ataxia 53, 54–56
atypical interstitial pneumonia (AIP) 84–87
babesiosis 48, 49, 272
bacillary hemoglobinuria 168–169, 273
Bacillus anthracis 271, 280–281
bacterial infections
  abortion 245–253, 257, 259
  bone 79, 208–210, 212–213
  brain/spinal cord 6, 23, 43–47
  calf sepsis 23–24
  cardiovascular 95, 97, 100–101, 106
  ear 378–379
  eye 372–374
  foot rot 351–352
  gastrointestinal 16–18, 21–22, 119–121, 131, 138, 145–147
  kidney 184–186, 189, 248–249
  liver 168–171, 273
  respiratory 9, 13, 70–81, 245, 251, 252
  seminal vesicle 228
  skeletal muscle 199–200
  skin 310–318
  udder 358, 359–362
  uterus 235
balanoposthitis 229
'barber pole' worm (*Haemonchus placei*) 139
benign peripheral nerve sheath tumor (schwannoma) 52
besnoitiosis 318, 319, 371, 372
beta-agonists 349–350

BHV *see* bovine herpesviruses
Bibersteinia trehalosi 80–81
blackleg (*Clostridium chauvoei*) 97, 121, 199, 317
bladder
  bracken fern toxicity 193, 413
  cystitis 191
  neoplasia 193
bleeding disorders
  Bovine leukocyte deficiency disease 267
  bovine neonatal pancytopenia 28–29
  BVDV thrombocytopenia 275
  plant toxins 282, 283, 335
  Simmental hereditary thrombopathy 267, 335
blepharitis 371–372
bloat (tympany) 21, 128–130, 335
blue-green algae toxicosis 164
bluetongue virus 116, 244, 364
BLV (bovine leukemia virus) 284–285, 376
bone *see* skeletal system
bone marrow
  infarction 270
  juvenile lymphoma 211, 286
  normal 265
  serous atrophy of fat 269
botulism 417–418
bovine herpes mammillitis (BHV-2) 309, 363–364
bovine herpesviruses (BHV) 40
  BHV-1
    abortion 240–242
    conjunctivitis 372
    encephalomyelitis 39
    gastrointestinal tract 14, 118, 125
    respiratory tract 57, 58, 60–62, 64–65
  BHV-2 309–310, 363–364
  BHV-5 39, 375
  BHV-6 39
  see also malignant catarrhal fever (MCF)
bovine leukemia virus (BLV) 284–285, 376
bovine leukocyte adhesion deficiency 267
bovine malignant catarrhal fever *see* malignant catarrhal fever (MCF)
bovine neonatal pancytopenia 28–29
bovine papular stomatitis (BPS) 118, 124, 307–308
bovine progressive degenerative myeloencephalopathy 53
bovine respiratory syncytial virus (BRSV) 12, 66–69
bovine spongiform encephalopathy (BSE) 37
bovine sporadic encephalomyelitis (BSE) 46–47
bovine vesicular stomatitis 118, 364
bovine viral diarrhea virus (BVDV) 112–114
  abortion 210–211, 242–244
  gastrointestinal tract 112–115, 124, 132, 147–149
  myocardium 97, 98
  ocular malformations 368
  Peyer's patches 148, 149, 275–276
  respiratory disease 69–70
  skin lesions 304–306
  skin test 151
  thrombocytopenia 275
  vasculitis 98, 149–151, 336
BPS (bovine papular stomatitis) 118, 124, 307–308
brachygnathia inferior 205
bracken fern (*Pteridium aquilinum*) 138, 193, 282, 413–414
brain *see* nervous system
Brangus calves, mechanobullous disease 299
Brassica spp. 282
brisket disease (high-altitude disease) 102–103, 382
bronchiectasis 64, 78, 81, 88
bronchiolitis obliterans 89
bronchitis/bronchiolitis
  BRSV 12, 67
  IBR 64–65
  lungworm 83
  Mycoplasma bovis 78
bronchopneumonia *see* pneumonia
BRSV (bovine respiratory syncytial virus) 12, 66–69
brucellosis 246–247
BSE (bovine spongiform encephalopathy) 37
buckwheat (*Fagopyrum* spp.) 413
Bunostomum phlebotomum (hookworm) 154
burns
  chemical 354
  thermal 339, 421
BVDV *see* bovine viral diarrhea virus

calcium
  calcification
    cardiovascular 100, 105
    kidney 181
    placenta 238
  calcinogenic plants 100, 408–409
  hypocalcemia 418
calves 1
  bovine neonatal pancytopenia 28–29
  BVDV infection in pregnant dams 210, 242–243
  calf sepsis (septicemia) 23–24, 220
  eye conditions 367–371
  floppy ear syndrome 29, 378
  gastrointestinal disease 14–22
  muscular disease 25, 195–197
  neoplasia 6–7, 26, 211, 286, 333, 334
  nervous system disease 6–8, 421
  respiratory disease 9–13
  skeletal disease 25–26, 202–205, 206–208, 212
  skin conditions 292–300
  thymus gland 262–263, 271–272
  thyroid disease 27–28, 292
  urinary system disease 4–5, 27
  see also congenital anomalies
calystegines 386
Campylobacter spp. 245, 251–252
cancer *see* neoplasia
candidiasis 11, 14
cardioglycosides 398–399, 421
cardiomegaly 101
cardiovascular system *see* aorta; heart
carotid rete mirabile 40, 218
Cassia (*Senna*) spp. 197–198, 402
castanospermine 386
cataracts 371
catarrhal enteritis 142, 154, 155
caudal vena cava thrombosis 89–90
cellulitis 317–318

central nervous system *see* nervous system
cerebellum
aplasia/hypoplasia 2, 3
herniation 6, 37
medulloblastoma 6–7
swainsonine poisoning 384, 385
ceroid-lipofuscinosis 55–56
cestode worms *see* tapeworms
Charolais cattle, ataxia 54–55
Chediak–Higashi disease 266–267
Chlamydophila pecorum 46–47
choke (esophageal obstruction) 123
chokecherry (*Prunus virginiana*) 411
cholecystitis 175
cholestasis, intrahepatic 175
chondrodysplasia 25, 26, 202–203
chorionitis 242, 245, 246, 251, 252, 254
chorioptic mange 322
Cicuta maculata (water hemlock) 390
citrullinemia 8
citrus pulp toxicosis 175, 187, 222
claw/claw horn capsule 343
coronary band 404
degloving injuries 349–350
heel horn erosion 353
laminitis 344–345, 404
non-healing lesions 348–349
screw claw 354–355
sepsis of the distal interphalangeal joint 348
sole trauma 347–348
sole ulcer 345–346
thin soles/thin sole toe ulcer 346–347
vertical wall crack 348
white line disease 346, 355
see also foot
cleft palate 3, 405
clostridial myositis 199
Clostridium botulinum 417–418
Clostridium chauvoei (blackleg) 97, 121, 199, 317
Clostridium haemolyticum (*Clostridium novyi*) 168–169, 273
Clostridium perfringens
gastrointestinal hemorrhage 17, 22, 144, 156
mastitis 359
Clostridium septicum 21, 199, 317
Clostridium tetani 418
clover 283, 335
coagulopathy *see* bleeding disorders
coccidiosis 19, 155, 421
cocklebur (*Xanthium strumarium*) 395–396
coenurosis, cerebral 51
cold injury 335, 336
coliform bacteria 16–17, 359
collagen dysplasia 295–296
coloboma 370
colon
coccidiosis 19, 155
displacement 14, 141
parasites 154
salmonellosis 18, 146
winter dysentery 142–143
congenital anomalies
arthrogryposis 244, 258, 405
chondrodysplasia 25, 26, 202–203
craniofacial 2, 3, 112, 205, 405
eye 367–371
heart 4, 94
hematological 266–268
intestines 3
nervous system 2–3, 244
skin 292–300
urinary system 4–5, 177–178
uterus 231–232
congenital erythropoietic porphyria 122, 268
coning (cerebellar herniation) 6, 37
Conium maculatum (poison hemlock) 389–390
conjunctivitis 372–373
contagious bovine pleuropneumonia 80
copper 282
cor pulmonale 103, 104
coriosis (laminitis) 344–345, 404
corkscrew claw 354–355
cornea 373
corns (interdigital fibroma) 353
coronavirus
enteritis 15, 142–143
pneumonia 9, 10
corpus cavernosum 229
cotyledonary placentation 237
cowdriosis 47
craniofacial duplication 2
crooked calf disease 405
cryptococcosis 47–48
cryptosporidiosis 19
cutaneous conditions *see* skin
cyanide-producing plants 410–411
cyanobacterial toxicosis 164
Cymopterus watsonii (spring parsley) 413
cysticercosis 200
cystitis 191

death camas (*Toxicoscordion venenosum*) 391–392
deer fluke 172
degloving injuries 349–350
dehydropyrrolizidine alkaloids 392–394
Delphinium spp. 387–388
dental diseases 121–122
dermatitis
allergic 337–338
of the foot/lower leg 305, 351, 352, 353–354
hairy vetch poisoning 414
idiopathic (ulcerative) 339–341
infectious 305, 308–317, 318–325, 326–327
photosensitivity 167–168, 338, 371, 394, 412–413
udder 357–358
dermatophilosis 310–311
dermatophytosis (ringworm) 326–327
dermoid, ocular 370
diaphragmatic hernia 158
dicoumarol 283, 335
Dictyocaulus viviparus (lungworm) 82–83
diet *see* nutritional and diet-related disorders

diprosopus 2
downer cow myopathy 198
dwarfism 25, 26, 202–203

ear 376
- floppy ear syndrome 29, 378
- necrosis 336
- neoplasia 379
- otitis externa/otitis media 377–379

Echinococcus granulosus 99, 172
ectopic heart 4
ectropion 370
Ehrlichia ruminantium 47
Eimeria spp. 19, 155, 421
embolic pneumonia 87
emphysema 87
encephalitis
- bacterial 43–47
- fungal 47–48
- parasitic 51
- prion disease (BSE) 37
- protozoal 48–50, 272, 421
- viral 38–43

encephalomyelopathy, breed-specific 53–56
endocardial calcification 100
endocardial fibrosis 99
endocarditis 100–101
endometritis 235
enteritis 142
- BVDV 147–151, 275–276
- in calves 14–20
- catarrhal 142, 154, 155
- fibrinonecrotic (salmonellosis) 18, 145–147
- granulomatous 152–153, 154
- hemorrhagic 17, 19, 142–144, 154, 155

enterotoxins 17, 144
entropion 370
eosinophilic dermatitis 337
eosinophilic intestinal droplets 158
eosinophils
- cuffing (salt intoxication) 35
- myositis 98, 200
- nasal granuloma 59
- in the skin 291, 320, 325

epidermolysis bullosa 299–300
epididymis 228
epitheliogenesis imperfecta 294
epizootic bovine abortion (EBA) 252–253
ergot poisoning 270, 336, 337
ergovaline (in tall fescue grass) 337, 349, 350
erythrocytes 262
- hemolytic anemia 272–274, 282, 413

Escherichia coli 16–17, 359
esophagus 123
- bloat line 128
- nematodes 125
- neoplasia 125
- obstruction 123
- trauma 123–124
- viral infections 124–125

eye 367
- albinism 370
- blepharitis 371–372
- cataracts 371
- colomba 370
- conjunctivitis/uveitis 372–374
- dermoid 370
- entropion/ectropion 370
- exophthalmos 284, 376
- hypopyon 23, 374
- intraocular hemorrhage 371
- lysosomal storage disease-related defects 369
- microphthalmia 367–368
- neoplasia 284, 374–376
- papilledema 369, 371
- remnant hyaloid artery 371
- vitamin A deficiency 368–369

Fagopyrum spp.(buckwheat) 413
fascioliasis 172, 270
fat
- hepatic lipidosis 161–162, 174
- necrosis (peritoneum) 159
- serous atrophy of bone marrow fat 269

fatigue syndrome 350
female reproductive system *see* reproductive system, female
fetal death 239
- *see also* abortion

fetal malformations *see* congenital anomalies
fiber, dietary 130
fibrinonecrotic enteritis (salmonellosis) 18, 145–147
fibroma 122, 334
- interdigital 353

fibropapilloma 125, 134, 229, 236
- *see also* papilloma

floppy ear syndrome 29, 378
flukes
- liver 172, 270
- rumen 133

fluorosis 121–122
foot 344
- abnormalities 205
- digital dermatitis 351
- foot rot 351–352
- foreign body trauma 352
- formalin burns 354
- interdigital dermatitis 305, 352
- interdigital fibroma 353
- mud fever 353–354
- necrosis 210, 336–337
- warts 353
- *see also* claw/claw horn capsule

foothill abortion (epizootic bovine abortion) 252–253
foreign bodies
- in the abomasum 21
- in the esophagus 123
- in the foot/claw 347–348, 352
- in the pericardium 95
- in the reticulum 131

forestomachs 126
bracken fern carcinoma 414
fibropapilloma 134
flukes 133
indigestion (obstruction) 130
inflammation 14, 131–133
lactic acidosis 126–127, 131–132
papillary hypertrophy 130
traumatic reticulitis 131
tympany (bloat) 128–130
unguiculliform papillae 134
urea toxicity 130, 419–420
formalin burns 354
freemartinism 230–231
frostbite 335, 336
fumonisins 397
fungal infections
abortion 254
brain 47–48
gastrointestinal 14, 20, 22, 131, 132
liver 171
lung 82
myocardium 98
skin 326–328
fungal toxins 397
aflatoxins 162–163
ergotamine 270, 336, 337
ergovaline (in tall fescue grass) 337, 349, 350
furocoumarins 413
Fusobacterium necrophorum 9, 131, 170, 171, 318, 359

gall bladder 175
gangrene
in the distal extremities 336–337, 349, 350
myositis 199
pneumonia 84
sinusitis 58
udder 358, 359–360
gastrointestinal tract 112
bacterial infections 16–18, 21–22, 119–121, 131, 138, 145–147
in calves 14–22
diaphragmatic hernia 158
displaced/rotated 14, 135, 141
fungal infections 14, 20, 22, 131, 132
obstruction 123, 130, 136
parasites 20, 125, 133, 139–140, 154–155
protozoal infections 19, 155
viral infections 15–16, 112–119, 124–125, 132, 142–143, 147–151
see also abomasum; esophagus; forestomachs; intestines; oral cavity; rectum
giardiasis 19
gingivitis 115, 116, 118
glossitis 116, 119–121
goats head (*Tribulus terrestris*) 394
goiter 27, 219, 292
gonadogenesis 230
Gongylonema pulchrum 125
granulomatous inflammation
enteritis 152–153, 154, 277–278
epididymal 228
hairy vetch poisoning 187, 222, 414–415
hepatitis 171, 175
lymphatic 108, 109, 278
mastitis 361–362
nephritis 187
pneumonia 81
rhinitis 59
skin 312, 328
granulosa cell tumor 234
grass tetany 419
greasewood (*Sarcobatus vermiculatus*) 407

haemonchosis 139
hair
alopecia 300–302, 304
hypotrichosis 292–294
hairballs 21
hairy vetch (*Vicia villosa*) 187, 222, 414–415
Halogeton glomeratus (saltlover) 407
hardware disease 95, 131
heart 93
aborted fetuses 252, 257
congenital anomalies 4, 94
congestive heart failure 101–104, 335, 382, 404
dissection 93–94
endocardial calcification 100
endocardial fibrosis 99
endocarditis 100–101
fibrovascular disease 106
myocardial degeneration 96, 398–399, 403
myocarditis 97–99, 257, 414
neoplasia 104, 285
pericardial effusion 94
plant toxins 96, 100, 398–399, 403, 414, 421
septic pericarditis 95
valvular cysts 100
heartwater (cowdriosis) 47
heavy metal poisoning
copper 282
lead 35, 180
mercury 36
heel horn erosion 353
Heinz bodies 282
hemal nodes 262, 263
hemangioma/hemangiosarcoma 109, 174
hematocele 228
hematocysts 100
hematopoietic and hemolymphatic system 262
anatomy and physiology 262–266
anemia 272–274, 282, 413
bleeding disorders 28–29, 267, 275, 282, 283, 335
bone marrow 265, 269–270
bovine leukocyte adhesion deficiency 267
Chediak–Higashi disease 266–267
degeneration 269–272
inflammation
anaplasmosis 175, 272
anthrax 271, 280–281

hematopoietic and hemolymphatic system (*continued*)
babesiosis 48, 49, 272
BVDV 148, 149, 243, 275–276
Clostridium novyi (*C. haemolyticum*) 168–169, 273
Mycoplasma bovis 278–279
Mycoplasma wenyonii 273
paratuberculosis 108, 152, 277–278
theileriosis 274
trypanosomiasis 273–274
tuberculosis 277
lymph nodes *see* lymph nodes
neonatal pancytopenia 28–29
neoplasia *see* lymphoma/lymphosarcoma
plant toxins 282–283, 411–412, 413
protoporphyria/porphyria 122, 268
Simmental hereditary thrombopathy 267, 335
spleen 253, 271, 280–281, 285, 415
thrombocytopenia 275, 282, 413
thymus gland 243, 244, 253, 262–263, 271–272, 286
hematuria 193, 413
hemlock 389–390
hemoglobinuria, bacillary 168–169, 273
hemoglobinuric nephrosis 181, 182
hemolytic anemia 272–274, 282, 413
hemorrhage, pulmonary 89–90
hemorrhagic abomasitis 21–22, 138
hemorrhagic bowel syndrome 156–157
hemorrhagic diathesis *see* bleeding disorders
hemorrhagic enteritis 17, 19, 142–144, 154, 155
hemorrhagic rumenitis 126–127
hepatic disease *see* liver
hepatocellular carcinoma 173
herpesviruses *see* bovine herpesviruses (BHVs); malignant catarrhal fever
high-altitude (brisket) disease 102–103, 382
Histophilus somni
encephalitis 45–46
laryngitis 9
myocarditis 97
myositis 199–200
nephritis 186
pneumonia 73–76
hock joint, calf sepsis 24
Hoflund syndrome 136
Honker's syndrome 62–63
hoof *see* claw/claw horn capsule
hydatid disease (echinococcosis) 77, 172
hydranencephaly 2
hydrocephalus 2, 244
hydronephrosis 192
hydrops amnii 383
hymen, persistent 236
Hypericum perforatum (St John's wort) 412
hypernatremia 35
hypocalcemia 418
hypodermosis 325
hypomagnesemia 419
hypopyon 23, 374
hypospadia 5
hypotrichosis 292–294

IBR *see* infectious bovine rhinotracheitis
ichthyosis, congenital 297
impetigo 314, 358, 365
infectious bovine keratoconjunctivitis 372, 373
infectious bovine rhinotracheitis (IBR, BHV-1)
abortion 240–242
conjunctivitis 372
encephalomyelitis 39
gastrointestinal tract 14, 118, 125
respiratory tract 57, 58, 60–62, 64–65
integument *see* skin
interdigital dermatitis 305, 352
interdigital fibroma 353
interdigital phlegmon (foot rot) 351–352
intestines 141
displacement 14, 141
enteritis 142
BVDV 147–151, 275–276
in calves 14–20
catarrhal 142, 154, 155
fibrinonecrotic (salmonellosis) 18, 145–147
granulomatous 152–153, 154
hemorrhagic 17, 19, 142–144, 154, 155
parasites 20, 154–155
protozoa 19, 155
eosinophilic droplets 158
hemorrhagic bowel syndrome 156–157
neoplasia 156
Peyer's patches 141, 148, 149, 265
segmental aplasia 3
intussusception 14, 141
iodine deficiency 27, 219
Ipomoea carnea (pink morning glory) 386
Isocoma pluriflora (rayless goldenrod) 399–400

jaw
brachygnathia inferior 205
mandibular osteomyelitis (lumpy jaw) 208, 209, 315–316
Johne's disease (paratuberculosis) 108, 152–153, 277–278
joints
arthrogryposis 244, 258, 405
degenerative disease 213
osteochondrosis 214–215
septic arthritis 23, 24, 26, 79, 212–213
jugular vein 107
juvenile bovine angiomatosis 333

keratoconjunctivitis 372–373
ketosis 419
kidney 177
in the aborted fetus 248–249, 250
amyloidosis 183
calculi 190, 192
congenital anomalies 4, 177–178
cysts 190
hemorrhage 178
hydronephrosis 192
infarcts 178–179
neoplasia 190

nephritis 184
chronic 188–189
granulomatous (toxic) 187
Histophilus somni 186
leptospirosis 184–185, 248–249
MCF 186–187
nephrosis 179–182, 406–408
nephrotoxic plants 179, 180, 181, 187, 406–408
pyelonephritis 189
white spotted kidney 27, 188
Kochia weed 396

lactic acidosis 126–127, 131–132
lameness *see* claw/claw horn capsule; foot
laminitis 344–345, 404
Lantana spp. 165–168, 397–398
larkspur (*Delphinium*) 387–388
laryngitis 9, 60
lead poisoning 35, 180
leiomyosarcoma 156
leptospirosis 169, 184–185, 247–249
leukocytes
congenital diseases 266–267
see also eosinophils
Leydig cell tumor 227
lice (pediculosis) 320
lightning strikes 339, 420–421
lipidosis, hepatic 161–162, 174
lipoma 334
listeriosis 43–45, 249–250, 372
liver 161
in the aborted fetus 240–241, 247–248, 249–250, 252, 253
cholestasis 175
citrus pulp toxicosis 175
in heart failure 103, 404
hepatitis 168
bacillary hemoglobinuria 168–169, 273
EBA 253
fungal 171
leptospirosis 169, 247–248
listeriosis 249–250
necrotizing/abscesses 170–171
parasitic 172, 270
hepatotoxins
aflatoxins 162–163
blue-green algae 164
cocklebur 395–396
dehydropyrrolizidine alkaloids 392–394
Kochia weed 396
lantadines 165–168, 397–398
saponins 394–395
lipidosis 161–162
vascular tension 174
neoplasia 173–174
telangiectasia 174
locoweed 382–385
Lolium spp. (ryegrass) 386–387
lumpy jaw 208, 209, 315–316
lung 63–64
in the aborted fetus 241, 245, 247, 251, 252, 255
abscesses 87
aspiration pneumonia 84
atypical interstitial pneumonia 84–87
bronchiectasis 64, 78, 81, 88
bronchiolitis obliterans 89
dysplasia 5
edema 88, 102
embolic pneumonia 87
emphysema 87
fibrosis 89
hemorrhage 89–90
inflammation (infections) 64, 79
Bibersteinia trehalosi 80–81
BRSV 12, 66–69
BVDV 69–70
in calves 9–13
coronavirus 9, 10
fungal 82
Histophilus somni 73–76
IBR 64–65
Mannheimia haemolytica 13, 70–72
Mycobacterium bovis 81
Mycoplasma bovis 77–79
Mycoplasma mycoides 80
parainfluenza-3 10–11
parasitic 82–83
Pasteurella multocida 13, 72–73
Trueperella pyogenes 76
neoplasia 83
vascular hyperconstriction in bloat 129
lungworm 82–83
lupines (*Lupinus* spp.) 390–391, 397, 405
lymphatic system/lymph nodes
in bloat 129
infarction 270
lymphoma 284
Mycoplasma bovis 278–279
paratuberculosis 108, 152, 277–278
reactive hyperplasia 266
trematodiasis 270
tuberculosis 277
lymphoma/lymphosarcoma
abomasum 140, 285
adrenal gland 221
bladder 193
brain/spinal cord 52
enzootic (caused by BLV) 284–285, 376
heart 104, 285
juvenile (of bone) 211, 286
kidney 190
liver 173, 174
lung 83
retrobulbar 284, 376
skin 287, 328
small intestine 156
spleen 271, 285
thymus 286
uterus 236
lysosomal storage diseases 369

mad cow disease (BSE) 37
magnesium (hypomagnesemia) 419
male reproductive system *see* reproductive system, male
malignant catarrhal fever (MCF) 40–41, 116
  brain 41
  esophagus 124
  eye 372, 373, 374
  kidney 186–187
  oral 116, 117
  sinonasal 58, 59
  skin 306–307
  vasculitis 40, 117, 307
malignant edema 199, 317
manganese deficiency 207–208
mange 321–323
Mannheimia haemolytica 13, 70–72
maple syrup urine disease 8
Marfan syndrome 106–107
mast cell tumor 330–332
mastitis
  chronic 361
  granulomatous 361–362
  necrotizing 359–360
  suppurative 360–361
MCF *see* malignant catarrhal fever
mechanobullous disease 299–300
medulloblastoma 6–7
megalocytes 163
melanoma 332
meningitis 6, 23, 47
mercury 36
mesothelioma
  peritoneal 26
  tunica albuginea 227
metabolic disorders
  inherited 8, 369
  nutritional *see* nutritional and diet-related disorders
methemoglobinemia 283, 388, 411–412
metritis 235
microphthalmia 367–368
milk fever 418
milk sickness 399–400
milk vein thrombophlebitis 358
mites
  ear infestations 377, 378
  mange 321–323
Moraxella bovis 372, 373
Mortellaro's disease 351
mouth *see* oral cavity
mucosal disease 113, 147, 304
  see also bovine viral diarrhea virus (BVDV)
mud fever 353–354
multifocal symmetrical encephalomyelopathy 53
Murray Grey cattle 54
muscular system 195
  hyperplasia 201
  myodegeneration
    downer cow 198
    nutritional (white muscle disease) 25, 96, 195–197
    plant toxins 96, 197–198, 398–404
  myositis
    bacterial 199–200
    cysticercosis 200
    iatrogenic 201
    sarcocystosis 200
mycobacteriosis, atypical (non-tuberculoid) 312–314
Mycobacterium avium subsp. *paratuberculosis* (paratuberculosis) 108, 152–153, 277–278
Mycobacterium bovis (tuberculosis) 81, 171, 277, 312
Mycoplasma bovis
  arthritis 79
  ear disease 29, 378
  lymphatic 278–279
  mastitis 361
  respiratory disease 77–79
Mycoplasma mycoides subsp. *mycoides* 80
Mycoplasma wenyonii 273
mycotic infections *see* fungal infections
mycotoxins
  aflatoxins 162–163
  ergotamine 270, 336, 337
  ergovaline (in tall fescue grass) 337, 349, 350
myocardial degeneration 96, 398–399, 403
myocarditis 97–99, 257, 414
myodegeneration (skeletal muscle)
  downer cow 198
  nutritional (white muscle disease) 25, 96, 195–197
  plant toxins 96, 197–198, 398–404
myoglobinuria 198, 400
myoglobinuric nephrosis 181, 182
myositis
  bacterial 199–200
  cysticercosis 200
  iatrogenic 201
  sarcocystosis 200

Naegleria fowleri 49–50
nasal conditions *see* nostrils; sinonasal conditions
Negri bodies 38
nematodes
  gastrointestinal 20, 125, 139–140, 154
  otitis 377, 378
  rhabditic dermatitis 324–325
  stephanofilariasis 323–324
neonates
  bovine neonatal pancytopenia 28–29
  see also congenital anomalies
neoplasia
  abomasum 140, 285
  adrenal gland 221
  bladder 193
  bone 211, 286
  brain/spinal cord 6–7, 52
  in calves 6–7, 26, 211, 286, 333, 334
  ear 379
  esophagus 125
  eye 284, 374–376
  heart 104, 285
  hemangioma/hemangiosarcoma 109, 174
  intestines 156

kidney 190
liver 173–174
lung 83
lymphoma *see* lymphoma/lymphosarcoma
mesothelioma 26, 227
oral cavity 122
ovary 233–234
penis 229
perineum 236
rumen 134, 414
sinonasal compartment 60, 109
skin 287, 328–334
testis 227
thyroid 219
udder 363
uterus 236
neosporiasis 255–257
nephritis 184
chronic 188–189
granulomatous (toxic) 187
Histophilus somni 186
leptospirosis 184–185, 248–249
MCF 186–187
pyelonephritis 189
nephrotoxicosis 179–182, 406–408
Nerium oleander 398
nervous system 31–32
botulism 417–418
breed-specific encephalomyelopathies 53–56
calves 6–8, 421
Clostridium perfringens enterotoxemia 144
congenital anomalies 2–3, 244
inflammation
bacterial 6, 23, 43–47
fungal 47–48
parasitic 51
prion disease (BSE) 37
protozoal 48–50, 272, 421
viral 38–43
metabolic disorders 8, 419
neoplasia 6–7, 52
neosporiasis (fetal) 257
neurotoxins
calystegines 386
castanospermine 386
death camas 391–392
Delphinium spp. 387–388
heavy metals 35, 36
hemlock 389–390
lupines 390–391
nitrotoxins 388–389
organophosphates 36, 420
ryegrass 386–387
salt 35
swainsonine (locoweed) 382–385
tetanus 418
trauma 51
vitamin A deficiency 36–37
neural tube defects 3
neurofibromatosis
brachial plexus 52
cardiac 104
neurotropic astrovirus 42–43
nitrate poisoning 283, 411–412
nitrotoxins 388–389
nits (pediculosis) 320
nocardiosis (udder) 362
nostrils 57, 58, 299, 307
nutritional and diet-related disorders
bloat 21, 128–130
citrus pulp toxicosis 175, 187, 222
hepatic lipidosis 151–162
hypocalcemia 418
hypomagnesemia 419
impaction of dry ingesta 130, 136
iodine deficiency 27, 219
manganese deficiency 207–208
nervous ketosis 419
osteoporosis 205–206
polioencephalomalacia 33–34
rickets/osteomalacia 206–207
rumen lactic acidosis 126–127
ruminal papillary hypertrophy 130
urea toxicity 130, 419–420
vitamin A deficiency 36–37, 368–369
white muscle disease 25, 96, 195–197

oak (*Quercus* spp.) 282, 406
Oesophagostomum radiatum 154
oleander 398
omasum 132, 134
omphalocele 5
optic disc swelling (papilledema) 369, 371
optic nerve degeneration 368–369
oral cavity
congenital anomalies 3, 112, 405
epizootic bovine abortion 252
inflammation
bacterial 119–121, 208, 209
viral 112–119
neoplasia 122
teeth 121–122
tonsils 264, 279
orchitis 226
organophosphates 36, 420
osteochondrosis 214–215
osteogenesis imperfecta 203–204
osteomalacia 206
osteomyelitis 208–209, 315
osteopetrosis 204
osteoporosis 205–206
Ostertagia ostertagii 139–140
otitis externa/otitis media 377–379
ovary 232
anatomy 232–233
cysts 233, 383
neoplasia 233–234
oviducts (uterine tubes) 234
oxalate nephrosis 180, 181, 406–408
Oxytropis spp. (locoweed) 382

palatoschisis (cleft palate) 3, 405
pancreolithiasis 176
pancytopenia
- bracken fern toxicity 282, 413
- neonatal 28–29

papilledema 369, 371
papilloma 302–304, 365, 374
- *see also* fibropapilloma

papular stomatitis 118, 124, 307–308
parainfluenza-3 virus 10, 11
Paramphistomum cervi 133
parasites
- brain 51
- ear 377–378
- gastrointestinal 20, 125, 133, 139–140, 154–155
- liver 172, 270
- lung 82–83
- myocardial 99
- skeletal muscle 200
- skin 320–325
- *see also* protozoa

parathyroid glands 217
paratuberculosis (Johne's disease) 108, 152–153, 277–278
Pasteurella multocida 13, 72–73
pediculosis (lice) 320
pelodera dermatitis 324–325
penis 229
pericardium
- effusion 94
- pericarditis in the aborted fetus 252
- septic pericarditis 95

perineal neoplasia 236
peritoneum 159
- fat necrosis 159
- peritonitis 137, 159

Peyer's patches 141, 265
- BVDV infection 148, 149, 275–276

pheasant's eye (*Adonis microcarpa*) 398–399
pheochromocytoma 174, 221
phomopsins 397
phosphorus deficiency 206–207
photosensitization 167–168, 338, 371
- congenital porphyria 268
- plant toxins 394, 412–413

pigweeds (*Amaranthus* spp.) 408
pine needles 409–410
pinkeye 372
pituitary gland 218
placenta
- chorionitis 242, 245, 246, 251, 252, 254
- normal 237–238
- retained 239

plants, toxic 382
- abortifacient 259, 383, 409–410
- calcinogenic 100, 408–409
- carcinogenic 193, 414
- cardiotoxic 96, 100, 398–399, 403, 414, 421
- cyanide-producing 410–411
- enzootic hematuria 193, 413
- foot necrosis 337, 349, 350
- gastrointestinal 138, 414
- granulomatous disease (due to hairy vetch) 187, 222, 414–415
- to the hematopoietic system 282–283, 411–412, 413
- hepatotoxic 165–168, 392–398
- myotoxic 96, 197–198, 398–404
- nephrotoxic 179, 180, 181, 187, 406–408
- neurotoxic 382–392
- nitrate-producing 411–412
- photosensitizing 394, 412–413
- reproduction 383
- teratogenic 5, 405

platelets
- Simmental hereditary thrombopathy 267, 335
- thrombocytopenia 275, 282, 413

pleural effusions 91
pleuritis 74, 75, 76, 91, 247
plumbism (lead poisoning) 35, 180
pneumonia 64, 79
- in the aborted fetus 245, 255
- aspiration 84
- atypical interstitial 84–87
- *Bibersteinia trehalosi* 80–81
- BRSV 12, 66–69
- BVDV 69–70
- in calves 9–13
- coronavirus 9, 10
- embolic 87
- fungal 82
- *Histophilus somni* 73–76
- *Mannheimia haemolytica* 13, 70–72
- *Mycobacterium bovis* 81
- *Mycoplasma bovis* 77–79
- *Mycoplasma mycoides* 80
- parainfluenza-3 10–11
- parasitic 82–83
- *Pasteurella multocida* 13, 72–73
- *Trueperella pyogenes* 76

poison hemlock (*Conium maculatum*) 389–390
poisoning *see* plants, toxic; toxins
polioencephalomalacia 33–34
polycystic kidney 4
polycystic ovary 233
polydactyly 205
porphyria 122, 268
prairie thermopsis (*Thermopsis rhombifolia*) 401
pregnancy 237
- fetal maceration/mummification 239
- hydrops amnii 383
- placentation 237–238
- prolonged gestation 258–259
- retained placenta 239
- uterine damage 239
- *see also* abortion

prion disease 37
progressive ataxia of Charolais cattle 54–55
progressive myelinopathy in Murray Grey cattle 54
Prototheca zopfii mastitis 362
protozoa
- abortion 254–257
- cerebral 48–50, 272, 421

eye/eyelid 373, 374
intestinal 19, 155
intraerythrocytic 48, 49, 272, 273–274
myocarditis 98, 99
skeletal muscle 200
skin 318–319
trypanosomiasis 50, 273–274
uterine 235
Prunus virginiana (chokecherry) 411
pseudocowpox 308, 364
pseudolumpy skin disease (BHV-2) 309–310
Pseudomonas aeruginosa mastitis 360
Pteridium aquilinum (bracken fern) 138, 193, 282, 413–414
pulmonary conditions *see* lung
pulmonary heart disease 102–104, 382
pyelonephritis 189
pyometra 235

Quercus spp. (oak) 282, 406

rabies 38
Raillietia auris 377, 378
rain scald (dermatophilosis) 310–311
rayless goldenrod (*Isocoma pluriflora*) 399–400
rectum
perforation 157
perirectal fat necrosis 159
red blood cells 262
hemolytic anemia 272–274, 282, 413
redwater (babesiosis) 48, 49, 272
renal disease *see* kidney
renal vein thrombosis 179
reproductive system 223–224
female
ovary 232–234, 383
perineum 236
plant toxins 383
uterine tubes 234
uterus 231–232, 235–236, 239
vagina/vulva 236
see also abortion; pregnancy
intersexes 230–231
male
epididymis 228
penis 229
seminal vesicle 228
testis 224–228
respiratory system 57
in calves 9–13
larynx 9, 60
lung *see* lung
nostrils 57, 58
pleura 74, 75, 76, 91, 247
sinonasal compartment 58–60, 109
trachea 60–63
reticulum 131, 132
retinopathy, BVDV-related 368
retrobulbar neoplasia 284, 376
Rhabditis bovis 324–325, 377, 378
rhinitis 58–59
rickets 206–207
Rickettsia
Anaplasma spp. 175, 272
cowdriosis 47
ringworm 326–327
rotavirus 16
round cell tumor, undifferentiated 334
rumen
bracken fern carcinoma 414
fibropapilloma 134
indigestion (obstruction) 130
lactic acidosis 126–127, 131, 132
papillary hypertrophy 130
rumenitis 14, 131, 132, 133
trichomoniasis 254–255
tympany (bloat) 128–130
urea toxicity 130, 419–420
Rusterholz ulcer (sole ulcer) 345–346
ryegrass (*Lolium*) 386–387

salmonellosis
abomasum 18, 138
enteric 18, 145–147
gall bladder 175
liver 170
stomatitis/glossitis 121
salt intoxication 35
saltlover (*Halogeton glomeratus*) 407
saponins 394–395
Sarcina ventriculi 22
Sarcobatus vermiculatus (greasewood) 407
Sarcocystis spp. 98, 99, 200
sarcoptic mange 321–322
Sarcosporidia spp. 318
SBE (sporadic bovine encephalomyelitis) 46–47
scald (interdigital dermatitis) 305, 352
schistosomus reflexus 259
Schmallenberg virus 244
schwannoma 52
scours 15
screw claw 354–355
scrotum, hematocele 228
selenium deficiency (white muscle disease) 25, 96, 195–197
selenium toxicity 402–404
seminal vesicle adenitis 228
Senecio longilobus (threadleaf) 393
Senna (*Cassia*) spp. 197–198, 402
sepsis of the distal interphalangeal joint 348
septic arthritis 23, 24, 26, 79, 212–213
septic pericarditis 95
septic peritonitis 137, 159
septic thrombosis of the jugular vein 107
septicemia (calf sepsis) 23–24
Sertoli cell tumor 227
shipping fever 64, 70–72
silage eye 372
Simmental cattle
hereditary thrombopathy 267, 335
multifocal symmetrical encephalomyelopathy 53

sinonasal conditions
  cysts 58
  inflammation 58–59
  neoplasia 60, 109
  see also nostrils
skeletal system 201
  calves 25–26, 202–205, 206–208, 212
  chondrodysplasia 25, 26, 202–203
  congenital anomalies 25, 26, 258, 405
  intrauterine BVDV infection 210–211
  localized abnormalities 205
  lymphoma (juvenile) 211, 286
  manganese deficiency 207–208
  osteochondrosis 214–215
  osteogenesis imperfecta 203–204
  osteomyelitis 208–209, 315
  osteopetrosis 204
  osteoporosis 205–206
  porphyria 268
  rickets and osteomalacia 206–207
  tetracycline deposition 212
  toe-tip necrosis 210
  see also bone marrow; joints
skin 289–291
  allergic dermatitis 337–338
  alopecia 300–302, 304
  bacterial infections
    actinobacillosis 316–317
    actinomycosis 209, 315–316
    atypical (non-tuberculoid) mycobacteriosis 312–314
    cellulitis 317–318
    dermatophilosis 310–311
    digital dermatitis 351
    foot rot 351–352
    interdigital dermatitis 352
    staphylococcal 314, 358, 365
    tuberculosis 312
  burns
    chemical 354
    thermal 339, 421
  congenital and genetic diseases
    cutaneous asthenia 295–296
    epitheliogenesis imperfecta 294
    familial acantholysis 298
    hypotrichosis 292–294
    ichthyosis 297
    mechanobullous disease 299–300
  fungal infections
    granuloma 328
    ringworm 326–327
  granulomatous dermatitis (hairy vetch toxicity) 414
  idiopathic ulcerative dermatitis 339–341
  infarcts 341
  mud fever (dermatitis of the lower leg) 353–354
  necrosis (gangrene) 336–337, 349, 350, 358
  neoplasia
    angiomatosis 333
    fibroma 334
    lipoma 334
    lymphoma 287, 328
    mast cell tumor 330–332
    melanoma 332
    squamous cell carcinoma 328–330
    undifferentiated round cell tumor 334
  parasitic infestations
    hypodermosis 325
    mange 321–323
    pediculosis (lice) 320
    pelodera (rhabditic) dermatitis 324–325
    stephanofilariasis 323–324
  photosensitization 167–168, 268, 338, 371, 394, 412–413
  protozoal infections 318–319
  subcutaneous swellings 335
  udder 357–358
  viral infections
    BPS 307–308
    BVDV 304–306
    MCF 306–307
    papillomatosis (warts) 302–304, 353, 365
    pseudocowpox 308, 364
    pseudolumpy skin disease 309–310
slurry heel (interdigital dermatitis) 305, 352
small intestine
  displacement 14, 141
  enteritis
    BVDV 147–150, 275–276
    in calves 14–20
    fibrinonecrotic (salmonellosis) 18, 145–146
    granulomatous 152–153
    hemorrhagic 17, 144, 154
  eosinophilic droplets 158
  hemorrhagic bowel syndrome 156–157
  neoplasia 156
  parasites 20, 154–155
  Peyer's patches 141, 148, 149, 265
Solanum spp. 386, 408–409
sole ulcer 345–346
  thin sole toe ulcer 346–347
spermatogenesis 225
spinal cord
  breed-specific myelopathies 53–56
  neoplasia 52
  removal 32
  spina bifida 3
  trauma 51
spinal muscular atrophy 53–54
spleen
  abscesses 281
  anthrax 271, 280–281
  epizootic bovine abortion 253
  granulomatous splenitis 415
  infarction 271
  splenomegaly 271, 281, 285
spondylitis 209
sporidesmin 397
spring parsley (*Cymopterus watsonii*) 413
squamous cell carcinoma 328–330, 375, 414
St John's wort (*Hypericum perforatum*) 412
Staphylococcus spp.
  dermatitis 314, 358, 365
  mastitis 361
stephanofilariasis 323–324

- stomach *see* abomasum; forestomachs
- stomatitis 112–121, 124–125
  - BPS 118, 124, 307–308
- *Streptococcus* mastitis 361
- streptothricosis (dermatophilosis) 310–311
- sulfur excess (polioencephalomalacia) 33–34
- sulfur granules 316, 317
- swainsonine intoxication 382–385
- sweet clover 283, 335
- syndactyly 205

- tail, gangrene 337
- tall fescue grass 337, 349, 350
- tapeworms
  - cerebral 51
  - intestinal 155
  - liver 172
  - myocardial 99
  - skeletal muscle 200
- *Taxus* spp. (yew) 404, 421
- teat 363
  - bluetongue virus 364
  - bovine herpes mammillitis (BHV-2) 309, 363–364
  - bovine papilloma virus 365
  - impetigo 365
  - pseudocowpox 308, 364
  - trauma 365
  - vesicular stomatitis 364
  - *see also* udder
- teeth 121–122
- telangiectasia, hepatic 174
- teratogens 5, 405
- testis
  - anatomy 224–225
  - degeneration 226
  - hematocele 228
  - hypoplasia 225
  - inflammation 226
  - neoplasia 227
- tetanus 418
- tetracycline deposition (in bone) 212
- theileriosis 48–49, 274
- thelitis
  - bluetongue 364
  - bovine herpes mammillitis (BHV-2) 309, 363–364
  - bovine papilloma virus 365
  - impetigo 365
  - pseudocowpox 308, 364
  - vesicular stomatitis 364
- *Thermopsis rhombifolia* (prairie thermopsis) 401
- threadleaf (*Senecio longilobus*) 393
- thrombocytopenia 275, 282, 413
- thrombosis
  - caudal vena cava 89–90
  - renal vein 179
  - septic, of the jugular vein 107
- thrombotic meningoencephalomyelitis 45–46
- thymus gland
  - atrophy 271–272
  - BVDV abortion 243, 244
  - epizootic bovine abortion 253
  - lymphoma 286
  - normal 262–263
- thyroid gland
  - in calves/stillborns 27–28, 292
  - goiter 27, 219, 292
  - neoplasia 219
- tick-borne diseases
  - babesiosis 48, 49, 272
  - cowdriosis 47
  - EBA 252–253
  - theileriosis 48–49, 274
- timber milkvetch (*Astragalus miser*) 388
- toe-tip necrosis 210
- tongue 116, 119–121
- tonsils 264, 279
- torsion, gastrointestinal 14, 135, 141
- toxic rumenitis/reticulitis 14
- *Toxicoscordion venenosum* (death camas) 391–392
- toxins
  - cyanobacterial 164
  - enterotoxins 17, 144
  - fungal 397
    - aflatoxins 162–163
    - ergotamine 270, 336, 337
    - ergovaline (in tall fescue grass) 337, 349, 350
  - heavy metals 35, 36, 180, 282
  - nitrate excess 283, 411–412
  - organophosphates 36, 420
  - plants *see* plants, toxic
  - salt excess 35
  - sulfur excess 33–34
  - urea 130, 419–420
- *Toxocara vitulorum* 20, 154
- trachea
  - Honker's syndrome 62–63
  - IBR 60–62
- transmissible serositis 46–47
- trauma
  - brain/spinal cord 51
  - claw 347–348, 349
  - esophagus 123–124
  - foot 352
  - penis 229
  - rectum 157
  - teat 365
  - vagina 236
- traumatic reticulopericarditis (hardware disease) 95, 131
- trematodiasis 172, 270
- *Tribulus terrestris* (goats head) 394
- trichobezoars 21
- trichomoniasis 235, 254–255
- *Trichostrongylus axei* 140
- *Trichuris discolor* 154
- *Trueperella pyogenes* 76, 361
- trypanosomiasis 50, 273–274
- tuberculosis (*Mycobacterium bovis*) 81, 171, 277, 312
- tumors *see* neoplasia
- twinning
  - freemartinism 230–231
  - incomplete (amorphous globosus) 238

two-grooved milkvetch (*Astragalus bisulcatus*) 403
tympany (bloat) 21, 128–130, 335
typhoid nodule 170

udder 357
  abscesses 358
  dermatitis 357–358
  impetigo 358
  mastitis 359–362
  milk vein thrombophlebitis 358
  neoplasia 363
  udder cleft syndrome 358
  see also teat
ulcers
  abomasum 21, 137
  foot 345–346, 346–347
  ulcerative dermatitis 339–341
umbilical hernia (omphalocele) 5
unguiculliform papillae 134
urea toxicity 130, 419–420
ureaplasmosis 251
urinary system
  bracken fern toxicity 193, 413
  congenital anomalies 4–5, 177–178
  cystitis 191
  enzootic hematuria 193, 413
  kidney *see* kidney
  neoplasia 190, 193
  ureteritis 189, 191
  urolithiasis 190, 191–192
uterine tubes 234
uterus 235
  congenital anomalies 231–232
  inflammation 235
  neoplasia 236
  segmental aplasia of the uterine horns 231
  torn 239
  torsion 239
  see also pregnancy
uveitis 372, 373–374

vagal indigestion 136
vagina 236
valvular cysts 100
valvular endocarditis 100–101
vasculitis
  aortic 105–106
  BVDV 98, 149–151, 336
  MCF 40, 117, 307
vena cava thrombosis 89–90
ventricular septal defect 4, 99
vertebral column 51, 209
see also spinal cord
vesicular stomatitis 118, 364
Vicia villosa (hairy vetch) 187, 222, 414–415
viral infections
  abortion 210–211, 240–245
  bone 210–211
  brain/spinal cord 38–43
  eye 372, 373, 374
  gastrointestinal 15–16, 112–119, 124–125, 132, 142–143, 147–151
  kidney 186–187
  myocardium 97, 98
  respiratory 9–12, 60–62, 64–70
  skin 302–310
  teat 308, 309, 363–365
  teratogenic 5
  vasculitis 105, 149–151, 307
vitamin A deficiency 36–37, 368–369
vitamin D deficiency 206–207
vitamin D excess 100, 408–409
vitamin E deficiency (white muscle disease) 25, 96, 195–197
volvulus 14, 135, 141
vulvovaginitis 236

warble grubs 325
warts 302–304, 353, 365
  'foot warts' (digital dermatitis) 351
water deprivation 35
water hemlock (*Cicuta maculata*) 390
Weaver syndrome 53
white blood cells
  congenital diseases 266–267
  see also eosinophils
white line disease 346, 355
white muscle disease 25, 96, 195–197
white snakeroot (*Ageratina altissima*) 399–400
white spotted kidney (thromboembolic glomerulonephritis) 27, 188
winter dysentery 142–143
wooden tongue 120

Xanthium strumarium (cocklebur) 395–396

yew (*Taxus* spp.) 404, 421

Zygomycetes spp. 82, 131, 171, 254